DATE DUE FOR RETURN

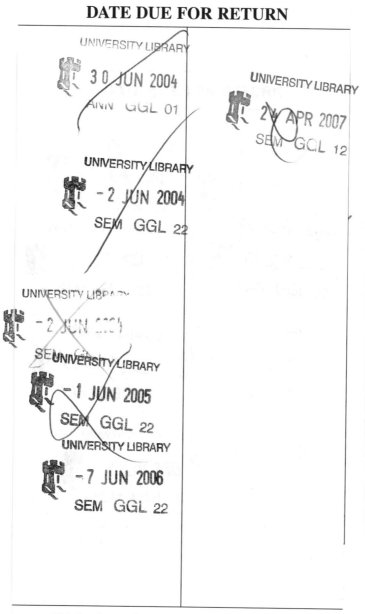
This book may be recalled before the above date.

Herbal Medicines

A Guide for Health-care Professionals

Herbal Medicines

A Guide for Health-care Professionals

Carol A. Newall

Linda A. Anderson

J. David Phillipson

London
THE PHARMACEUTICAL PRESS
1996

Published by the Pharmaceutical Press
1 Lambeth High Street, London SE1 7JN

First published 1996
Reprinted 1996, 1997 (twice), 1998 (twice)

© 1996 Pharmaceutical Press

Printed and bound in Great Britain at the University Press, Cambridge

ISBN 0 85369 289 0

A catalogue record for this book is available from the British Library.

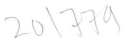

Dedication

This book is dedicated to the memory of the late Dr W Gwynne Thomas, former Director of Pharmaceutical Sciences at the Royal Pharmaceutical Society of Great Britain. The inspiration for the book came from him and it is due to his efforts that the necessary funding was obtained.

Affiliations

Carol A. Newall (née Baldwin) BPharm, DipInfSc, MRPharmS

Linda A. Anderson BPharm, PhD, MRPharmS

J. David Phillipson DSc, PhD, MSc, BSc(Pharm), FRPharmS, FLS

Department of Pharmacognosy, The School of Pharmacy, University of London

CONTENTS

Preface and Acknowledgements, viii

How To Use This Book, 1
Introduction to the Monographs, 3
General References, 17
Monographs, 19

Agnus Castus, 19
Agrimony, 21
Alfalfa, 23
Aloe vera, 25
Aloes, 27
Angelica, 28
Aniseed, 30
Apricot, 32
Arnica, 34
Artichoke, 36
Asafoetida, 38
Avens, 40
Bayberry , 41
Bloodroot, 42
Blue Flag, 44
Bogbean, 45
Boldo, 46
Boneset, 48
Borage, 49
Broom, 50
Buchu, 51
Burdock, 52
Burnet, 54
Calamus, 55
Calendula, 58
Capsicum, 60
Cascara, 62
Cassia, 63
Celery, 65
Centaury, 67
Cereus, 68
Chamomile, German, 69
Chamomile, Roman, 72
Chaparral, 74
Cinnamon, 76
Clivers, 78
Clove, 79
Cohosh, Black, 80
Cohosh, Blue, 82
Cola, 84
Coltsfoot, 85

Comfrey, 87
Corn Silk, 90
Couchgrass, 91
Cowslip, 92
Damiana, 94
Dandelion, 96
Devil's Claw, 98
Drosera, 100
Echinacea, 101
Elder, 104
Elecampane, 106
Eucalyptus, 108
Euphorbia, 109
Evening Primrose, 110
Eyebright, 114
False Unicorn, 116
Fenugreek, 117
Feverfew, 119
Figwort, 122
Frangula, 123
Fucus, 124
Fumitory, 127
Garlic, 129
Gentian, 134
Ginger, 135
Ginkgo, 138
Ginseng, Eleutherococcus, 141
Ginseng, Panax, 145
Golden Seal, 151
Gravel Root, 153
Ground Ivy, 154
Guaiacum, 156
Hawthorn, 157
Holy Thistle, 160
Hops, 162
Horehound, Black, 164
Horehound, White, 165
Horse-chestnut, 166
Horseradish, 168
Hydrangea, 169
Hydrocotyle, 170
Ispaghula, 173
Jamaica Dogwood, 174
Juniper, 176
Lady's Slipper, 178
Lemon Verbena, 179
Liferoot, 180
Lime Flower, 181
Liquorice, 183
Lobelia, 187

Marshmallow, 188
Maté, 189
Meadowsweet, 191
Mistletoe, 193
Motherwort, 197
Myrrh, 199
Nettle, 201
Parsley, 203
Parsley Piert, 205
Passionflower, 206
Pennyroyal, 208
Pilewort, 209
Plantain, 210
Pleurisy Root, 213
Pokeroot, 215
Poplar, 218
Prickly Ash, Northern, 219
Prickly Ash, Southern, 220
Pulsatilla, 222
Quassia, 223
Queen's Delight, 225
Raspberry, 226
Red Clover, 227
Rhubarb, 228
Rosemary, 229
Sage, 231
Sarsaparilla, 233
Sassafras, 235
Saw Palmetto, 237
Scullcap, 239
Senega, 241
Senna, 243
Shepherd's Purse, 245
Skunk Cabbage, 247
Slippery Elm, 248
Squill, 249
St. John's Wort, 250
Stone Root, 253
Tansy, 254
Thyme, 256

Uva-Ursi, 258
Valerian, 260
Vervain, 263
Wild Carrot, 264
Wild Lettuce, 266
Willow, 268
Witch Hazel, 270
Yarrow, 271
Yellow Dock, 274
Yucca, 275

Appendixes, 277

1   Potential Drug/Herb Interactions, 277
2   Laxative Herbal Ingredients, 280
3   Cardioactive Herbal Ingredients, 280
4   Diuretic Herbal Ingredients, 281
5   Hypotensive and Hypertensive Herbal
    Ingredients, 281
6   Anticoagulant or Coagulant Herbal Ingredients, 282
7   Hypolipidaemic and Hyperlipidaemic Herbal
    Ingredients, 282
8   Sedative Herbal Ingredients, 283
9   Hypoglycaemic and Hyperglycaemic Herbal
    Ingredient, 283
10 Hormonally Active Herbal Ingredients, 283
11 Immunostimulating Herbal Ingredients, 284
12 Allergenic Herbal Ingredients, 284
13 Irritant Herbal Ingredients, 284
14 Herbal Ingredients with Amines, Alkaloids or
    Sympathomimetic Action, 285
15 Herbal Ingredients containing Coumarins, 286
16 Herbal Ingredients containing Flavonoids, 286
17 Herbal Ingredients containing Iridoids, 286
18 Herbal Ingredients containing Saponins, 286
19 Herbal Ingredients containing Tannins, 286
20 Herbal Ingredients containing Volatile Oils, 286

Index, 287

PREFACE

Not so many years ago the advances being made in medicine and the innovations of the pharmaceutical industry made it seem inevitable that the use of herbal remedies in developed countries would decline to insignificance. It is somewhat of a paradox therefore, that at a time when there is such an unprecedented number of therapeutic drugs available for the treatment of all forms of disease, that herbal remedies continue to be demanded by the general public. In fact, this demand has steadily increased over the past decade and as a result of enquiries from practising pharmacists, the Royal Pharmaceutical Society of Great Britain commissioned this volume in order to provide factual information on medicinal herbs.

The chapter 'Introduction to the Monographs' sets the herbal scene in the light of complementary therapies and goes on to consider UK and European legislation. The control of herbal remedies is a matter of concern to the Royal Pharmaceutical Society who have pointed out that the public may be at risk due to the sale of herbal products which are not licensed as medicines. All medicines are assessed for their quality, safety and efficacy and these parameters should be used to assess all herbs and herbal products which are intended for medical use.

The majority of herbal products sold in the UK are not licensed as medicines and because herbs are 'natural' some people consider that they must be safe. This is simply not true and some herbs are capable of causing adverse effects. With herbs, as with all medicines, it is necessary to consider precautions for specific patient groups, contra-indications, warnings and the potential for interaction with other medicines. Summary tables giving examples of herbal ingredients with potential adverse reactions, or those which are best avoided during pregnancy, are included in the chapter 'Introduction to the Monographs'.

Sensitive scientific methods for investigating the chemical constituents of herbs and for determining their biological activities are now available and a number of herbs are currently being subjected to detailed scientific scrutiny. A short account of such work and some relevant examples are given.

The major part of the text deals with 141 herbs which have been selected on the basis that they are ingredients of herbal remedies which are on sale in UK pharmacies. There is a brief section on 'How to Use this Handbook' on p. 1. The purpose and scope of the handbook, background on the the standard monograph sections is given. The reader is advised to consult this section before referring to specific monographs.

Each herb is the subject of a monograph which is in a datasheet-type format. In addition to the names, synonyms and plant part used, each monograph indicates whether the herb is, or has been, the subject of a monograph in the European or a national pharmacopoeia. The legal category, food use and herbal doses are given where known, the constituents are listed briefly together with any documented pharmacology and human use. For some herbs, little pharmacology and particularly clinical information is available, and the reader may need to ascertain the current state of medical and scientific evidence. Any side-effects and toxicity are listed together with contra-indications and warnings. Each monograph carries a section on 'Pharmaceutical Comment' in which there is a brief comment on the advisability of using the particular herb for medicinal purposes. In some instances, the literature clearly indicates that the risk to benefit ratio precludes the use of the herb and if this is the case then it is clearly stated in the monograph.

A set of literature references is included with each monograph but some judgement has had to be exercised in the extent to which references are cited. In an attempt to overcome the vast numbers of references which could be included for some of the monographs, the references have been divided into two categories, general and specific. There are some 35 general references which include review books of herbal use, pharmacopoeial descriptions, chemistry, pharmacology and toxicology. For well known medicinal herbs such as Cascara, only general references are cited whereas for lesser known herbs or for herbs undergoing recent investigation, every attempt has been made to cite original literature references in order to help those readers wishing to delve more deeply into the subject.

As the book has developed, it has become obvious that it would be of wider use as a reference book not only to pharmacists but to other health-care professionals who can use their own clinical and professional judgement. It is our hope that this text will prove to be of benefit to all who deal professionally with herbs which are used for medical treatment.

Dr Linda Anderson was involved in the preparation of this book during her previous employment as a Research Fellow at the School of Pharmacy, University of London. The views expressed in this book are those of the authors and do not represent those of the Medicines Control Agency.

Acknowledgements
We are grateful to the Royal Pharmaceutical Society of Great Britain for their financial support and the interest which they have shown during the preparation of the book. Particular thanks are due to Ainley Wade and, in earlier years, John Martin of RPSGB for their strong editorial involvement. Our thanks to Linda Lisgarten, Librarian, The School of Pharmacy, University of London and to her staff for their continued cheerful help through the many queries which we have put to them.

November 1995

HOW TO USE THIS HANDBOOK

PURPOSE AND SCOPE

This handbook is intended to serve as a reference work for pharmacists, doctors and other health-care professionals, assisting in their provision of advice on the use of herbal remedies to members of the public. The book is not intended to represent a guide to self-diagnosis and self-treatment with herbal remedies, and should not be used as such.

The term 'herbal remedy' is used to describe a marketed product, whereas 'herbal ingredient' refers to an individual herb that is present in a herbal remedy. 'Herbal constituent' is used to describe a specific chemical constituent of a herbal ingredient. Thus, as examples, Valerian Tablets are a herbal remedy, valerian is a herbal ingredient, and valtrate is a herbal constituent of valerian.

The main criterion for inclusion of a herbal ingredient in the text is its presence in herbal remedies that are used in the UK, particularly those which are sold through pharmacies. In addition, herbs which have recently been the subject of media or scientific interest, such as Ginkgo, have also been included. The aim of the handbook is to draw the attention of the reader to the reputed actions and uses of herbal ingredients and, to whether or not, these have been substantiated by animal or human studies. In addition, any known or potential toxicities of herbal ingredients, and how these may influence the suitability for inclusion in herbal remedies or for use with conventional medicines, are also discussed.

INTRODUCTION TO THE MONOGRAPHS

The introductory section to the 141 monographs on the individual herbal ingredients contained in this handbook discusses the legal aspects of herbal remedies including licensed medicines and non-licensed products in the UK and within the European Community (EC). All medicines are assessed for their quality, safety and efficacy, and in the context of herbal remedies there are often specific criteria which are not encountered in the assessment of other medicines. As a first line in ensuring the safety and efficacy of herbal remedies there are a series of guidelines for quality assessment and these are briefly discussed. In terms of safety, it is a popular conception that just because herbs are 'natural' then they must also be safe. This is a misconception and within this section it is pointed out that some herbal ingredients have the capability to cause adverse effects whilst some are decidedly toxic. Within the context of the 141 monographs on herbal ingredients, most have documented adverse effects or the potential to interact with other medication and hardly any could be recommended for use during pregnancy.

Three Tables in the Introduction and 20 Appendixes after the Monographs summarise the safety aspects of these herbal ingredients and give information on biologically active herbal ingredients and their active principles. Clinical efficacy has not been established for the majority of the herbal ingredients described in this handbook and in some instances there is a lack of documentation for chemical constituents and for pharmacological actions.

THE HERBAL MONOGRAPHS

Some 141 monographs on individual herbal ingredients found in herbal remedies comprise the bulk of this handbook and they are presented in alphabetical order with respect to their preferred common name. The index includes preferred common names, other synonyms and the Latin binomial names, and should be used to assist in the location of a particular monograph. A data sheet-type format was chosen for the monographs because it was felt important to arrange the relevant information in a format familiar to pharmacists and doctors. Although conventional data sheets are written for products, it was decided to draw up the data sheets for herbal ingredients and not for products.

The headings used in the herbal monographs are listed below with a brief explanation of the information held under them.

Monograph title	Common name for the herbal ingredient; if more than one common name exists, this is the chosen preferred name
Species (Family)	Preferred botanical name with authority, together with the plant family
Synonyms	Other common or botanical names
Part(s) Used	Plant part(s) traditionally used in herbal medicine
Pharmacopoeial Monographs	Key pharmacopoeial monographs, with special emphasis on European national pharmacopoeias
Legal Category	Legal category of the herb with respect to licensed products. For the majority of herbal ingredients this will be GSL

Constituents Main documented chemical constituents grouped into categories such as alkaloids (type specified), flavonoids, iridoid glycosides, saponins, tannins, triterpenes, volatile oil and other constituents for miscellaneous and minor chemical components

Food Use Provides an indication as to whether the herbal ingredient is used in foods. Council of Europe (COE) category (N1 to N4) is quoted where applicable which reflects the opinion of the COE on the suitability of the herbal ingredient for use as a food flavouring.
Also where applicable, the FDA listing is stated, e.g. 'Generally Regarded as Safe' (GRAS), and 'Herb of Undefined Safety'.

Herbal Use States the reputed actions and uses of the herbal ingredients. For many of the monographs this section refers to the British Herbal Pharmacopoeia (BHP). In some instances current investigations of particular interest are included

Dose States the traditional dose of the herbal ingredient, mainly from the BHP, giving doses for plant part used (herb, rhizome, leaf), liquid extract and infusion

Pharmacological Actions Describes any documented pharmacological actions for the herbal ingredient.
The sections on Animal Studies refer to studies with animals, either *in vivo* or *in vitro*.
The Human Studies refer to studies performed with human subjects although very few of these can be classed as clinical trials.

Side-effects, Toxicity Details any documented side-effects to the herbal ingredient and any toxicological studies. If side-effects or toxicity are generally associated with any of the constituents in the herbal ingredient or with its plant family, then these are mentioned here. See also Table 1 (p. 8) and Table 2 (pp. 15–16) in the Introduction to the Monographs

Contra-indications, Warnings Describes any potential contra-indications and, warns against any potential side-effects and any individuals who may be more susceptible to a side-effect. This section should be used in conjunction with Appendixes 1 to 20 which are placed after the monographs on pp. 277–86.
Comments on Pregnancy and lactation are included; a summary is provided in Table 3 of the Introduction to the Monographs, pp. 13–14.

Pharmaceutical Comment This section is designed to give the reader an overall summary of the monograph contents, indicating the extent of phytochemical and pharmacological data available for the herbal ingredient, whether or not proposed herbal uses are justified, any concerns over safety, and, based on the above information, whether or not the herbal ingredient is considered suitable for use as a herbal remedy

References References are included at the end of the text on each monograph. There is considerable literature on herbal plants and some 35 general references have been selected for use with the handbook. These General References, referred to as G1 to G35, are listed after the Introduction on p. 17. For some well known herbal ingredients, e.g. Cascara, only general references are cited. The majority of the monographs also contain specific references which are cited at the end of each monograph

INTRODUCTION TO THE MONOGRAPHS

A general disillusionment with conventional medicines, coupled with the desire for a 'natural' life style has resulted in an increasing utilisation of alternative or complementary therapies. During 1990, sales of OTC phytomedicines in 7 EC countries were estimated to represent US$2.4 billion at their selling price[1], highlighting the enormous popularity of complementary therapies in Europe.

In the UK, many complementary therapies are available ranging from acupuncture and Alexander Technique to reflexology and sound therapy.[2]

Homoeopathy and herbal medicine are two complementary therapies often mistaken by the layperson to be one and the same. Homoeopathy is based on the principle of 'like should be treated by like' and involves the administration of minute doses of those remedies that, in larger doses, produce symptoms in a healthy person mimicking those expressed by the patient. By contrast, herbal medicine involves the use of plants, dried or as an extract in therapeutic doses to treat the symptoms exhibited, and in this respect is similar to orthodox medicine.

Herbal medicine is being increasingly used by the general public on a self-selection basis to either replace or complement conventional medicines. Medicinal herbs are therefore of particular interest to pharmacists, doctors and other health-care professionals. A pharmacist should be able to advise the consumer on the rational and safe use of all medicines. To fulfil this role with respect to herbal medicines, a pharmacist should be reliably informed of their quality, safety and efficacy. Many doctors are becoming increasingly aware of their patients' use of herbal remedies and need to be informed of the suitability of these remedies for use as medicines.

In response to this need for information, a series of articles on herbal remedies was published in *The Pharmaceutical Journal* during the 1980s.[3–15] Topics covered in these articles included counter-prescribing of herbal remedies, pharmacologically active compounds in herbal remedies, sedative and antirheumatic herbal remedies, and specific articles on ginseng, feverfew and mistletoe. More recently, review articles have been published in the *Journal* on aloe vera, evening primrose, valerian, gingko, echinacea, agnus castus, feverfew, chamomile, guarana, ginseng and others.[16-25]

This handbook brings together in one text a series of data-sheet-style monographs on 141 herbs commonly present in herbal remedies sold through pharmacies in the UK. Various appendixes are also presented grouping together herbs with specific actions, and highlighting potential interactions with conventional medicines.

As preface to the monographs, an overview of UK and European legislation concerning herbal products is provided, together with issues pertaining to their quality, safety and efficacy.

In addition to retail purchase, herbs can be obtained by picking the wild plant or from a herbal practitioner. This handbook does not discuss the self-collection of plant material for use as a herbal remedy or the prescribing of herbal remedies by herbal practitioners.

UK and European Legislation

Herbal products are available in the UK through various retail outlets such as pharmacies, health food shops, mail order companies, supermarkets and departmental stores. Some herbal products consist solely of loose, dried plant material; others are presented as prepackaged formulated products in a variety of pharmaceutical forms for both internal (tablets, capsules, liquids) and external use (creams, ointments) and may contain 4–5 herbal ingredients which may be dried herbs or their extracts.

The legal status of herbal products is complicated by the fact that in most EC member states they are available both as medicinal products and as food supplements.[26] In the UK the majority of herbal products are marketed without medical claims as food supplements and are controlled under food legislation by MAFF (Ministry of Agriculture, Fisheries and Foods). This situation has arisen because of the difficulties in defining the status of products occupying the borderline between medicines and foods. Provided the products were marketed without reference to medicinal claims the Medicines Control Agency (MCA), the body responsible for regulating medicinal products, has in the past generally been satisfied that the products were not subject to medicines legislation.[27] However, changing circumstances including implementation of the definition of a medicinal product in accordance with EC Directives (see below), together with European Court of Justice (ECJ) judgements are likely to result in greater emphasis being placed on the nature of the herbal ingredients and whether the product is medicinal by function[27]. Article 1 of Directive 65/65 EEC [28] defines a 'medicinal product' as:

> 'any substance or combination of substances presented for treating, or preventing disease in human beings or animals'

> 'any substance or combination of substances which may be administered to human beings or animals with a view to making diagnosis or to restoring, correcting or modifying physiological functions in human beings or animals is likewise considered a medicinal product'.

The first part of the definition describes a product which is medicinal by presentation while the second describes a product which is medicinal by function.

Licensed Herbal Remedies

Almost all of the licensed herbal medicines on the UK market have been available for some time and most originally held Product Licences of Right (PLR) (see Review of Herbal Medicines below). The MCA regulates medicinal products for human use in accordance with the Medicines for Human Use (Marketing Authorisations Etc.) Regulations 1994 SI 3144 (The Regulations)[29] and the Medicines Act 1968.[30] The Regulations which took effect from January 1995 arose out of the need to implement EC legislation establishing the new EC marketing authorisation procedures (Future Systems). The Regulations effectively implement the full range of controls set out in Directive 65/65 EEC which apply to 'relevant medicinal products' (as defined in the Regulations). The main controls include application requirements and procedures for the grant, variation and renewal of UK licences, requirements in relation to pharmacovigilance, labelling and package leaflets as well as provisions for suspension, compulsory variation or revocation and related enforcement measures.

The Medicines Act and secondary legislation made under it remain the legal basis for other aspects of medicines control including manufacturer and wholesale dealers' authorisations, controls on sale and supply and controls on promotion. Further explanation may be obtained by reference to the chapter on herbal remedies in Dale and Appelbe's Pharmacy Law and Ethics.[31]

Prior to marketing therefore all new licensed herbal products are assessed by MCA for safety, quality and efficacy in accordance with EC and UK legislation. Specific EC guidelines exist on the 'Quality of Herbal Remedies'[32] and 'Manufacture of Herbal Medicinal Products'.[33]

Herbal Remedies Exempt from Licensing

Under the Medicines Act, herbal remedies manufactured and sold or supplied in accordance with specific exemptions set out in Sections 12(1) or (2) or Article 2 of the Medicines (Exemptions from Licences) (Special and Transitional Cases) Order 1971 (SI 1450)[34] are exempt from the requirement to hold product licences. The exempt products are those compounded and supplied by herbalists on their own recommendation, those which comprise solely of dried, crushed or comminuted plants sold under their botanical name with no written recommendations as to their use, and those made by a holder of a Specials Manufacturing Licence on behalf of a herbalist.

The exemptions are intended for example to give herbal practitioners the flexibility they need to prepare their own remedies for individual patients without the burden of licensing, and to enable simple dried herbs to be readily available to the public. During consideration of the UK legislation to implement the EC Future Systems legislation, the question arose as to whether or not herbal medicines exempted under the Medicines Act were eligible for exemption under Directive 65/65 EEC as amended. The Directive requires herbal medicinal products to possess marketing authorisations if they are 'industrially produced' but this term is not defined in UK or EC law. The UK Government has, however, adopted the view that herbal medicines currently exempted under the Medicines Act are manufactured or supplied on a small scale or by traditional processes which take them outside the meaning of 'industrially produced'. As a result these products fall outside the scope of the new Regulations and retain their exempt status.[35]

It has been suggested that this situation is not ideal and that special licensing requirements should be made in order to control all herbal medicine-like products.[36] This view has been endorsed by two UK medical practitioners following hepatic failure and subsequent death of a 32-year-old man attributed to a herbal ingredient in a Chinese herbal remedy.[37]

Most of the herbal ingredients used in licensed herbal medicines have been used as traditional remedies for centuries without major safety problems and the majority are included in the General Sales List (GSL).[38] Potentially hazardous plants such as digitalis, rauwolfia and nux vomica are specifically controlled under the Medicines Act as Prescription Only Medicines (POM)[39] and thus are not available other than via a registered medical practitioner. In addition, certain herbal ingredients are controlled under The Medicines (Retail Sale and Supply of Herbal Remedies) Order 1977 SI 2130.[40] This Order specifies 25 plants (Part I) which cannot be supplied except via a pharmacy and includes well known toxic species such as areca, crotalaria, dryopteris and strophanthus. The Order also specifies in Part II plants species which can be supplied by herbal practitioners such as aconite species, belladonna, ephedra, and hyoscyamus and in Part III defines the dosage and route of administration permitted.

Review of Herbal Remedies in the UK

The majority of licensed herbal remedies available in the UK have been marketed for a long time, in fact, for many from before the Medicines Act or any medicines licensing system. In September 1971 a registration exercise issued all medicinal products already on the market with a Product Licence of Right (PLR) and no scientific assessment was undertaken. In order to be issued with PLRs for their products, pharmaceutical companies had simply to provide details of the products and evidence that the products had been marketed prior to 1971. This procedure applied to all medicinal products including herbal remedies and in total some 39000 PLRs were granted. It was obvious that at some future date all PLR products (including herbal remedies) would have to be assessed by the Licensing Authority (LA) for their quality, safety, and efficacy in the same manner as those products which had applied for a product licence after 1971. European Community (EC) legislation required that this review of all PLR products be completed by May 1990.

During the UK review of herbal remedies holding a PLR, the Licensing Authority agreed to accept bibliographic evidence of efficacy for herbal remedies which were indicated for minor, self-limiting conditions.[41] No evidence would be required from new clinical trials provided the manufacturers agreed to label their products as 'a traditional herbal remedy for the symptomatic relief of...' and to include the statement 'if symptoms persist consult your doctor'. The Licensing Authority considered it inappropriate to relax the requirements for proof of efficacy for herbal remedies indicated for more serious conditions. Thus, evidence was required from controlled clinical trials for herbal remedies indicated for conditions considered to be inappropriate for self-diagnosis and treatment.

In its assessment of the safety of herbal remedies, the Licensing Authority agreed to rely as far as possible on the work of other agencies. Thus, supporting evidence of safety included, for example, acceptance of a herbal ingredient for food use, or inclusion of a herbal ingredient on Schedule 1 of the General Sales List (GSL).

Herbal Remedies in Europe

The legal status of herbal remedies within Europe and the problems involved in harmonising their assessment have been reviewed.[1,26,42] The advent of the new pan-European marketing authorisation system has raised a number of questions about herbal remedies and their possible transfer to other European markets. The new systems for marketing authorisations involve three procedures: centralised, decentralised (mutual recognition) and national.[43]

The centralised procedure is mandatory for biotechnology products and optional for high-technology products and medicinal products containing new active substances. The decentralised procedure or mutual recognition system involves agreement of assessment between the member states involved and will remain optional until January 1, 1998 for products requesting authorisation in more than one member state. Thereafter, simultaneous national applications will be possible but the mutual recognition system will automatically be involved once an authorisation has been granted in the first member state. Existing national procedures will remain for medicinal products requesting authorisation in a single member state.

National procedures implemented by member states to comply with the earlier EC requirements to review all licensed herbal products by May 1990 have differed from state to state as a herbal remedy may have a well-established use in one country but not in another. Clearly, European harmonisation on what is acceptable for the assessment of quality, safety and efficacy for these products is required to enable the mutual recognition system to operate. An important initiative in this harmonisation process has been the formation of ESCOP (European Scientific Cooperative for Phytotherapy) an umbrella organisation representing national associations for phytotherapy. Since 1990, ESCOP has produced a series of monographs on herbal drugs drawn from published scientific literature and experience of national delegates.[44] A number of the ESCOP monographs (frangula bark, senna fruit, senna leaf) have been adopted by the European CPMP (Committee on Proprietary Medicinal Products) as core-SPCs (Summary of Product Characteristics) for herbal medicinal products.

QUALITY, SAFETY AND EFFICACY OF HERBAL REMEDIES

In order to obtain a marketing authorisation (product licence) manufacturers of medicinal herbal remedies are required to demonstrate that their products meet acceptable standards of quality, safety and efficacy.

QUALITY

Compared with conventional preparations, herbal products present a number of unique problems when quality aspects are considered. These arise because of the nature of the herbal ingredients, which are complex mixtures of constituents, and it is well documented that levels of plant constituents can vary considerably depending on environmental and genetic factors. Furthermore, the constituents responsible for the claimed therapeutic effects are frequently unknown or only partly explained and this precludes the level of control which can routinely be achieved with synthetic drug substances in conventional pharmaceuticals. The position is further complicated by the traditional practice of using combinations of herbal ingredients, and it is not uncommon to have as many as 5 herbal ingredients in one product.

In recognition of the special problems associated with the herbal remedies the CPMP have issued specific guidelines dealing with quality aspects and manufacture.[32,33]

These guidelines have been reviewed[43] and comprehensive articles dealing with the quality of herbal remedies have been published.[45-48] The CPMP Guidelines highlight the need for good control of the starting materials and the finished product and emphasise the importance of good manufacturing practice in the manufacture of herbal products.

Herbal Ingredients

Control of starting material is essential in order to ensure reproducible quality of a herbal remedy.[45-48] The following are to be considered in the control of starting materials.

Authentication and Reproducibility of Herbal Ingredients[44,48] Herbal ingredients must be accurately identified by macroscopical and microscopical comparison with authentic material or accurate descriptions of authentic herbs. It is essential that herbal ingredients are referred to by their binomial Latin names of genus and species; only permitted synonyms should be used. Even when correctly authenticated, it is important to realise that different batches of the same herbal ingredient may differ in quality due to a number of factors.

Inter/Intra- Species Variation For many plants, there is considerable inter- and intraspecies variation in constituents, which is genetically controlled and may be related to the country of origin.

Environmental Factors The quality of a herbal ingredient can be affected by environmental factors, such as climate, altitude and growing conditions.

Time of Harvesting For some herbs the optimum time of harvesting should be specified as it is known that the level of constituents in a plant can vary during the growing cycle or even during the course of a day.

Plant Part Used   Active constituents usually vary between plant parts and it is not uncommon for a herbal ingredient to be adulterated with parts of the plant not normally utilised. In addition, plant material that has been previously subjected to extraction and is therefore 'exhausted' is sometimes used to increase the weight of a batch of herbal ingredient.

Post-harvesting Factors   Storage conditions and processing treatments can greatly affect the quality of a herbal ingredient. Inappropriate storage after harvesting can result in microbial contamination, and processes such as drying may result in a loss of thermolabile active constituents.

Adulteration/Substitution   Instances of herbal remedies adulterated with other plant material and even with conventional medicines have been documented.[46] Reports of herbal products devoid of known active constituents have reinforced the need for adequate quality control of herbal remedies.

Misidentification of a Chinese plant included in a slimming preparation is believed to be responsible for serious toxicity experienced by some 70 Belgian women, 30 of whom have needed dialysis or kidney transplants.[49,50] Confusion between *Stephania tetrandra* and the nephrotoxic and potentially carcinogenic plant *Aristolochia fangchi* has been linked with the toxicity and is thought to have arisen because of similarities in the common Chinese names used for the two plants.

Identity Tests   In order to try and ensure the quality of licensed herbal remedies, it is essential therefore not only to establish the botanical identity of a herbal ingredient but also to ensure batch-to-batch reproducibility. Thus, in addition to macroscopical and microscopical evaluation, identity tests are necessary. Such tests include simple chemical tests, e.g. colour or precipitation and chromatographic tests. Thin-layer chromatography is commonly used for identification purposes but for herbal ingredients containing volatile oils a gas-liquid chromatographic test may be used. Although the aim of such tests is to confirm the presence of active principle(s), it is frequently the case that the nature of the active principle has not been established. In such instances chemical and chromatographic tests help to provide batch-to-batch comparability and the chromatogram may be used as a 'fingerprint' for the herbal ingredient by demonstrating the profile of some common plant constituents such as flavonoids.

Assay   For those herbal ingredients with known active principles, an assay should be established in order to set the criterion for the minimum accepted percentage of active substance(s). Such assays should, wherever possible, be specific for individual chemical substances and high pressure liquid chromatography or gas liquid chromatography are the methods of choice. Where such assays have not been established then non-specific methods such as titration or colorimetric assays may be used to determine the total content of a group of closely related compounds.

Contaminants of Herbal Ingredients   Herbal ingredients should be of high quality and free from insect, other animal matter and excreta. It is not possible to remove completely all contaminants and hence specifications should be set in order to limit them:

Ash values   Incineration of a herbal ingredient produces ash which constitutes inorganic matter. Treatment of the ash with hydrochloric acid results in acid-insoluble ash which consists mainly of silica and may be used to act as a measure of soil present. Limits may be set for ash and acid-insoluble ash of herbal ingredients.

Foreign Organic Matter   It is not possible to collect a herbal ingredient without small amounts of related parts of plant or other plants. Standards should be set in order to limit the percentage of such unwanted plant contaminants.

Microbial Contamination   Aerobic bacteria and fungi are normally present in plant material and may increase due to faulty growing, harvesting, storage or processing. Herbal ingredients, particularly those with high starch content may be prone to increased microbial growth.[46] It is not uncommon for herbal ingredients to have aerobic bacteria present at 10^2–10^8 colony forming units per gram. Pathogenic organisms including *Enterobacter*, *Enterococcus*, *Clostridium*, *Pseudomonas*, *Shigella* and *Streptococcus* have been shown to contaminate herbal ingredients. It is essential that limits be set for microbial contamination.

Pesticides   Herbal ingredients, particularly those grown as cultivated crops, may be contaminated by DDT or other chlorinated hydrocarbons, organophosphates, carbamates or polychlorinated biphenyls. Limit tests are necessary for acceptable levels of pesticide contamination of herbal ingredients.

Fumigants   Ethylene oxide, methyl bromide and phosphine have been used to control pests which contaminate herbal ingredients. The use of such substances is no longer permitted in Europe.

Toxic Metals   Lead, cadmium. mercury, thallium and arsenic have been shown to be contaminants of some herbal ingredients. Limit tests for such toxic metals are essential for herbal ingredients.

Other Contaminants   As standards increase for the quality of herbal ingredients it is possible that tests to limit other contaminants such as endotoxins, mycotoxins and radionuclides will be utilised to ensure high quality for medicinal purposes.

Herbal Products

Quality assurance of herbal products may be ensured by control of the herbal ingredients and by means of good manufacturing practice. Some herbal products have many herbal ingredients with only small amounts of individual herbs being present. Chemical and chromatographic tests are useful for developing finished product specifications. Stability and shelf life of herbal products should be established by manufacturers. There should be no differences in standards set for the quality of dosage forms, such as tablets or capsules, of herbal remedies from those of other pharmaceutical preparations.

For licensed herbal remedies the ESCOP monographs are an important development in establishing EC-wide specification of herbal ingredients and hence of products. The Review of Medicines (*see* p. 4) has resulted in a rationalisation of some products, and the reduction of the number of herbal ingredients in any one product has been encouraged by Licensing Authorities.

The quality of an unlicensed herbal remedy will not have been assessed by a Licensing Authority and may thus potentially affect the safety and efficacy of the product. In view of this, it may be concluded that a pharmacist should only sell or recommend herbal remedies that hold a product licence. However, the majority of herbal remedies are only available as unlicensed products. When deciding upon the suitability of such products, a pharmacist should consider the intended use and the manufacturer. It is highly likely that unlicensed herbal remedies manufactured by an established pharmaceutical company will have been subjected to suitable in-house quality control procedures.

SAFETY

As with all forms of self-treatment, the use of herbal remedies presents a potential risk to human health.[1,46,47,51–55] Self-administration of any therapy in preference to orthodox treatment may delay a patient seeking qualified advice, or cause a patient to abandon conventional treatment without first seeking qualified advice.

The safety of all medicinal products is of the utmost importance. All product licence applications for new medicines undergo extensive evaluation of their risk-to-benefit ratio and, once granted, licensed products are closely monitored for the occurrence of adverse effects. The safety of herbal remedies is of particular importance in that the majority of these products are self- prescribed and are used to treat minor and often chronic conditions.

The extensive traditional use of plants as medicines has enabled those medicines with acute and obvious signs of toxicity to be well recognised and their use avoided. However, the premise that traditional use of a plant for perhaps many hundreds of years establishes its safety does not necessarily hold true. The more subtle and chronic forms of toxicity, such as carcinogenicity, mutagenicity, and hepatotoxicity, may well have been overlooked by previous generations and it is these types of toxicities that are of most concern when assessing the safety of herbal remedies.

Intrinsically Toxic Constituents of Herbal Ingredients

Limited toxicological data are available on medicinal plants. However, there exists a considerable overlap between those herbs used for medicinal purposes and those used for cosmetic or culinary purposes, for which a significant body of information exists. For many culinary herbs used in herbal remedies, there is no reason to doubt their safety providing the intended dose and route of administration is in line with their food use. When intended for use in larger therapeutic doses the safety of culinary herbs requires re-evaluation.

Culinary Herbs

Some culinary herbs contain potentially toxic constituents. The safe use of these herbs is ensured by limiting the level of constituent permitted in a food product to a level not considered to represent a health hazard.

Apiole The irritant principle present in the volatile oil of parsley is held to be responsible for the abortifacient action.[54] Apiole is also hepatotoxic and liver damage has been documented as a result of excessive ingestion of parsley, far exceeding normal dietary consumption, over a prolonged period.[54] See Parsley monograph.

β-Asarone Calamus rhizome oil contains β-asarone as the major component, which has been shown to be carcinogenic in animal studies.[54] Many other culinary herbs contain low levels of β-asarone in their volatile oils and therefore the level of β-asarone permitted in foods as a flavouring is restricted.

Estragole (Methylchavicol) Estragole is a constituent of many culinary herbs but is a major component of the oils of tarragon, fennel, sweet basil, and chervil. Estragole has been reported to be carcinogenic in animals.[54] The level of estragole permitted in food products as a flavouring is restricted.

Safrole Animal studies involving safrole, the major component of sassafras oil, have shown it to be hepatotoxic.[54] The permitted level of safrole in foods is 0.1 mg/kg.

Other Intrinsically Toxic Constituents

Pyrrolizidine Alkaloids (PAs) are present in a number of plant species, notably *Crotalaria, Heliotropium and Senecio*. Many of these plants have been used in African, Caribbean and South American countries as food sources and as medicinal 'bush teas'. Hepatotoxicity associated with their consumption is well documented and has been attributed to the pyrrolizidine alkaloid constituents.[46,52,55] Pyrrolizidine alkaloids can be divided into two categories based on their structure, namely those with an unsaturated nucleus (toxic) and those with a saturated nucleus (considered to be non-toxic).

A number of herbs currently used in herbal remedies contain pyrrolizidines; they include liferoot (*Senecio aureus*), borage, comfrey, coltsfoot, and echinacea (see individual monographs).

In addition to various animal studies, two cases of human hepatotoxicity associated with the ingestion of comfrey have been documented (*see* Comfrey monograph). The levels of pyrrolizidine alkaloid present in borage and coltsfoot are thought to be too low to be of clinical significance, although the dangers associated with low-dose exposure are unclear. The use of borage oil as a source of gamma-linolenic acid and as an alternative to evening primrose oil is currently very popular. Whether or not pyrrolizidine alkaloids are present in the borage oil is unclear from published data. The pyrrolizidine alkaloids identified in echinacea to-date have been of the non-toxic saturated type.

Benzophenanthridine Alkaloids are present in bloodroot and in prickly ash. Although some of these alkaloids have exhibited cytotoxic properties in animal studies, their toxicity to humans has been refuted (see Bloodroot monograph).

Proteins

Lectins are plant proteins which possess haemagglutinating and potent mitogenic properties. Both mistletoe and pokeroot contain lectins. Systemic exposure to pokeroot has resulted in haematological aberrations. Mistletoe lectins may also inhibit protein synthesis[4] (see Mistletoe and Pokeroot monographs).

Viscotoxins, constituents of mistletoe, are low molecular weight proteins which possess cytotoxic and cardiotoxic properties.[4] For many years, mistletoe preparations have been used in Europe as cancer treatments. Clinical trials carried out with Iscador™, a product produced from the naturally fermented plant juice of mistletoe, have concluded that Iscador™ may exhibit some weak antitumour effects but should only be used alongside conventional therapy in the long term treatment of cancer.

Lignans   Hepatotoxic reactions reported for chaparral have been associated with the lignan constituents (*see* Chaparral monograph).

Saponins   Pokeroot also contains irritant saponins which have produced severe gastrointestinal irritation involving intense abdominal cramping and haematemesis. Systemic exposure to these saponins has resulted in hypotension and tachycardia. In May 1979, the US Herb Trade Association requested that all its members should stop selling pokeroot as a herbal beverage or food because of its toxicity. [56]

Diterpenes   The irritant properties of many diterpenes are well documented and queen's delight contains diterpene esters which are extremely irritant to all mucosal surfaces (see Queen's Delight monograph).

Cyanogenetic Glycosides   Cyanogenetic glycosides are present in the kernels of a number of fruits including apricot, bitter almond, cherry, pear, and plum seeds. Gastric hydrolysis of these compounds following oral ingestion results in the release of hydrogen cyanide (HCN), which is rapidly absorbed from the upper gastrointestinal tract and which can lead to respiratory failure. It has been estimated that oral doses of 50 mg of HCN can be fatal, equivalent to about 50-60 apricot kernels[7] (see Apricot monograph). However, variation in cyanogenetic glycoside content of the kernels could reduce or increase the number required for a fatal reaction. In the early 1980s a substance called amygdalin was promoted as a 'natural' non-toxic cure for cancer. Amygdalin is a cyanogenetic glycoside that is also referred to as laetrile and vitamin B_{17}. Two near-fatal episodes of HCN poisoning were recorded in which the patients had consumed apricot kernels as an alternative source of amygdalin, due to the poor availability of laetrile. Scientific research did not support the claims made for laetrile, although a small number of anecdotal reports suggested that laetrile may have some slight anticancer activity. As a result, legislation drawn up in 1984[57] restricted the availability of cyanogenetic substances so that amygdalin can only be administered under medical supervision.

Volatile oils   See below, p. 9.

Herbal Ingredients that may cause Adverse Effects

Examples of adverse effects that have been documented in humans or animals for the herbal ingredients described in the monographs are summarised in **Table 1**. These adverse effects include allergic, cardiac, hepatic, hormonal, irritant, and purgative effects, and a range of toxicities. Some of the potential adverse effects of the herbal ingredients which are the subject of the 141 monographs are listed in **Table 2** (pp. 13–14). For further detailed information, including literature references, the reader should consult individual monographs. The following few examples are illustrative of some of the adverse effects caused by herbal ingredients.

Comfrey, Coltsfoot   Hepatotoxic reactions have been documented for comfrey and coltsfoot. Both of these herbal ingredients contain pyrrolizidine alkaloids, compounds known to be hepatotoxic. However, it was later reported that the reaction documented for coltsfoot may have in fact involved a herbal tea containing a *Senecio* species rather than coltsfoot.[46] The *Senecio* genus is characterized by its pyrrolizidine alkaloid constituents.

Table 1   Examples of Adverse Effects that may occur with Herbal Ingredients

Potential Adverse Effect	Constituent/Herbal Ingredient
Allergic (*see* Appendix 12)	
Hypersensitive	Sesquiterpene lactones: arnica, chamomile, feverfew, yarrow
Phototoxic	Furanocoumarins: angelica, celery, wild carrot
Immune	Canavanine: alfalfa
Cardiac (see Appendix 3)	Cardiac glycosides: pleurisy root, squill
Endocrine	
Hypoglycaemic (*see* Appendix 9)	Alfalfa, fenugreek
Hyperthyroid	Iodine: fucus
Hormonal (*see* Appendix 10)	
Mineralocorticoid	Triterpenoids: liquorice
Oestrogenic	Isoflavonoids: alfalfa, red clover Saponins: ginseng
Anti-androgen	Saw palmetto
Irritant (*see* Appendix 13)	
Gastrointestinal	Numerous compounds including anthraquinones (purgative), capsaicinoids, diterpenes, saponins, terpene-rich volatile oils
Renal	Aescin: horse-chestnut; terpene-rich volatile oils
Toxic	
Hepatotoxic/carcinogenic	Pyrrolizidine alkaloids: comfrey, liferoot; β-asarone: calamus; lignans: chaparral; safrole:sassafras
Mitogenic	Proteins: mistletoe, pokeroot
Cyanide poisoning	Cyanogenetic glycosides: apricot
Convulsant	Camphor/thujone-rich volatile oils

Mistletoe, Scullcap A case of hepatitis has been reported for a woman who was taking a multi-constituent herbal product (see Mistletoe monograph). Based on the known toxic constituents of mistletoe and other herbal ingredients present in the product, it was concluded that mistletoe was the component responsible for the hepatitis. Lectins and viscotoxins, the toxic constituents in mistletoe, are not known to be hepatotoxic and no other reports of liver damage associated with mistletoe ingestion have been documented. The product also contained scullcap, which is recognised to be frequently adulterated with a *Teucrium* species. Recently, hepatotoxic reactions have been associated with germander (*Teucrium chamaedrys*) (*see* Scullcap monograph).

Pokeroot Severe gastrointestinal irritation and haematological abnormalities documented for pokeroot can be directly related to the saponin and lectin constituents of pokeroot.[46]

Sassafras Hepatotoxicity has been associated with the consumption of a herbal tea containing sassafras. The principal component of sassafras volatile oil is safrole, which is known to be hepatotoxic.[54]

Excessive Ingestion

Ginseng Excessive doses of ginseng have been reported to cause agitation, insomnia, and raised blood pressure and have been referred to as abuse of the remedy. However, side-effects have also been reported for ginseng following the ingestion of recommended doses, and include mastalgia and vaginal bleeding.[13]

Liquorice Excessive ingestion of liquorice has resulted in typical corticosteroid-type side-effects of oedema and hypertension.[52]

Parsley Parsley volatile oil contains apiole which is structurally related to the recognised hepatocarcinogen, safrole. Ingestion of apiole has resulted in a number of cases of fatal poisoning.[54]

Hypersensitivity Reactions

Chamomile Sesquiterpene lactones are known to possess allergenic properties.[42] They occur predominantly in herbs of the Compositae (Asteraceae) family, of which chamomile is a member. Hypersensitivity reactions have been reported for chamomile and other plants from the same family. Cross-sensitivity to other members of the Compositae family is well recognised.

Feverfew The sesquiterpene lactones present in feverfew are considered to be the active principles in the herb. It is unknown whether documented side-effects for feverfew, such as mouth ulcers and swollen tongue, are also attributable to these constituents.[14]

Phototoxic Reactions

Parsley Furanocoumarins, compounds known to cause phototoxic reactions, are constituents of parsley. Excessive ingestion of parsley has been associated with the development of photosensitive rash which resolved once parsley consumption ceased.[54]

Precautions in Specific Patient Groups

Pregnant/Nursing Mothers

Few conventional medicines have been established as safe to take during pregnancy and it is generally recognised that no drug substance should be taken unless the perceived benefit outweighs the possible risk. This rule is also applicable to herbal remedies which are often mistakenly considered to be natural and completely safe alternatives to conventional medicines.

Table 3 (p. 15–16) lists some herbal ingredients taken from the following 141 monographs that are specifically best avoided or used with caution during pregnancy. As with conventional medicines, no herbal remedies should be taken during pregnancy unless the benefit outweighs the potential risk.

Volatile Oils Many herbs are traditionally reputed to be abortifacient and for some this reputation can be attributed to their volatile oil component.[54] A number of volatile oils are irritant to the genito-urinary tract if ingested and may induce uterine contractions. Herbs that contain irritant volatile oils include ground ivy, juniper, parsley, pennyroyal, sage, tansy and yarrow. Some of these oils contain the terpenoid constituent thujone which is known to be abortifacient. Pennyroyal oil also contains the hepatotoxic terpenoid constituent pulegone. A case of liver failure in a woman who ingested pennyroyal oil as an abortifacient has been documented (see Pennyroyal monograph).

Uteroactivity A stimulant or spasmolytic action on uterine muscle has been documented for some herbal ingredients including blue cohosh, burdock, fenugreek, golden seal, hawthorn, jamaica dogwood, motherwort, nettle, raspberry, and vervain. Raspberry is a popular remedy taken during pregnancy to help promote an easier labour by relaxing the uterine muscles. The pharmacological activity exhibited by raspberry may vary between different preparations and from one individual to another. Raspberry should not be used during pregnancy unless under medical supervision.

Herbal Teas Increased awareness of the harmful effects associated with excessive tea and coffee consumption has prompted many individuals to switch to herbal teas. Whilst some herbal teas may offer pleasant alternatives to tea and coffee, some contain pharmacologically active herbal ingredients, which may have unpredictable effects depending on the quantity of tea consumed and strength of the brew. Some herbal teas contain laxative herbal ingredients such as senna, frangula, and cascara. In general stimulant laxative preparations are not recommended during pregnancy and the use of unstandardised laxative preparations is particularly unsuitable. A case of hepatotoxicity in a newborn baby has been documented in which the mother consumed a herbal tea during pregnancy as an expectorant.[58] Following analysis the herbal tea was reported to contain pyrrolizidine alkaloids which are known to be hepatotoxic.

Nursing Mothers A drug substance taken by a nursing mother presents a hazard if it is transferred to the breast milk in pharmacologically or toxicologically significant amounts. Limited information is available regarding the safety of conventional medicines taken during breastfeeding. Much less information exists for herbal ingredients, and generally the use of herbal remedies is not recommended during lactation.

Paediatric Use

Herbal remedies have traditionally been used to treat both adults and children. Herbal remedies may offer a milder alternative to some conventional medicines, although the suitability of a herbal remedy needs to be considered with respect to quality, safety and efficacy. Herbal remedies should be used with caution in children and medical advice should be sought if in doubt. Chamomile is a popular remedy used to treat teething pains in babies. However, chamomile is known to contain allergenic sesquiterpene lactones and should therefore be used with caution. The administration of herbal teas to children is generally unwise unless used according to professional advice.

Contra-indications, Warnings, Drug Interactions

Limited information has been documented concerning the interaction of herbal remedies with conventional medicines. [12,53] Instances of drug interactions have been tentatively linked, retrospectively, to the concurrent use of herbal remedies, although the rationale for such interactions is often difficult to justify if knowledge regarding the pharmacological activity of the herbal remedy is in question. An attempt can be made, however, to identify herbal ingredients that have the potential to interfere with specific categories of conventional drugs, based on known phytochemical and pharmacological properties of the herb, and on any documented side-effects.

For example, herbs containing substantial levels of coumarins may potentially increase blood coagulation time if taken in large doses. St John's Wort contains hypericin, a known photosensitiser, and celery and parsley contain furanocoumarins which may also precipitate a photosensitive allergic reaction. Some herbs, such as juniper, sage, tansy and yarrow, contain irritant volatile oils and may be toxic if ingested in large quantities. Prolonged or excessive use of a herbal diuretic may potentiate existing diuretic therapy, interfere with existing hypo/hypertensive therapy, or potentiate the effect of certain cardioactive drugs due to hypokalaemia. Herbs which have been documented to lower blood sugar levels may cause hypoglycaemia if taken in sufficient amounts and interfere with existing hypoglycaemic therapy. An individual receiving antihypertensive therapy may be more susceptible to the hypertensive side-effects that have been documented with, for example, ginseng or which are associated with the excessive ingestion of plants such as liquorice.

This approach has been used in drawing up Appendixes 1–13 which are to be found on pp. 277–84, after the monographs. These Appendixes provide information on **potential** drug-herb interactions. Appendix 1 groups together various therapeutic categories of medical drugs that may be affected by a particular herb or group of herbs. Appendixes 2–13 list herbal ingredients which are claimed to have a specific activity alphabetically within each Appendix, including laxative, cardioactive, diuretic, hypo/hypertensive, anticoagulant/coagulant, hypo/hyperlipidaemic, seda-

tive, hypo/hyperglycaemic, hormonal, immunostimulant, allergenic or irritant. Some commonly occurring groups of natural products found within these 141 herbal ingredients contribute towards their activities, toxicities or adverse effects. Appendixes 14–20 (pp. 285–6) list those herbal ingredients which contain amines, alkaloids or have sympathomimetic activity, coumarins, flavonoids, iridoids, saponins, tannins or volatile oils.

EFFICACY

Many of the herbs which are used medicinally in Europe have a traditional reputation for their uses, but there is little scientific or medical documentation in respect of their active constituents, pharmacological actions or clinical efficacy. Examples of this group include avens, boneset, burdock, clivers, damiana, jamaica dogwood, parsley piert, pulsatilla, and wild lettuce. For other herbs, documented phytochemical or animal data may support traditional uses, but evidence of human efficacy is limited.

Relatively few herbal ingredients have been subjected to rigorous scientific study, with their pharmacological activities and active principles successfully investigated. Examples of herbs that have been subject to such study include chamomile, feverfew, ginkgo, ginseng, hawthorn, hops, uva-ursi, and valerian.

A number of factors specific to herbs need to be considered when attempting scientific validation of efficacy.

Lack of Phytochemical Data   The chemical constituents of a herb can provide a useful indication of its pharmacological properties.

In vivo and In vitro Relevance   In terms of efficacy the relevance of *in-vivo* or *in-vitro* animal studies, often the only information available, is questionable for any pharmacologically active substance.

Lack of Clinical Data   Clinical trials require considerable resources, normally far beyond the budget of most herbal remedy manufacturers. Of those studies that are performed, many are of inadequate trial design and therefore provide limited valid information.

Formulated Product versus Crude Extract   A formulated product containing, for example, an aqueous plant extract, equivalent to the same weight of a crude aqueous plant extract may not necessarily be bioequivalent. Most pharmacological studies *in vivo* involve the administration of a crude plant extract and not a formulated product. Many herbal remedies contain milligram doses of herbal ingredients which would appear sub-therapeutic when compared to therapeutic doses recommended in various herbal pharmacopoeias. Despite the dearth of documented clinical data for the majority of herbal ingredients, there is no reason why they should not be available for **minor** conditions providing that these are consistent with traditional uses and that the herbal ingredients are of suitable quality and safety. It would seem to be more appropriate to use those herbal ingredients for which documented phytochemical and pharmacological data support the traditional use. Herbal remedies intended for use in more serious medical conditions require full clinical data to support their use.

Herbal Remedies of Current Interest

Evening Primrose Use of the oil in varying conditions such as premenstrual tension, eczema, and hyperactivity in children has been under recent investigation.[15,17]

Feverfew Clinical trials have reported feverfew to be an effective prophylactic for the treatment of migraine in patients refractory to conventional treatment.[14] However, there are currently no licensed feverfew products available in the UK.

Garlic Numerous studies have documented the hypocholesterolaemic and antimicrobial properties of garlic. However, the efficacy of formulated products compared with the raw bulb has not been established.

Ginger Human studies indicated ginger to be an effective prophylactic against motion sickness, although subsequent researchers have concluded ginger to be ineffective.

Ginkgo Ginkgo is widely used in France and Germany in licensed herbal remedies for the treatment of circulatory insufficiencies (peripheral and cerebral). Numerous studies have documented the anti-inflammatory actions of Ginkgo.[19] Currently, no licensed herbal remedies containing Ginkgo are available in the UK.

Ginseng Ginseng is widely renowned for its adaptogenic properties in Eastern countries, where it is used to help the body cope with stress and fatigue, and to promote recovery from illness or imbalance such as hypertension or hypoglycaemia. generally it is only recommended to be used for certain individuals with specific illnesses. By comparison, in the UK ginseng is mainly self-administered and taken in the form of tablets or capsules containing dried extracts of the root. Ginseng products available in the UK are sold as food supplements, often in combination with vitamins and minerals. A wealth of research has been documented for ginseng describing an incredible range of pharmacological activities, particularly on the hypothalamic and pituitary regions of the brain.[6,13,25]

Valerian and Hops Human studies have reported valerian to be effective in improving sleep disturbances.[8,18] It is unclear whether the active principles in valerian are associated with volatile oil, the iridoid components termed valepotriates or with some other, as yet unidentified, group of constituents. Valerian has been recommended as an alternative to orthodox sedatives, particularly to assist in the withdrawal of patients from benzodiazepine dependence.[59] Sedative properties have been documented for hops in animals and, when given in combination with valerian, hops have also been reported to improve sleep quality in humans.

Immunostimulant Activity High molecular weight polysaccharide components are thought to be responsible for the immunostimulant activity of certain plants including arnica, calendula, chamomile, echinacea, ginseng, and saw palmetto.

Antihepatotoxic Activity One of the best studied groups of plant substances with respect to their hepatoprotective properties is the silymarin mixture of *Silybum marianum*. Other plants reported to exhibit antihepatotoxic activity include

artichoke, *Schizandra* species and plantain. Results of these investigations have indicated that activity is associated with the phenolic constituents such as flavonoids and lignans.

Antiviral Activity Hypericin isolated from St. John's Wort is currently under investigation for antiviral activity, particularly against the HIV virus.

Conclusion

This handbook provides the reader with factual information on a number of herbal ingredients present in herbal remedies in the United Kingdom. Herbal remedies can offer an alternative to conventional medicines in non-life-threatening conditions, providing they are of adequate quality and safety, and are used in an appropriate manner by suitable individuals.

References

1. Keller K. Phytotherapy on the European level. *European Phytotelegram* 1994; **6:** 40-9.

2. Fulder S. *The handbook of complementary medicine.* Sevenoaks: Coronet, 1984.

3. Phillipson JD. The pros and cons of herbal remedies. *Pharm J* 1981; **227:** 387-92.

4. Anderson LA and Phillipson JD. Mistletoe – the magic herb. *Pharm J* 1982; **229:** 437-9.

5. Phillipson JD and Anderson LA. Pharmacologically active compounds in herbal remedies. *Pharm J* 1984; **232:** 41-4.

6. Phillipson JD and Anderson LA. Ginseng – quality, safety and efficacy? *Pharm J* 1984; **232:** 161-5.

7. Chandler RF, Phillipson JD and Anderson LA. Controversial laetrile. *Pharm J* 1984; **232:** 330-2.

8. Phillipson JD and Anderson LA. Herbal remedies used in sedative and antirheumatic preparations. Part 1. *Pharm J* 1984; **233:** 80-2.

9. Phillipson JD and Anderson LA. Herbal remedies used in sedative and antirheumatic preparations. Part 2. *Pharm J* 1984; **233:** 111-15.

10. Phillipson JD and Anderson LA. Counterprescribing of herbal remedies. Part 1. *Pharm J* 1984; **233:** 235-8.

11. Phillipson JD and Anderson LA. Counterprescribing of herbal remedies. Part 2. *Pharm J* 1984; **233:** 272-4.

12. Anderson LA and Phillipson JD. Herbal medicine. education and the pharmacist. *Pharm J* 1985; **236:** 303-5.

13. Baldwin CA, Anderson LA and Phillipson JD. What pharmacists should know about ginseng. *Pharm J* 1986; **237:** 583-6.

14. Baldwin CA, Anderson LA and Phillipson JD. What pharmacists should know about feverfew. *Pharm J* 1987; **239:** 237-8.

15. Barber AJ. Evening primrose oil: a panacea? *Pharm J* 1988; **240:** 723-5.

16. Marshall JM. Aloe vera gel: what is the evidence? *Pharm J* 1990; **24:** 360-2.

17. Li Wan Po A. Evening primrose oil. *Pharm J* 1991; **246:** 670-6.

18.   Houghton PJ. Valerian. *Pharm J* 1994; **253:** 95-6

19.   Houghton PJ. Ginkgo. *Pharm J* 1994; **253:** 122-3.

20.   Houghton PJ. Echinacea. *Pharm J* 1994; **253:** 342-3.

21.   Houghton PJ. Agnus castus. *Pharm J* 1994; **253:** 720-1.

22.   Berry M. Feverfew. *Pharm J* 1994; **253:** 806-8.

23.   Berry M. The chamomiles. *Pharm J* 1995; **254:** 191-3

24.   Houghton PJ. Guarana. *Pharm J* 1995; **254:** 435-6.

25.   Raman A and Houghton PJ. Ginseng. *Pharm J* 1995; **254:** 150-1.

26.   Cranz H. Medicinal Plants and phytomedicines within the European Community. *Herbalgram* 1994; **30:** 50-3.

27.   Medicines Act Leaflet (MAL) 8. A Guide to the Status under the Medicines Act of Borderline Products for Human Use. London: Medicines Control Agency.

28.   Council Directive 65/65/EEC. *Off J EC* 1965; **22:** 369.

29.   Statutory Instrument (SI) 1994:3144, The Medicines for Human Use (Marketing Authorisations Etc) Regulations.

30.   The Medicines Act, l968. London: HM Stationery Office.

31.   Appelbe GE and Wingfield J. *Dale and Appelbe's Pharmacy Law and Ethics*, 5th Ed.., Herbal Remedies, Chapter 11 pp.104–9. London: The Pharmaceutical Press 1993.

32.   Quality of Herbal Remedies. *The Rules Governing Medicinal Products in the European Community* 1989, vol. III; 31-7.

33.   Manufacture of Herbal Products. *The Rules Governing Medicinal Products in the European Community* 1992, vol. IV: 127–9.

34.   Statutory Instrument (SI) 1971: 1450, The Medicines (Exemptions from Licences) (Special and Transitional Cases) Order.

35.   Anon. Herbal licensing position confirmed. *Pharm J* 1994; **253:** 746.

36.   De Smet PAGM. Should herbal medicine-like products be licensed as medicines? *Br Med J* 1995; **310:** 1023-4.

37.   Vautier G, Spiller RC. Safety of complementary medicines should be monitored. *Br Med J* 1995; **311:** 633.

38.   Statutory Instrument (SI) 1984: 769, The Medicines (Products Other than Veterinary Drugs) (General Sales List) Order, 1984, as amended by SI 1985:1540, SI 1987: 910, SI 1989: 969 and SI 1990: 1129.

39.   Statutory Instrument (SI) 1983: 1212, The Medicines (Products Other than Veterinary Drugs) (Prescription Only) Order 1983, as amended.

40.   Statutory Instrument (SI) 1977: 2130, (The Medicines Retail Sale or Supply of Herbal Remedies) Order, 1977.

41.   Medicines Act Leaflet (MAL) 2. Guidelines on Safety and Efficacy Requirements for Herbal Medicinal Products. *Guidance Notes on Applications for Product Licences*; 1989, 53-4

42.   Deboyser P. Traditional herbal medicines around the globe: modern perspectives. *Swiss Pharma* 1991; 13: 86-9.

43.   Britt R . The New EC Systems in the UK, *Regulatory Affairs J* 1995; **6:** 380-4.

44.   European Scientific Cooperative for Phytotherapy (ESCOP). *Proposals for European Monographs*, vol. 1 1990, vol. 2 1992, vol. 3 1992. Meppel, Netherlands: ESCOP.

45.   Phillipson JD. Quality assurance of medicinal plants. In: Franz C, Seitz R and Verlet N. First World Congress on medicinal and aromatic plants for human welfare, WOCMAP, quality, phytochemistry, industrial aspects, economic aspects. *Acta Horticulturae* 1993; **333:** 117-22.

46.   De Smet PAGM (ed.) *et al. Adverse effects of herbal drugs* vol. 1. Berlin: Springer Verlag, 1992.

47.   Der Smet PAGM (ed.) *et al.* Adverse effects of herbal drugs vol. 2. Berlin: Springer Verlag, 1993.

48.   Evans WC. *Trease and Evans' Pharmacognosy*, 13th Ed. London: Bailliere Tindall, 1989.

49.   Vanhaelen M, Vanhaelen-Fastre R, But P, Vennerwegnem J-L. Identification of aristolochic acid in Chinese herbs. *Lancet* 1994; **343:** 174.

50.   Cosyns J-P, Jadoul M. Squifflet J-P, DePlaen J-F, Ferluga D, van Ypersele de Strihou, C. Chinese herbs nephropathy: a clue to Balkan endemic nephropathy. *Kidney International* 1994; **45:** 1680-8.

51.   Dukes MNG. Remedies used in non-orthodox medicine. Dukes MNG (Ed.) *Side effects of drugs annual*. 1. Amsterdam: Excerpta Medica 1977; 317-8.

52.   D'Arcy PF. Adverse reactions and interactions with herbal medicines. Part 1. Adverse reactions. *Adverse Drug React Toxicol Rev* 1991; **10:** 189-208.

53.   D'Arcy PF. Adverse reactions and interactions with herbal medicines. Part 2. Drug interactions. *Adverse Drug React Toxicol Rev* 1993; **12:** 147-62.

54.   Tisserand R and Balacs T. *Essential oil safety.* Edinburgh: Churchill Livingstone, 1995.

55.   Mattocks AR. *Chemistry and toxicology of pyrrolizidine alkaloids.* New York: Academic Press 1986.

56.   Tyler VE. *The Honest Herbal*, 3rd Edn. New York: Howarth Press, 1993.

57.   Statutory Instrument (SI) 1984:87. The Medicines (Cyanogenetic Substances) Order 1984.

58.   Roulet M et al. Hepatic veno-occlusive disease in newborn infant of a woman drinking herbal tea. *J Pediatr* 1988; **112:** 433-6.

59.   Hoffman D. How herbs help in benzodiazepine dependence. *J Alternative Medicine* 1985; **27:** 10-11.

TABLE 2   ADVERSE EFFECTS   13

Table 2   Potential Adverse Effects of Herbal Ingredients Listed in theMonographs

Herb	Adverse effect	Reasons/Comments
Agnus Castus	Allergic reactions	—
Alfalfa	Systemic lupus erythematosus syndrome	Canavanine, toxic amino acid
Aloes	Purgative, irritant to GI tract	Anthraquinones
Angelica	Phototoxic dermatitis	Furanocoumarins
Aniseed	Contact dermatitis	Anethole in volatile oil
Apricot[1]	Cyanide poisoning, seed	Cyanogenetic glycosides
Arnica[1]	Dermatitis, irritant to GI tract	Sesquiterpene lactones
Artichoke	Allergenic, dermatitis	Sesquiterpene lactones
Asafoetida	Dermatitis, irritant	Gum, related species
Bayberry	Carcinogenic to rats	—
Blue Flag	Nausea, vomiting, irritant to GI tract and eyes	Fresh root, furfural (volatile oil)
Bogbean	Purgative, vomiting	In large doses
Boldo	Toxicity, irritant	Volatile oil
Boneset	Dermatitis, cytotoxic	Sesquiterpene lactones
Borage[1]	Genotoxic, carcinogenic, hepatotoxic	Pyrrolizidine alkaloids
Broom	Cardiac depressant	Sparteine (alkaloid)
Buchu	Irritant to GI tract, kidney	Volatile oil
Calamus[1]	Carcinogenic, nephrotoxic, convulsions	β-Asarone in oil
Capsicum	Irritant	Capsaicinoids
Cascara	Purgative, irritant to GI tract	Anthraquinones
Cassia	Allergenic, irritant	Cinnamaldehyde in volatile oil
Celery	Phototoxic, dermatitis	Furanocoumarins
Cereus	Irritant to GI tract	Fresh juice
Chamomile, German	Allergic reactions	Sesquiterpene lactones
Chamomile, Roman	Allergic reactions	Sesquiterpene lactones
Chaparral	Dermatitis, hepatotoxic	Lignans
Cinnamon	Allergenic, irritant	Cinnamaldehyde in volatile oil
Clove	Irritant	Eugenol in volatile oil
Cohosh, Black	Nausea, vomiting	High doses
Cohosh, Blue	Irritant to GI tract	Seeds poisonous
Cola	Sleeplessness, anxiety, tremor	Caffeine
Coltsfoot[1]	Genotoxic, carcinogenic, hepatotoxic	Pyrrolizidine alkaloids
Comfrey[1]	Genotoxic, carcinogenic, hepatotoxic	Pyrrolizidine alkaloids
Corn Silk	Allergenic, dermatitis	—
Cowslip	Allergenic	Quinones
Damiana	Convulsions	High dose (one report only), quinones, cyano-genetic glycosides
Dandelion	Allergenic, dermatitis	Sesquiterpene lactones
Echinacea	Allergenic, irritant	Polysaccharide
Elecampane	Allergenic, irritant	Sesquiterpene lactones
Eucalyptus	Nausea, vomiting	Oil
Evening Primrose Oil	Mild indigestion, increased risk of epilepsy	Schizophrenic patients on phenothiazines
Eyebright	Mental confusion, raised intraocular pressure	Tincture
Feverfew	Allergenic, dermatitis	Sesquiterpene lactones
Frangula	Purgative, irritant to GI tract	Anthraquinones
Fucus	Hyperthyroidism	Iodine content
Garlic	Irritant to GI tract, dermatitis	Sulphides
Ginkgo	Gastric upset, headache	—

Herb	Adverse effect	Reasons/Comments
Ginseng	Mastalgia, vaginal bleeding , insomnia	Various effects, *see* Monographs
Golden Seal	Gastric upset	Berberine, potentially poisonous
Gravel Root[1]	Genotoxic, carcinogenic, hepatotoxic	Pyrrolizidine alkaloids
Ground Ivy	Irritant to GI tract, kidneys	Pulegone in volatile oil
Guaiacum	Allergenic, dermatitis	Lignans
Hops	Allergenic, dermatitis	Oleo-resin
Horehound, White	Dermatitis, irritant	Plant juice
Horse-chestnut	Nephrotoxic	Aescin
Horseradish	Allergenic, irritant	Glucosinolates
Hydrangea	Dermatitis, irritant to GI tract	—
Hydrocotyle	Phototoxic, dermatitis	—
Ispaghula	Oesophageal obstruction, flatulence	If swallowed dry
Jamaica Dogwood	Irritant, numbness, tremors	High doses
Juniper	Irritant, abortifacient	Volatile oil, confusion with savin
Lady's Slipper	Allergenic, dermatitis, hallucinations	—
Liferoot[1]	Genotoxic, carcinogenic, hepatotoxic	Pyrrolizidine alkaloids
Liquorice	Hyperaldosteronism	Excessive ingestion
Lobelia	Nausea, vomiting, diarrhoea	Lobeline (alkaloid)
Maté	Sleeplessness, anxiety, tremor	Caffeine
Mistletoe	Hepatitis, hypotension, poisonous	Mixed herbal preparation
Motherwort	Phototoxic dermatitis	Volatile oil
Nettle	Irritant	Amines
Parsley	Irritant, hepatitis, phototoxic, abortifacient	Apiole in volatile oil, excessive ingestion
Pennyroyal	Irritant, nephrotoxic, hepatotoxic	Pulegone in volatile oil
Pilewort[1]	Irritant	Protoanemonin
Plantain	Allergenic, dermatitis, irritant	Mustard-type oil
Pleurisy Root	Dermatitis, irritant, cardiac activity	Cardenolides
Pokeroot	Mitogenic, toxic, nausea, vomiting, cramp	Lectins
Prickly Ash, Southern	Toxic to animals	—
Pulsatilla[1]	Allergenic, irritant	Protanemonin
Queen's Delight[1]	Irritant to GI tract	Diterpenes
Red Clover	Oestrogenic	Isoflavonoids
Rhubarb	Purgative, irritant to GI tract	Anthraquinones
Rosemary	Convulsions	Camphor in volatile oil
Sage	Toxic, convulsant	Thujone, camphor in volatile oil
Sassafras[1]	Carcinogenic, genotoxic	Safrole in volatile oil
Scullcap	Hepatotoxicity	Mixed product; adulteration with *Teucrium* spp.
Senega	Irritant to GI tract	Saponins
Senna	Purgative, irritant to GI tract	Anthraquinones
Shepherd's Purse	Irritant	Isothiocyanates
Skunk Cabbage	Itch, inflammation	—
Squill	Irritant, cardioactive	Saponins
St. John's Wort	Phototoxic	Hypericin
Tansy[1]	Severe gastritis, convulsions	Thujone in volatile oil
Thyme	Irritant to GI tract	Thymol in volatile oil
Wild Carrot	Phototoxic, dermatitis	Furanocoumarins
Yarrow	Allergenic, dermatitis	Sesquiterpene lactones
Yellow Dock	Purgative, irritant to G1 tract	Anthraquinones

[1] Not recommended for internal use

TABLE 3   PREGNANCY   15

Table 3   Herbal Ingredients Best Avoided or used with Caution during Pregnancy

Absence of a herbal ingredient from this list does not signify safety and as with all medicines, herbal remedies should only be used where the perceived benefit outweighs any possible risk. For a number of herbs the chemistry and pharmacology are poorly documented and their use in pregnancy should be avoided. Some of the herbs listed are reputed to be abortifacient or to affect the menstrual cycle although no recent clinical or experimental data exists. In view of the potential serious effects caution in their use is advised.

Herb	Effect
Agnus Castus	Hormonal action
Aloes	Cathartic, reputed abortifacient
Apricot	Cyanide toxicity
Asafoetida	Reputed abortifacient and to affect menstrual cycle
Avens	Reputed to affect menstrual cycle
Blue Flag	Irritant oil
Bogbean	Irritant, possible purgative
Boldo	Irritant oil
Boneset	Cytotoxic constituents (related species)
Borage	Pyrrolizidine alkaloids
Broom	Sparteine is oxytoxic
Buchu	Irritant oil
Burdock	Uterine stimulant, *in vivo*
Calendula	Reputed to affect menstrual cycle, uterine stimulant, *in vitro*
Cascara	Anthraquinones, non-standardised preparations to be avoided
Chamomile, German	Reputed to affect menstrual cycle, uterine stimulant with excessive use
Chamomile, Roman	Reputed abortifacient and to affect menstrual cycle with excessive use
Chaparral	Uterine activity, hepatotoxic
Cohosh, Black	Uterine oestrogen receptor binding *in vitro*
Cohosh, Blue	Reputed abortifacient and to affect menstrual cycle
Cola	Caffeine, consumption should be restricted
Coltsfoot	Pyrrolizidine alkaloids
Comfrey	Pyrrolizidine alkaloids
Cornsilk	Uterine stimulant, *in vivo*
Damiana	Cyanogenetic glycosides, risk of cyanide toxicity in high doses
Devil's Claw	Oxytoxic
Eucalyptus	Oil should not be taken internally during pregnancy
Euphorbia	Smooth muscle activity, *in vitro*
Fenugreek	Oxytoxic, uterine stimulant, *in vitro*
Feverfew	Reputed abortifacient and to affect menstrual cycle
Frangula	Anthraquinones, non-standardised preparations to be avoided

Herb	Effect
Fucus	Thyroid gland activity, possible heavy metal contamination
Gentian	Reputed to affect menstrual cycle
Ginseng, Eleutherococcus	Hormonal activity
Ginseng, Panax	Hormonal activity
Golden Seal	Alkaloids with uterine stimulant activity, *in vitro*
Ground Ivy	Irritant oil
Hawthorn	Uterine activity, *in vivo*, *in vitro*
Hops	Uterine activity, *in vitro*
Horehound, Black	Reputed to affect menstrual cycle
Horehound, White	Reputed abortifacient and to affect menstrual cycle
Horseradish	Irritant oil; avoid excessive ingestion
Hydrocotyle	Reputed abortifacient and to affect menstrual cycle
Jamaica Dogwood	Uterine activity, *in vitro*, *in vivo*; irritant
Juniper	Reputed abortifacient and to affect menstrual cycle. Confusion over whether oil is toxic
Liferoot	Pyrrolizidine alkaloids
Liquorice	Oestrogenic activity, reputed abortifacient
Lobelia	Lobeline, toxicity
Maté	Caffeine, consumption should be restricted
Meadowsweet	Uterine activity, *in vitro*
Mistletoe	Toxic constituents, uterine stimulant, animal
Motherwort	Uterine activity, *in vitro*, reputed to affect menstrual cycle
Myrrh	Reputed to affect menstrual cycle
Nettle	Reputed abortifacient and to affect menstrual cycle
Passionflower	Harman, harmaline uterine stimulants, animal
Pennyroyal	Abortifacient, irritant oil (pulegone)
Plantain	Uterine activity, *in vitro*; laxative
Pleurisy Root	Uterine activity, *in vivo*; cardioactive constituents
Pokeroot	Toxic constituents, uterine stimulant, reputed to affect menstrual cycle

Herb	Effect	Herb	Effect
Poplar	Conflicting reports over use of aspirin in pregnancy; salicylates excreted in breast milk may cause rashes in babies	Shepherd's Purse	Reputed abortifacient and to affect menstrual cycle
Prickly Ash, Northern	Pharmacologically active alkaloids and coumarins	Skunk Cabbage	Reputed to affect menstrual cycle
Prickly Ash, Southern	Pharmacologically active alkaloids	Squill	Reputed abortifacient and to affect menstrual cycle
Pulsatilla	Reputed to affect menstrual cycle, uterine activity,, *in vitro*, *in vivo;* irritant (fresh plant)	St. John's Wort	Slight uterine activity, *in vitro*
Queen's Delight	Irritant diterpenes	Tansy	Uterine activity, abortifacient (thujone in oil)
Raspberry	Uterine activity, *in vitro*, traditional use to ease parturition	Uva-Ursi	Large doses, oxytocic
Red Clover	Oestrogenic activity	Vervain	Reputed abortifacient, oxytocic, uteroactivity *in vivo*
Rhubarb	Anthraquinones, non-standardised preparations to be avoided	Wild Carrot	Oestrogenic activity, irritant oil
Sassafras	Abortifacient (oil), hepatotoxic (safrole)	Willow	Conflicting reports over use of aspirin in pregnancy; salicylates excreted in breast milk may cause rashes in babies
Scullcap	Traditional use to eliminate afterbirth and promote menstruation; potential hepatotoxicity	Yarrow	Reputed abortifacient and to affect menstrual cycle (thujone in oil)
Senna	Anthraquinones, non-standardised preparations to be avoided	Yellow Dock	Anthraquinones, non-standardised preparations to be avoided

GENERAL REFERENCES

G1 Bisset NG, editor. *Herbal drugs and phytopharmaceuticals* (Wichtl M, editor, German edition). Stuttgart: Medpharm, 1994.

G2 Bradley PR, editor. *British Herbal Compendium*, Vol 1. Bournemouth: British Herbal Medicine Association, 1992.

G3 *British Herbal Pharmacopoeia.* Keighley: British Herbal Medicine Association, 1983.

G4 *British Herbal Pharmacopoeia 1990*, Vol 1. Bournemouth: British Herbal Medicine Association, 1990.

G5 *British Pharmaceutical Codex 1934.* London: Pharmaceutical Press, 1934.

G6 *British Pharmaceutical Codex 1949.* London: Pharmaceutical Press, 1949.

G7 *British Pharmaceutical Codex 1973.* London: Pharmaceutical Press, 1973.

G8 *British Pharmacopoeia 1993.* London: HMSO, 1993.

G9 Council of Europe. *Flavouring substances and natural sources of flavourings*, 3rd ed. Strasbourg: Maisonneuve, 1981.

G10 Duke JA. *Handbook of medicinal herbs.* Boca Raton: CRC, 1985.

G11 *European Pharmacopoeia*, 2nd edition. Strasbourg: Maisonneuve, 1980.

G12 Farnsworth NR. Potential value of plants as sources of new antifertility agents I. *J Pharm Sci* 1975; **64**: 535-98.

G13 Frohne D, Pfänder HJ. *A colour atlas of poisonous plants.* London: Wolfe, 1984.

G14 The Medicines (Products other than Veterinary Drugs) (General Sales List), SI No.769: 1984, as amended SI No.1540: 1985; SI No.1129: 1990; and SI No.2410: 1994.

G15 Grieve M. *A modern herbal.* Thetford, Norfolk: Lowe and Brydon, 1979.

G16 Guenther E. *The essential oils*, 6 volumes. New York: Van Nostrand, 1948-1952.

G17 Hamon NW, Blackburn JL. *Herbal products – a factual appraisal for the health care professional.* Winnipeg: Cantext, 1985.

G18 Hoppe HA. *Taschenbuch der drogenkunde.* Berlin: de Gruyter, 1981.

G19 Leung AY. *Encyclopedia of common natural ingredients used in food, drugs and cosmetics.* New York-Chichester: Wiley, 1980

G20 Mabey, R (editor). *The complete new herbal.* London: Elm Tree Books, 1988.

G21 *Martindale: The Extra Pharmacopoeia*, 28th edition. (Reynolds JEF, editor). London: The Pharmaceutical Press, 1982.

G22 *Martindale: The Extra Pharmacopoeia*, 29th edition. (Reynolds JEF, editor). London: The Pharmaceutical Press, 1989.

G23 *Martindale, The Extra Pharmacopoeia*: 30th edition. (Reynolds JEF, editor). London: The Pharmaceutical Press, 1993.

G24 *The Merck Index.* An encyclopedia of chemicals, drugs and biologicals, 11th edition. Rahway NJ: Merck, 1989.

G25 Mills SY. *The dictionary of modern herbalism.* Wellingborough: Thorsons, 1985.

G26 Mitchell J, Rook A. *Botanical dermatology – plants and plant products injurious to the skin.* Vancouver: Greengrass, 1979.

G27 Morelli I *et al. Selected medicinal plants.* Rome: FAO, 1983.

G28 Simon JE *et al. Herbs – an indexed bibliography, 1971-80.* Oxford: Elsevier, 1984.

G29 Trease GE, Evans WC. *Pharmacognosy*, 13th edition. London: Baillière Tindall, 1989.

G30 Tyler VE. *The honest herbal*, 3rd edition. Philadelphia: Strickley, 1993.

G31 Wagner H *et al. Plant drug analysis.* Berlin : Springer-Verlag, 1983.

G32 Wren RC. *Potter's new cyclopedia of botanical drugs and preparations* (revised, Williamson EW, Evans FJ). Saffron Walden: Daniel, 1988.

G33 De Smet PAGM (ed.) et al. *Adverse effects of herbal drugs* vol. 1. Berlin: Springer Verlag, 1992.

G34 De Smet PAGM (ed.) et al. *Adverse effects of herbal drugs* vol. 2. Berlin: Springer Verlag, 1993.

G35 Tisserand R and Balacs T. *Essential oil safety.* Edinburgh: Churchill Livingstone, 1995.

AGNUS CASTUS

Species (Family)
Vitex agnus-castus L. (Verbenaceae)

Synonym(s)
Chasteberry, Chaste tree, Monk's pepper

Part(s)Used
Fruit

Pharmacopoeial Monographs
None

Legal Category (Licensed Products)
GSL[G14]

Constituents[G18]
Alkaloids Viticin
Flavonoids Flavonol (kaempferol, quercetagetin) derivatives, the major constituent being casticin . Other identified flavonoids include penduletin and chrysophanol D.[1–3]
Iridoids (leaf). Aucubin 0.3%, its *p*-hydroxybenzoyl derivative, agnuside 0.6%, and 0.07% unidentified glycosides.[2,4]
Other constituents Volatile oil 0.5% with cineol and pinene as main components; castine (a bitter principle).[5,6]

Food Use
Agnus castus is not used in foods.

Herbal Use
Traditionally, agnus castus has been used for menstrual problems resulting from corpus luteum deficiency, including premenstrual symptoms and spasmodic dysmenorrhoea, for certain menopausal conditions, and for insufficient lactation.[G25]

Dose
Fruit 0.5–1.0 g three times daily[G25]

Pharmacological Actions
Animal studies Agnus castus does not contain any oestrogenic constituents but has been reported to diminish release of follicle stimulating hormone from the anterior pituitary whilst increasing the release of luteinising hormone and prolactin.[7,8]
Human studies A proprietary preparation containing an alcoholic extract of agnus castus (0.2% w/w) has been available in Germany since the 1950s. It is used in the treatment of breast disease and pain, ovarian insufficiency, and dysfunctional uterine bleeding.[7,9–13] Numerous studies have been documented, mainly in Germany,[9–12] which investigated the use of this product to treat symptoms of corpus luteum deficiency such as irregular menstrual cycles, dysfunctional uterine bleeding, mastopathy, premenstrual syn-

drome, and acne. Results of studies have indicated that agnus castus can have a beneficial effect (in some cases resulting in pregnancy) when administered to women aged 20 to 40 years of normal weight, whose ovarian function is not too impaired (progesterone concentration 7 to 12 ng/mL) and who do not have any additional hormonal imbalances such as disorders of thyroid function or prolactin metabolism, or adrenocortical abnormalities.[9,10] Agnus castus has been found to restore progesterone concentrations, prolong the hyperthermic phase in the basal temperature curve, and restore the LH-RH test to normal when given for at least 3 months at a daily dose of 40 drops.[14] The drops are usually taken on an empty stomach in the morning, although the alcohol content of the preparation may necessitate the drops to be taken in divided doses after meals. It has been recommended that agnus castus therapy should be tried before commencing alternative treatments such as oestrogen or antioestrogen preparations[14].

Agnus castus has also been reported to be effective in the treatment of endocrine disorders such as menstrual neuroses and dermatoses [14] and has been used for the treatment of acne.[15,16].

A lactogenic action has been documented for agnus castus;[17] chemical analysis of the breast milk revealed no changes in composition.

The precise mode of action of agnus castus and the active constituents has not been established. However, it is thought to act on the pituitary-hypothalamic axis rather than directly on the ovaries.

Side-effects, Toxicity
Agnus castus has been reported to be free from side-effects[8,14] although allergic reactions, which resolved following discontinuation of agnus castus therapy, have been reported;[14] headaches, increase in menstrual flow.[7]

Contra-indications, Warnings
In view of the documented action on the pituitary gland and the hypothalamus, agnus castus may interfere with other endocrine therapies (e.g. hormone replacement therapy, oral contraceptives, sex hormones). The use of agnus castus to treat symptoms of corpus luteum deficiency has only been recommended in a specific group of patients who are not on any other hormonal therapy (*see* Human studies).

Pregnancy and lactation In view of the documented pharmacological actions and lack of toxicity data, the use of agnus castus during pregnancy should be avoided. Agnus castus has been reported to stimulate milk secretion without altering the composition of the breast milk.[14,17] Nevertheless, agnus castus should be avoided during lactation until further information is available.

Pharmaceutical Comment

The chemistry of agnus castus is poorly documented. However, proprietary preparations containing extracts of agnus castus have been available in Germany since the 1950s and many documented studies have investigated the use of these products to treat various gynaecological disorders. The results of these studies have indicated that agnus castus is beneficial in the treatment of symptoms associated with corpus luteum deficiency in a specific group of patients, although the mode of action and active constituents have not been determined. [18]

References

See General References G18 and G25.

1   Belic I *et al*. Constituents of *Vitex agnus castus* seeds. Part 1. Casticin. *J Chem Soc* 1961; 2523–5.

2   Gomaa CS *et al*. Flavonoids and iridoids from *Vitex agnus castus*. *Planta Medica* 1978; **33**: 277.

3   Wollenweber E and Mann K. Flavonols from fruits of *Vitex agnus castus*. *Planta Medica* 1983; **48**: 126–7.

4   Rimpler H. Verbenaceae. Iridoids and ecdysones from *Vitex* species. *Phytochemistry* 1972; **11**: 2653–4.

5   Kustrak D *et al*. The composition of the volatile oil of *Vitex agnus castus*. *Planta Medica* 1992; **58** (Suppl.1): A681.

6   Zwaving JH and Bos R. Composition of the essential fruit oil of *Vitex agnus castus*. *Pharmacy World and Science* 1993; **15** (6, Suppl.H): H15.

7   Houghton PJ. Agnus castus. *Pharm J* 1994; **253**: 720–1.

8   Amann W. Umkehrung der pharmakologischen wirkung von *Agnus castus* bei niedriger dosierung. (Gleichzeitig ein beitrag zur endokrinologie der sexualhormone). *Z Forsch Praxis Fortbildung (Med)* 1966; **7**: 229–33.

9   Amann W. Prämenstruelle Wasserretention. Günstige wirkung von *Agnus castus* (Agnolyt[R]) auf prämenstruelle wasserretention. *Z Allg Med* 1979; **55**: 48–51.

10   Amann W. Das "prämenstruelle syndrom" hat viele gesichter. Häufig bringt schon die gezielte anamnese aufschluss. *Arztl Praxis* 1979; **31**: 3091–2.

11   Amann W. Amenorrhoe. Günstige wirkung von *Agnus castus* (Agnolyt[R]) auf amenorrhoea. *Z Allg Med* 1982; **58**: 228–31.

12   Turner S and Mills S. A double-blind clinical trial on a herbal remedy for premenstrual syndrome; a case study. *Complementary Therapies in Medicine* 1993; **1**: 73–7.

13   Milewicz A *et al*. *Vitex agnus castus* extract in the treatment of luteal phase defects due to latent hyperprolactinaemia. Results of a randomized placebo-controlled double blind study. *ArnzneimittelForsch* 1993; **43(II)**: 752-6.

14   Kartnig T. *Vitex agnus-castus* — Mönchspfeffer oder Keuschlamm. Ein arneipflanze mit indirekt-luteotroper wirkung. *Z Phytotherapie* 1986; **7**: 119–22.

15   Amann W. Akne vulgaris und *Angus castus* (Agnolyt[R]). *Z Allg Med* 1975; **51**: 1645–48.

16   Amann W. Ist die acne vulgaris eine psychosomatische erkrankung? Versuch einer klärung: Der psychosomatische aspekt der acne vulgaris. *Artzliche Kosmetologie* 1984 **14**: 162–70.

17   Bruckner C. In mitteleuropa genutzte heilpflanzen mit milchsekretionsfördernder wirkung (galactagoga). *Gleditschia* 1989; **17**: 189–201.

18   Bohnert K-J, Hahn G. Phytotherapie in gynäkologie und geburtshilfe : *Vitex agnus-castus* (keuschlamm). *Erfahrungsheilkunde*. 1990; **39**: 494–502.

AGRIMONY

Species (Family)
Agrimonia eupatoria L. (Rosaceae)

Synonym(s)
Agrimonia

Part(s) Used
Herb

Pharmacopoeial Monographs
BHP 1983

Legal Category (Licensed Products)
GSL[G14]

Constituents[G1,G10,G18,G32]
Acids Palmitic acid, salicylic acid, silicic acid, stearic acid
Flavonoids Apigenin, luteolin, luteolin-7-glucoside, quercetin, quercitrin[1]
Tannins (3–21%). Condensed tannins in herb; hydrolysable tannins (e.g. ellagitannin)
Vitamins Ascorbic acid (vitamin C), nicotinamide complex (about 100–300 µg/g leaf), thiamine (about 2 µg/g leaf), vitamin K
Other constituents Bitter principle, triterpenes (e.g. α-amyrin, ursolic acid), phytosterols, volatile oil 0.2%.

Food Use
Agrimony is listed by the Council of Europe as a natural source of food flavouring (category N2). This category indicates that agrimony can be added to foodstuffs in small quantities, with a possible limitation of an active principle (as yet unspecified) in the final product.[G9]

Herbal Use
Agrimony is stated to possess mild astringent and diuretic properties. It has been used for diarrhoea in children, mucous colitis, grumbling appendicitis, urinary incontinence, cystitis, and as a gargle for acute sore throat and chronic nasopharyngeal catarrh.[G1,G3]

Dose
Dried herb 2–4 g or by infusion three times daily[G3]
Liquid extract (1:1 in 25% alcohol) 1–3 mL three times daily[G3]
Tincture (1:5 in 45% alcohol) 1–4 mL three times daily[G3]

Pharmacological Actions
Animal studies Significant uricolytic activity has been documented for agrimony infusions and decoctions (15%w/v), following their oral administration to male rats at a dose of 20 mL/kg body-weight (equivalent to 3 g dry drug).[4] Diuretic activity was stated to be minimal and elimination of urea unchanged. A hypotensive effect in anaesthetised cats has been documented for an agrimony extract by intravenous injection; blood pressure was lowered by more than 40%.[5]

Marked antibacterial activity against *Staphylococcus aureus* and α-haemolytic streptococci has been reported for agrimony.[6]

Tannins are known to possess astringent properties.

In-vivo antitumour activity in mice, documented for a related species *A. pilosa*, has been attributed to a tannin constituent, agrimoniin.[2] *In-vivo* antitumour activity against ascites-type and solid-type tumours in mice has also been documented for agrimoniin.[7] The mode of action was thought to involve immunostimulation of the host animal. Agrimoniin has not been documented as a constituent of *A. eupatoria*.

Human studies The successful treatment of cutaneous porphyria in a group of 20 patients receiving agrimony infusions has been described.[8] An improvement in skin eruptions together with a decrease of serum-iron concentrations and of urinary porphyrins was noted.

A compound herb preparation containing agrimony has been used to treat 35 patients suffering from chronic gastroduodenitis.[9] After 25 days of therapy, 75% of patients claimed to be free from pain, 95% from dyspeptic symptoms and 76% from palpitation pains. Gastroscopy was said to indicate that previous erosion and haemorrhagic mucous changes had healed. No side-effects or signs of toxicity were documented.

Research in China has indicated that agrimony can increase blood coagulation by up to 50%.[G20]

Side-effects, Toxicity
None documented for *A. eupatoria*.

In mice, agrimoniin has been documented to cause stretching and writhing reactions when administered by intraperitoneal injection, and cyanosis and necrosis at the site of intravenous injection.[7] These reactions were considered to be inflammatory reactions. The LD_{50} of agrimoniin in mice has been estimated as 33 mg/kg (intravenous injection), 101 mg/kg (intraperitoneal injection), and greater then 1 g/kg (by mouth).[7] Cytotoxic activity has been reported for *A. pilosa*[2] (*see* Animal studies).

Contra-indications, Warnings
Excessive doses may interfere with existing drug treatment for high or low blood pressure, and anticoagulant therapy. In view of the tannin constituents, excessive use should be avoided.

Pregnancy and lactation Agrimony is reputed to affect the menstrual cycle.[G10] In view of the lack of toxicity data, excessive use of agrimony should be avoided during pregnancy and lactation.

Pharmaceutical Comment

Relatively limited information is available on the chemistry of agrimony. Human studies have indicated that agrimony may be useful in the treatment of certain cutaneous and gastro-intestinal disorders, although further studies are needed to confirm these reports. The tannin constituents may justify the astringent activity attributed to the herb. In view of the lack of toxicity data, excessive use of agrimony should be avoided.

References

See General References G1, G3, G9, G10, G14, G18, G20 and G32.

1.   Sendra J and Zieba J. Flavonoids from *Agrimonia eupatoria* L. *Diss Pharm Pharmacol* 1971; **24:** 79–83.

2.   Miyamoto K *et al.* Isolation of agrimoniin, an antitumour constituent, from the roots of *Agrimonia pilosa* Ledeb. *Chem Pharm Bull* 1985; **33:** 3977–81.

3.   Péter MH and Racz G. Der gerstoffgehalt verschiedener agrimoniaarten. *Pharmazie* 1973; **28:** 539–41

4.   Giachetti D *et al.* Ricerche sull'attivita diuretica ed uricosurica di *Agrimonia eupatoria. Boll Soc Ital Biol Sper* 1986; **62:** 705–11

5.   Petkov V. Plants with hypotensive, antiatheromatous and coronarodilatating action. *Am J Chin Med* 1979; **7:** 197–236.

6.   Petkov V. Bulgarian traditional medicine: A source of ideas for phytopharmacological investigations. *J Ethnopharmacol* 1986; **15:** 121–32.

7.   Miyamoto K *et al.* Antitumour effect of agrimoniin, a tannin of *Agrimonia pilosa* Ledeb., on transplantable rodent tumors. *Jpn J Pharmacol* 1987; **43:** 187–95.

8.   Patrascu V *et al.* Rezultate terapeutice favorabile in porfiria cutanata cu *Agrimonia eupatoria. Dermato-venerologia* 1984; **29:** 153–7.

9.   Chakarski I *et al.* Clinical study of a herb combination consisting of Agrimonia eupatoria, Hipericum perforatum, Plantago major, Mentha piperita, Matricaria chamomila for the treatment of patients with chronic gastroduodenitis. *Probl Vatr Med* 1982; **10:** 78–84.

ALFALFA

Species (Family)
Medicago sativa L. (Fabaceae/Leguminosae)

Synonym(s)
Lucerne, Medicago, Purple Medick

Part(s) Used
Herb

Pharmacopoeial Monographs
BHP 1983
Martindale 30th edition

Legal Category (Licensed Products)
GSL[G14]

Constituents[G10,G19,G32]

Acids Lauric acid, maleic acid, malic acid, malonic acid, myristic acid, oxalic acid, palmitic acid, quinic acid

Alkaloids Pyrrolidine-type (e.g. stachydrine, homostachydrine); pyridine-type (e.g. trigonelline) in the seeds only

Amino acids Arginine, asparagine (high concentration in seeds), cystine, histidine, isoleucine, leucine, lysine, methionine, phenylalanine, threonine, tryptophan, valine. The non-protein amino acid, canavanine is in high concentrations in the seed and low concentrations in the aerial parts.

Coumarins Medicagol

Isoflavonoids Coumestrol, biochanin A, daidzein, formononetin, genistein

Saponins (2–3%). Hydrolysis yields aglycones medicagenic acid, soyasapogenols A-F and hederagenin.[1] Sugar chain components include arabinose, galactose, glucuronic acid, glucose, rhamnose and xylose.

Steroids Campesterol, cycloartenol, β-sitosterol (major component), α-spinasterol, stigmasterol

Other constituents Carbohydrates (e.g. arabinose, fructose, sucrose, xylose), vitamins (A, B_1, B_6, B_{12}, C, E, K), pectin methylesterase, pigments (e.g. chlorophyll, xanthophyll, β-carotene, anthocyanins), proteins, minerals, trace elements. *See* reference G10 for more detailed chemical information.

Food Use

Alfalfa is widely used in foods and is listed by the Council of Europe as a source of natural food flavouring (category N2 and N3). These categories indicate that alfalfa can be added to foodstuffs in small quantities, with a possible limitation of an active principle (as yet unspecified) in the final product.[G9] In the USA, alfalfa is listed as GRAS (Generally Regarded As Safe).[G19]

Herbal Use

Alfalfa is stated to be a source of vitamins A, C, E, and K, and of the minerals calcium, potassium, phosphorous, and iron. It has been used for avitaminosis A, C, E, or K, hypo-prothrombinaemic purpura, and debility of convalescence.[G3,G32]

Dose
Dried herb 5–10 g or as an infusion three times daily[G3]
Liquid Extract (1:1 in 25% alcohol) 5–10 mL three times daily[G3]

Pharmacological Actions

Animal studies Alfalfa top (stem and leaves) saponins have been reported to decrease plasma-cholesterol levels without changing high-density lipoprotein cholesterol
levels, decrease intestinal absorption of cholesterol, increase excretion of neutral steroids and bile acids, prevent atherosclerosis and induce the regression of atherosclerosis.[2]

Hypocholesterolaemic activity has been reported for root saponins, when given to monkeys receiving a high cholesterol diet.[3]

Oestrogenic activity in ruminants has been documented for coumestrol and the isoflavone constituents.[G10,G19]

An investigation into the effect of various herbs on hepatic drug metabolising enzymes in the rat, showed that alfalfa potentiated the activity of aminopyrine *N*-demethylase but had no effect on glutathione *S*-transferase or epoxide hydrolase activities.[4]

The seeds are reported to contain trypsin inhibitors.[G19]

Alfalfa root saponins have been documented to exhibit selective toxicity towards fungi.[1,5] A medicagenic acid glycoside with low haemolytic activity, isolated from alfalfa root, was found to exhibit both strong inhibitory and fungitoxic activities towards several medically important yeasts including *Candida* species, *Torulopsis* species, *Geotrichum canadidum*, and *Rhodotorula glutinis*.[5] It has been proposed that the antimycotic activity of alfalfa saponins is related to their ability to complex steroids and that fungi sensitive to the saponins may contain relatively more steroids in their membranes.[5] Antifungal properties have also been documented for medicagol.[G19]

The saponin constituents are documented to be haemolytic and to interfere with vitamin E utilisation, and are believed to be one of the causes of ruminant bloat.[G19] Haemolytic activity is associated with the medicagenic acid glycosides (HI 3000) and not the hederagenin and soyasapogenol glycosides.

Human studies Results of a study involving 15 patients with hyperlipoproteinaemia, who were given 40 g of heat-treated alfalfa seeds three times a day for eight weeks, concluded that alfalfa seeds added to the diet of patients with type II hyperlipoproteinaemia could help to normalise serum-cholesterol concentrations.[6]

The manganese content of alfalfa (45.5 mg/kg) is reported to be the active principle responsible for a hypoglycaemic effect documented for the herb.[7] A diabetic patient, treated with soluble insulin but poorly controlled, found that an alfalfa extract adequately controlled his diabetes. When administered separately, only small doses of manganese chloride (5 to 10 mg) were required to have a hypoglycaemic effect. However, no effect was seen on the blood-sugar levels of non-diabetic controls or other diabetic patients, who were also administered manganese. It was concluded that manganese lowered the blood-sugar concentration in this particular diabetic patient because he was unable to utilise manganese stored in his body.

Side-effects, Toxicity

Both alfalfa seed and herb have been reported to induce a systemic lupus erythematosus (SLE)-like syndrome in female monkeys.[2,8] This activity has been attributed to canavanine, a nonprotein amino acid constituent which has been found to have effects on human immunoregulatory cells *in vitro*.[9] Reactivation of quiescent SLE in humans has been associated with the ingestion of alfalfa tablets which, following analysis, were found to contain canavanine.[10] It was not stated whether the tablets contained seed or herb material. Canavanine is known to be toxic to all animal species because of its structural similarity to arginine. Alfalfa seeds are reported to contain substantial quantities of canavanine (8.33–13.6 mg/kg), whereas the herb is stated to contain considerably lesser amounts.[11,12]

Pancytopenia has been associated with human ingestion of ground alfalfa seeds (80–160 g/day), which were taken to lower plasma-cholesterol concentrations.[13]

Dietary studies using alfalfa top saponins (ATS) in the diet of rats and monkeys, showed no evidence of toxicity and serum lipid levels were lowered.[2,14,15] In addition, when ATS were given to cholesterol-fed animals, a reduction in serum-lipid concentrations was observed.[2,14,15] ATS are reported to be free of the SLE-inducing substance that is present in the seeds.[2]

Negative results were documented for alfalfa when tested for mutagenicity using *Salmonella* strains TA98 and TA100.[2]

Contra-indications, Warnings

Individuals with a history of SLE should avoid ingesting alfalfa. Ingestion of large amounts of alfalfa (exceeding amounts normally consumed in the diet) should be avoided in view of the documented oestrogenic activity and potential anticoagulant activity. Excessive doses may interfere with anticoagulant therapy and with hormonal therapy, including the oral contraceptive pill and hormone replacement therapy. Alfalfa may affect blood-sugar concentrations in diabetic patients because of the manganese content. *Pregnancy and lactation* Alfalfa seeds are reputed to affect the menstrual cycle and to be lactogenic.[G12] Although the safety of alfalfa herb has not been established, it is probably acceptable for use during pregnancy and lactation provided that doses do not exceed the amounts normally ingested as a food. Alfalfa seeds should not be ingested during pregnancy or lactation.

Pharmaceutical Comment

The chemistry of alfalfa is well documented and it does appear to be a good source of vitamins and minerals,

thereby supporting the herbal uses. However, normal human dietary intake of alfalfa is low and excessive ingestion should be avoided in view of the many pharmacologically active constituents (e.g. canavanine, coumarins, isoflavones, saponins), which may give rise to unwanted effects if taken in excess. Oestrogenic effects are generally associated with the ingestion of large amounts of the herb such as in fodder for poultry and cattle. Reports of a possible SLE-inducing capacity of alfalfa, particularly the seeds, also suggests that excessive ingestion is not advisable.

References

See General References G3, G9, G10, G11, G12, G14, G19, G22, G23, G32 and G33.

1. Oleszek W and Jurzysta M. Isolation, chemical characterization and biological activity of alfalfa (*Medicago media* Pers.) root saponins. *Acta Soc Bot Pol* 1986; **55**: 23–33.

2. Malinow MR *et al*. Lack of toxicity of alfalfa saponins in cynomolgus macaques. *J Med Primatol* 1982; **11**: 106–18.

3. Malinow MR *et al*. Prevention of elevated cholesterolemia in monkeys by alfalfa saponins. *Steroids* 1977; **29**: 105–110.

4. Garrett BJ *et al*. Consumption of poisonous plants (*Senecio jacobaea, Symphytum officinale, Pteridium aquilinum, Hypericum perforatum*) by rats: chronic toxicity, mineral metabolism, and hepatic drug-metabolizing enzymes. *Toxicol Lett* 1982; **10**: 183–8.

5. Polacheck I *et al*. Activity of compound G2 isolated from alfalfa roots against medically important yeasts. *Antimicrob Agents Chemother* 1986; **30**: 290–4.

6. Mölgaard J *et al*. Alfalfa seeds lower low density lipoprotein cholesterol and apolipoprotein B concentrations in patients with type II hyperlipoproteinemia. *Atherosclerosis* 1987 **65**: 173–9.

7. Rubenstein AH *et al*. Manganese-induced hypoglycaemia. *Lancet* 1962; **ii**: 1348–51.

8. Malinow MR *et al*. Systemic lupus erythematosus-like syndrome in monkeys fed alfalfa sprouts: role of a nonprotein amino acid. *Science* 1982; **216**: 415–7.

9. Alcocer-Varela J *et al*. Effects of L-canavanine on T cells may explain the induction of systemic lupus erythematosus by alfalfa. *Arthritis Rheum* 1985; **28**: 52–7.

10. Roberts JL and Hayashi JA. Exacerbation of SLE associated with alfalfa ingestion. *New Engl J Med* 1983; **308**: 1361.

11. Natelson S. Canavanine to arginine ratio in alfalfa (*Medicago sativa*), clover (*Trifolium*), and the jack bean (*Canavalia ensiformis*). *J Agric Food Chem* 1985; **33**: 413–419.

12. Natelson S. Canavanine in alfalfa (*Medicago sativa*). *Experentia* 1985; **41**: 257–59.

13. Malinow MR *et al*. Pancytopenia during ingestion of alfalfa seeds. *Lancet* 1981; **i**: 615.

14. Malinow MR *et al*. The toxicity of alfalfa saponins in rats. *Fd Cosmet Toxicol* 1981; **19**: 443–5.

15. René M *et al*. Lack of toxicity of alfalfa saponins in rats. *Cholesterol Metabolism* 1981 **40**: 349.

16. White RD *et al*. An evaluation of acetone extracts from six plants in the Ames mutagenicity test. *Toxicol Lett* 1983; **15**: 25–31.

ALOE VERA

Species (Family)
Aloe barbadensis Mill., *Aloe ferox* Mill., and hybrids with *Aloe africana* Mill. and *Aloe spicata* Baker (Liliaceae)

Synonyms
Aloe gel, *Aloe vera* Tourn. ex L., *Aloe vera* (L.) Webb

Parts Used
Leaf gel

Pharmacopoeial Monographs
Martindale 30th edition (Aloes)

Legal Category (Licensed Products)
Aloe vera is not included in the GSL.

Constituents[G1,G2,G10,G19]
Aloe vera is reported to contain mono- and polysaccharides, tannins, sterols, organic acids, enzymes (including cyclooxygenase),[1] saponins, vitamins, and minerals.[2]
Carbohydrates Glucomannan and other polysaccharides containing arabinose, galactose, and xylose.
Lipids Includes cholesterol, gamolenic acid, and arachidonic acid.[1] The polar, non-polar, and fatty acid composition has been investigated.[1]

Food Use
Aloe vera is not used in foods

Herbal Use
Traditionally, aloe vera has been used in ointments and creams to assist the healing of wounds, burns, eczema, and psoriasis.[G1,G2,G19,G32]

Dose
None documented.

Pharmacological Actions
Aloe vera refers to the mucilaginous tissue located in the leaf parenchyma of *Aloe vera* or related *Aloe* species. However, many documented studies for *Aloe vera* have utilised homogenised leaf extracts which therefore combine aloe vera with aloes, the laxative preparation obtained from the bitter, yellow juice also found in the leaf (*see* Aloes). Unless otherwise specified, the following studies will refer to a total leaf extract.
Animal studies Gel preparations have been reported to be effective against radiation burns, skin ulcers, and peptic ulcers.[2] However, the gel was also found to be ineffective against drug- and stress-induced gastric and peptic ulcers in rats.[2]
Anti-inflammatory activity has been observed in various rat and mouse models that received subcutaneous injections of *Aloe vera* leaf extract.[3] A positive response was noted in wound healing (10 mg/kg, rat; 100 mg/kg, mouse), mustard oedema (10 mg/kg, rat) and polymorphonuclear leucocyte infiltration (2 mg/kg, mouse) tests, although no activity was demonstrated in the antifibrosis test (cotton pellet granuloma) (400 mg/kg, rat).

Anti-arthritic and anti-inflammatory activity has been documented for a cream containing homogenised *Aloe africana* leaves, ribonucleic acid, and ascorbic acid, following topical application to rats who had been injected (day 0) with *Mycobacterium butyricum* to cause adjuvant arthritis.[4] This model is considered a good experimental tool for studying rheumatoid arthritis.[4] The cream was found to be active when applied both as a prevention (days 1 to 13) and as a regression (day 21 to 35) treatment.[4] Subsequent work suggested that anthraquinone compounds (anthraquinone, anthracene, anthranilic acid) may be the active components in the aloe leaf mixture.[5] These compounds are however constituents of aloes rather than aloe vera (*see* Aloes). Aloe vera juice (presumably containing the anthraquinones contained in aloe preparation) has been applied directly to open pressure sores to assist in their healing.[6] The aloe vera extract exhibited an anaesthetic reaction, antibacterial action, and increased local micro-circulation.[6]

Endogenous cyclooxygenase in *Aloe vera* has been found to convert endogenous arachidonate to various prostanoids, namely PGE_2 (major), TXB_2, PGD_2, PGF_2, and 6-keto-PGF_{1b}.[1] The production of these compounds, especially PGE_2, has been associated with the beneficial effect of an aloe extract on human bronchial asthma[8] (see below).

Hypoglycaemic actions have been documented for Aloes extracts (*see* Aloes)

Human studies Enhancement of phagocytosis in adult bronchial asthma has been attributed to a non-dialysable fraction of the extract, consisting of active components that are a mixture of polysaccharide, and protein or glycoprotein.[7] Despite the nature of these proposed active components, it has been proposed that activity of the fraction may be related to the previous observation that aloe vera synthesises prostaglandins from endogenous arachidonic acid using endogenous cyclo-oxygenase.[1] In this current study,[7] activity of the aloe vera extract required dark storage at 4 to 30°C, for a period of 3 to 10 days.[3] These conditions are reported to be favourable for the hydrolysis of phospholipids thus releasing arachidonic acid for synthesis of prostanoids.[1] In addition, activity was dependent on patients not having received prior treatment with a corticosteroid.[8] The gel has been reported to be effective in the treatment of mouth ulcers.[8]

Side-effects, Toxicity

None documented.

Contra-indications, Warnings

Hypoglycaemic activity has been documented for an aloe vera extract, although it is unclear whether this is associated with the true aloe vera gel or the aloes extract.[9]

Pregnancy and lactation The external application of aloe vera gel during pregnancy is not thought to be any cause for concern. However, products stated to contain aloe extracts or aloe vera may well contain gastrointestinal stimulant anthraquinone components that are well recognised as the active constituents in aloes (laxative). As such, ingestion of such preparations during pregnancy and lactation should be avoided.

Pharmaceutical Comment

Aloe vera is obtained from the mucilaginous tissue in the centre of the *Aloe vera* leaf and consists mainly of polysaccharides and lipids. It should not be confused with aloes, which is obtained by evaporation of water from the bitter yellow juice that is drained from the leaf. Unlike aloes, aloe vera does not contain any anthraquinone compounds and does not therefore, exert any laxative action. Studies have reported an anti-inflammatory and anti-arthritic action for total leaf extracts but the activity seems to be associated with anthraquinone compounds. Hypoglycaemic activity has been reported for aloe vera extract. Aloe vera is a source of gamolenic acid. The literature on burn management with aloe vera gel preparations is confused and further studies are required.[10]

References

See General References G1, G2, G10, G19, G22, G23 and G32.

1. Afzal M *et al*. Identification of some prostanoids in *Aloe vera* extracts. *Planta Med* 1991; **57**: 38–40.

2. Parmar NS *et al*. Evaluation of *Aloe vera* leaf exudate and gel for gastric and duodenal anti-ulcer activity. *Fitoterapia* 1986; **57**: 380–1.

3. Davis RH *et al*. Biological activity of *Aloe vera*. *Med Sci Res* 1987; **15**: 235.

4. Davis RH *et al*. Topical effect of aloe with ribonucleic and vitamin C on adjuvant arthritis. *J Am Pod Med Assoc* 1985; **75**: 229–237.

5. Davis RH *et al*. Antiarthritic activity of anthraquinones found in aloe for podiatric medicine. *J Am Pod Med Assoc* 1986; **76**: 61–66.

6. Cuzzell JZ. Readers' remedies for pressure sores. *Am J Nurs* 1986; **86**: 923–4.

7. Shida T *et al*. Effect of Aloe extract on peripheral phagocytosis in adult bronchial asthma. *Planta Med* 1985; **51**: 273–5.

8. Plemons JM *et al*. Evaluation of acemannan in the treatment of aphthous stomatitis. *Wounds* 1994; **6**: 40–45.

9. Ghanam N *et al*. The antidiabetic activity of aloes: preliminary clinical and experimental observations. *Hormone Res* 1986; **24**: 288–94.

10. Marshall JM. Aloe vera gel: What is the evidence? *Pharm J* 1990; **244**: 360–2.

ALOES

Species (Family)
(i) *Aloe barbadensis* Mill. (Liliaceae)
(ii) *Aloe ferox* Mill. and its hybrids with *Aloe africana* Mill. and *Aloe spicata* Baker.

Synonym(s)
Aloe vera Tourn. ex. L. and *A. vera* (L.) Webb ford.

Part(s) Used
Dried leaf juice

Pharmacopoeial Monographs
BHP 1990 (*Aloe barbadensis* and *Aloe capensis*)
Martindale 30th edition
Pharmacopoeias—Aust., Br., Braz., Egypt., Eur., Fr., Ger., Gr., Hung., It., Jpn, Neth., Nord., Pol., Port., Rom., Swiss, Turk., and U.S. Br. also includes Powdered Aloes. Braz. and Egypt. also allow Socotrine aloes.

Legal Category (Licensed Products)
GSL[G14]

Constituents[G1,G10,G19,G32]
Anthraquinones (Up to 30%, mainly *C*-glucosides). Collectively known as aloin, the mixture contains barbaloin, isobarbaloin, and emodin (glycosides), and free anthraquinones (e.g. aloe-emodin)
Other constituents Resins, aloesin and its aglycone aloesone (a chromene)

Food Use
Aloes is listed by the Council of Europe as a natural source of food flavouring (category N3)[G9]. This category indicates that aloes can be added to foodstuffs in the traditionally accepted manner, although there is insufficient information available for an adequate assessment of potential toxicity. The concentration of aloin present in the final product is limited to 0.1 mg/kg; 50 mg/kg in alcoholic beverages.[G9]

Herbal Use
Aloes is recommended for the treatment of atonic constipation and suppressed menstruation.[G1,G25,G32]

Dose
Dried juice 50–200 mg or equivalent thrice daily[G2,G25]

Pharmacological Actions
The activity of aloes can be attributed to the anthraquinone glycoside constituents of the leaf juice or latex.
Animal studies Aloe-emodin and an alcoholic extract of aloes have been reported to possess antitumour activity.[G19] Hypoglycaemic activity has been shown in alloxan-diabetic mice for aloes[1] and in diabetic rats for an aloe gum extract[2,3].
Human studies The purgative action of the anthraquinone glycosides is well recognised (*see* Senna), although aloes is reported to be more potent than both senna and cascara.[G19,G22]. An aloes extract in doses too small to cause abdominal cramps or diarrhoea had a significant hypoglycaemic effect in 5 non-insulin-dependent diabetics.[1]

Side-effects, Toxicity
Aloes is a potent purgative that may cause abdominal pains, gastro-intestinal irritation leading to pelvic congestion and, in large doses, may result in nephritis, bloody diarrhoea, and haemorrhagic gastritis.[G19,G21] Like all stimulant purgatives, prolonged use of aloes may produce watery diarrhoea with excessive loss of water and electrolytes (particularly potassium), muscular weakness, and weight loss.[G21]
Tests of the possible carcinogenicity of hydroxyanthraquinones and their glycosides showed that exposure to certain aglycones and glycosides may represent a human cancer risk.[4] Most of the aglycones tested were found to be mutagenic and some, such as emodin and aloe-emodin, were genotoxic in mammalian cells.

Contra-indications, Warnings
Aloes has been superseded by less toxic laxatives.[G22] The drastic purgative action of aloes contra-indicates its use in individuals with haemorrhoids and existing kidney disease. In common with all purgatives, aloes should not be given to patients with intestinal obstruction, abdominal pain, nausea, or vomiting. Aloes colours alkaline urine red.
Pregnancy and lactation In view of the irritant and cathartic properties documented for aloes, its use is contra-indicated during pregnancy.[G21] Anthraquinones may be secreted into breast milk and, therefore, aloes should be avoided during lactation (*see* Senna).
Aloes is reputed to be an abortifacient and to affect the menstrual cycle.[G10]

Pharmaceutical Comment
Aloes and aloe gel are often confused with each other. Aloes is obtained by evaporation of water from the bitter yellow juice drained from the leaves of *A. vera*. Commercial 'aloin' is a concentrated form of aloes.[G19] Aloe gel is prepared by many methods, but is obtained from the mucilaginous tissue in the centre of the leaf and does not contain anthraquinones (*see* Aloe Vera). Aloes is a potent purgative which has been superseded by less toxic drugs such as senna and cascara. Generally, the use of unstandardised preparations containing anthraquinone glycosides should be avoided, since their pharmacological effect is unpredictable and they may cause abdominal cramp and diarrhoea. In particular, the use of products containing combinations of anthraquinone laxatives should be avoided.

References
See General References G1, G2, G4, G9, G10, G14, G19, G21, G22, G23, G25, G32 and G34.

1.   Ghannam N *et al.* The antidiabetic activity of aloes: preliminary and experimental observations. *Hormone Res* 1986; **24:** 288–94.

2.   Al-Awadi FM, Gumaa KA. Studies on the activity of individual plants of an antidiabetic plant mixture. *Acta Diabetol Lat* 1987; **24:** 37–41.

3.   Al-Awadi FM *et al.* On the mechanism of the hypoglycaemic effect of a plant extract. *Diabetalogia* 1985; **28:** 432–4.

4. Westendorf J, *et al.* Possible carcinogenicity of anthraquinone-containing medical plants. *Planta Med* 1988; 54: 562.

ANGELICA

Species (Family)
Angelica archangelica L. (Apiaceae/Umbelliferae)

Synonym(s)
Archangelica officinalis Moench or Hoffm.

Part(s) Used
Fruit, Leaf, Rhizome, Root

Pharmacopoeial Monographs
BHP 1983
BPC 1934
Martindale 28th edition

Legal Category (Licensed Products)
GSL[G14]

Constituents[G1,G10,G19,G24,G28,G32,G35]
Coumarins Angelicin, osthol (major constituent in rhizome/root at 0.2%), bergapten, imperatorin (major constituents in fruit at 0.1% and 0.5% respectively), oreoselone, oxypeucedanin, umbelliferone, xanthotoxin, xanthotoxol

Volatile oils (0.3–1.0%, highest in fruit). Major components include α- and β-phellandrene, α-pinene, α-thujene, limonene, β-caryophyllene, linalool, borneol, acetaldehyde, and four macrocyclic lactones.

Other constituents Archangelenone (a flavonoid), palmitic acid, sugars (fructose, glucose, sucrose, umbelliferose)

Food Use
Angelica is widely used in foods. The related species *Angelica silvestris* is listed by the Council of Europe as a source of natural food flavouring (category N3). This category indicates that *A. silvestris* can be added to foodstuffs in the traditionally accepted manner, although there is insufficient information available for an adequate assessment of potential toxicity.[G9] In the USA, angelica is listed as GRAS (Generally Regarded As Safe).[G19]

Herbal Use
Angelica is stated to possess antispasmodic, diaphoretic, expectorant, bitter aromatic, carminative, diuretic, and local anti-inflammatory properties. It has been used for respiratory catarrh, psychogenic asthma, flatulent dyspepsia, anorexia nervosa, rheumatic diseases, peripheral vascular disease, and specifically for pleurisy and bronchitis, applied as a compress, and for bronchitis associated with vascular deficiency.[G1,G3,G25,G32]

Dose
Dried leaf 2–5 g or by infusion three times daily[G3]
Leaf liquid extract (1:1 in 25% alcohol) 2–5 mL three times daily[G3]
Leaf tincture (1:5 in 45% alcohol) 2–5 mL three times daily[G3]
Dried rhizome/root 1–2 g or by infusion three times daily[G3]
Rhizome/Root liquid extract (1:1 in 25% alcohol) 0.5–2.0 mL three times daily[G3]
Rhizome/Root tincture (1:5 in 50% alcohol) 0.5–2 mL three times daily[G3]
Fruit 1–2 g[G25]

Pharmacological Actions
Animal studies Minimal anti-inflammatory activity (1% inhibition of carrageenan-induced rat paw oedema) has been documented for fruit extracts (100 mg/kg body-weight by mouth) given 45 minutes before eliciting oedema.[1] This was compared to 45% inhibition by indomethacin (5 mg/kg by mouth). Angelica is reported to possess antibacterial and antifungal properties.[G19,G23] Antibacterial activity against *Mycobacterium avium* has been documented, with no activity exhibited against *Escherichia coli*, *Bacillus subtilis*, *Streptococcus faecalis*, or *Salmonella typhi*.[2] Antifungal activity was reported in 14 of 15 fungi tested.[2]

Furanocoumarins isolated from a related Chinese species, *Angelica koreana*, have been reported to affect the hepatic metabolism of hexobarbitone. The compounds were found to cause a marked inhibition of drug metabolism in the first phase and an acceleration in the second phase, and were thought to be drug-metabolising enzyme inhibitors rather than enzyme inducers. Furanocoumarins investigated included imperatorin and oxypeucedanin, which are also documented as constituents of *A. archangelica*. It has been reported that a related Chinese species, *Angelica sinensis*, may be hepatoprotective and prevent the reduction of hepatic glycogen.

In the rabbit, a uterotonic action has been documented for Japanese angelica root following intraduodenal administration of a methanolic extract (3 g/kg).[3] *A. sinensis* is reported to have induced uterine contraction and relaxation.[G28]

Human studies None documented for angelica (*A. archangelica*). Many related species are traditionally used in Chinese medicine.[G28] *A. sinensis* has been reported to be effective in improving abnormal protein metabolism in patients with chronic hepatitis or hepatic cirrhosis.[4]

The furanocoumarin constituent bergapten (5-methoxypsoralen) has been used in the PUVA treatment of psoriasis.[G22]

Side-effects, Toxicity
Both angelica and the root oil have been reported to cause photodermatitis and phototoxicity, respectively, following

external contact.[2,G10,G13,G35] Angelica contains furanocoumarin constituents which are known to cause photosensitisation. Concern has been expressed at the possible carcinogenic risk of the furanocoumarin bergapten.

The root oil has been reported to be non-irritant and non-sensitising on animal and human skin.[2]

Root and fruit oils obtained by steam distillation are claimed to be devoid of furanocoumarins, although extracts may contain them.[G19]

Toxicity studies have been documented for the root oil.[2] Acute LD_{50} values have been reported as 2.2 g/kg bodyweight (mouse, by mouth) and 11.16 g/kg (rat, by mouth). Death was attributed to liver and kidney damage, although animals surviving for three days completely recovered with a reversal of organ damage. An acute LD_{50} (rabbit, dermal) value was reported to be greater than 5 g/kg. Subacute toxicity studies lasting eight weeks, suggested that the tolerated dose in the rat was 1.5 g/kg, although at lower doses the animals weighed less than the controls.[2]

Contra-indications, Warnings

Angelica may provoke a photosensitive allergic reaction, because of the furanocoumarin constituents. Excessive doses may interfere with anticoagulant therapy, because of the coumarin constituents.

The use of bergapten in cosmetic and suntan preparations is stated to be ill-advised by some regulatory authorities,[G22] in view of the concerns regarding the risk of cancer. The International Fragrance Association recommends that Angelica root oil be limited to a maximum of 0.78% in products applied to skin which is then exposed to sunshine.[G35]

Pregnancy and lactation Angelica root is reputed to be an abortifacient and to affect the menstrual cycle. In view of this and the photosensitising constituents, the use of angelica during pregnancy and lactation in amounts exceeding those used in foods should be avoided.

Pharmaceutical Comment

The chemistry of angelica is well documented. Although the traditional use of Chinese angelica species, such as *A. sinensis* and *A. acutiloba,* is well established in oriental medicine, there is limited documented pharmacological information available for *A. archangelica*, the species commonly used in Europe, to justify its herbal uses. In view of the presence of known pharmacologically active constituents, especially bergapten, consumption of amounts exceeding normal human dietary intake should be avoided. Angelica contains furanocoumarins which are known to possess photosensitising properties.

References

See General References G1, G3, G5, G9, G10, G13, G14, G19, G21, G22, G24, G25, G28, G32 and G35.

1. Zielinska-Jenczylik J *et al.* Effect of plant extracts on the *in vitro* interferon synthesis. *Arch Immunologiae et Therapiae Experimentalis* 1984; **32:** 577.

2. Opdyke DLJ. Angelica root oil. *Food Cosmet Toxicol* 1975; **13:** (Suppl.) 713.

3. Harada M *et al.* Effect of Japanese angelica root and peony root on uterine contraction in the rabbit *in situ. J Pharm Dyn* 1984; **7:** 304–11.

4. Chang HM *et al.* Advances in Chinese medicinal materials research. Philadelphia: World Scientific, 1985.

ANISEED

Species (Family)
Pimpinella anisum L. (Apiaceae/Umbelliferae)

Synonym(s)
Anise, Anisi Fructus, Anisum, *Anisum officinarum* Moench., *Anisum vulgare* Gaertn.

Part(s) Used
Fruit

Pharmacopoeial Monographs
BHP 1983
Martindale 30th edition
Pharmacopoeias—Aust., Br., Cz., Egypt., Eur., Fr., Ger., Gr., Hung., It., Neth., Rom., Rus., and Swiss. Aust., Braz., Chin., and Fr. also include a monograph for Star Anise, the dried ripe fruit of *Illicium verum* (Magnoliaceae).

Legal Category (Licensed Products)
GSL[G14]

Constituents[G1,G10,G19,G32,G35]
Coumarins Scopoletin, umbelliferone, umbelliprenine; bergapten (furanocoumarin).
Flavonoids Flavonol (quercetin) and flavone (apigenin, luteolin) glycosides, e.g. quercetin-3-glucuronide, rutin, luteolin-7-glucoside, apigenin-7-glucoside; isoorientin and isovitexin (*C*-glucosides).
Volatile oils (14%). Major components are *trans*-anethole (75–90%), estragole (methyl chavicol), anise ketone (*p*-methoxyphenylacetone) and β-caryophyllene. Minor components include anisaldehyde and anisic acid (oxidation products of anethole), linalool, limonene, α-pinene, acetaldehyde, *p*-cresol, cresol, hydroquinone, β-farnesene, α-, β-, and γ-himachalene, bisabolene, *d*-elemene, *ar*-curcumene and myristicin.[1]
Other constituents. Carbohydrate (50%), lipids 16% (saturated and unsaturated), β-amyrin (triterpene), stigmasterol (phytosterol) and its palmitate and stearate salts.

Food Use
Aniseed is used extensively as a spice and is listed by the Council of Europe as a natural source of food flavouring (category N2). This category allows small quantities of aniseed to be added to foodstuffs, with a possible limitation of an active principle (as yet unspecified) in the final product.[G9] In the USA, aniseed is listed as GRAS (Generally Regarded As Safe).[G19]

Herbal Use
Aniseed is stated to possess expectorant, antispasmodic, carminative, and parasiticide properties. Traditionally, it has been used for bronchial catarrh, pertussis, spasmodic cough, flatulent colic, topically for pediculosis and scabies, and specifically for bronchitis, tracheitis with persistent cough, and as an aromatic adjuvant to prevent colic from cathartics.[G1,G3,G32]
Aniseed has been used as an oestrogenic agent.[2] It has been reputed to increase milk secretion, promote menstruation, facilitate birth, alleviate symptoms of the male climacteric, and increase libido.[2]

Dose
Dried fruit 0.5–1.0 g or by infusion three times daily[G3]
Oil 0.05–0.2 mL three times daily[G3]
Spirit of Anise (BPC 1949) 0.3–1.0 mL three times daily
Distilled Anise Water (BPC 1934) 15–30 mL three times daily

Pharmacological Actions
The pharmacological effects of aniseed are largely due to the presence of anethole, which is structurally related to the catecholamines adrenaline, noradrenaline, and dopamine. Anethole dimers closely resemble oestrogenic agents stilbene and stilboestrol.[2]
Animal studies Anethole, anisaldehyde, and myristicin have exhibited mild insecticidal properties.[G19] Whole plant aqueous infusions have been reported to delay (but not prevent) the onset of picrotoxin-induced seizures and reduce the mortality rate in mice following intraperitoneal injection.[1] Aniseed was also found to slightly elevate gamma-aminobutyric acid concentrations in brain tissue.[1] However, the anticonvulsant effect demonstrated by aniseed was much weaker compared to conventional treatment and was therefore not considered to justify its Arabic folkloric use.[1]
Human studies Aniseed oil is reported to be carminative and expectorant.[G19] Sympathomimetic type effects have been attributed to anethole.[2] The reputed lactogogic action of anise has been attributed to anethole, which exerts a competitive antagonism at dopamine receptor sites (dopamine inhibits prolactin secretion), and to the action of polymerised anethole, which is structurally related to the oestrogenic compounds stilbene and stilboestrol.[2] Anethole is also structurally related to the hallucinogenic compound myristicin. Bergapten, in combination with ultraviolet light, has been used in the treatment of psoriasis.[G22]

Side-effects, Toxicity
Contact dermatitis reactions to aniseed and aniseed oil have been attributed to anethole.[4,G26,G35] Reactions have been reported with products such as creams and toothpastes flavoured with aniseed oil.[G26] The volatile oil and anethole have been stated to be both irritant and sensitising.[G26] Bergapten is known to cause photosensitivity reactions and concern has been expressed over the possible carcinogenic risk of bergapten.[G22]

Ingestion of as little as 1-5 mL of anise oil can result in nausea, vomiting, seizures, and pulmonary oedema.[4]

Anethole is reported to be a moderate acute toxin with an acute oral LD_{50} value in rats of 2090 mg/kg.[1] Mild liver lesions were observed in rats fed repeated anethole doses (695 mg/kg) for an unspecified duration.[1] Hepatic changes have been described in rats fed anethole in their daily diet (1%) for 15 weeks,[G10] although at a level of 0.25% there were no changes after one year. In therapeutic doses, anethole is reported to cause minimal hepatotoxicity.[G10]

Contra-indications, Warnings

Aniseed may cause an allergic reaction. It is recommended that the use of aniseed oil should be avoided in dermatitis, or any inflammatory or allergic skin condition.[5] Bergapten may cause photosensitivity in sensitive individuals. Excessive doses may interfere with anticoagulant and MAOI therapy. The documented oestrogenic activity of anethole and its dimers may affect existing hormone therapy, including the oral contraceptive pill and hormone replacement therapy, if excessive doses are ingested. In view of the structural similarity reported between anethole and myristicin, consumption of large amounts of aniseed may cause neurological effects similar to those documented for nutmeg.

Pregnancy and lactation. Traditionally, aniseed is reputed to be an abortifacient[G10] and also to promote lactation. The safety of aniseed taken during pregnancy and lactation has not been established; however, there are no known problems provided that doses taken do not greatly exceed the amounts used in foods.

Pharmaceutical Comment

The chemistry of aniseed is well studied and documented pharmacological activities support some of the herbal uses. Aniseed is used extensively as a spice and is widely used in conventional pharmaceuticals for its carminative, expectorant, and flavouring properties. Aniseed contains anethole and estragole which are structurally related to safrole, a known hepatotoxin and carcinogen. Although both anethole and estragole have been shown to cause hepatotoxicity in rodents, aniseed is not thought to represent a risk to human health when it is consumed in amounts normally encountered in foods.

References

See General References G1, G3, G8, G9, G10, G14, G19, G22, G23, G26, G32 and G35.

1. Burkhardt G *et al*. Terpene hydrocarbons in *Pimpinella anisum* L. *Pharm Weekbl (Sci)* 1986; **8:** 190–3.

2. Albert-Puleo M. Fennel and anise as estrogenic agents. *J Ethnopharmacol* 1980; **2:** 337–344.

3. Abdul-Ghani A-S *et al*. Anticonvulsant effects of some Arab medicinal plants. *Int J Crude Drug Res* 1987; **25:** 39–43.

4. Chandler RF, Hawkes D. Aniseed — a spice, a flavor, a drug. *Can Pharm J* 1984; **117:** 28–9.

APRICOT

Species (Family)

Prunus armeniaca L. (Rosaceae)

Synonym(s)

—

Part(s) Used

Kernel (seed), expressed oil

Pharmacopoeial Monographs

BPC 1934

Martindale 30th edition (Persic oil and Laetrile)

Pharmacopoeias—Chin. and Jpn. Rus. and USNF include Persic Oil

Legal Category (Licensed Products)

Apricot is not listed in the GSL. Amygdalin (a cyanogenetic glycoside) is classified as a POM.[7]

Constituents

Acids (phenolic). Various quinic acid esters of caffeic, *p*-coumaric and ferulic acids. Neochlorogenic acid major in kernel, chlorogenic in fruit.[2]

Glycosides (cyanogenetic). Amygdalin (mandelonitrile diglucoside). Cyanide content of kernel varies from 2 to 200 mg/100 g.[2]

Tannins Catechins, proanthocyanidins (condensed)[1]

Other constituents Cholesterol, an oestrogenic fraction (0.09%) containing oestrone (both free and conjugated) and α-oestradiol.[3]

Other plant parts (leaves and fruit). Various flavonol (kaempferol, quercetin) glycosides including rutin (major).[4]

Food Use

Apricot fruit is commonly eaten. Apricot is listed by the Council of Europe as a natural source of food flavouring (category N1 and N2). These categories limit the total amount of hydrocyanic acid permitted in the final product to 1 mg/kg. Exceptions to this are 25 mg/kg for confectionery, 50 mg/kg for marzipan, and 5 mg/kg for fruit juices.[G9]

Herbal Use

Traditionally, the oil has been incorporated into cosmetic and perfumery products such as soaps and creams.[G15]

Dose

None documented. Traditionally, apricot kernels have not been utilised as a herbal remedy.

Pharmacological Actions

During the late 1970s and early 1980s considerable interest was generated in apricot from claims that laetrile (a semi-synthetic derivative of amygdalin) was an effective treatment for cancer. Two review papers[5,6] discuss these claims for laetrile together with its chemistry, metabolism, and potential toxicity.

The claims for laetrile were based on three different theories. The first theory claimed that cancerous cells contained abundant quantities of β-glucosidases, enzymes which release hydrogen cyanide from the laetrile molecule as a result of hydrolysis. Normal cells were said to be protected because they contained low concentrations of β-glucosidases and high concentrations of rhodanese, an enzyme which converts cyanide to the less toxic thiocyanate. However, this theory was disproved when it was shown that both cancerous and normal cells contain only trace amounts of β-glucosidases, and similar amounts of rhodanese. In addition, it was thought that amygdalin was not absorbed intact from the gastro-intestinal tract.[5,6]

The second theory proposed that following ingestion, amygdalin was hydrolysed to mandelonitrile, transported intact to the liver and converted to a β-glucuronide complex. This complex was then carried to the cancerous cells, hydrolysed by β-glucuronidases to release mandelonitrile and subsequently hydrogen cyanide. This theory was considered to be untenable.[6]

A third theory proposed that laetrile is vitamin B_{17}, that cancer is a result of a deficiency of this vitamin, and that chronic administration of laetrile would prevent cancer. Again this was not substantiated by any scientific evidence.[6]

A retrospective analysis of the use of laetrile by cancer patients reported that it may have slight activity.[5,6] However, a subsequent clinical trial concluded that laetrile was ineffective in cancer treatment. Furthermore, it was claimed that patients taking laetrile reduced their life expectancy as a result of lack of proper medical care and chronic cyanide poisoning.[5,6]

In order to reduce potential risks to the general public, amygdalin was made a prescription-only medicine in 1984.[7]

Side-effects, Toxicity

Laetrile and apricot kernel ingestion are the most common sources of cyanide poisoning, with more than 20 deaths reported.[5,6] Apricot kernels are toxic because of their amygdalin content. Hydrolysis of the amygdalin molecule by β-glucosidases, heat, mineral acids or high doses of ascorbic acid (vitamin C) yields hydrogen cyanide (HCN), benzaldehyde, and glucose. β-Glucosidases are not generally abundant in the gastro-intestinal tract, but they are present in the kernels themselves as well as certain foods including beansprouts, carrots, celery, green peppers, lettuce, mushrooms, and sweet almonds. Hydrolysis of the amygdalin molecule is slow in an acid environment but much more rapid in an alkaline pH. There may therefore be a delay in the onset of symptoms of HCN poisoning as a result of the transit time from the acid pH of the stomach to the alkaline environment of the small intestine.

Acute poisoning Cyanide is rapidly absorbed from the upper gastro-intestinal tract, diffuses readily throughout the body and promptly causes respiratory failure if untreated. Symptoms of cyanide toxicity progress rapidly from dizziness, headache, nausea, vomiting and drowsiness to dyspnoea, palpitations, marked hypotension, convulsions, paralysis, coma and death, which may occur from 1 to 15 minutes after ingestion. Antidotes for cyanide poisoning include nitrite, thiosulphate, hydroxocobalamin, cobalt edetate, and aminophenol.[5,6]

Chronic poisoning Principal symptoms include increased blood thiocyanate, goitre, thyroid cancer, lesions of the optic nerve, blindness, ataxia, hypertonia, cretinism, and mental retardation.[5] These symptoms may develop as a result of ingesting significant amounts of cyanide, cyanogenetic precursors in the diet, or cyanogenetic drugs such as laetrile. Demyelinating lesions and other neuromyopathies reportedly occur secondary to chronic cyanide exposure, including long-term therapy with laetrile. Agranulocytosis has also been attributed to long-term laetrile therapy.[5,6]

For individual reports of adverse reactions and cyanide poisoning in patients using laetrile *see* reference G22.

Normally, low concentrations of ingested cyanide are controlled naturally by exhalation or by rapid conversion to the less toxic thiocyanate by the enzyme rhodanese. Oral doses of 50 mg of hydrogen cyanide (HCN) can be fatal. This is equivalent to approximately 30 g kernels which represents about 50 to 60 kernels, and approximately 2 mg HCN/g kernel. Apricot seed has also been reported to contain 2.92 mg HCN/g.[8] A 500 mg laetrile tablet was found to contain between 5 to 51 mg HCN/g.

There may be considerable variation in the number of kernels required to be toxic, depending on the concentration of amygdalin and β-glucosidases present in the kernels, the time-span of ingestion, the degree of maceration of the kernels, individual variation in hydrolysing, and detoxifying abilities.

Systemic concentrations of β-glucosidases are low and therefore toxicity following parenteral absorption of amygdalin is low. However, cyanide poisoning has been reported in rats following intraperitoneal administration of laetrile, suggesting another mechanism of hydrolysis had occurred.[5,6]

It is thought that cyanogenetic glycosides may possess carcinogenic properties. Mandelonitrile (amygdalin = mandelonitrile diglucoside) is mutagenic and stimulates guanylate cyclase.[5,6]

Contra-indications, Warnings

Apricot kernels are toxic due to their amygdalin content. Following ingestion hydrogen cyanide is released and may result in cyanide poisoning. Fatalities have been reported following the ingestion of apricot kernels. Contact dermatitis has been reported for apricot kernels.[9]

Pregnancy and lactation. Apricot kernels are toxic and should not be ingested. The ingestion of cyanogenetic substances may result in teratogenic effects.[5] However, one case has been reported where no acute toxicity was noted in the infant when laetrile was used during the third term of pregnancy. It was unknown whether chronic effects would be manifested at a later date.[5] Breeding rats fed ground apricot kernels had pups with normal birth weights, but with lower survival rates and lower weaning weights.[2]

Pharmaceutical Comment

Interest in apricot kernels was generated as a result of claims in the late 1970s that laetrile, a semi-synthetic derivative of the naturally occurring constituent amygdalin, was a natural, non-toxic cure for cancer. Apricot kernels were seen as an alternative source for this miracle cure. These claims have since been disproved and it has been established that laetrile (amygdalin) is far from non-toxic, particularly if administered orally. Fatal cases of cyanide poisoning have been reported following the ingestion of apricot kernels.

References

See General References G5, G9, G15, G22 and G28.

1. Möller B, Herrmann K. Quinic acid esters of hydroxycinnamic acids in stone and pome fruit. *Phytochemistry* 1983; **22:** 477–81.

2. Miller KW *et al.* Amygdalin metabolism and effect on reproduction of rats fed apricot kernels. *J Toxicol Environ Health* 1981; **7:** 457–67.

3. Awad O. Steroidal estrogens of *Prunus armeniaca* seeds. *Phytochemistry* 1973; **13:** 678–90.

4. Henning W, Herrmann K. Flavonol glycosides of apricots (*Prunus armeniaca* L.) and peaches (*Prunus persica* Batch). 13. Phenolics of fruits. *Z Lebensm Unters Forsch* 1980; **171:** 183–8.

5. Chandler RF *et al.* Laetrile in perspective. *Can Pharm J* 1984; **117:** 517–20.

6. Chandler RF *et al.* Controversial laetrile. *Pharm J* 1984; **232:** 330–332

7. The Medicines (Cyanogenetic Substances) Order, SI 1984 No. 187, London: HMSO, 1984.

8. Holzbecher MD *et al.* The cyanide content of laetrile preparations, apricot, peach and apple seeds. *Clin Toxicol* 1984; **22:** 341–7.

9. Göransson K. Contact urticaria to apricot stone. *Contact Dermatitis* 1981; **7:** 282.

ARNICA

Species (Family)
Arnica montana (Asteraceae/Compositae)

Synonym(s)
Leopard's Bane, Wolf's Bane, Mountain Tobacco

Part(s) Used
Flower

Pharmacopoeial Monographs
BHP 1983
BPC 1949
Martindale 30th edition
Pharmacopoeias—Aust., Braz., Fr., Ger., Rom., and Swiss. Aust. also includes Arnica Root.

Legal Category (Licensed Products)
GSL, for external use only[G14]

Constituents[G1,G10,G19,G32]

Amines Betaine, choline, trimethylamine
Carbohydrates Mucilage, polysaccharides including inulin
Coumarins Scopoletin, umbelliferone
Flavonoids Betuletol, eupafolin, flavonol glucuronides,(1-3) hispidulin, isorhamnetin, kaempferol, laciniatin, luteolin, patuletin, quercetin, spinacetin, tricin, 3,5,7-trihydroxy-6,3', 4'-trimethoxyflavone
Terpenoids Sesquiterpenes including helenalin and dihydrohelenalin derivatives (about 0.5%),[4] arnifolin and the arnicolides
Volatile oils (up to 1%, normally about 0.3%). Thymol and thymol derivatives.
Other constituents Bitter principle (arnicin), caffeic acid, carotenoids, phytosterols, resin, tannin (unspecified)

Food Use
Arnica is listed by the Council of Europe as a natural source of food flavouring (category N2). This category indicates that arnica can be added to foodstuffs in small quantities, with a possible limitation of an active principle (as yet unspecified) in the final product.[G9] In the USA, arnica is listed by the FDA as an 'unsafe herb'[G10] and is only approved for food use in alcoholic beverages.[G19]

Herbal Use
Arnica is stated to possess topical counter-irritant properties. It has been used for unbroken chilblains, alopecia neurotica, and specifically for sprains and bruises.[G1,G3,G32]

Arnica is mainly used in homoeopathic preparations; it is used to a lesser extent in herbal products.

Dose
Tincture of Arnica Flower (BPC 1949) 2–4 mL for external application only

Pharmacological Actions
Animal studies Arnica has been reported to exhibit bactericidal properties against *Listeria monocytogenes* and *Salmonella typhimurium*.[G19] Moderate (29%) anti-inflammatory activity in the carrageenan rat paw model has been reported for arnica.[5] Helenalin and dihydrohelenalin are documented to possess analgesic, antibiotic, and anti-inflammatory properties.[G10] Helenalin has also been reported to possess immunostimulant activity *in vitro*,[6] while high molecular-weight polysaccharides have been found to exhibit immunostimulant activity *in vivo* in the carbon clearance test in mice.[6,7]
Arnica contains an adrenaline-like pressor substance and a cardiotonic substance.[G11]

Side-effects, Toxicity
Arnica is poisonous if taken internally. It is irritant to mucous membranes and ingestion may result in fatal gastroenteritis, muscle paralysis (voluntary and cardiac), increase or decrease in pulse rate, palpitation of the heart, shortness of breath, and may even lead to death.[G13,G19] Helenalin is stated to be the toxic principle responsible for these effects.[G13] Thirty millilitres of a 20% arnica tincture, taken by mouth, was reported to produce serious, but not fatal, symptoms.[G19] The topical application of arnica has been documented to cause dermatitis.[8,G26] Arnica is a strong sensitiser, with the sesquiterpene lactone constituents implicated as the contact allergens: they possess an α-methylene group exocyclic to a γ-lactone ring, which is recognised as an immunological prerequisite for contact allergy.[8,9] Helenalin is also reported to possess cytotoxic activity and this has been attributed to its ability to alkylate with sulphydryl groups.[G13]

Contra-indications, Warnings
Arnica should not be taken internally except in suitable homoeopathic dilutions.[G20]
Externally, arnica is poorly tolerated by some people, precipitating allergic reactions in sensitive individuals.[G20] It should only be applied to unbroken skin and withdrawn at the first sign of reaction.[G3] Toxic allergic skin reactions have occurred following application of the tincture.[G13]

Pharmaceutical Comment
The chemistry of arnica is well studied. Anti-inflammatory properties associated with sesquiterpene lactones justify the herbal uses, although allergenic and cytotoxic properties are also associated with this class of constituents. Arnica is not suitable for internal use, although it is present in some homoeopathic products. External use of arnica tincture,

which is included as an ingredient in some cosmetics, hair shampoos and bath preparations, may cause an allergic reaction.

References

See General References G1, G3, G6, G9, G10, G14, G19, G20, G22, G23, G24, G26, G32 and G33

1. Merfort I and Wendisch D. Flavonoidglycoside aus *Arnica montana* und *Arnica chamissonis. Planta Med* 1987; **53:** 434–437.

2. Merfort I. Flavonol glycosides of Arnicae flos DAB 9. *Planta Med* 1986; **52:** 427.

3. Merfort I and Wendisch D. Flavonolglucuronide aus den blüten von *Arnica montana. Planta Med* 1988; **54:** 247–250.

4. Leven W and Willuhn G. Spectrophotometric determination sesquiterpenlactone (S1) in "Arnicae flos DAB 9" with m-dinitrobenzene. *Planta Med* 1986; **52:** 537–538.

5. Mascolo N *et al.* Biological screening of Italian medicinal plants for anti-inflammatory. *Phytotherapy Res* 1987; **1:** 28–31.

6. Chang HM *et al.* Advances in Chinese medicinal materials research. Phildelphia: World Scientific, 1985.

7. Puhlmann J and Wagner H. Immunologically active polysaccharides from *Arnica montana* herbs and tissue cultures. *Planta Med* 1989; **55:** 99.

8. Rudzki E and Grzywa Z. Dermatitis from *Arnica montana. Contact Dermatitis* 1977; **3:** 281–2.

9. Hausen BM. Identification of the allergens of *Arnica montana* L. *Contact Dermatitis* 1978; **4:** 308.

ARTICHOKE

Species (Family)

Cynara scolymus L. (Asteraceae/Compositae)

Synonym(s)

Globe Artichoke.

Jerusalem artichoke is the tuber of *Helianthus tuberosa* L.

Part(s) Used

Aerial parts, Root

Pharmacopoeial Monographs

Martindale 30th edition

Pharmacopoeias—Braz., Fr., and Rom.

Legal Category (Licensed Products)

GSL[G14]

Constituents[G1,G19,G25,G32]

Acids (phenolic, up to 2%). Caffeic acid, mono- and di-caffeoylquinic acid (CQA) derivatives (e.g. cynarin (1,5-di-*O*-CQA), chlorogenic acid (mono derivative))

Flavonoids (0.1–1%). Flavone glycosides (e.g. luteolin-7-β-rutinoside (scolymoside), luteolin-7β-D-glucoside and luteolin-4β-D-glucoside

Volatile oils Sesquiterpenes β-selinene and caryophyllene (major); also eugenol, phenylacetaldehyde, decanal, oct-1-en-3-one, hex-1-en-3-one, and non-*trans*-2-enal

Other constituents Phytosterols (taraxasterol and β-taraxasterol), tannins, glycolic and glyceric acids, sugars, inulin, enzymes including peroxidases,[1] cynaropicrin (bitter, sesquiterpene lactone).[2] The root and fully developed fruits and flowers are devoid of cynaropicrin; highest content reported in young leaves.[3]

Food Use

Artichoke is listed by the Council of Europe as a natural source of food flavouring (category N2). This category indicates that artichoke can be added to foodstuffs in small quantities, with a possible limitation of an active principle (as yet unspecified) in the final product.[G9] In the USA, artichoke leaves are approved for use in alcoholic beverages only, with an average maximum concentration of 0.0016% (16 ppm).[G19]

Herbal Use

Artichoke is stated to possess diuretic, choleretic, hypocholesterolaemic, hypolipidaemic, and hepatostimulating properties.[4,5,6, G1,G32]

Dose

Leaf, **stem**, or **root** 1–4 g three times daily[G25]

Pharmacological Actions

Animal studies Hypocholesterolaemic, hypolipidaemic, and choleretic effects have been described in rats for both purified and total artichoke extracts.[4] The purified extract was found to exhibit more potent activity compared to the total artichoke extract; this was attributed to the higher concentration of mono-CQA (e.g. chlorogenic, neochlorogenic) compared to di-CQA (e.g. cynarin) present in the purified extract.

In-vivo hepatoprotectivity against tetrachloromethane-induced hepatitis has been documented for artichoke extracts administered orally to rats before intoxication.[6] A hepatoregenerating effect has also been described for an aqueous artichoke extract administered orally to rats following partial hepatectomy.[7] The leaf extract was found to be more potent compared to the root extract.[8] The hepatoprotective effect of polyphenolic compounds isolated from artichoke has been investigated *in vitro* using rat hepatocytes.[5] Cynarin was the only compound reported to exhibit significant cytoprotective activity, with a lesser action demonstrated by caffeic acid.

Human studies Cynarin has been administered to 17 patients with familial type IIa or type IIb hyperlipoproteinaemia for whom blood-lipid concentrations were maintained with dietary treatment alone.[9] Cynarin was taken 15 minutes before meals at either 250 mg or 750 mg daily dose. Over a period of 3 months cynarin was reported to have no effect on mean serum cholesterol and triglyceride concentrations.[9] The results were in agreement with the findings of some previous workers, but also in contrast to other studies that have reported cynarin to be effective in lowering serum concentrations of cholesterol and triglycerides when taken in daily doses ranging from 60 mg to 1500 mg.[9]

Side-effects, Toxicity

Allergic contact dermatitis, with cross-sensitivity to other Compositae plants, has been documented for artichoke.[10, G26] Cynaropicrin and other sesquiterpene lactones with allergenic potential have been isolated form artichoke.[10,G27] Purified artichoke extract is more toxic than a total extract. LD_{50} values (rat, by intraperitoneal injection) have been documented as greater than 1000 mg/kg (total extract) and 265 mg/kg (purified extract).[4]

Contra-indications, Warnings

Artichoke yields cynaropicrin, a potentially allergenic sesquiterpene lactone.[G26]. Individuals with an existing hypersensitivity to any member of the Compositae family may develop an allergic reaction to artichoke.

Pregnancy and lactation In view of the lack of toxicity data, excessive use of artichoke should be avoided during pregnancy and lactation.

Pharmaceutical Comment

Artichoke is characterised by the phenolic acid constituents, in particular cynarin (a di-CQA). Documented studies support some of the reputed uses of artichoke. Traditionally, the choleretic and cholesterol lowering activities of artichoke have been attributed to cynarin.[4] However, studies in animals and humans have suggested that these effects may in fact be due to the mono-CQAs present in artichoke (e.g. chlorogenic and neochlorogenic acids). Conflicting results have been documented from human studies investigating the use of artichoke and cynarin in the treatment of hyperlipidaemia. Hepatoprotective and hepatoregenerating activities have been documented for cynarin in animals. Further studies are required to establish the benefit of artichoke as a lipid and cholesterol lowering agent and as a hepatostimulant and protectant.

References

See General References G1, G9, G14, G19, G22, G23, G25, G26 G32 and G33.

1. Kamel MY, Ghazy AM. Peroxidases of *Cyanara scolymus* (global artichoke) leaves: Purification and properties. *Acta Biol Med Germ* 1973; **31:** 39–49.

2. Jouany JM *et al*. Dosage indirect de la cynaropicrine dans la *Cynara scolymus* (Compositae) par libération de sa chaîne latérale hydroxyméthylacrylique. *Plant Méd Phytothér* 1975; **9:** 72–8.

3. Schneider G, Thiele Kl. Die Verteilung des Bitterstoffes Cynaropicrin in der Artischocke. *Planta Med* 1974; **26:** 174–83.

4. Lietti A. Choleretic and cholesterol lowering properties of two artichoke extracts. *Fitoterapia* 1977; **48:** 153–8.

5. Adzet T *et al*. Hepatoprotective activity of polyphenolic compounds from *Cynara scolymus* against CCl_4 toxicity in isolated rat hepatocytes. *J Nat Prod* 1987; **50:** 612–17.

6. Adzet T *et al*. Action of an artichoke extract against CCl_4-induced heptotoxicity in rats. *Acta Pharm Jugosl* 1987; **37:** 183–7.

7. Maros T *et al*. Wirkungen der *Cynara scolymus*-Extrakte auf die Regeneration der Rattenleber. *Arzneimittelforschung* 1966; **16:** 127–9.

8. Maros T *et al*. Wirkungen der *Cynara scolymus*-extrakte auf die Regeneration der Rattenleber. *Arzneimittelforschung* 1968; **18:** 884–6.

9. Heckers H *et al*. Inefficiency of cynarin as therapeutic regimen in familial type II hyperlipoproteinaemia. *Atherosclerosis* 1977; **26:** 249–53.

10. Meding B. Allergic contract dermatitis from artichoke, *Cynara scolymus*. *Contact Dermatitis* 1983; **9:** 314.

ASAFOETIDA

Species (Family)
Ferula species including
(i) *Ferula assafoetida* L. (*Ferula rubricaulis* Boiss)
(ii) *Ferula foetida* (Bunge) Regel (Apiaceae/Umbelliferae)

Synonym(s)
Asant, Asafetida, Devil's Dung, Gum Asafetida

Part(s) Used
Oleo-gum resin obtained by incising the living rhizomes and roots

Pharmacopoeial Monographs
BHP 1983
BHP 1990
BPC 1949
Martindale 30th edition

Legal Category (Licensed Products)
GSL [G14]

Constituents [G2,G19,G23,G24,G29,G31,G32,G35]
Gum fraction (25%). Glucose, galactose, L-arabinose, rhamnose, and glucuronic acid.
Resins (40–64%). Ferulic acid esters (60%), free ferulic acid (1.3%), asaresinotannols and farnesiferols A, B, and C, coumarin derivatives (e.g. umbelliferone), coumarin-sesquiterpene complexes (e.g. asacoumarin A and asacoumarin B).[1] Free ferulic acid is converted to coumarin during dry distillation.
Volatile oils (3–17%). Sulphur containing compounds with disulphides as major components, various monoterpenes.[1]
The oleo-gum-resins of different *Ferula* species are not identical and many papers have documented their phytochemistry,[2–11] reporting polysulphanes,[2–11] complex acetylenes,[3] phenylpropanoids,[7] and many sesquiterpene derivatives.[2,4,5,6,8,9]
C-3 prenylated 4-hydroxycoumarin derivatives (e.g. ferulenol) are thought to represent the toxic principles in the species *Ferula communis*.[12]

Food Use
Asafoetida is used widely in foods and is listed by the Council of Europe as a source of natural food flavouring (category N2). This category allows for asafoetida to be added to foodstuffs in small quantities, with a possible limitation of an active principle (as yet unspecified) in the final product. [G9] Asafoetida is approved for food use in the USA.[G19]

Herbal Use
Asafoetida is stated to possess carminative, antispasmodic, and expectorant properties. It has been used for chronic bronchitis, pertussis, laryngismus stridulus, hysteria, and specifically for intestinal flatulent colic.[G2,G3]

Dose
Powdered resin 0.3–1 g three times daily[G2,G3]
Tincture of Asafoetida (BPC 1949) 2–4 mL

Pharmacological Actions
Animal studies Asafoetida has been reported to possess anticoagulant and hypotensive properties.[G19] Asafoetida is an ingredient of a plant mixture reported to have antidiabetic properties in rats.[13] However, when the individual components of the mixture were studied asafoetida was devoid of antidiabetic effect with myrrh and aloe gum extracts representing the active hypoglycaemic principles.[14]
Oestrogenic activity in rats has been documented for carotane sesquiterpenes and ferujol (a coumarin) isolated from *Ferula jaeschkeana*.[15,16]
Human studies A protective action against fat-induced hyperlipidaemia has been documented for asafoetida and attributed to the sulphur compounds in the volatile oil fraction of the resin.[17] Two double-blind studies have reported the efficacy of asafoetida in the treatment of irritable bowel syndrome to be just below the 5% significance level in one study[18] and at 1% in the other.[19]

Side-effects, Toxicity
Asafoetida is documented to be relatively non-toxic; ingestion of 15 g produced no untoward effects.[G22] A report of methaemoglobinaemia has been associated with the administration of asafoetida (in milk) to a five-week old infant for the treatment of colic.[20] Asafoetida was found to exert an oxidising effect on foetal haemoglobin but not on adult haemoglobin.
Toxic coumarin constituents of a related species, *Ferula communis*, have been documented to reduce prothrombin concentrations and to cause haemorrhaging in livestock.[21, G26]
Two other species, *Ferula galbaniflua* and *Ferula rubicaulis*, are stated to contain a gum that is rubefacient and irritant causing contact dermatitis in sensitive individuals.[G26, G35]
A weak sister chromatid exchange-inducing effect in mouse spermatogonia[22] and clastogenicity in mouse spermatocytes [23] has been documented for asafoetida. Chromosomal damage by asafoetida has been associated with the coumarin constituents.

Contra-indications, Warnings
Asafoetida should not be given to infants because of the oxidising effect on foetal haemoglobin resulting in methaemoglobinaemia.[20] The gum of some *Ferula* species is reported to be irritant and therefore may cause gastro-intestinal irritation or induce contact dermatitis in some individ-

uals. Excessive doses may interfere with anticoagulant therapy and with hypertensive and hypotensive therapy.

Pregnancy and lactation Asafoetida has a folkloric reputation as an abortifacient and an emmenagogue.[G12] However the use of asafoetida during pregnancy is probably acceptable, provided doses do not exceed amounts normally ingested in foods. In view of the toxic effect to infants (e.g. methaemoglobinaemia), asafoetida should be avoided during breast-feeding.

Pharmaceutical Comment

Asafoetida is a complex oleo-gum resin consisting of many constituents that vary according to the different species used. Asafoetida is commonly used in foods but little scientific evidence is available to justify the herbal uses. In view of the known pharmacologically active constituents, asafoetida should not be taken in amounts exceeding those used in foods.

References

See General References G2, G3, G9, G12, G14, G19, G23, G24, G26, G29, G31, G32, G33 and G35.

1. Kajimoto T *et al*. Sesquiterpenoid and disulphide derivatives from *Ferula assa-foetida*. *Phytochemistry* 1989; **28**: 1761–3.

2. Dawidar A-A *et al*. Marmaricin, a new sesquiterpenoid coumarin from *Ferula marmarica* L. *Chem Pharm Bull* 1979; **27**: 3153–5.

3. de Pascual Teresa J *et al*. Complex acetylenes from the roots of *Ferula communis*. *Planta Med* 1986; **52**: 458–62.

4. Miski M. Fercoperol, an unusual cyclic-endoperoxynerolidol derivative from *Ferula communis* subsp. *communis*. *J Nat Prod* 1986; **49**: 916–18.

5. Garg SN *et al*. Feruginidin and ferugin, two new sesquiterpenoids based on the carotane skeleton from *Ferula jaeschkeana*. *J Nat Prod* 1987; **50**: 253–5.

6. Garg SN *et al*. New sesquiterpenes from *Ferula jaeschkeana*. *Planta Med* 1987; **53**: 341–2.

7. Gonzalez AG *et al*. Phenylpropanoid and stilbene compounds from *Ferula latipinna*. *Planta Med* 1988; **54**: 184–5.

8. Miski M. New daucane and germacrane esters from *Ferula orientalis* var. *orientalis*. *J Nat Prod* 1987; **50**: 829–34.

9. Miski M. New daucane esters from *Ferula tingitana*. *J Nat Prod* 1986; **49**: 657–60.

10. Samimi MN and Unger W. Die gummiharze afghanischer asa foetida-liefernder ferula-arten. Beobachtungen zur herkunft und qualität afghanischer asa foetida. *Planta Med* 1979; **36**: 128–33.

11. Zhi-da M *et al*. Polysulfanes in the volatile oils of *Ferula* species. *Planta Med* 1987; **53**: 300–302.

12. Valle MG *et al*. Prenylated coumarins and sesquiterpenoids from *Ferula communis*. *Phytochemistry* 1987; **26**: 253–6.

13. Al-Awadi FM *et al*. On the mechanism of the hypoglycaemic effect of a plant extract. *Diabetologia* 1985; **28**: 432–4.

14. Al-Awadi FM and Gumaa KA. Studies on the activity of individual plants of an antidiabetic plant mixture. *Acta Diabetol Lat* 1987; **24**: 37–41.

15. Singh MM *et al*. Contraceptive efficacy and hormonal profile of ferujol: a new coumarin from *Ferula jaeschkeana*. *Planta Med* 1985; **51**: 268–70.

16. Singh MM *et al*. Antifertility and hormonal properties of certain carotane sesquiterpenes of *Ferula jaeschkeana*. *Planta Med* 1988; **54**: 492–4.

17. Bordia A and Arora SK. The effect of essential oil (active principle) of asafoetida on alimentary lipemia. *Indian J Med Res* 1975; **63**: 707–711.

18. Rahlfs VW and Mössinger P. Zur Behandlung des Colon irritabile. *ArzneimittelForsch* 1976; **26**: 2230–4.

19. Rahlfs VW and Mössinger P. Asa foetida bei colon irritabile. *Dtsch med Wochenschr* 1978; **104**: 140–3.

20. Kelly KJ *et al*. Methemoglobinemia in an infant treated with the folk remedy glycerited asafoetida. *Pediatrics* 1984; **73**: 717—9.

21. Aragno M *et al*. Experimental studies on the toxicity of *Ferula communis* in the rat. *Res Commun Chem Pathol Pharmacol* 1973; **59**: 399–402.

22. Abraham SK and Kesavan PC. Genotoxicity of garlic, turmeric and asafoetida in mice. *Mutat Res* 1984; **136**: 85–8.

23. Walia K. Effect of asafoetida (7-hydroxycoumarin) on mouse spermatocytes. *Cytologia* 1973; **38**: 719–24.

AVENS

Species (Family)
Geum urbanum L. (Rosaceae)

Synonym(s)
Benedict's Herb, Colewort, Geum, Herb Bennet

Part(s) Used
Herb

Pharmacopoeial Monographs
BHP 1983

Legal Category (Licensed Products)
Avens is not listed in the GSL.[G14]

Constituents[G18,G25,G32]
Limited information is available on the herb. Constituents reported include bitter principles, resin, tannins, and volatile oil.
Other plant parts The root has been more extensively studied and is reported to contain a phenolic glycoside (gein), yielding eugenol as the aglycone and vicianose (disaccharide) as the sugar component;[1] 30% tannin, including gallic, caffeic and chlorogenic acids (pseudotannins generally associated with condensed tannins);[1] a bitter substance, a flavonoid, and volatile oil.

Food Use
Avens is listed by the Council of Europe as a natural source of food flavouring (category N2). This category indicates that avens can be added to foodstuffs in small quantities, with a possible limitation of an active principle (as yet unspecified) in the final product.[G9]

Herbal Use
Avens is stated to possess antidiarrhoeal, antihaemorrhagic, and febrifugal properties. It has been used for diarrhoea, catarrhal colitis, passive uterine haemorrhage, intermittent fevers, and specifically for ulcerative colitis.[G3,G32]

Dose
Dried herb 1–4 g or by infusion three times daily[G3]

Liquid extract (1:1 in 25% alcohol) 1–4 mL three times daily[G3]

Pharmacological Actions
Animal studies A 20% aqueous decoction of avens, administered by intravenous injection, has been reported to produce a reduction in blood pressure in cats.[2] Tannins are generally known to possess astringent properties.

Side-effects, Toxicity
None documented.

Contra-indications, Warnings
In view of the reported tannin constituents and the lack of toxicity data, it is advisable to avoid excessive use of avens.
Pregnancy and lactation Avens is reputed to affect the menstrual cycle.[G12] In view of the lack of phytochemical, pharmacological, and toxicological data, the use of avens during pregnancy should be avoided.

Pharmaceutical Comment
Limited phytochemical or pharmacological data are available for avens, although reported tannin constituents would indicate an astringent action thus supporting the traditional use in diarrhoea and haemorrhage. In view of the lack of toxicity data, excessive use should be avoided.

References
See General References G3, G9, G12, G14, G18,and G25 and G32.

1. Psenák M *et al*. Biochemical Study on *Geum urbanum*. *Planta Med* 1970; **19:** 154–9.

2. Petkov V. Plants with hypotensive, antithrombotous and coronadilating. *Am J Chin Med* 1979; **7:** 197–236.

BAYBERRY

Species (Family)
Myrica cerifera L. (Myricaceae)

Synonym(s)
Candleberry Bark, Myrica, Wax Myrtle Bark

Part(s) Used
Root bark

Pharmacopoeial Monographs
BHP 1983
BPC 1949
Martindale 28th edition

Legal Category (Licensed Products)
GSL[G14]

Constituents[G10,G19,G24,G32]
Flavonoids Myricitrin
Tannins 3.9% (bark), 34.82% (total aqueous extract)
Terpenoids Myricadiol, taraxerol, taraxerone[1]
Other constituents Albumen, red dye, gum, resin, starch, wax containing palmitic, myristic, and lauric acid esters

Food Use
Bayberry is not used in foods.

Herbal Use
Bayberry is stated to possess antipyretic, circulatory stimulant, emetic, and mild diaphoretic properties. It has been used for diarrhoea, colds, and specifically for mucous colitis. An infusion has been used as a gargle for a sore throat, and as a douche for leucorrhoea. Powdered root bark has been applied topically for the management of indolent ulcers.[G3,G19,G32]

Dose
Powdered bark 0.6–2.0 g by infusion or decoction three times daily[G3]
Liquid extract (1:1 in 45% alcohol) 0.6–2.0 mL three times daily[G3]

Pharmacological Actions
Animal studies Myricitrin has been reported to exhibit choleretic, bactericidal, paramecicidal, and spermatocidal activity; myricadiol has mineralocorticoid activity.[G19] Tannins are known to possess astringent properties.

Side-effects, Toxicity
A total aqueous extract, tannin fraction, and tannin-free fraction from bayberry were all reported to produce tumours in NIH black rats, following weekly subcutaneous injections for up to 75 weeks[2,3]. The number of tumours that developed were stated to be statistically significant for the tannin fraction and tannin-free fraction. Analysis of the tannin-free fraction revealed the presence of four phenolic compounds, one of which was identified as myricitrin. No tumours were reported in a later study, in which rats were given subcutaneous injections of total aqueous extract for 78 weeks.

Large doses may cause typical mineralocorticoid side-effects (e.g. sodium and water retention, hypertension).

Contra-indications, Warnings
Large doses may interfere with existing hypertensive, hypotensive, or steroid therapy. Excessive use of tannin-containing herbs is not recommended.

Pregnancy and lactation The safety of bayberry has not been established. In view of the possible mineralocorticoid activity and the reported carcinogenic activity, the use of bayberry during pregnancy and lactation should be avoided.

Pharmaceutical Comment
Limited chemical information is available for bayberry. Documented tannin constituents justify some of the herbal uses. In addition, mineralocorticoid activity has been reported for one of the triterpene constituents. In view of this and the tannin constituents, excessive use of bayberry should be avoided.

References
See General References G3, G6, G10, G14, G19, G21, G24 and G32.

1. Paul BD *et al.* Isolation of myricadiol, myricitrin, taraxerol, and taraxerone from *Myrica cerifera* L. root bark. *J Pharm Sci* 1974; **63**: 958–9.

2. Kapadia GJ *et al.* Carcinogenicity of *Camellia sinensis* (tea) and some tannin-containing folk medicinal herbs administered subcutaneously in rats. *J Natl Cancer Inst* 1976; **57**: 207–9.

3. Kapadia GJ *et al.* Carcinogenicity of some folk medicinal herbs in rats. *J Natl Cancer Inst* 1978; **60**: 683–6.

BLOODROOT

Species (Family)

Sanguinaria canadensis L. (Papaveraceae)

Synonym(s)

Red Indian Paint, Red Root, Sanguinaria, Tetterwort

Part(s) Used

Rhizome

Pharmacopoeial Monographs

BHP 1983
Martindale 30th edition

Legal Category (Licensed Products)

Bloodroot is not included on the GSL[G14]

Constituents[G10,G19]

Alkaloids (isoquinoline type) 3.0–7.0%.[1] Sanguinarine (ca. 1%), sanguidimerine, chelerythrine, protopine; others include oxysanguinarine, α- and β-allocryptopine, sanguilutine, dihydrosanguilutine, berberine, coptisine, and homochelidonine.

Other Constituents Resin, starch, organic acids (citric, malic)

Alkaloid content of other plant parts recorded as 0.08% (leaf), 1.8% (root).

Food Use

Bloodroot is listed by the Council of Europe as a natural source of food flavouring (category N3). This category indicates that bloodroot can be added to foodstuffs in the traditionally accepted manner, although there is insufficient information available for an adequate assessment of potential toxicity.[G9]

Herbal Use

Bloodroot is stated to act as an expectorant, spasmolytic, emetic, cathartic, antiseptic, cardioactive, topical irritant and escharotic (scab-producing). Traditionally it is indicated for bronchitis (sub-acute or chronic), asthma, croup, laryngitis, pharyngitis, deficient capillary circulation, nasal polypus (as a snuff), and specifically for asthma and bronchitis with feeble peripheral circulation. [G3]

Dose

Rhizome 0.06–0.5 g (1–2 g for emetic dose) three times daily.[G3]

Liquid Extract 0.06–0.3 mL (1:1 in 60% alcohol) (1–2 mL for emetic dose) three times daily.[G3]

Tincture 0.3–2 mL (1:5 in 60% alcohol) (2–8 mL for emetic dose) three times daily.[G3]

Pharmacological Actions

Activities documented for bloodroot are principally attributable to the isoquinoline alkaloid constituents, in particular sanguinarine. In the last 10 years, interest has focused on the use of sanguinarine in dental hygiene products. Unless otherwise stated, the following actions refer to sanguinarine:

Animal studies Considerable antimicrobial activity has been documented against both Gram-positive and Gram-negative bacteria, *Candida* and dermatophytes (fungi), and *Trichomonas* (protozoa).[2] In addition, anti-inflammatory activity has been described against carrageenan-induced rat paw oedema.[3]

Prolongation of the ventricular refractory period has been attributed to an inhibition of Na^+-K^+ ATP-ase.[4,5] However, a single intravenous injection of sanguinarine to anaesthetised dogs reportedly exerted no effect on cardiovascular parameters monitored.[4]

In-vitro inhibition of bone resorption and collagenase has been documented.[2]

Human studies Many studies have investigated the efficacy of bloodroot extracts in oral hygiene.[2] Preparations containing bloodroot extracts, such as oral rinses and toothpastes, have been reported to significantly lower plaque, gingival, and bleeding indices.[2] Alteration of the oral microbial flora, or development of resistant microbial strains has not been observed with the use of bloodroot extracts.[2]

Side-Effects, Toxicity

None documented for bloodroot. Much has been documented concerning the potential toxicity of the alkaloid constituents in bloodroot, in particular of sanguinarine.

In the 1920s contamination of cooking oil with *Argemone mexicana* seed oil was proposed as the causative factor for epidemic dropsy and associated glaucoma, with sanguinarine considered the toxic component of the seed oil.[1,6,7] However, subsequent workers disputed this theory and the toxicity of *A. mexicana* oil has been attributed to a fatty acid constituent.[1,7]

Conclusions reached in the 1960s over the carcinogenic potential of sanguinarine have more recently been disproved.[8] In addition, negative mutagenic activity has been observed in the Ames test (microbial, with and without activation).[8]

Sanguinarine is poorly absorbed from the gastro-intestinal tract. This is reflected in stated acute oral LD_{50} values (rat) of 1.7 g/kg (sanguinarine) and 1.4 g/kg (sanguinaria extract), compared with an acute intravenous LD_{50} (rat) value of 28.7 mg/kg (sanguinarine).[1] Symptoms of diarrhoea, ataxia and reduced activity were observed in animals receiving high oral doses of sanguinarine.[5] The acute dermal toxicity (LD_{50}) of sanguinarine is stated to be greater than 200 mg/kg in rabbits.[1] The first experimental study of sanguinarine toxicity (1876) reported prostration and severe respiratory distress as the most marked signs of oral toxicity.[1] However, in more recent short-term toxicity studies no toxic signs were observed in the fetuses of rats following maternal administration of 5–30 mg/kg/day of sanguinarine [1]

The reproductive and developmental toxicity potential of an *S. canadensis* extract has been evaluated in rats and rabbits.[8] Developmental toxicity (increase in postimplantation loss, slight decrease in foetal and pup body weights) was only evident at maternally toxic doses. No effect was reported on reproductive capabilities, on parturition or on lactation. It was concluded that oral ingestion of sanguinaria extract has no selective effect on fertility, reproduction, or on foetal or neonatal development.[8]

Hepatotoxicity has been documented in rats following a single intraperitoneal administration (10 mg/kg) of sanguinarine.[5] Toxicity was indicated by an increase in SGPT and SGOT activity, and by a significant reduction in microsomal cytochrome P-450 and benzphetamine *N*-demethylase activities.[5] Macroscopic lesions were also observed but the authors stated that the two events could not be conclusively directly related.[5] No hepatotoxicity has been observed in short-term toxicity studies involving oral administration of sanguinarine.[1]

Animal studies have indicated sanguinarine to be non-irritant and to exhibit no allergenic or anaphylactic potential.[4] *Human* patch tests have shown sanguinarine to be non-irritant and non-sensitising.[4]

Contra-indications, Warnings

None documented.

Pregnancy and lactation Animal studies have indicated bloodroot to be non-toxic during pregnancy (see above). However, in view of its pharmacologically active constituents, use of bloodroot during pregnancy and lactation is best avoided.

Pharmaceutical Comment

Bloodroot is characterised by isoquinoline alkaloid constituents (benzophenanthridine-type), predominantly sanguinarine. A wide-range of pharmacological activities has been documented for this class of compounds including antimicrobual, anti-inflammatory, antihistaminic, cardiotonic, and anti-plaque.[1,8] Other benzophenanthridine alkaloids have been associated with cytotoxic activities. However, recent interest over the potential use of bloodroot in oral hygiene has stimulated considerable research into both sanguinarine and bloodroot extracts. Results have indicated that products such as oral rinses and toothpastes containing either sanguinaria extracts or sanguinarine may be of value in dental hygiene, and are of low toxicity.

References

See General References G3, G9, G10, G14, G19, and G23

1. Becci PJ *et al.* Short-term toxicity studies of sanguinarine and of two alkaloid extracts of *Sanguinaria canadensis.* J Toxicol Environ Health 1987; **20:** 199–208.

2. Godowski KC. Antimicrobial action of sanguinarine. *J Clin Dentistry* 1989; **1:** 96–101.

3. Lenfield J *et al.* Antiinflammatory activity of quaternary benzophenanthridine alkaloids from *Chelidonium majus. Planta Med* 1981; **43:** 161–5

4. Schwartz HG. Safety profile of sanguinarine and Sanguinaria extract. *Compend Cont Ed Dent Suppl* 1986; **7:** S212–S217.

5. Dalvi RR. Sanguinarine: its potential as a liver toxic alkaloid present in the seeds of *Argemone mexicana. Experientia* 1985; **41:** 77–8.

6. Sood NN *et al.* Epidemic dropsy following transcutaneous absorption of *Argemone mexicana* oil. *Trans Roy Soc Trop Med Hyg* 1985; **79:** 510-2.

7. Lord G *et al.* Sanguinarine and the controversy concerning its relationship to glaucoma in epidemic dropsy. *J Clin Dentistry* 1989; **1:** 110-5.

8. Keller KA. Reproductive and developmental toxicological evaluation of Sanguinaria extract. *J Clin Dentistry* 1989; **1:** 59–66.

BLUE FLAG

Species (Family)
Iris versicolor L. or *Iris caroliniana* Watson (Iridaceae)

Part(s) Used
Rhizome

Pharmacopoeial Monographs
BHP 1990
BPC 1934

Legal Category (Licensed Products)
GSL[G14]

Constituents[G10,G18,G24,G32]
Acids Isophthalic acid 0.002%, salicylic acid, lauric acid, stearic acid, palmitic acid, and 1-triacontanol
Volatile oils (0.025%). Furfural
Other constituents Iridin, β-sitosterol, iriversical,[1] tannin

Food Use
Blue flag is not used in foods.

Herbal Use
Blue flag is stated to possess cholagogue, laxative, diuretic, dermatological, anti-inflammatory, and anti-emetic properties. It has been used for skin diseases, biliousness with constipation and liver dysfunction, and specifically for cutaneous eruptions.[G3,G32]

Dose
Dried rhizome 0.6–2.0 g or by decoction three times daily[G2,G3,G5]
Liquid extract (1:1 in 45% alcohol) 1–2 mL three times daily[G2,G3,G5]

Pharmacological Actions
None documented.

Side-effects, Toxicity
It has been stated that the fresh root of blue flag can cause nausea and vomiting.[G20]

Furfural, a volatile oil constituent, is known to be irritant to mucous membranes causing lachrymation, inflammation of the eyes, irritation of the throat, and headache.[G24] Whether these irritant properties are attributable to the volatile oil of blue flag has not been established. Acute oral toxicity (rat, LD_{50}) for furfural has been documented as 127 mg/kg bodyweight.[G24] Iridin has been reported to be poisonous in both humans and livestock.[G10] However, it is unclear whether this substance is the same iridin documented as a constituent of blue flag.

Contra-indications, Warnings
Only small doses of the dried root are advisable, because of the risk of nausea and vomiting.[G20] In view of the possible irritant nature of the volatile oil, blue flag may not be suitable for internal use, especially in sensitive individuals.

Pregnancy and lactation The safety of blue flag has not been established. In view of this, together with the documented irritant properties of some of the constituents, blue flag should not be taken during pregnancy.

Pharmaceutical Comment
Little is known about the phytochemical, pharmacological or toxicological properties of blue flag and its constituents, although related species are known to be toxic. In view of these factors, the use of blue flag is best avoided.

References
See General References G2, G3, G5, G10, G14, G18, G20, G24 and G32.

1. Krick W *et al* Isolation and structural determination of a new methylated triterpenoid from rhizomes of *Iris versicolor* L. Z *Naturforsch* 1983; **38**: 689–92.

BOGBEAN

Species (Family)
Menyanthes trifoliata L. (Menyanthaceae)

Synonym(s)
Buckbean, Marsh Trefoil, Menyanthes

Part(s) Used
Leaf

Pharmacopoeial Monographs
BHP 1983
BHP 1990
Martindale 30th edition
National pharmacopoeias—Aust., Cz., Fr., Hung., and Rus.

Legal Category (Licensed Products)
GSL[G14]

Constituents[G1,G31,G32]
Acids Caffeic acid, chlorogenic acid, ferulic acid, *p*-hydroxybenzoic acid, protocatechuic acid, salicylic acid, vanillic acid;[1,2] folic acid and palmitic acid[2]
Alkaloids Gentianin and gentianidine (pyridine-type); choline[2]
Coumarins Scopoletin[2]
Flavonoids Hyperin, kaempferol, quercetin, rutin, trifolioside[1,2]
Iridoids 7',8'-Dihydrofoliamenthin, foliamenthin, loganin, menthiafolin, sweroside[2,3,4]
Other constituents Carotene, ceryl alcohol, enzymes (e.g. emulsin, invertin), α-spinasterol, an unidentified substance with haemolytic properties.[2] α-Spinasterol has been reported to be a mixture of five sterols with α-spinasterol and stigmast-7-enol as major components.[5]

Food Use
Bogbean is listed by the Council of Europe as a natural source of food flavouring (category N2). This category indicates that bogbean can be added to foodstuffs in small quantities, with a possible limitation of an active principle (as yet unspecified) in the final product.[G9]

Herbal Use
Bogbean is stated to possess bitter and diuretic properties. It has been used for rheumatism, rheumatoid arthritis, and specifically for muscular rheumatism associated with general asthenia.[G1,G3,G4,G32]

Dose
Dried leaf 1–2 g or by infusion three times daily[G3]
Liquid extract (1:1 in 25% alcohol) 1–2 mL three times daily[G3]
Tincture (1:5 in 45% alcohol) 1–3 mL three times daily[G3]

Pharmacological Actions
Animal studies A choleretic action has been described for caffeic acid and ferulic acid; a stomachic secretive action has been reported for protocatechuic acid and *p*-hydroxybenzoic acid. The iridoids possess bitter properties.[1] The bitter index (BI) of bogbean is stated to be 4000–10 000 (compared to gentian BI 10 000–30 000).[G31] Bogbean extracts have antibacterial activities.[6,7]

Side-effects, Toxicity
Large doses of bogbean are stated to be purgative and may cause vomiting.[8] An unidentified substance with haemolytic activity has been isolated from bogbean.[2]

Contra-indications, Warnings
Excessive doses may be irritant to the gastro-intestinal tract causing diarrhoea, griping pains, nausea, and vomiting.[8]
Pregnancy and lactation The safety of bogbean has not been established. In view of the lack of toxicity data and possible purgative action, the use of bogbean during pregnancy and lactation should be avoided.

Pharmaceutical Comment
The chemistry of bogbean is well studied, but no pharmacological information is available to justify the herbal uses. In view of the lack of toxicity data, excessive doses should be avoided.

References
See General References G1, G3, G4, G9, G14, G31 and G32.

1. Swiatek L *et al.* Content of phenolic acids in leaves of Menyanthes trifoliata. *Planta Med* 1986; **52:** 530.

2. Giaceri G. Chromatographic identification of coumarin derivatives in Menyanthes trifoliata L. *Fitoterapia* 1972; **43:** 134–8.

3. Battersby AR *et al.* Seco-cyclopentane glucosides from *Menyanthes trifoliata*: foliamenthin, dihydrofoliamenthin, and menthiafolin. *Chemical Communications* 1968;1277–80.

4. Loew P *et al.* The structure and biosynthesis of foliamenthin. *Chemical Communications* 1968; 1276–7.

5. Popov S. Sterols of the Gentianaceae family. *Dokl Bolg Akad Nauk* 1969; **22:** 293–6.

6. Moskalenko SA. Preliminary screening of Far-Eastern ethnomedicinal plants for antibacterial activity. *J Ethnopharmacol* 1986; **15:** 231–59.

7. Bishop CJ and MacDonald RE. A survey of higher plants for antibacterial substances. *Can J Botany* 1951; **29:** 260–9.

8. Todd RG (ed). *Martindale: The Extra Pharmacopoeia* 25th Edn. London: Pharmaceutical Press, 1967.

BOLDO

Species (Family)
Peumus boldus Molina (Monimiaceae)

Synonym(s)
Boldus, *Boldus boldus* (Mol.) Lyons

Part(s) Used
Leaf

Pharmacopoeial Monographs
BHP 1983
BPC 1934
Martindale 30th edition
National pharmacopoeias—Cz., Egypt., Fr., It., Rom., and Swiss.

Legal Category (Licensed Products)
GSL[G14]

Constituents[G1,G10,G19,G31,G32,G35]
Alkaloids (isoquinoline-type) 0.25–0.7%. Boldine 0.06% (major, disputed), isoboldine, 6a,7-dehydroboldine, isocorydine, isocorydine-*N*-oxide, norisocorydine, laurolitsine, laurotetanine, *N*-methyllaurotetanine, reticuline (aporphines); (–)-pronuciferine (proaporphine), sinoacutine (morphinandienone)[1–4]

Flavonoids Flavonols (e.g. isorhamnetin) and their glycosides[5,6]

Volatile oils (2.5%). Some 38 components have been identified including *p*-cymene 28.6%, ascaridole 16.1%, 1,8-cineole 16.0%, linalool 9.1%, terpinen-4-ol 2.6%, α-terpineol 0.9%, fenchone 0.8%, terpinolene 0.4%

Other constituents Coumarin 0.5%, resin, tannin

Food Use
Boldo is listed by the Council of Europe as a natural source of food flavouring (category N3). This category indicates that boldo can be added to foodstuffs in the traditionally accepted manner, although insufficient information is available for an adequate assessment of potential toxicity.[G9]

Herbal Use
Boldo is stated to possess cholagogue, liver stimulant, sedative, diuretic, mild urinary demulcent, and antiseptic properties. It has been used for gallstones, pain in the liver or gall bladder, cystitis, rheumatism, and specifically for cholelithiasis with pain.[G1,G3,G32]

Dose
Dried leaf 60–200 mg or by infusion three times daily[G3]
Liquid extract (1:1 in 45% alcohol) 0.1–0.3 mL three times daily[G3]

Tincture (1:10 in 60% alcohol) 0.5–2.0 mL three times daily[G3]

Pharmacological Actions
Animal studies Boldo has exhibited choleretic (highest activity in rats), diuretic, stomachic, and cholagogic properties.[G19] The choleretic activity of boldo has been attributed to the alkaloidal constituents.[7] Boldo essential oil contains terpinen-4-ol, the irritant and diuretic principle in juniper oil.

Human studies Boldo, in combination with cascara, rhubarb, and gentian, has been reported to exhibit a beneficial effect on a variety of symptoms such as loss of appetite, digestion difficulties, constipation, flatulence, and itching.[7, 8] Rhubarb and gentian were found to be more effective with respect to appetite-loss related symptoms, and boldo and cascara more effective in constipation-related symptoms.

Two preparations containing extracts of boldo and cascara have been documented to increase biliary flow without altering the lithogenic index or bile composition.[9]

Ascaridole, a component of the volatile oil, previously found a clinical use as an anthelmintic agent.[10] However, this use has declined with the development of synthetic compounds with lower toxicity and a wider range of activity.

Boldo leaf oil has been used as a remedy for gonorrhoea and liver diseases.[11]

Side-effects, Toxicity
No reported side-effects to boldo were located. Boldo volatile oil is stated to be one of the most toxic oils.[G35] Application of the undiluted oil to the hairless backs of mice has an irritant effect.[11] The oil contains irritant terpenes including terpinen-4-ol, the irritant principle in juniper oil.

An acute oral LD_{50} value for boldo oil has been detailed as 0.13 g/kg body-weight in rats, with doses of 0.07 g/kg causing convulsions.[11] The acute dermal LD_{50} in rabbits has been reported as 0.625–1.25 g/kg.[11]

Contra-indications, Warnings
Excessive doses of boldo may cause renal irritation, because of the volatile oil, and should be avoided by individuals with an existing kidney disorder. Ascaridole is toxic and use of the oil is not recommended.[G35]

Pregnancy and lactation The safety of boldo taken during pregnancy has not been established. In view of the potential irritant nature of the volatile oil, the use of boldo during pregnancy should be avoided.

Pharmaceutical Comment
The chemistry of boldo is well documented, but limited pharmacological data are available. Human studies have described various properties including choleretic activity, but have only involved boldo given in combination with

other herbs. The reputed diuretic and mild urinary antiseptic properties of boldo are probably attributable to the irritant volatile oil. In view of the toxicity data and the irritant nature of the volatile oil, excessive use of boldo should be avoided.

References

See General References G1, G3, G5, G9, G10, G14, G19, G22, G23, G28, G31, G32 and G35.

1. Urzúa A, Acuña P. Alkaloids from the bark of *Peumus boldus*. *Fitoterapia* 1983; **4:** 175–7.

2. Urzúa A, Torres R. 6a,7-Dehydroboldine from the bark of *Peumus boldus*. *J Nat Prod* 1984; **47:** 525–6.

3. Hughes DW *et al*. Alkaloids of *Peumus boldus*. Isolation of laurotetatine and laurolitsine. *J Pharm Sci* 1968; **57:** 1619–20.

4. Hughes DW *et al*. Alkaloids of *Peumus boldus*. Isolation of (+) reticuline and isoboldine. *J Pharm Sci* 1968; **57:** 1023–5.

5. Bombardelli E *et al*. A new flavonol glycoside from *Peumus boldus*. *Fitoterapia* 1976; **46:** 3–5.

6. Krug H, Borkowski B. Neue Flavonol-Glykoside aus den Blättern von Peumus boldus Molina. *Pharmazie* 1965; **20:** 692–8.

7. Borgia M *et al*. Pharmacological activity of a herbs extract: A controlled clinical study. *Curr Ther Res* 1981; **29:** 525–36.

8. Borgia M *et al*. Studio policentrico doppio-cieco doppio-controllato sull'attività terapeutica di una nota associazione di erbe medicamentose. *Clin Ter* 1985; **114:** 401–409.

9. Salati R *et al*. Valutazione delle proprietà coleretiche di due preparati contenenti estratti di boldo e cascara. *Minerva Dietol Gastroenterol* 1984; **30:** 269–72.

10. Wagner H, Wolff P, editors. New natural products and plant drugs with pharmacological, biological or therapeutical activity. Berlin: Springer-Verlag, 1977.

11. Boldo leaf oil. *Food Chem Toxicol* 1982; **20**(Suppl B): 643.

BONESET

Species (Family)

Eupatorium perfoliatum L. (Asteraceae/Compositae)

Synonym(s)

Feverwort, Thoroughwort. Snakeroot has been used to describe poisonous *Eupatorium* species.

Part(s) Used

Herb

Pharmacopoeial Monographs

BHP 1983

Legal Category

GSL — as Boneset and Eupatorium[G14]

Constituents[G10,G19,G24,G32]

Flavonoids Flavonol (kaempferol, quercetin) glycosides including astragalin, hyperoside, rutin; eupatorin (flavone), dihydroflavonols.[1]

Terpenoids Sesquiterpene lactones including euperfolin and euperfolitin (germacranolides), eufoliatin (guianolide), eufoliatorin (dilactone guaiane), euperfolide.[2] Sesquiterpenes, diterpenes (dendroidinic acid, hebeclinolide), triterpenes (α-amyrin, dotriacontane), sterols (sitosterol, stigmasterol).

Other constituents Volatile oil, resin, wax, tannic and gallic acids, bitter glucoside, inulin, polysaccharides, sugars.

Food Use

Boneset is not used in foods

Herbal Use

Boneset is stated to possess diaphoretic and aperient properties. Traditionally, it has been used for influenza, acute bronchitis, nasopharyngeal catarrh, and specifically for influenza with deep aching, and congestion of the respiratory mucosa.[G3,G32]

Dose

Herb 1–2 g or by infusion three times daily[G3]

Liquid extract (1:1 in 25% alcohol) 1–2 mL three times daily[G3]

Tincture (1:5 in 45% alcohol) 1–4 mL three times daily[G3]

Pharmacological Actions

Animal studies Immunostimulant activity (*in-vitro* stimulation of granulocyte phagocytic activity) has been demonstrated by high dilutions (10^{-5}–10^{-7} g/100 mL) of various sesquiterpene lactones isolated from *E. perfoliatum*.[3] In addition, immunostimulating actions (granulocyte, macrophage, and carbon clearance tests) have been documented for polysaccharide fractions from *E. perfoliatum*.[3,4]

An ethanol extract of the whole plant has exhibited weak anti-inflammatory activity in rats.[G19] Many activities have been documented for flavonoid compounds including anti-inflammatory activity.

Side-effects, Toxicity

Contact dermatitis has been reported for *Eupatorium* species but not specifically for boneset (*E. perfoliatum*).[G26]

Cytotoxic properties have been documented for a related species *E. cannabinum* and are attributed to the sesquiterpene lactone eupatoriopicrin. This compound has not been documented as a constituent of boneset. Hepatotoxic pyrrolizidine alkaloids (PAs) have been isolated from various *Eupatorium* species although none have been documented as constituents of boneset (*E. perfoliatum*).[5]

Instances of allergic and anaphylactic reactions have been associated with the sesquiterpene lactone constituents in German chamomile, although no reactions specifically involving boneset have been documented.

The FDA has classified boneset as a herb of undefined safety.[G10]

Contra-indications, Warnings

The allergenic potential of sesquiterpene lactones is well recognised. Individuals with a known hypersensitivity to other members of the Asteraceae family (e.g. chamomile, feverfew, ragwort, tansy) should avoid using boneset. Individuals with existing hypersensitivities/allergies should use boneset with caution.

Pregnancy and lactation The safety of boneset taken during pregnancy has not been established. In view of the lack of toxicity data and the possibility of constituents with allergenic activity, the use of boneset during pregnancy and lactation should be avoided.

Pharmaceutical Comment

The constituents of boneset are fairly well documented and include many pharmacologically active classes such as flavonoids, sesquiterpene lactones (typical for the Asteraceae family), and triterpenes. Immunostimulant activity (*in vitro*) has been reported for sesquiterpene lactone and polysaccharide components, possibly supporting the traditional use of boneset in influenza. Many pharmacological studies have focussed on the cytotoxic/antitumour actions of sesquiterpene lactone components of various *Eupatorium* species, although these actions have not been reported for sesquiterpene lactones isolated from boneset. Little is known regarding the toxicity of boneset. Hepatotoxic pyrrolizidine alkaloids, which have been documented for other *Eupatorium* species, have not been reported for boneset.

References

See General References G3, G10, G14, G19, G24, G26, G32 and G34.

1. Herz W *et al*. Dihydroflavonols and other flavonoids of *Eupatorium* species. *Phytochemistry* 1972; **11**: 2859–63.

2. Herz W *et al*. Sesquiterpene lactones of *Eupatorium perfoliatum*. *J Org Chem* 1977; **42**: 2264–71.

3. Wagner, H. Immunostimulants from Medicinal Plants. In: Chang HM *et al*. Advances in chinese medicinal materials research. Singapore: World Scientific, 1985: 159–70.

4. Wagner H *et al*. Immunostimulating polysaccharides (heteroglycans) of higher plants. *Arzneimittelforschung* 1985; **35**: 1069.

5. Pyrrolizidine alkaloids. Environmental Health Criteria 80. Geneva: WHO, 1988.

BORAGE

Species (Family)
Borago officinalis L. (Boraginaceae)

Synonym(s)
Beebread, Bee Plant, Burrage, Starflower (oil)

Part(s) Used
Herb

Legal Category
Not included in the GSL.

Constituents[G10,G32]
Alkaloids (pyrrolizidine-type) Lycopsamine, intermedine, acetyllycopsamine, acetylintermedine, amabiline, supinine, thesinine (unsaturated).[1,2] Concentrations reported as 0.01% and 2 to 10 ppm for commercial dried samples. Alkaloid concentrations reportedly the same for fresh and dried samples; fresh samples revealed alkaloids as the free base in the roots and mainly as *N*-oxides in the leaves.
Mucilages (11.1%). Yielding glucose, galactose, and arabinose.
Oil Rich in fatty acids, in particular gamolenic acid.
Other constituents Acids (acetic, lactic, malic, silicic), cyanogenetic compounds, saponins,[6] tannins (up to 3%).

Food Use
Borage is occasionally used in salads and soups.

Herbal Use[G32]
Borage is stated to possess diaphoretic, expectorant, tonic, anti-inflammatory, and galactogogue properties.[3] Traditionally, borage has been used to treat many ailments including fevers, coughs, and depression.[3,G20] Borage is also reputed to act as a restorative agent on the adrenal cortex.[3] Borage oil (starflower oil) is used as an alternative source to evening primrose oil for gamolenic acid.

Dose
Infusion Two 5-mL spoonfuls of dried herb to 1 cup boiling water three times daily[3]
Tincture 1–4 mL three times daily[3]

Pharmacological Actions
Animal studies Borage oil has been reported to attenuate cardiovascular reactivity to stress in rats.[4]
Human studies The effect of borage seed oil on the cardiovascular reactivity of man to acute stress has been studied in 10 individuals, who each received a total daily dose of 1.3 g for 28 days.[4] The individuals were required to undertake an acute psychological task requiring sensory intake and vigilance (Stroop colour test). Borage oil was found to attenuate cardiovascular reactivity to stress indicated by a reduction in systolic blood pressure and heart rate, and by increased task performance. The specific mechanisms by which borage exerts this effect were unknown but a central mechanism of action of the fatty acids was suggested in view of the simultaneous reduction in heart rate and blood pressure.[4]

Side-effects, Toxicity
No side-effects of borage have been located. Borage contains low concentrations of unsaturated pyrrolizidine alkaloids, which are known to be hepatotoxic in both animals and man (*see* Comfrey).[5]

Contra-indications, Warnings
Evening primrose oil is recommended to be used with caution in epileptic patients especially in those with schizophrenia and/or those taking phenothiazines (*see* Evening Primrose); as borage oil is used similarly it should also be used with caution. In view of the known toxic pyrrolizidine alkaloid constituents, excessive or prolonged ingestion of borage should be avoided. In particular, infusions (e.g. herbal teas) containing borage should be avoided.

Pregnancy and lactation In view of the documented pyrrolizidine constituents and lack of toxicity data, borage should not be used during pregnancy or lactation.

Pharmaceutical Comment
Limited information is available on the constituents of borage. No documented pharmacological data were located to support the traditional uses, although the mucilage content supports the use of borage as a demulcent. Interest has focused on the volatile oil as a source of gamolenic acid. Borage contains known toxic pyrrolizidine alkaloids, although at concentrations considerably lower than comfrey for which human toxicity has been documented. However, it would seem wise to avoid excessive or prolonged ingestion of borage. It is unclear whether borage oil, currently available in food supplements, contains any pyrrolizidine alkaloids.

References
See General References G10, G20, and G34.

1. Luthry J *et al*. Pyrrolizidin-Alkaloide in Arzneipflanzen der Boraginaceen: *Borago officinalis* and *Pulmonaria officinalis*. *Pharma Acta Helv* 1984; **59**: 242–6.

2. Larsen *et al*. Unsaturated pyrrolizidines from Borage (*Borage officinalis*) a common garden herb. *J Nat Prod* 1984; **47**: 747–8.

3. Hoffman D. The herb users guide, the basic skills of medical herbalism. Wellingborough: Thorsons, 1987.

4. Mills DE. Dietary fatty acid supplementation alters stress reactivity and performance in man. *J Human Hypertension* 1989; **3**: 111–6.

5. Mattock AR. Chemistry and toxicology of pyrrolizidine alkaloids. London: Academic Press 1986, pp.1–393.

BROOM

Species (Family)

Sarothamnus scoparius (L.) Koch. (Leguminosae/Papilionaceae)

Synonym(s)

Hogweed, Scoparius, *Cytisus scoparius* (L.) Link, *Spartium scoparium* L.

Part(s) Used

Flowerhead

Pharmacopoeial Monographs

BHP 1983
BPC 1949
Martindale 30th edition
National Pharmacopoeias—Fr.

Legal Category (Licensed Products)

Broom is not included on the GSL[G14]

Constituents[G1,G18,G19,G24,G31,G32]

Alkaloids (quinolizidine-type) 0.8–1.5%. Sparteine 0.3–0.8% (major component); minor alkaloids include cytisine (presence disputed), genisteine (*d*-α-isosparteine), lupanine, oxysparteine, and sarothamine.
Amines Epinine, hydroxytyramine, tyramine
Flavonoids Scoparin, vitexin
Other constituents Amino acids, bitter principles, carotenoids, fat, resin, sugars, tannin, wax, volatile oil

Food Use

Broom is listed by the Council of Europe as a natural source of food flavouring (category N3). This category indicates that broom can be added to foodstuffs in the traditionally accepted manner, although there is insufficient information available for an adequate assessment of potential toxicity.[G9]

Herbal Use

Broom is stated to possess cardioactive, diuretic, peripheral vasoconstrictor, and antihaemorrhagic properties. It has been used for cardiac dropsy, myocardial weakness, tachycardia, profuse menstruation, and specifically for functional palpitation with lowered blood pressure.[G1,G3,G32] Broom is also reported to possess emetic and cathartic properties.[G19]

Dose

Dried tops 1–2 g as a decoction[G3]
Liquid extract (1:1 in 25% alcohol) 1–2 mL[G3]
Tincture (1:5 in 45% alcohol) 0.5–2.0 mL[G3]

Pharmacological Actions

The pharmacological actions of broom are primarily due to the alkaloid constituents.

Animal studies Sparteine is reported to exhibit pharmacological actions similar to those of quinidine. Low doses administered to animals result in tachycardia, whereas high doses cause bradycardia and may lead to ventricular arrest. Sparteine has little effect on the CNS, but peripherally, paralyses motor nerve terminals and sympathetic ganglia as a result of a curare-like action.[G21]

The flowers, seeds, root, and whole herb have been used to treat tumours.[G19]

Human studies None documented for broom. However, sparteine is known to decrease the irritability and conductivity of cardiac muscle and has been used to treat cardiac arrhythmias,[G21] restoring normal rhythm in previously arrhythmic patients.[G1] Sparteine is reported to have a quinidine-like action rather than a digitalis-like action.[G1] Sparteine is also stated to be a powerful oxytocic drug, which was once used to stimulate uterine contractions.

Side-effects, Toxicity

The alkaloid constituents in broom are toxic. Sparteine sulphate has been reported to be a cardiac depressant and can also produce respiratory arrest.[G21] Symptoms of poisoning are characterised by tachycardia with circulatory collapse, nausea, diarrhoea, vertigo, and stupor.

Contra-indications, Warnings

Broom is stated to be inappropriate for non-professional use.[G25] Its use is contra-indicated in individuals with high blood pressure[G25] or a cardiac disorder, because of the alkaloid constituents.

Pregnancy and lactation The use of sparteine is contra-indicated during pregnancy.[G20] Sparteine is stated to be a powerful oxytocic drug and is cardiotoxic. Broom should not be taken during lactation.

Pharmaceutical Comment

The chemistry of broom is well documented. The pharmacological actions of broom are primarily due to the alkaloid constituents. Sparteine, the major alkaloid component, is a cardiac depressant with actions similar to those of quinidine. Although these actions support the documented traditional herbal uses, broom is not suitable for self-medication.

References

See General References G1, G3, G6, G9, G14, G18, G19, G20, G21, G23, G24, G25, G31 and G32.

BUCHU

Species (Family)

Agathosma betulina (Berg.) Pillans (Rutaceae)

Synonym(s)

Short Buchu, Round Buchu, *Barosma betulina* Bart. & Wendl.

Note. Oval buchu refers to *Agathosma crenulata* (L.) Pillans (synonym *Barosma serratifolia* (Curt.) Willd.). Long buchu refers to *Agathosma crenulata* (L.) Pillans (synonym *Barosma crenulata* (L.) Hook).[G7]

Part(s) Used

Leaf

Pharmacopoeial Monographs

BHP 1990
BPC 1963
Martindale 30th edition
National pharmacopoeias—Egypt. and Fr.

Legal Category (Licensed Products)

GSL[G14]

Constituents[G1,G10,G19,G24,G32]

Flavonoids Diosmetin, quercetin, diosmin, quercetin-3,7-diglucoside, rutin

Volatile oils (1.0–3.5%). Over 100 identified compounds, including diosphenol, limonene, menthone, and pulegone as the major components.

Other constituents Mucilage, resin. Coumarins have been reported for many other *Agathosma* species.[1]

Food Use

Buchu is listed by the Council of Europe as a natural source of food flavouring (category N3). This category allows buchu to be added to foodstuffs in the traditionally accepted manner, although there is insufficient information available for an adequate assessment of potential toxicity.[G9] In the USA, buchu volatile oil is approved for food use with concentrations usually up to about 0.002% (15.4 ppm).[G9,G19]

Herbal Use

Buchu is stated to possess urinary antiseptic and diuretic properties. It has been used for cystitis urethritis, prostatitis, and specifically for acute catarrhal cystitis.[G1,G3,G4,G32]

Dose

Dried leaf 1–2 g by infusion three times daily[G2,G3]
Liquid extract (1:1 in 90% alcohol) 0.3–1.2 mL[G2,G3]
Tincture (1:5 in 60% alcohol) 2–4 mL[G2,G3]

Pharmacological Actions

Animal studies None documented for buchu. Diosmin has documented anti-inflammatory activity against carrageenan-induced rat paw oedema, at a dose of 600 mg/kg body-weight.[2]

Side-effects, Toxicity

None documented for buchu. The volatile oil contains pulegone, a known hepatotoxin (*see* Pennyroyal)[G34]. The oil may cause gastro-intestinal and renal irritation.

Contra-indications, Warnings

Excessive doses of buchu should not be taken in view of the potential toxicity of the volatile oil. Buchu should be avoided in kidney infections.[G20]

Pregnancy and lactation The safety of buchu has not been established. In view of this, together with the potential toxicity and irritant action of the volatile oil, the use of buchu during pregnancy and lactation should be avoided.

Pharmaceutical Comment

Limited chemical data are available for buchu. No scientific evidence was found to justify the herbal uses, although reputed diuretic and anti-inflammatory activities are probably attributable to the irritant nature of the volatile oil and the flavonoid components, respectively. In view of the lack of documented toxicity data, together with the presence of pulegone in the volatile oil, excessive use of buchu should be avoided.

References

See General References G1, G2, G3, G4, G9, G10, G14, G19, G20, G22, G24, G32 and G35.

1. Campbell WE *et al.* Coumarins of the Rutoideae: tribe Diosmeae. *Phytochemistry* 1986; **25**: 655–7.

2. Farnsworth NR and Cordell GA. A review of some biologically active compounds isolated from plants as reported in the 1974–1975 literature. *Lloydia* 1976, **39**: 420–55.

BURDOCK

Species (Family)

Arctium majus Bernh. (Asteraceae/Compositae)

Synonym(s)

Lappa, *Arctium lappa* L. and other *Arctium* species

Part(s) Used

Root

Pharmacopoeial Monographs

BHP 1983
BHP 1990
BPC 1934
Martindale 30th edition
National pharmacopoeias—Chin. and Fr.

Legal Category (Licensed Products)

GSL[G14]

Constituents[G1,G2,G10,G19,G24,G32]

Acids Acetic acid, butyric acid, caffeic acid, chlorogenic acid, gamma-guanidino-*n*-butyric acid, α-guanidino-*n*-isovaleric acid, *trans*-2-hexenoic acid, isovaleric acid, lauric acid, linoleic acid, linolenic acid, myristic acid, oleic acid, palmitic acid, propionic acid, stearic acid, tiglic acid[1,2,3]

Aldehydes Acetaldehyde, benzaldehyde, butyraldehyde, caproicaldehyde, isovaleraldehyde, propionaldehyde, valeraldehyde.[1]

Carbohydrates Inulin (up to 45–50%), mucilage, pectin, sugars

Polyacetylenes (0.001–0.002% dry weight). Fourteen identified compounds include 1,11-tridecadiene-3,5,7,9-tetrayne (50%), 1,3,11-tridecatriene-5,7,9-triyne (30%), and 1-tridecen-3,5,7,9,11-pentayne as the major components[4]; arctinone-a, arctinone-b, arctinol-a, arctinol-b, arctinal, arctic acid-b, arctic acid-c, methyl arctate-b, arctinone-a acetate (sulphur-containing acetylenic compounds)[5,6]

Other constituents Fats (0.4–0.8%), fixed and volatile oils (0.07–0.18%) oils, sesquiterpene lactones (arctiopicrin),[7] bitters (lappatin), resin, phytosterols (sitosterol and stigmasterol), tannin[8], lignan-type compound[9,10,11]

Other species Flavonol (kaempferol, quercetin) glycosides, *Arctium minus* (Hill) Bernh.[3]

Food Use

Burdock is listed by the Council of Europe as a natural source of food flavouring (category N2). This category indicates that burdock can be added to foodstuffs in small quantities, with a possible limitation of an active principle (as yet unspecified) in the final product.[G9]

Herbal Use

Burdock is stated to possess diuretic and orexigenic properties. It has been used for cutaneous eruptions, rheumatism, cystitis, gout, anorexia nervosa, and specifically for eczema and psoriasis.[G1,G2,G3,G4,G30]

Dose

Dried root 2–6 g or by infusion three times daily[G3]

Liquid extract (1:1 in 25% alcohol) 2–8 mL three times daily[G3]

Tincture (1:10 in 45% alcohol) 8–12 mL three times daily[G3]

Decoction (1:20) 500 mL per day[G3]

Pharmacological Actions

Animal studies The roots and leaves of burdock plants not yet flowering are stated to possess diuretic, hypoglycaemic, and antifurunculous properties.[7] A burdock extract (plant part not stated) was reported to cause a sharp, long-lasting reduction in the blood-sugar concentration in rats, together with an increase in carbohydrate tolerance and a reduction in toxicity.[12] The antimicrobial activity documented for burdock has been attributed to the polyacetylene constituents,[4] although only traces of these compounds are found in the dried commercial herb.[G31] Furthermore, arctiopicrin is stated to be a bitter with antibiotic activity against Gram-positive bacteria.[7,13] Antibacterial activity against Gram-positive (e.g. *Staphylococcus aureus*, *Bacillus subtilis*, *Mycobacterium smegmatis*) and Gram-negative (*Escherichia coli*, *Shigella flexneri*, *Shigella sonnei*) bacteria has been documented for burdock leaf and flower, whereas the root was only found to be active towards Gram-negative strains.[14]

In-vivo uterine stimulant activity has been reported.[G12]

Protection against mutagenic activity has also been documented for burdock.[9,15,16]

Burdock reduced the mutagenicity to *Salmonella typhimurium* (TA98, TA100) of mutagens both requiring and not requiring S9 metabolic activation.[10] A lignan-like structure was proposed for the desmutagenic factor.[9] *In-vivo* studies have shown that fresh or boiled plant juice from burdock may cause a significant reduction in DMBA-induced chromosome aberrations.[16]

Burdock has been reported to exhibit antitumour activity.[17] The addition of dietary fibre (5%) from burdock roots to the diet of rats has been documented to provide protection against the toxicity of various artificial food colours.[18]

Side-effects, Toxicity

A single report of human poisoning with burdock has been documented.[19] The patient exhibited symptoms of atropine-like poisoning following the ingestion of a commercially-packaged burdock root tea. Atropine is not a constituent of burdock, and subsequent analysis indicated that the tea was contaminated with a herbal source of solanaceous alkaloids, possibly belladonna leaf. This report served to highlight the problems which may arise with inadequate quality control of herbal preparations.

The carcinogenicity of burdock was investigated in 12 rats fed dried roots (33% of diet) for 120 days, followed by a normal diet until 480 days.[20] Ten of the 12 rats survived 480 days and no tumours were detected. A urinary bladder papilloma and an oligodendroglioma were observed in one rat but these were considered to have been induced spontaneously.

Burdock has been reported to exhibit antitumour properties (*see* Animal studies).

Contra-indications, Warnings

Excessive doses may interfere with existing hypoglycaemic therapy (*see* Animal studies).

Pregnancy and lactation In-vivo uterine stimulant action has been reported.[G12] In view of this, and the lack of toxicity data, the use of burdock during pregnancy and lactation should be avoided.

Pharmaceutical Comment

The chemistry of burdock and related *Arctium* species has been well studied. Various pharmacological activities have been reported in animals although none support the reputed herbal uses. Documented bitter constituents, however, may explain the traditional use of burdock as an orexigenic. In view of the lack of toxicity data, excessive use of burdock should be avoided.

References

See General References G1, G2, G3, G4, G5, G9, G10, G12, G14, G19, G22, G23, G24, G30, G31, G32 and G34.

1. Obata S *et al.* Studies on the components of the roots of *Arctium lappa* L. *Agric Biol Chem* 1970; **34**: A31.

2. Yamada Y *et al.* γ-Guanidino-*n*-butyric acid from *Arctium lappa*. *Phytochemistry* 1975; **14**: 582.

3. Saleh NAM, Bohm BA. Flavonoids of *Arctium minus* (Compositae). *Experientia* 1971; **27**: 1494.

4. Schulte KE *et al.* Polyacetylenes in burdock root. *ArzneimittelForsch* 1967; **17**: 829–33.

5. Washino T *et al.* New sulfur-containing acetylenic compounds from *Arctium lappa*. *Agric Biol Chem* 1986; **50**: 263–9.

6. Washino T *et al.* Structures of lappaphen-a and Lappahen-b, new guaianolides linked with a sulfur-containing acetylenic compound, from *Arctium lappa* L. *Agric Biol Chem* 1987; **51**: 1475–80.

7. Bever BO, Zahnd GR. Plants with oral hypoglycaemic action. *Quart J Crude Drug Res* 1979; **17**: 139–96.

8. Nakabayashi T. Tannin of fruits and vegetables. III. Polyphenolic compounds and phenol-oxidising enzymes of edible burdock. *Nippon Shokuhin Kogyo Gakkaishi* 1968; **15**: 199–206.

9. Morita K *et al.* Chemical nature of a desmutagenic factor from burdock (*A. lappa* L.). *Agric Biol Chem* 1985; **49**: 925–32.

10. Ichihara A *et al.* Lappaol A and B, novel lignans from *Arctium lappa* L. *Tetrahedron Lett* 1976; **44**: 3961–4.

11. Ichihara A *et al.* New sesquilignans from *Arctium lappa* L. The structure of lappaol C, D and E. *Agric Biol Chem* 1977; **41**: 1813–14.

12. Lapinina LO, Sisoeva TF. Investigation of some plants to determine their sugar lowering action. *Farmatsevt Zh* 1964; **19**: 52–8.

13. Cappelletti EM *et al.* External antirheumatic and antineuralgic herbal remedies in the traditional medicine of North-eastern Italy. *J Ethnopharmacol* 1982; **6**: 161–90.

14. Moskalenko SA. Preliminary screening of far-eastern ethnomedicinal plants for antibacterial activity. *J Ethnopharmacol* 1986; **15**: 231–59.

15. Morita K *et al.* Desmutagenic factor isolated from burdock (*Arctium lappa* L.) *Mutat Res* 1984; **129**: 25–31.

16. Ito Y *et al.* Suppression of 7,12-dimethylbenz(a)anthracene-induced chromosome aberrations in rat bone marrow cells by vegetable juices. *Mutat Res* 1986; **172**: 55–60.

17. Dombradi CA, Foldeak S. Anti-tumor activity of *A. lappa* ext. *Tumori* 1966; **52**: 173–5.

18. Tsujita J *et al.* Comparison of protective activity of dietary fiber against the toxicities of various food colors in rats. *Nutr Rep Int* 1979; **20**: 635–42.

19. Bryson PD *et al.* Burdock root tea poisoning. Case report involving a commercial preparation. *JAMA* 1978; **239**: 2157–8.

20. Hirono I *et al.* Safety examination of some edible plants, Part 2. *J Environ Path Toxicol* 1977; **1**: 72–4.

BURNET

Species (Family)
Sanguisorba officinalis L. (Rosaceae)

Synonym(s)
Garden Burnet, Greater Burnet, Sanguisorba

Part(s) Used
Herb

Pharmacopoeial Monographs
BHP 1983

Legal Category (Licensed Products)
GSL (Sanguisorba)[G14]

Constituents[G18,G32]
All phytochemical data located refer to the underground plant parts and not to the herb.
Flavonoids Flavones, unstable flavonol derivatives
Saponins Ziyu glycosides I and II (major glycosides),[2] pomolic acid as aglycone (not tomentosolic acid as documented in earlier work), sanguisorbin 2.5–4.0%
Tannins Numerous compounds (condensed and hydrolysable) have been isolated including 3,3,4-tri-*O*-methylellagic acid.[1,3–6]
Other constituents Volatile oil, ascorbic acid (vitamin C) in the fresh plant

Food Use
Burnet is not used in foods.

Herbal Use
Burnet is stated to possess astringent, antihaemorrhagic, styptic, and antihaemorrhoidal properties. It has been used for ulcerative colitis, metrorrhagia, and specifically for acute diarrhoea.[G3,G32]

Dose
Dried herb 2–6 g or by infusion three times daily[G3]
Liquid extract (1:1 in 25% alcohol) 2–6 mL three times daily[G3]
Tincture (1:5 in 45% alcohol) 2–8 mL three times daily[G3]

Pharmacological Actions
Animal studies None documented for burnet. The roots have been reported to contain an antihaemorrhagic principle 3,3,4-tri-*O*-methylellagic acid.[3]

Side-effects, Toxicity
None documented.

Contra-indications, Warnings
None documented.

Pregnancy and lactation In view of the lack of phytochemical, pharmacological, and toxicity data, the use of burnet during pregnancy and lactation should be avoided.

Pharmaceutical Comment
The chemistry of burnet herb does not appear to have been studied, although data are available for the underground plant parts. If present in the herb as well as the root, the tannin constituents would support the reputed astringent and antihaemorrhagic actions of burnet. In view of the lack of toxicity data and the possible high tannin content of the herb, excessive use of burnet should be avoided.

References
See General References G3, G14, G18, G21 and G32.

1. Kosuge T *et al.* Studies on antihemorrhagic substances in herbs classified as hemostatics in Chinese medicine. III. On the antihemorrhagic principle in *Sanguisorba officinallis* L. *Chem Pharm Bull* 1984; **32:** 4478–81.

2. Yosioka I *et al.* Soil bacterial hydrolysis leading to genuine aglycone. III. The structures of glycosides and genuine aglycone of Sanguisorbae radix. *Chem Pharm Bull* 1971; **19:** 1700–1707.

3. Nonaka G-I *et al.* Tannins and related compounds. XVII. Galloylhamameloses from *Castanea crenata* L. and *Sanguisorba officinalis* L. *Chem Pharm Bull* 1984; **32:** 483–9.

4. Nonaka G-I *et al.* A dimeric hydrolyzable tannin, sanguiin H-6 from *Sanguisorba officinalis* L. *Chem Pharm Bull* 1982; **30:** 2255–7.

5. Tanaka T *et al.* Tannins and related compounds. XVI. Isolation and characterization of six methyl glucoside gallates and a gallic acid glucoside gallate from *Sanguisorba officinalis* L. *Chem Pharm Bull* 1984; **32:** 117–21.

6. Tanaka T *et al.* 7-*O*-galloyl-(+)-catechin and 3-*O*-galloylprocyanidin B-3 from *Sanguisorba officinalis*. *Phytochemistry* 1983; **22:** 2575–8.

CALAMUS

Species (Family)

Acorus calamus L. (Araceae)

Various genetic species (n=12): diploid North American, triploid European, tetraploid Asian, Eastern, Indian.

Synonym(s)

Sweet Flag

Part(s) Used

Rhizome

Pharmacopoeial Monographs

BHP 1983
BPC 1934
Martindale 30th edition

Legal Category (Licensed Products)

GSL[G14]

Constituents[G10,G19,G33,G35]

Amines Dimethylamine, methylamine, trimethylamine, choline.

Volatile oil (1.5–3.5%) β-asarone content varies between genetic species: 96% in tetraploid (Indian), 5% in triploid (European) and 0% in the diploid (N. American) species.[1,2,3,4] Other identified components include calamenol (5%), calamene (4%), calamone (1%), methyl eugenol (1%), eugenol (0.3%) and the sesquiterpenes acolamone, acoragermacrone and isoacolamone. Considerable qualitative and quantitative differences have been reported between the volatile oil from different genetic species, and between the volatile fraction of an alcoholic extract and the essential oil from the same variety (European).[3,4]

Tannin 1.5%

Other constituents Bitter principles (eg. acorin), acoric and palmitic acids, resin (2.5%), mucilage, starch (25–40%), sugars.

Food Use

The level of β-asarone permitted in foods is restricted to 0.1 mg/kg in foods and beverages, 1 mg/kg in alcoholic beverages and in foods containing *A. calamus* or *Asarum europaeum*.[G9] Calamus is listed by the Council of Europe as a source of natural food flavouring (category N3). This category indicates that calamus can be added to foodstuffs in the traditionally accepted manner, although there is insufficient information available for an adequate assessment of potential toxicity.[G9] Calamus is classified as an 'unsafe herb' by the FDA[G10], and the use of the rhizome and its derivatives (oil, extracts) are prohibited from use in human food.[G19]

Herbal Use

Calamus is stated to act as a carminative, spasmolytic, and diaphoretic. Traditionally it has been indicated for acute and chronic dyspepsia, gastritis and gastric ulcer, intestinal colic, and anorexia.[G3]

Dose

Rhizome 1–3 g or by infusion three times daily[G3].
Liquid Extract 1–3 mL (1:1 in 60% alcohol) three times daily[G3]
Tincture 2–4 mL (1:5 in 60% alcohol) three times daily[G3]

Pharmacological Actions

Animal studies Numerous documented studies have concentrated on activities associated with the oil. The pharmacology and toxicology of calamus oil have been reviewed.[5] Unless specified, all of the following actions refer to those exhibited by the oil.

Spasmolytic action *in vitro* versus various spasmogens in different smooth muscle preparations including tracheal, intestinal, uterine, bronchial and vascular has been reported for European and Indian varieties.[5,6,7,8] In one study activity was associated with a lack of β-asarone[6], whereas oils with either low or high levels of β-asarone have also exhibited activity.[5,7] The pattern of spasmolytic activity has been compared to that of papaverine and a direct musculotropic action has been proposed.[8] Unlike papaverine an acetylcholine-like action has also been observed with low dilutions of the oil and asarone.[8]

Inhibition of monoamine oxidase activity and a stimulation of D- and L-amino oxidase has been reported.[5] The mechanism for this activity, involving serotonin and adrenaline, has been disputed with an alternative mechanism involving depression of hypothalamic function proposed.[9]

In vitro oil rich in β-asarone has been reported to reduce phenylbutazone-induced ulcers in the rat by 5–60%, although no effect was observed on stress- or ethanol-induced ulcers.[7] No spasmolytic activity was reported for oil free from or with low levels of β-asarone.[7]

A sedative action and a potentiation of barbiturate effect (increased sleeping time, reduction in body temperature) have been described in a number of small animals (mice, rats, rabbits and cats) following intravenous or intraperitoneal administration of European (alcoholic and aqueous extracts) and Indian varieties.[5] Dexamphetamine has been found to block the potentiating action of the Indian variety on barbiturate sleeping time.[5] Potentiation of morphine activity has been reported for the European variety.

The Indian oil has been reported to deplete levels of serotonin and noradrenaline in the rat brain following intraperitoneal administration.[5] The mechanism of action was suggested as similar to that of reserpine, and a potentiation of the amphetamine-detoxifying effect of reserpine has also been described.[5] In contrast, the central action of the European variety has been stated to not resemble that of reserpine.[5] Anti-adrenergic activity demonstrated by antagonism of dexamphetamine-induced agitational symptoms has been reported for the Indian variety in various small animals.[5]

Anticonvulsant, anti-arrhythmic (like quinidine), and hypotensive (apparently not due to a nervous mechanism) activities in small animals have also been reported for the Indian variety.[5]

α-Asarone, isolated from *Asarun europaeum* (Aristolochiaceae), has a local anaesthetic activity similar to that of benzocaine.[10]

Antifungal activity has been documented for β-asarone[11] and for the oil (weak).[5] Insecticidal and leech repellant properties have been reported for the oil and may be synergised by synthetic pine oil.[5] Antibacterial activity primarily versus organisms responsible for gut and throat infections has been documented[12], although a lack of antibacterial activity has also been reported.[5]

Side-Effects, Toxicity[G33,G35]

Concerns over the toxicity of calamus centre around the volatile oil and in particular on the β-asarone content. The level of β-asarone in the oil varies considerably between the different genetic species of calamus (see Constituents).

Feeding studies (rat) using the Indian oil (high β-asarone) have shown death, growth depression, hepatic and heart abnormalities, and serous effusion in abdominal and/or peritoneal cavities.[13,14] A two-year study involving diet supplemented with calamus oil at 0, 500, 1000, 2500 and 5000 ppm, reported growth depression, and malignant duodenal tumours after 59 weeks at all levels of dietary supplementation.[13,14] Tumours of the same type were not noted in the controls.

Genotoxic activity (strong induction of chromosomal aberrations, slight increase in the rate of sister chromatid exchanges) has been exhibited by β-asarone in human lymphocyte cultures in the presence of microsomal activation.[15] Mutagenic activity (Ames) has been documented for root extracts, a tincture and β-asarone in one (TA100) of the various *Salmonella typhimurium* strains (TA98, 100, 1535, 1537, 1538) tested, but only in the presence of a microsomal activation mix.[16] Lack of mutagenicity has also been reported for an organic extract, when tested in the above *Salmonella typhimurium* strains (except TA1538) with and without activation.[17]

Acute toxicities (LD_{50}) quoted for the volatile oil from the Indian variety (high β-asarone content) include 777 mg/kg (rat, oral), >5 g/kg (guinea pig, dermal), 221 mg/kg (rat, intraperitoneal).[5] The oleoresin is stated to be toxic at 400 and 800 mg/kg (mouse, intraperitoneal).[5] The LD_{50} of asarone in mice is stated to be 417 mg/kg (oral) and 310 mg/kg (intraperitoneal).[9]

Generally the oil is considered to be non-irritant, non-sensitising and non-phototoxic.[5,G35] However, bath preparations containing the oil have reportedly caused erythema, and dermatitis has been reported in hypersensitive individuals.[5]

Contra-indications, Warnings

The toxicity of calamus oil has been associated with the β-asarone content.[16] It has therefore been advised that only roots free from, or with a low content of β-asarone should be used in human phytotherapy.[16] In foods and beverages, the level of β-asarone permitted in the final product is restricted (see Food Use above).

Use of the isolated oil is not recommended.[G25,G35] External contact with the oil may cause an irritant reaction in sensitive individuals.

Calamus may potentiate MAOI therapy (*in-vitro* MAOI activity, amine constituents) although any clinical significance of the *in-vitro* action has not been established.

Pregnancy and lactation In view of the toxic properties associated with calamus, it should not be used during pregnancy or lactation. It is not known whether β-asarone is excreted into the breast milk. In general, the topical application of any undiluted oil is not recommended. Application of preparations containing calamus oil may provoke an irritant reaction and is therefore best avoided.

Pharmaceutical Comment

The phytochemistry of calamus, especially the oil, has been extensively investigated. Three genotypes (diploid, triploid, tetraploid) have been identified which are chemically distinctive with respect to the β-asarone content. Spasmolytic and anti-ulcer effects documented for the oil support the traditional herbal uses of calamus. In addition, bitter principles documented as constituents may account for the use of the root in anorexia. However, in view of the toxic properties documented for the oil and associated with β-asarone, it has been recommended that only β-asarone-free calamus root should be used in phytotherapy. Use of the oil is not recommended due its carcinogenic activity and its ability to cause kidney damage, tremors and convulsions.[G35] Studies carried out to investigate the mutagenic potential of calamus have produced conflicting results.

References

See General References G3, G5, G9, G10, G14, G19, G33 and G35.

1.   Stahl E and Keller K. Zur Klassifizierung handelsüblicher Kalmusdrogen. *Planta Med* 1981; **43**: 128–40.

2.   Keller K and Stahl E. Zusammensetzung des ätherischen Öles von β-asaronfreiem Kalmus. *Planta Med* 1983; **47**: 71–4.

3.   Mazza G. Gas chromatographic and mass spectrometric studies of the constituents of the rhizome of calamus. I. The volatile constituents of the essential oil. *J Chromatogr* 1985; **328**: 179–94.

4.   Mazza G. Gas chromatographic and mass spectrometric studies of the constituents of the rhizome of calamus. II. The volatile constituents of alcoholic extracts. *J Chromatogr* 1985; **328**: 195–206.

5.   Opdyke DJL. Calamus Oil. *Food Cosmet Toxicol* 1977; **15**: 623–6.

6.   Keller K *et al.* Spasmolytische wirkung des isoasaronfreien kalmus. *Planta Med* 1985; 6–9.

7.   Keller K *et al.* Pharmacological activity of calamus oil with different amount of cis-isoasaron. *Naunyn Schmiedeberg's Arch Pharmacol* 1983; **324:** suppl R55.

8.   Das PK *et al.* Spasmolytic activity of asarone and essential oil of Acorus calamus, Linn. *Arch int Pharmacodyn* 1962; **135:** 167–77.

9.   Calamus. *Lawrence Review of Natural Products* 1989.

10.   Gracza L. The active substances of Asarum europaeum. 16. The local anaesthetic activity of the phenylpropanoids. *Planta Med* 1983; **48:** 153–7.

11.   Ohmoto T and Sung Y-I. Antimycotic substances in the crude drugs II. *Shoyakugaku Zasshi* 1982; **36:** 307–14

12.   Jain SR *et al.* Antibacterial evaluation of some indigenous volatile oils. *Planta Med* 1974; **26:** 196-9.

13.   Taylor JM *et al.* Toxicity of oil of calamus (Jammu Variety). *Tox & Appl Pharmacol* 1967; **10:** 405.

14.   Gross MA et al. Carcinogenicity of oil of calamus. *Proc Amer Ass Cancer Res* 1967; **8:** 24.

15.   Abel G. Chromosome damaging effect on human lymphocytes by β-asarone. *Planta Med* 1987; 251–3.

16.   Göggelmann W and Schimmer O. Mutagenicity testing of β-asarone and commercial calamus drugs with *Salmonella typhimurium. Mutat Res* 1983; **121:** 191–4.

17.   Riazuddin S *et al.* Mutagenicity testing of some medicinal herbs. *Environmental and Molecular Mutagensis* 1987; 10: 141–8.

CALENDULA

Species (Family)
Calendula officinalis L. (Compositae)

Synonym(s)
Gold-bloom, Marigold, Marybud, Pot Marigold

Part(s) Used
Flower

Pharmacopoeial Monographs
BHP 1983
BPC 1934

Legal Category (Licensed Products)
GSL (external use only)[G14]

Constituents[G1,G24,G27,G31,G32]
Flavonoids Flavonol (isorhamnetin, quercetin) glycosides including isoquercitrin, narcissin, neohesperidoside, and rutin.[1]
Terpenoids Many components include α- and β-amyrin, lupeol, longispinogenin, oleanolic acid, arnidiol, brein, calenduladiol, erythrodiol, faradiol, helantriols A1, B0, B1, and B2, lupeol, maniladiol, urs-12-en-3,16,21-triol, ursadiol; oleanolic acid saponins including calendulosides C-H;[2] campesterol, cholesterol, sitosterol, stigmasterol, and taraxasterol (sterols).
Volatile oils Terpenoid components include menthone, isomenthone, caryophyllene, and an epoxide and ketone derivative, pedunculatine, α- and β-ionone, a β-ionone epoxide derivative, dihydroactinidiolide.[3]
Other constituents Bitter (loliolide),[4] arvoside A (sesquiterpene glycoside),[5] carotenoid pigments,[6] calendulin (gum),[6] polysaccharide.

Food Use
Calendula is not used in foods.

Herbal Use
Calendula is stated to possess antispasmodic, mild diaphoretic, anti-inflammatory, anti-haemorrhagic, emmenagogue, vulnerary, styptic, and antiseptic properties. Traditionally, it has been used to treat gastric and duodenal ulcers, amenorrhoea, dysmenorrhoea, and epistaxis; crural ulcers, varicose veins, haemorrhoids, anal eczema, proctitis, lymphadenoma, inflamed cutaneous lesions (topically), and conjunctivitis (as an eye lotion).[G1,G3,G32]

Dose
Dried florets 1–4 g or by infusion three times daily.[G3]
Liquid extract 0.5–1.0 mL (1:1 in 40% alcohol) three times daily.[G3]

Calendula Tincture (BPC 1934) 0.3–1.2 mL (1:5 in 90% alcohol) three times daily.[G3]

Pharmacological Actions
Animal studies Anti-inflammatory, antibacterial, and antiviral activities have been reported for calendula.[7] Weak anti-inflammatory activity in rats (carrageenan-induced oedema) has been reported.[8,9]
A combination of allantoin and calendula extract applied to surgically-induced skin wounds in rats has been reported to stimulate physiological regeneration and epithelisation.[10] This effect was attributed to a more intensive metabolism of glycoproteins, nucleoproteins, and collagen proteins during the regenerative period in the tissues.[10] Allantoin applied on its own was found to exert a much weaker action.[10]
A proprietary cream containing a combination of plant extracts, including calendula, has been reported to be effective in dextran and burn oedemas and in acute lymphoedema in rats. Activity against lymphoedema was primarily attributed to an enhancement of macrophage proteolytic activity.[11] Slight increases in foot oedema were attributed to a vasodilatory action.
The trichomonacidal activity of calendula has been associated with the essential oil terpenoid fraction.[3]
An *in-vitro* uterotonic effect has been described for calendula extract on rabbit and guinea-pig preparations.[12]
Immunostimulant activity, assayed using granulocyte and carbon clearance tests, of calendula extracts has been attributed to polysaccharide fractions of high molecular weight.[13]
The triterpenoid constituents of calendula are reported to be effective as spermicides and as antiblastocyst and abortion agents.[G27]
In-vitro cytotoxic activity and *in-vivo* antitumour activity (against mouse Ehrlich carcinoma) have been documented for calendula extracts.[7] The most active fraction *in vivo* (saponin-rich) was not the most active *in vitro*.[7]
Human studies A proprietary cream preparation containing various plant extracts, including calendula, has been reported to reduce pain associated with post-mastectomy lymphoedema, although there was no significant clinical difference in the reduction of oedema between controls and experimental groups.[11] Calendula tincture 20% has been reported to be useful in the treatment of chronic suppurative otitis.[14] Calendula extracts are used to accelerate healing and to reduce inflammation.[6]

Side-effects, Toxicity
No reported side-effects or documented toxicity studies were located for calendula. *In-vitro* cytotoxic activity has been reported.[7]

Contra-indications, Warnings
None known.

Pregnancy and lactation Calendula is traditionally reputed to affect the menstrual cycle. An uterotonic effect (*in vitro*) has been reported, and the triterpenoid constituents are reported to be effective as spermatocides and as antiblastocyst and abortion agents. In view of the lack of toxicity data, the use of calendula is best avoided during pregnancy and lactation.

Pharmaceutical Comment

Phytochemical studies have reported three main groups of constituents for calendula, namely flavonoids, volatile oil and triterpenes. The latter seems to represent the principal group, with many compounds isolated including pentacyclic alcohols, glycosides (saponins), and sterols. Animal studies have reported wound healing and anti-inflammatory effects, supporting the traditional uses of calendula in various dermatological conditions. Flavonoid constituents may contribute to the anti-inflammatory effect, whilst the reputed antispasmodic effect may be attributable to the volatile oil fraction. In addition, immunostimulant activity has been reported for high molecular weight polysaccharide components.

References

See General References G1, G3, G5, G14, G24, G27, G31 and G32.

1.   Vidal-Ollivier E *et al*. Flavonol glycosides from *Calendula officinalis* flowers. *Planta Med* 1989; **55**: 73.

2   Pizza C *et al*. Plant metabolites. Triterpenoid saponins from *Calendula arvensis*. *J Nat Prod* 1987; **50:** 927–31.

3.   Gracza L. Oxygen-containing terpene derivatives from *Calendula officinalis*. *Planta Med* 1987; **53:** 227.

4.   Willuhn G, Westhaus R-G. Loliolide (Calendin) from *Calendula officinalis*. *Planta Med* 1987; **53:** 304.

5.   Pizza C, de Tommasi N. Plants metabolites. A new sesquiterpene glycoside from *Calendula arvensis*. *J Nat Prod* 1987; **50:** 784–9.

6.   Fleischner AM. Plant extracts: To accelerate healing and reduce inflammation. *Cosmet Toilet* 1985; **100:** 45.

7.   Boucard-Maitre Y *et al*. Cytotoxic and antitumoral activity of *Calendula officinalis* extracts. *Pharmazie* 1988; **43:** 220.

8.   Peyroux J *et al*. Propriétés anti-oedémateuses et anti-hyperhémiantes du *Calendula officinalis* L. *Plant Méd Phytothér* 1981; **15:** 210–16.

9.   Mascolo N *et al*. Biological screening of Italian medicinal plants for anti-inflammatory activity. *Phytotherapy Res* 1987; **1:** 28–31.

10.   Kioucek-Popova E *et al*. Influence of the physiological regeneration and epithelization using fractions isolated from *Calendula officinalis*. *Acta Physiol Pharmacol Bulg* 1982; **8:**:63–7

11.   Casley-Smith JR, Casley-Smith JR. The effect of "Unguentum lymphaticum" on acute experimental lymphedema and other high-protein edemas. *Lymphology* 1983; **16:** 150–6.

12.   Shipochliev T. Extracts from a group of medicinal plants enhancing the uterine tonus. *Vet Med Nauki* 1981; **4:** 94–8.

13.   Wagner H *et al*. Immunostimulating polysaccharides (heteroglycans) of higher plants. *Arzneimittelforsch* 1985; **35:** 1069.

14.   Shaparenko BA. On use of medicinal plants for treatment of patients with chronic suppurative otitis. *Zh Ushn Gorl Bolezn* 1979; **39:** 48–51.

CAPSICUM

Species (Family)
Capsicum species (Solanaceae) including *C. annum* L., *C. baccatum* L., *C. chinense* Jacq., *C. frutescens* L., *C. pubescens* Ruiz. et Pavon, *C. minimum* Roxb.

Synonym(s)
Cayenne, Chilli Pepper, Hot Pepper, Paprika, Red Pepper, Tabasco Pepper

Part(s) Use
Fruit

Pharmacopoeial Monographs
BHP 1983
BPC 1973
Martindale 30th edition
Pharmacopoeias—Aust., Egypt, Ger., Hung., It., Jpn, and Swiss. Belg. includes capsicum oleoresin.

Legal Category (Licensed Products)
GSL[G14]

Constituents[G10,G19,G32]
Capsaicinoids (up to 1.5%, usually 0.11%). Major components capsaicin (48.6%), 6,7-dihydrocapsaicin (36%), nordihydrocapsaicin (7.4%), homodihydrocapsaicin (2%), and homocapsaicin (2%)
Volatile oils (trace). Over 125 components have been isolated with at least 24 characterised.
Other constituents Carotenoid pigments (capsanthin, capsorubin, carotene, lutein), proteins (12–15%), fats (9–17%), vitamins including A and C
Other plant parts The plant material contains solanidine, solanine and solasodine (steroidal alkaloidal glycosides), and scopoletin (coumarin).

Food Use
Capsicum (chilli) peppers are widely used as a spice. Capsicum is listed by the Council of Europe as a natural source of food flavouring (category N2). This category indicates that capsicum can be added to foodstuffs in small quantities, with a possible limitation of an active principle (as yet unspecified) in the final product.[G9] In the USA, capsicum is stated to be GRAS (Generally Regarded As Safe).[G19]

Herbal Use
Capsicum is stated to possess stimulant, antispasmodic, carminative, diaphoretic, counterirritant, antiseptic, and rubefacient properties. Traditionally, it has been used for colic, flatulent dyspepsia without inflammation, chronic laryngitis (as a gargle), insufficiency of peripheral circulation and externally for neuralgia including rheumatic pains and unbroken chilblains (as a lotion/ointment).[G3,G32]

Dose
Fruit 30–120 mg three times daily[G3]
Capsicum Tincture (BPC 1968) 0.3–1.0 mL
Stronger Tincture of Capsicum (BPC 1934) 0.06–2.0 mL
Oleoresin 0.6–2.0 mg[G21]
Oleoresin, internal, 1.2 mg (MD), 1.8 mg (MDD)[G14]
Oleoresin, external, 2.5% maximum strength[G14]

Pharmacological Actions
The action of capsaicin on nervous, cardiovascular, respiratory, thermoregulatory, and gastro-intestinal systems has been reviewed.[1] Capsaicin has been used as a neurochemical tool for studying sensory neurotransmission.[1]
Animal studies Infusion of capsaicin (200 µg/kg, by intravenous injection) has been reported to evoke dose-dependent catecholamine secretion (adrenaline, noradrenaline) from the adrenal medulla of pentobarbitone-anaesthetised rats.[2]
The addition of capsaicin (0.014%) to a high-fat (30%) diet fed to rats was found to reduce serum-triglyceride concentrations but to have no effect on serum cholesterol or pre-β-lipoprotein concentrations.[3] Capsaicin was thought to stimulate lipid mobilisation from adipose tissue. Lipid absorption was unaffected by capsaicin supplementation.[3]
Activities of two hepatic enzymes, glucose-6-phosphate dehydrogenase and adipose lipoprotein lipase, were elevated in rats when capsaicin was added to the diet.[3] Capsicum extracts fed orally to hamsters have been reported to significantly decrease hepatic vitamin A concentrations.[4] Serum vitamin A concentrations were not affected.[4]
Both the gastric and duodenal mucosae are thought to contain 'capsaicin-sensitive' areas which afford protection against acid- and drug-induced ulcers when stimulated by hydrochloric acid or by capsaicin itself. Stimulation causes an increase in mucosal blood flow and/or vascular permeability, inhibits gastric motility, and activates duodenal motility.[5] Desensitisation of these areas, using a regimen involving subcutaneous or oral administration of capsaicin, is thought to remove the protection.[5] However, capsaicin desensitisation was found to have little effect on peripheral responses to stress (i.e. ulcer formation) but did enhance central responses (increase in plasma-corticosterone concentration) in rats.[6] The increase in plasma-corticosterone concentration observed in capsaicin-desensitised rats was similar in stressed and non-stressed animals.[6]
Capsaicin was found to influence adrenal cortical activity independently of the presence of a stress factor and may represent a stressor in itself.[6] Capsaicin desensitisation was not found to influence basal gastric acid secretion in non-stressed rats but did lower pentagastrin-stimulated gastric output.[6] However, other results have reported that capsaicin-desensitisation does increase acid secretion.[6]
Capsicum (leaf and stem) has been reported to exhibit uterine stimulant activity in animal studies.[G12]

Pharmacokinetic studies in rats have reported that capsaicin is readily transported via the gastro-intestinal tract and absorbed through non-active transport into the portal vein.[2] Capsaicin is partly hydrolysed during absorption and the majority is excreted in the urine within 48 hours.[2,7] Dihydrocapsaicin-hydrolysing enzyme is present in various organs of the rat but principally in the gastro-intestinal tract and the liver. The biotransformation pathway of dihydrocapsaicin in the rat has been studied.[7] Metabolites are mainly excreted as glucuronide conjugates in the urine.[7]

Human studies Capsicum is applied externally as a counter-irritant in many preparations used for rheumatism, arthritis, neuralgia, and lumbago.

Ingestion of red chillies (10 g in wheatmeal) by controls and duodenal ulcer sufferers has been reported to have no significant effect on acid or pepsin secretion, or on sodium, potassium, and chloride concentrations in the gastric aspirate.[8] There was reported to be no apparent change (qualitative or quantitative) in mucous and no gastric mucosal erosion was evident.[8] However, in contrast, capsicum has been shown to increase acid concentration and DNA content (indicating exfoliation of epithelial cells) of gastric aspirates in both control subjects and patients with duodenal ulcers.[1]

Side-effects, Toxicity

Capsicum contains pungent principles (capsaicinoids) that are strongly irritant to mucosal membranes. Inhalation of paprika can produce a form of allergic alveolitis.[G26] Chronic administration of capsicum extract (0.5 µg capsaicin/kg body-weight) to hamsters has been reported to be toxic.[4] Treated animals did not survive beyond 17 months whereas all untreated controls survived beyond this period. In addition, eye abnormalities were observed in the treated animals. This effect was attributed to the depletion of substance P in primary afferent neurones by capsaicin, causing a loss of corneal pain sensation and subsequently the loss of protective corneal reflexes.[4]

It is thought that metabolism of capsaicin and related analogues may reduce their acute toxicity.[7] LD_{50} values (mg/kg) stated for capsaicin in mice include 0.56 (intravenous), 7.56 (intraperitoneal), 9.00 (subcutaneous), and 190 (oral). In rats, an intraperitoneal LD_{50} of 10 mg/kg has been reported for capsaicin.[7] The toxicity of capsaicinoids has reportedly not been ascribed to any one specific action but may be due to their causing respiratory failure, bradycardia, and hypotension.[7]

Contra-indications, Warnings

Capsicum may cause gastro-intestinal irritation, although it has been stated that capsicum does not influence the healing of duodenal ulcers and does not need to be avoided by patients with this condition.[1] Excessive ingestion may cause gastro-enteritis, hepatic or renal damage.[G20] Capsicum may interfere with MAOIs and antihypertensive therapy (increased catecholamine secretion), and may increase the hepatic metabolism of drugs (glucose-6-phosphate dehydrogenase and adipose lipoprotein lipase activity elevated).

Pregnancy and lactation There are no known problems with the use of capsicum during pregnancy, although it may cause gastro-intestinal irritation and should therefore be used with caution. Doses should not greatly exceed amounts normally ingested in foods. It is not known whether the pungent components in capsicum are secreted into the breast milk.

Pharmaceutical Comment

Capsicum is commonly used in both foods and in medicinal products. The capsaicinoids are principally responsible for the biological activity of capsicum. These pungent principles are thought to stimulate and aid digestion and to act as a counter-irritant when applied externally. Capsaicin has also been used as a neurochemical tool for studying sensory neurotransmission.

Conflicting reports have been documented concerning the effect of capsicum on acid secretion and on ulcer healing. Capsaicin-sensitive areas of the gastric and duodenal mucosa are thought to provide protection against mucosal damage. It has been suggested that this protection is lost if these sensory fibres are desensitised. Whether oral consumption of capsicum by humans can cause desensitisation is unclear. The toxicity of capsicum extracts observed in animals is considered to be due to the capsaicinoid components. However, ingestion of capsicum in the diet is not thought to represent a health risk. Capsicum should not be ingested in doses greatly exceeding amounts normally used in foods.

References

See General References G3, G7, G9, G10, G12, G13, G14, G19, G21, G22, G23, G24, G26 and G32.

1. Locock RA. Capsicum. *Can Pharm J* 1985; **118:** 517–19.

2. Watanabe T *et al*. Capsaicin, a pungent principle of hot red pepper, evokes catecholamine secretion from the adrenal medulla of anesthetized rats. *Biochem Biophys Res Comm* 1987; **142:** 259–64.

3. Kawada T *et al*. Effects of capsaicin on lipid mtetabolism in rats fed a high fat diet. *J Nutr* 1986; **116:** 1272–8.

4. Agrawal RC *et al*. Chilli extract treatment and induction of eye lesions in hamsters. *Toxicol Lett* 1985; **28:** 1–7.

5. Maggi CA *et al*. Capsaicin-sensitive mechanisms and experimentally induced duodenal ulcers in rats. *J Pharm Pharmacol* 1987; **39:** 559–61.

6. Dugani A, Glavin GB. Capsaicin effects on stress pathology and gastric acid secretion in rats. *Life Sci* 1986; **39:** 1531–8.

7. Kawada T, Iwai K. *In vivo* and *in vitro* metabolism of dihydrocapsaicin, a pungent principle of hot pepper in rats. *Agric Biol Chem* 1985; **49:** 441–8.

8. Pimparkar BND *et al*. Effects of commonly used spices on human gastric secretion. *J Assoc Physicians India* 1972: **20:** 901–10.

CASCARA

Species (Family)

(*Rhamnus purshiana* DC (*Frangula purshiana* (DC) A Gray ex JC Cooper) (Rhamnaceae)

Synonym(s)

Cascara Sagrada, Rhamni Purshianae Cortex, Rhamnus

Part(s) Used

Bark

Pharmacopoeial Monographs

BHP 1990
BPC 1973
Martindale 30th edition
Pharmacopoeias—Aust., Belg., Br., Braz., Egypt., Eur., Fr., Ger., Gr., It., Neth., Nord., Port., Swiss, Turk., and U.S. Br. and Turk. also describe Powdered Cascara.

Legal Category (Licensed Products)

GSL[G14]

Constituents[G1,G2,G19,G24,G29,G31,G32]

Anthraquinones Cascarosides A and B (aloin *O*- and *C*-glycosides) and cascarosides C and D (deoxyaloin *O*- and *C*-glycosides) as major components; others include barbaloin and chrysaloin (*C*-glycosides), *O*-glycosides of emodin (e.g. frangulin), emosin oxanthrone, aloe-emodin, and chrysophanol, dianthrones including those of emodin, aloe-emodin, and chrysophanol, and palmidin A, B and C (see Rhubarb), and free aglycones including aloe-emodin, chrysophanol, and emodin.
Other constituents Linoleic acid, myristic acid, syringic acid, lipids, resin, tannin

Food Use

Cascara is listed by the Council of Europe as a natural source of food flavouring (category N4). This category indicates that while the use of cascara for flavouring purposes is recognised, it cannot be classified into the categories N1, N2, or N3 because of insufficient information.[G9]

Herbal Use

Cascara is stated to possess mild purgative properties and has been used for constipation.[G1,G2,G4,G32]

Dose

Cascara Liquid Extract (BP 1980) 2–5 mL

Pharmacological Actions

The laxative action of anthraquinone glycosides is well recognised (*see* Senna). Cascara has a laxative action.[G22]

Side-effects, Toxicity

The side-effects and toxicity documented for anthraquinone glycosides are applicable. [G10] *See* Senna

Contra-indications, Warnings

The contra-indications and warnings documented for anthraquinone glycosides are applicable. *See* Senna.

Pregnancy and lactation See Senna.

Pharmaceutical Comment

The chemistry of cascara is characterised by the anthraquinone derivatives, especially the cascarosides. The laxative action of these compounds is well recognised. Cascara has been used extensively in conventional pharmaceutical preparations. Stimulant laxatives have largely been superseded by bulk-forming laxatives. However, the use of non-standardised anthraquinone-containing preparations should be avoided since their pharmacological effects will be variable and unpredictable. In particular, the use of products containing combinations of anthraquinone laxatives is not advisable.

References

See General References G1, G2, G4, G7, G9, G10, G11, G14, G19, G22, G23, G24, G29, G31, G32 and G34.

CASSIA

Species (Family)

Cinnamomum cassia Blume (Lauraceae)

Synonym(s)

Cinnamomum aromaticum Nees, Cassia Bark, Cassia Lignea, Chinese Cinnamon, False Cinnamon

Part(s) Used

Bark

Pharmacopoeial Monographs

BPC 1949

BHP 1983

Martindale 28th edition

Martindale 30th edition (Cassia oil)

Pharmacopoeias—Chin., Egypt., Hung., Jpn, and Mex. describe Cassia Oil. Chin., Hung., Jpn, and Rom. include Cassia Bark, which may be known as cinnamon bark.

Legal Category (Licensed Products)

GSL (oil)[G14]

Constituents[G19,G29,G31,G32,G35]

Volatile oils (1-2%). Mainly composed of cinnamaldehyde (75-90%). Other major components include salicylaldehyde, methylsalicylaldehyde, and methyleugenol. Eugenol is reported to be absent. Cassia oil contains no monoterpenoids or sesquiterpenoids.[1]

Other constituents Calcium oxalate, coumarin, mucilage (higher content compared to cinnamon), resins, sugars, tannins (condensed). Complex diterpenoids have been isolated from Cinnamomi Cortex, for which *C. cassia* is used as a source.[1]

Food Use

Cassia bark and oil are extensively used as food flavourings. A temporary estimated acceptable daily intake of cinnamaldehyde is 700 µg/kg body-weight. In the USA, cassia is listed as GRAS (Generally Regarded As Safe).[G19]

Herbal Use

Cassia is stated to possess carminative, antispasmodic, antiemetic, antidiarrhoeal and antimicrobial properties. It has been used for flatulent dyspepsia, flatulent colic, diarrhoea, the common cold, and specifically for colic or dyspepsia with flatulent distension and nausea.[G3] Cassia bark is also documented to possess astringent properties.[G19,G32] Carminative and antiseptic properties are documented for the oil.[G19]

Dose

Dried bark 0.5-1 g or by infusion three times daily[G3]

Oil of Cassia (BPC 1949) 0.05-0.2 mL three times daily[G3]

Pharmacological Actions

Animal studies Anti-ulcerogenic properties have been described for two propionic derivatives isolated from cassia.[2] An *in-vivo* study using rats reported activity against a variety of ulcerogens including serotonin, phenylbutazone, ethanol, water immersion, and stress. The compounds were thought to act by improving gastric blood flow rather than by inhibiting gastric secretion.

Many pharmacological investigations have been carried out on Cinnamomi Cortex for which sources include *C. cassia* (cassia) and *Cinnamomum zeylanicum* (cinnamon). These studies have either looked at the volatile oil, in particular the major constituent cinnamaldehyde, or at parts excluding the oil.[1]

Activities documented for cinnamaldehyde include CNS stimulation (low dose), sedation (high dose), hypothermic and antipyretic actions;[1,G19] antibacterial and antifungal activity, acceleration of catecholamine (mainly adrenaline) release from the adrenal glands, weak papaverine-like action, increase in peripheral blood flow, hypotension, bradycardia, and hyperglycaemia have also been reported.[1] However, these actions are of low potency and, in addition, much of the cinnamaldehyde content of cassia is thought to be lost by evaporation and auto-oxidation during decoction of the crude drug. The contribution of cinnamaldehyde to the overall therapeutic efficacy of cassia has therefore been doubted.[1]

Actions observed for essential oil-free aqueous extracts have been reported to be weak, and the only appreciable effects are prolongation of barbiturate-induced sedation and a slight reduction of acetic acid-induced writhing.[1]

In-vivo inhibitory activity against complement formation has been documented and attributed to the diterpenoid and condensed tannin constituents.[1] Anti-inflammatory activity exhibited by the Japanese plant *Cinnamomum sieboldii* Meisn (also used as a source for Cassia bark), has been attributed to a series of condensed tannin constituents.[1] Antiplatelet aggregation and antithrombotic actions have also been reported. These actions, together with the documented anti-inflammatory activity, are thought to contribute to the suppression of thrombus formation in certain diseases.[1]

Antitumour activity has been described and the activity depends on the plant source used.[1]

Side-effects, Toxicity

Allergic reactions, mainly contact sensitivity, to cassia oil and bark have been reported.[G26,G35] Cinnamaldehyde in toothpastes and perfumes has also been reported to cause contact sensitivity.[G26] Cassia oil is stated to cause dermal and mucous membrane irritation.[3] The irritant and sensitising properties of cassia oil have been attributed to cinnamaldehyde.[3] The dermal LD_{50} value for cassia oil is stated as 320 mg/kg body-weight.[G35]

Contra-indications, Warnings

Contact with cassia bark or oil may cause an allergic reaction. Cassia oil is stated to be one of the most hazardous oils and should not be used on the skin in concentrations of more than 0.2%.[G35]

Pregnancy and lactation. There are no known problems with the use of cassia during pregnancy, provided that amounts taken do not exceed those generally used in foods.

Pharmaceutical Comment

Cassia is similar in composition to cinnamon and both are widely used as flavouring agents in foods, and in pharmaceutical and cosmetic preparations. Cassia oil is stated to be inferior in flavour to cinnamon oil. The reputed herbal uses of cassia have been attributed to the oil. Cassia contains an irritant and sensitising principle in the oil, cinnamaldehyde, and should not be used in amounts generally exceeding those used in foods. It has been recommended that the oil should never be applied topically.

References

See General References G3, G6, G14, G19, G21, G22, G23, G26, G29, G31, G32, G33, G34 and G35.

1.   Hikino H.   Oriental medicinal plants.   In Economic and Medicinal Plants. (Wagner H, Hikino H, Farnsworth NR, editors). London: Academic Press Vol.1, pp. 69–70, 1985.

2.   Tanaka S *et al.* Antiulcerogenic compounds isolated from Chinese Cinnamon. *Planta Med* 1989; **55:** 245–8.

CELERY

Species (Family)
Apium graveolens L. (Apiaceae/Umbelliferae)

Synonym(s)
Apii Fructus, Celery Fruit, Celery Seed, Smallage

Part(s) Used
Fruit

Pharmacopoeial Monographs
BHP 1983
BHP 1990
BPC 1949
Martindale 28th edition

Legal Category (Licensed Products)
GSL[G14]

Constituents[G1,G2,G10,G16,G19,G24,G28,G32,G35]
Flavonoids Apigenin, apiin, isoquercitrin, and others[1]
Furanocoumarins Apigravin, apiumetin, apiumoside, bergapten, celerin, celereoside, isoimperatorin, isopimpinellin, osthenol, rutaretin, seselin, umbelliferone, 8-hydroxy-5-methoxypsoralen.[1-8,17]
Low concentrations (not exceeding 1.3 ppm) of furanocoumarins have been identified in commercial celery,[9] although concentrations are reported to rise considerably in diseased stems.[10]
Volatile oils (2–3%) Many components including limonene (60%) and selenine (10–15%), and various sesquiterpene alcohols (1–3%), e.g. α-eudesmol and β-eudesmol, santalol.[11,12] Phthalide compounds, 3-*n*-butyl phthalide and sedanenolide, provide the characteristic odour of the oil (presence of sedanolide and sedanonic anhydride disputed).[13,14]
Other constituents Choline, ascorbate,[15] fatty acids (e.g linoleic, myristic, myristicic, myristoleic, oleic, palmitic, palmitoleic, petroselinic, and stearic acids)

Food Use
Celery is listed by the Council of Europe as a natural source of food flavouring (category N2). This category indicates that celery can be added to foodstuffs in small quantities, with a possible limitation of an active principle (as yet unspecified) in the final product.[G9] Celery stem (not the fruit) is commonly used in foods.

Herbal Use
Celery is stated to possess antirheumatic, sedative, mild diuretic and urinary antiseptic properties. It has been used for arthritis, rheumatism, gout, urinary tract inflammation, and specifically for rheumatoid arthritis with mental depression.[G1,G2,G3,G4,G32]

Dose
Dried fruits 0.5–2.0 g or by decoction 1:5 three times daily[G3]
Liquid Extract 0.3–1.2 mL (1:1 in 60% alcohol) three times daily[G3]
Liquid Extract of Celery (BPC 1934) 0.3–1.2 mL

Pharmacological Actions
Animal studies In mice, sedative and antispasmodic activities have been documented for the phthalide constituents.[16,G10] Celery seed oil has been reported to exhibit bacteriostatic activity against *Bacillus subtilis*, *Vibrio cholerae*, *Staphylococcus aureus*, *Staphylococcus albus*, *Shigella dysenteriae*, *Corynebacterium diphtheriae*, *Salmonella typhi*, *Streptococcus faecalis*, *Bacillus pumilus*, *Streptococcus pyogenes*, and *Pseudomonas solanacearum*.[17] No activity was observed against *Escherichia coli*, *Sarcina lutea* or *Pseudomonas aeruginosa*.

Apigenin has exhibited potent antiplatelet activity *in vitro*, inhibiting the aggregation of rabbit platelets induced by collagen, ADP, arachidonic acid, and platelet-activating factor (PAF), but not that induced by thrombin or ionophore A23187.[18]

Studies with celery plant extracts have demonstrated antiinflammatory activity in the mouse ear test and against carrageenan-induced rat paw oedema,[19] and a hypotensive effect in rabbits and dogs after intravenous administration.[G19] In addition, hypoglycaemic activity has been documented.[G10]

Celery juice has been reported to exhibit choleretic activity and the phthalide constituents are stated to possess diuretic activity.[12]

Human studies None documented for celery fruit. Hypotensive activity was reported in 14 of the 16 hypertensive patients given a celery plant extract.[G19]

Side-effects, Toxicity
None documented for celery fruit. Photosensitivity reactions have been reported as a result of external contact with celery stems.[20,21,G26] These reactions have been attributed to the furanocoumarin constituents which are known to possess photosensitising properties.[10,22] The concentrations of these compounds are reported to increase considerably in diseased celery stems.[10,22] It is thought that psoralen, the most potent phototoxic furanocoumarin, acts as a transient precursor for other furanocoumarins and does not accumulate in celery.[5,10]

Instances of allergic and anaphylactic reactions to celery have also been documented[23] following oral ingestion of the stems.[24] Celery allergy is reported to be mediated by IgE antibodies and an association between pollen and celery allergy has been postulated, although the common antigen had not been determined.[25]

Cross-sensitivities to celery have been documented in patients with existing allergies to dandelion and wild carrot.[G26]

Acute LD$_{50}$ values (rats, by mouth; rabbits, dermal) have been reported as greater than 5 g/kg body-weight.[26] Celery seed oil is stated to be non-irritant, non-phototoxic, and non-sensitising in humans.[26,G35]

Contra-indications, Warnings

Celery fruit contains phototoxic compounds, furanocoumarins, which may cause photosensitive reactions. Celery fruit may precipitate allergic reactions, particularly in individuals with existing plant, pollen, or food allergies. Diseased celery stems (indicated by a browning of the stem) should not be ingested.

Pregnancy and lactation Celery fruit is reputed to affect the menstrual cycle and to be abortifacient.[G12] Uterine stimulant activity has been documented for the oil,[G10,G12] and the use of celery fruits is contra-indicated during pregnancy.[G25] This does not refer to celery stems that are commonly ingested as a food, although excessive consumption should be avoided.

Pharmaceutical Comment

Celery fruit should not be confused with the commercial celery stem, which is commonly eaten as a food. The chemistry of celery fruit is well studied and the phototoxic furanocoumarin constituents are well documented. Phototoxicity appears to be associated with the handling of the celery stems, especially diseased plant material. Limited scientific evidence is available to justify the herbal uses of celery, although bacteriostatic activity has been documented for the oil. Celery fruit should be used cautiously in view of the documented allergic reactions.

References

See General References G1, G2, G3, G4, G6, G9, G10, G12, G14, G16, G19, G21, G24, G25, G26, G28, G32 and G35.

1.   Garg SK *et al*. Glucosides of Apium graveolens. *Planta Med*; 1980; **38:** 363–5.

2.   Garg SK *et al*. Apiumetin—a new furanocoumarin from the seeds of *Apium graveolens*. *Phytochemistry* 1978; **17:** 2135–6.

3.   Garg SK *et al*. Celerin, a new coumarin from Apium graveolens. *Planta Med* 1980; **38:** 186–8.

4.   Garg SK *et al*. Minor phenolics of *Apium graveolens* seeds. *Phytochemistry* 1979; **18:** 352.

5.   Dall'Acqua *et al*. Biosynthesis of O-alkylfurocoumarins. *Planta Med* 1975; **27:** 343–8.

6.   Garg SK *et al*. Apiumoside, a new furanocoumarin glucoside from the seeds of *Apium graveolens*. *Phytochemistry* 1979; **18:** 1764–5.

7.   Garg SK *et al*. Coumarins from *Apium graveolens* seeds. *Phytochemistry* 1979; **18:** 1580–81.

8.   Innocenti G *et al*. Investigations of the content of furocoumarins in *Apium graveolens* and in *Petroselinum sativum*. *Planta Med* 1976; **29:** 165–70.

9.   Beier RC *et al*. Hplc analysis of linear furocoumarins (psoralens) in healthy celery (*Apium graveolens*). *Food Chem Toxicol* 1983; **21:** 163–5.

10.   Chaudhary SK *et al*. Increased furocoumarin content of celery during storage. *J Agric Food Chem* 1985; **33:** 1153–7.

11.   Fehr D. Untersuchung über aromastoffe von sellerie (Apium graveolens L.). *Pharmazie* 1979; **34:** 658–662.

12.   Stahl E. Drug analysis by chromatography and microscopy. Ann Arbor, Michigan: Ann Arbor Science, 1973.

13.   Bjeldanes LF and Kim I-S. Phthalide components of celery essential oil. *J Org Chem* 1977; **42:** 2333–5.

14.   Bos R *et al*. Composition of the volatile oils from the roots, leaves and fruits of different taxa of Apium graveolens. *Planta Med* 1986; **52:** 531.

15.   Kavalali G and Akcasu A. Isolation of choline ascorbate from *Apium graveolens*. *J Nat Prod* 1985; **48:** 495.

16.   Gijbels MJM *et al*. Phthalides in roots of *Apium graveolens*, *A. graveolens* var. *rapaceum*, *Bifora testiculata* and *Petroselinum crispum* var. *tuberosum*. *Fitoterapia* 1985; **56:** 17–23.

17.   Kar A and Jain SR. Investigations on the antibacterial activity of some Indian indigenous aromatic plants. *Flavour Industry* Feb 1971.

18.   Teng CM *et al*. Inhibition of platelet aggregation by apigenin from Apium graveolens. Asia Pacific J Pharmacol 1988; **1:** 85–9.

19.   Lewis DA *et al*. The anti-inflammatory activity of celery *Apium graveolens* L. (Fam. Umbelliferae). *Int J Crude Drug Res* 1985; **23:** 27–32.

20.   Berkley SF *et al*. Dermatitis in grocery workers associated with high natural concentrations of furanocoumarins in celery. *Ann Intern Med* 1986; **105;** 351–5.

21.   Austad J and Kavli G. Phototoxic dermatitis caused by celery infected by *Sclerotinia sclerotiorum*. *Contact Dermatitis* 1983; **9:** 448–51.

22.   Ashwood-Smith MJ *et al*. Mechanisms of photosensitivity reactions to diseased celery. *Br Med J* 1985; **290:** 1249.

23.   Déchamp C *et al*. Choc anaphylactique au céleri et sensibilisation à l'ambroisie et à l'armoise. Allergie croisée ou allergie concomitante? *Presse Med* 1984; **13:** 871–4.

24.   Forsbeck M and Ros A-M. Anaphylactoid reaction to celery. *Contact Dermatitis* 1979; **5:** 191.

25.   Pauli G *et al*. Celery sensitivity: clinical and immunological correlations with pollen energy. *Clin Allergy* 1985; **15:** 273–9.

26.   Opdyke DLJ. Celery Seed Oil. *Food Cosmet Toxicol* 1974; **12:** 849–50.

CENTAURY

Species (Family)
Centaurium erythraea Rafin. (Gentianaceae)

Synonyms
Minor Centaury, *Erythraea centaurium* Pers., *C. umbellatum* Gilib, *C. minus* Moench[G22]

Part(s) Used
Herb

Pharmacopoeial Monographs
BHP 1983
Martindale 30th edition
Pharmacopoeias—Aust., Cz., Fr., Ger., Hung., Pol., Rom., Span., Swiss, and Yug.

Legal Category (Licensed Products)
GSL[G14]

Constituents[G1,G19,G32]
Acids (phenolic). Protocatechuic, *m*- and *p*-hydroxybenzoic, vanillic, syringic, β-coumaric, ferulic, sinapic, and caffeic acids among others.
Alkaloids (pyridine-type). Traces of gentianine, gentianidine, gentioflavine and others.
Monoterpenoids Iridoids (bitters)[1,2]. Gentiopicroside (about 2%) as major, others include centapicrin, gentioflavoside, sweroside, and swertiamarin.
Triterpenoids Includes α- and β-amyrin, erythrodiol, crataegolic acid, oleanolic acid, sitosterol.
Other constituents Flavonoids, xanthones, fatty acids, alkanes, waxes.

Food Use
Centaury is listed by the Council of Europe as a natural source of food flavouring (category N2). This category indicates that centaury can be added to foodstuffs in small quantities, with a possible limitation of an active principle (as yet unspecified) in the final product.[G9] In the USA, the bitter properties of centaury are utilised in alcoholic and non-alcoholic beverages with maximum permitted doses between 0.0002% and 0.0008%.[G19]

Herbal Use
Centaury is reputed to act as a bitter, aromatic and stomachic. Traditionally, it has been used for anorexia and dyspepsia.[G3]

Dose
Herb 2–4 g or by infusion three times daily[G3]
Liquid extract (1:1 in 25% alcohol) 2–4 mL three times daily[G3]

Pharmacological Actions
Centaury is stated to have bitter tonic, sedative, and antipyretic properties.[G19] The antipyretic activity is stated to be due to the phenolic acids.[G22] Gentiopicrin is stated to have antimalarial properties.[G24]
Animal studies Anti-inflammatory activity has been documented in two rat models; subchronic inflammation (air pouch granuloma and polyarthritis) test,[3] and the carrageenan rat paw oedema test (19% compared to 45% with indomethacin).[4] Antipyretic activity has also been exhibited by a centaury extract against experimentally induced hyperthermia in rats, although pretreatment with the extract did not prevent hyperthermia.[3] In the same study, no analgesic activity could be demonstrated in mice (writhing syndrome and hot plate models).[3]

Side-effects, Toxicity
No reported side-effects or documented toxicity data were located for centaury (*C. erythraea*).

Contra-indications, Warnings
None known.
Pregnancy and lactation The safety of centaury taken during pregnancy has not been established. In view of the lack of toxicity data, use of centaury during pregnancy and lactation is best avoided.

Pharmaceutical Comment
There is little published information specifically concerning *C. erythraea*. Bitter components support the traditional use of centaury as an appetite stimulant, although it is said to be less active than comparable bitter herbs such as Gentian.[G1] In view of the lack of pharmacological and toxicological data, excessive use should be avoided.

References
See General References G1, G3, G9, G14, G22, G23, G24 and G32.

1. Van der Sluis WG and Labadie RP. Onderzok naar en van secoiridoid glucosiden en zanthonen in het gescglacht *Centautium*. *Pharm Weekbl* 1978; **113**: 21–32.

2. Van der Sluis WG and Labadie RP. Secoiridoids and xanthones in the genus *Centaurium*. Part 3. Decentapicrins A, B and C, new *m*-hydroxybenzoyl esters of sweroside from *Centaurium littorale*. *Planta Med* 1981; **41**: 150–60.

3. Berkan T *et al.* Antiinflammatory, analgesic, and antipyretic effects of an aqueous extract of *Erythraea centaurium*. *Planta Med* 1991; **57**: 34–7.

4. Mascolo N *et al.* Biological screening of Italian medicinal plants for anti-inflammatory activity. *Phytotherapy Res* 1987; **1**: 28–31.

CEREUS

Species (Family)

Selenicereus grandiflorus (L.) Britt. and Rose (Cactaceae)

Synonym(s)

Night Blooming Cereus, *Cactus grandiflorus*, *Cereus grandiflorus* Mill.

Part(s) Used

Stem

Pharmacopoeial Monographs

BPC 1934

Legal Category (Licensed Products)

Cereus is not included on the GSL.[G14]

Constituents[G10,G18,G32]

Alkaloids (Isoquinoline-type). Unidentified alkaloids[1]

Amines Tyramine[2], hordenine,[3] previously referred to as cactine

Flavonoids Rutin, kaempferitrin, hyperoside, isorhamnetin-3-β-(galactosyl)-rutinoside

Other constituents Resin

Food Use

Cereus is not used in foods.

Herbal Use

Cereus is reputed to act as a cardiac stimulant and as a partial substitute for digitalis, although there is no proof of its therapeutic value. Cereus has been used in cases of dropsy and various cardiac affections.[G5,G32]

Dose

Liquid Extract of Cereus (BPC 1934) 0.06–0.6 mL
Tincture of Cereus (BPC 1934) 0.12–2.0 mL

Pharmacological Actions

Animal studies None documented for cereus. Cereus is reported to contain a cardiotonic amine, tyramine, which has positive inotropic activity.

Side-effects, Toxicity

The fresh juice of cereus is irritant to the oral mucosa, causing a burning sensation, nausea, and vomiting. Diarrhoea has also been reported following cereus consumption.[G10]

Contra-indications, Warnings

In view of the documented tyramine content, excessive doses of cereus may interact with concurrent monoamine oxidase inhibitor (MAOI) treatment and may affect patients with an existing cardiac disorder.

Pregnancy and lactation The safety of cereus has not been established. In view of the limited information available on cereus, its use during pregnancy and lactation should be avoided.

Pharmaceutical Comment

Little phytochemical or pharmacological information has been documented for cereus, although the presence of tyramine, a cardiotonic amine, may support the traditional use of cereus as a cardiac stimulant. Cardiac complaints are not considered for self-medication.

References

See General References G5, G10, G14, G18, G24 and G32

1. Brown SD *et al*. Cactus alkaloids. *Phytochemistry* 1968; **7**: 2031–36.

2. Wagner H and Grevel J. Neue herzwirksame drogen II, nachweis und isolierung herzwirksamer amine durch ionenpaar-HPLC. *Planta Med* 1982; **44**: 36–40.

3. Petershofer-Halbmayer H *et al*. Isolierung von Hordenin (Cactin) aus *Selenicereus grandiflorus* (L.) Britt. & Rose und *Selenicereus pteranthus* (Link & Otto) Britt. & Rose. *Sci Pharm* 1982; **50**: 29–34.

CHAMOMILE, GERMAN

Species (Family)
Matricaria recutita L. (Asteraceae/Compositae)

Synonym(s)
Hungarian Chamomile, Sweet False Chamomile, Wild Chamomile, *Chamomilla recutita* (L.) Rauschert, *Matricaria chamomilla* L.

Part(s) Used
Flowerhead

Pharmacopoeial Monographs
BHP 1983
BHP 1990
BPC 1949
Martindale 30th edition
Pharmacopoeias—Aust., Br., Cz., Egypt., Eur., Fr., Ger., Gr., Hung., It., Neth., Rom., Rus., Swiss, and Yug. include chamomile from *Matricaria recutita*. Aust. and Hung. also include Matricaria Oil.

Legal Category (Licensed Products)
GSL[G14]

Constituents[G1,G2,G10,G16,G19,G24,G32]
Coumarins Umbelliferone and its methyl ether, heniarin
Flavonoids Apigenin, apigetrin, apiin, luteolin, quercetin, quercimeritrin, rutin
Volatile oils (0.24–1.9%) Main components as (–)-α-bisabolol (up to 50%)[1] and chamazulene (1–15%).[2] Others include (–)-α-bisabolol oxide A and B, (–)-α-bisabolone oxide A, spiroethers (e.g. *cis*- and *trans*-en-yn-dicycloether), sesquiterpenes (e.g. anthecotulid), cadinene, farnesene, furfural, spanthulenol, and proazulenes (e.g. matricarin and matricin).
Chamazulene is formed from a natural precursor during steam distillation of the oil. It varies in yield depending on the origin and age of the flowers.[2]
Other constituents Amino acids, anthemic acid (bitter), choline, polysaccharide, plant and fatty acids, tannin, triterpene hydrocarbons (e.g. triacontane)

Food Use
German chamomile is listed by the Council of Europe as a natural source of food flavouring (category N2). This category indicates that chamomile can be added to foodstuffs in small quantities, with a possible limitation of an active principle (as yet unspecified) in the final product.[G9] German chamomile is commonly used in herbal teas.

Herbal Use
German chamomile is stated to possess carminative, antispasmodic, mild sedative, anti-inflammatory, antiseptic, and anticatarrhal properties. It has been used for flatulent nervous dyspepsia, travel sickness, nasal catarrh, nervous diarrhoea, restlessness, and specifically for gastro-intestinal disturbance with associated nervous irritability in children. It has been used topically for haemorrhoids, mastitis, and leg ulcers[G1,G2,G3,G4,G32]

Dose
Dried flowerheads 2–8 g or by infusion three times daily[G3]
Liquid extract (1:1 in 45% alcohol) 1–4 mL three times daily[G3]

Pharmacological Actions
Animal studies A wide range of pharmacological activities have been documented for German chamomile[24] including antibacterial, anti-inflammatory, antispasmodic, anti-ulcer, antiviral, and hypouraemic activities.

Anti-allergic and anti-inflammatory activities[2,3] are well documented for German chamomile. The azulene components of the volatile oil are thought to contribute by inhibiting histamine release and they have been reported to prevent allergic seizures in guinea-pigs.[2] Matricin, the precursor to chamazulene, is reported to be a more effective anti-inflammatory agent than chamazulene.[2,4] Anti-inflammatory activity has also been documented for the sesquiterpene bisabolol compounds, with greatest activity reported for (–)-α-bisabolol,[2,5] and for *cis*-spiroether.[2] Anti-inflammatory activity (rat paw carrageenan test) has also been documented for a *cis*-spiroether against dextran induced oedema; no activity was observed against oedema induced by serotonin, histamine, or bradykinin.[6] In addition, flavonoids are known to possess anti-inflammatory activity.

Anti-ulcerogenic activity in rats has been reported for (–)-α-bisabolol; the development of ulcers induced by indomethacin, stress, or ethanol was inhibited.[2,7]

Antibacterial activity has been documented for the coumarin constituents.[2] High molecular-weight polysaccharides with immunostimulating activity have been isolated from German chamomile.[8]

The oil has been reported to increase bile secretion and concentration of cholesterol in the bile, following the administration of 0.1 mL/kg by mouth to cats and dogs.[9] A dose of 0.2 mL/kg was stated to exhibit hypotensive, and cardiac and respiratory depressant properties.[9]

Antispasmodic activity on the isolated guinea-pig ileum has been documented for the flavonoid and bisabolol constituents.[2,10] Greatest activity was exhibited by the flavonoids, especially apigenin which was found to be more than three times as potent as papaverine.[2] (–)-α-Bisabolol activity was found to be comparable to that of papaverine, while the total volatile oil was considerably less active.[2] Smooth muscle relaxant properties have also been documented for a *cis*-spiroether.[2,6,11]

Enhancement of uterine tone in the guinea-pig and rabbit has been reported for an aqueous extract at a concentration of 1–2 mg extract/cm³.[12]

An ethanolic extract of the entire plant has been reported to inhibit the growth of poliovirus and herpesvirus.[13]

The ability of the volatile oil to regenerate liver tissue in partially hepatectomised rats has been attributed to the azulene constituents.[2]

The volatile oil has been documented to reduce the serum concentration of urea in rabbits with experimentally induced uraemic conditions.[14]

Human studies German chamomile extracts have been reported to exhibit anti-inflammatory, antipeptic, and antispasmodic activities on the human stomach and duodenum.[2]

A sedative effect has been documented for German chamomile. Oral administration of an extract induced a deep sleep in 10 of 12 patients undergoing cardiac catheterisation.[2]

German chamomile has been reported to be an effective treatment for mucosal infections. Diluted extracts administered as a mouthwash 5 or 6 times daily provided cooling and astringent effects.[2]

A cream containing German chamomile has produced additional anti-inflammatory, slight anaesthetic, cooling, and deodorant effects in patients with cutaneous leg infections, when used in conjunction with existing treatment.[2]

Side-effects, Toxicity

Reports of allergic reactions to chamomile are common, although in the majority of cases the plant species is not specified.[15] Two reports of anaphylactic reactions to chamomile (species unspecified) have been documented[16,17] and in both cases the individuals concerned had an existing hypersensitivity to ragweed (member of Asteraceae/Compositae). The symptoms they experienced included abdominal cramps, thickness of the tongue and a tight sensation in the throat,[17] angioedema of the lips and eyes, diffuse pruritus, a full sensation of the ears, generalised urticaria, upper airway obstruction, and pharyngeal oedema.[16] Both patients made a full recovery following medical treatment. Patients with an existing hypersensitivity to German chamomile have demonstrated cross-sensitivities to other members of the family Asteraceae/Compositae[18,G26], and also to celery (family Umbelliferae).[G26]

Allergic skin reactions have been documented following external contact with German chamomile.[2,19,G26] Consumption of chamomile tea may exacerbate existing allergic conditions and the use of a chamomile enema has been documented to cause asthma and urticaria.[G26]

The allergenic properties documented for chamomile have been attributed to anthecotulid, a sesquiterpene lactone present in low concentrations,[15] and to matricarin, a proazulene which has produced positive patch tests in patients with an existing sesquiterpene lactone hypersensitivity.[G26]

Sesquiterpene lactones have been implicated in the allergenic activity of many plants, especially those belonging to the Asteraceae/Compositae family (*see* Feverfew). The prerequisite for allergenic activity is thought to be an exocyclic α-methylene group.[20]

The flowerheads contain anthemic acid, which is reported to act as an emetic in large doses.[G10]

The acute toxicity of chamomile oil (German and Roman) is reported to be low.[21] Oral and dermal LD_{50} values in rabbits have been documented as greater than 5 g/kg,[21] and the application of undiluted oil to the hairless backs of mice, to rabbit skin, and to human skin was not found to produce any observable irritation.[21] An LD_{50} value (mouse, by mouth) for German chamomile oil has been documented as 2.5 mL /kg.[9] The acute oral toxicity of (−)-α-bisabolol in mice and rats is reported to be low at approximately 15 mL/ kg.[22] The subacute oral toxicity of (−)-α-bisabolol has been estimated to be between 1.0 and 2.0 mL/kg in rats and dogs.[22] An LD_{50} value (mouse, intraperitoneal injection) for *cis*-spiroether has been stated as 670 mg/kg.[6]

Contra-indications, Warnings

In view of the documented allergic reactions and cross-sensitivities, German chamomile should be avoided by individuals with a known hypersensitivity to any members of the Asteraceae/Compositae family. In addition, German chamomile may precipitate an allergic reaction or exacerbate existing symptoms in susceptible individuals (e.g. asthmatics). Excessive doses may interfere with existing anticoagulant therapy, because of the coumarin constituents.

The use of chamomile preparations for teething babies is not recommended.

Pregnancy and lactation German chamomile is reputed to affect the menstrual cycle[G12] and extracts are reported to be uterotonic.[2,12] Teratogenicity studies in rats, rabbits, and dogs have been documented for (−)-α-bisabolol, with the oral toxic dose stated as 1–3 mL/kg.[22] A dose of 3 mL/kg was found to increase the number of foetuses reabsorbed and reduce the body-weight of live offspring.[22] (−)-α-Bisabolol administered orally (250 and 500 mg/kg) to pregnant rats has been reported to have no effect on the foetus.[1] In view of the documented information, the excessive use of chamomile during pregnancy and lactation should be avoided.

Pharmaceutical Comment

The chemistry of German chamomile, especially of the volatile oil component, is well documented and is similar to that of Roman chamomile.[24] Pharmacological activity is associated with the flavonoid and volatile oil fractions. A wide range of pharmacological actions have been documented (e.g. anti-inflammatory and antispasmodic activities) and many of these support the reputed herbal uses[23,24]. Toxicity studies to-date have indicated chamomile to be of low toxicity, although allergic reactions are documented.

References

See General References G1, G2, G3, G4, G6, G8, G9, G10, G11, G12, G14, G16, G19, G23, G24, G26, G32 and G33.

1. Isaac O. Pharmacological investigations with compounds of chamomile I. On the pharmacology of (–)-α-bisabolol and bisabolol oxides (review). *Planta Med* 1979; **35:** 118–24.

2. Mann C, Staba EJ. The chemistry, pharmacology, and commercial formulations of chamomile. In: Herbs, spices, and medicinal plants: Recent advances in botany, horticulture, and pharmacology; vol 1. Craker LE, Simon JE, editors. Arizona: Oryx Press, 1986:235–80.

3. Tubaro A *et al*. Evaluation of antiinflammatory activity of a chamomile extract after topical application. *Planta Med* 1984; **50:** 359.

4. Jakovlev V *et al*. Pharmacological investigations with compounds of chamomile VI. Investigations on the antiphlogistic effects of chamazulene and matricine. *Planta Med* 1983; **49:** 67–73

5. Jacovlev V *et al*. Pharmacological investigations with compounds of chamomile II. New investigations on the antiphlogistic effects of (–)-α-bisabolol and bisabolol oxides. *Planta Med* 1979; **35:** 125–40.

6. Breinlich VJ, Scharnagel K. Pharmakologische Eigenschaften des EN-IN-dicycloäthers aus *Matricaria chamomilla*. *Arzneimittelforschung* 1968; **18:** 429–31.

7. Szelenyi I *et al*. Pharmacological experiments with compounds of chamomile III. Experimental studies of the ulcerprotective effect of chamomile. *Planta Med* 1979; **35:** 218–27.

8. Wagner VH *et al*. Immunstimulierend wirkende polysaccharide (heteroglykane) aus höheren pflanzen. *Arzneimittelforschung* 1985; **35:** 1069.

9. Ikram M. Medicinal plants as hypocholesterolemic agents. *JPMA* 1980; **30:** 278–82.

10. Achterrath-Tuckermann U *et al*. Pharmacological investigations with compounds of chamomile. V. Investigations on the spasmolytic effect of compounds of chamomile and Kamillosan on the isolated guinea pig ileum. *Planta Med* 1980; **39:** 38–50.

11. Hölzl, J *et al*. Preparation of ^{14}C-spiro ethers by chamomile and their use by an investigation of absorption. *Planta Med* 1986 **52:** 533.

12. Shipochliev T. Extracts from a group of medicinal plants enhancng the uterine tonus. *Vet Med Nauki* 1981; **18:** 94–8.

13. Suganda AG *et al*. Effets inhibiteurs de quelques extraits bruts et semi purifiés de plantes indigènes françaises sur la multiplication de l'herpesvirus humain 1 et du poliovirus humain 2 en culture cellulaire. *J Nat Prod* 1983; **46:** 626–32.

14. Grochulski VA, Borkowski B. Influence of chamomile oil on experimental glomerulonephritis in rabbits. *Planta Med* 1972; **21:** 289–92.

15. Hausen BM *et al*. The sensitizing capacity of Compositae plants. *Planta Med* 1984; **50:** 229–34.

16. Casterline CL. Allergy to chamomile tea. *JAMA* 1980; **4:** 330–1.

17. Benner MH, Lee HJ. Anaphylactic reaction to chamomile tea. *J Allergy Clin Immunol* 1973; **52:** 307–8.

18. Hausen BM. The sensitising capacity of Compositae plants. III. Test results and cross-reactions in Compositae-sensitive patients. *Dermatologica* 1979; **159:** 1–11.

19. Kettel WG. Allergy to *Matricaria chamomilla*. *Contact Dermatitis* 1987; **16:** 50–1.

20. Mitchell JC, Dupuis G. Allergic contact dermatitis from sesquiterpenoids of the Compositae family of plants. *Br J Derm* 1971; **84:** 139–50.

21 Opdyke DLJ. Chamomile oil German. *Food Cosmet Toxicol* 1974; **12:** 851–2.

22. Habersang S *et al*. Pharmacological studies with compounds of chamomile IV. Studies on toxicity of (–)-α-bisabolol. *Planta Med* 1979; **37:** 115–23.

23. Harris B, Lewis R. Chamomile—Part 1. *Int J Alternative Complementary Medicine* 1994; September; 12.

24. Berry M. The chamomiles. *Pharm J* 1995; **254:** 191–3.

CHAMOMILE, ROMAN

Species (Family)
Chamaemelum nobile (L.) All. (Asteraceae/Compositae)

Synonym(s)
Anthemis nobilis L.

Part(s) Used
Flowerhead

Pharmacopoeial Monographs
BHP 1983
BHP 1990
BPC 1954
Martindale 30th edition
Pharmacopoeias—Aust., Br., Eur., Fr., Ger., Gr., It., Neth., and Swiss include chamomile from *Anthemis nobilis*.

Legal Category (Licensed Products)
GSL[G14]

Constituents[G1,G2,G10,G19,G24,G32]
Coumarins Scopoletin-7-glucoside
Flavonoids Apigenin, luteolin, quercetin and their glycosides (e.g. apiin, luteolin-7-glucoside, and rutin)
Volatile oils (0.4–1.75%). Angelic and tiglic acid esters (85%);[1] others include 1,8-cineole, *l-trans*-pinocarveol, *l-trans*-pinocarvone, chamazulene, farnesol, nerolidol; germacranolide-type sesquiterpene lactones (0.6%)[2] including nobilin, 3-epinobilin, 1,10-epoxynobilin, 3-dehydronobilin; various alcohols including amyl and isobutyl alcohols, anthemol.[1–4] Chamazulene is formed from a natural precursor during steam distillation of the oil, and varies in yield depending on the origin and the age of flowers.[1]
Other constituents Anthemic acid (bitter), phenolic and fatty acids, phytosterol, choline, inositol.

Food Use
Roman chamomile is listed by the Council of Europe as natural source of food flavouring (category N2). This category indicates that Roman chamomile can be added to foodstuffs in small quantities, with a possible limitation of an active principle (as yet unspecified) in the final product.[G9] Chamomile is commonly used as an ingredient of herbal teas.

Herbal Use
Roman chamomile is stated to possess carminative, antiemetic, antispasmodic, and sedative properties. It has been used for dyspepsia, nausea and vomiting, anorexia, vomiting of pregnancy, dysmenorrhoea, and specifically for flatulent dyspepsia associated with mental stress.[G1,G2,G3,G4,G32]

Dose
Dried flowerheads 1–4 g or by infusion three times daily[G3]
Liquid extract (1:1 in 70% alcohol) 1–4 mL three times daily[G3]

Pharmacological Actions
German and Roman chamomile possess similar pharmacological activities. *See* the monograph for German chamomile for a fuller description of documented pharma-cological actions.
Animal studies Few studies have been documented specifically for Roman chamomile. The azulene compounds are reported to possess anti-allergic and anti-inflammatory properties; their mechanism of action is thought to involve inhibition of histamine release (*see* German chamomile). The volatile oil has been documented as having anti-inflammatory activity (carrageenan rat paw oedema test), and antidiuretic and sedative effects following intraperitoneal administration of doses up to 350 mg/kg body-weight to rats.[5]
The azulenes have been reported to stimulate liver regeneration following oral, but not subcutaneous, administration.
The sesquiterpenoids nobilin, 1,10-epoxynobilin, and 3-dehydronobilin have demonstrated *in-vitro* antitumour activity against human cells.[1] The concentration of hydroxyisonobilin required for cytotoxic activity is reported to be low enough to warrant further investigations (ED_{50} = 0.56 µg/mL vs HeLa; ED_{50} = 1.23 µg/mL vs KB; arbitrary acceptable test level = 4 µg/mL).

Side-effects, Toxicity
Instances of allergic and anaphylactic reactions to chamomile have been documented (*see* Chamomile, German) The allergenic principles in chamomile are thought to be the sesquiterpene lactones.[1] Roman chamomile yields nobilin, a sesquiterpene lactone that is reported to be potentially allergenic.[1] However, Roman chamomile oil has also been reported to be non-irritant and non-sensitising to human skin.[2] Animal studies have indicated the oil to be either mildly or non-irritant, and to lack any phototoxic effects.[2]
Large doses of Roman chamomile are stated to act as an emetic[G21] and this has been attributed to the anthemic acid content.[6]
The acute toxicity of Roman chamomile in animals is reported to be relatively low.[1] Acute LD_{50} values in rabbits (dermal) and rats (by mouth) have been stated to exceed 5 g/kg.[2]

Contra-indications, Warnings
In view of the documented allergic reactions and cross-sensitivities (*see* Chamomile, German), Roman chamomile should be avoided by individuals with a known hypersensitivity to any members of the Asteraceae/Compositae family.

In addition, Roman chamomile may precipitate an allergic reaction or exacerbate existing symptoms in susceptible individuals (e.g. asthmatics). Excessive doses may interfere with anticoagulant therapy because of the coumarin constituents.

The use of chamomile preparations in teething babies is not recommended.

Pregnancy and lactation Roman chamomile is reputed to be an abortifacient and to affect the menstrual cycle.[G12] In view of this and the potential for allergic reactions, the excessive use of chamomile during pregnancy and lactation should be avoided.

Pharmaceutical Comment

The chemistry of Roman chamomile, particularly of the volatile oil, is well documented and is similar to that of German chamomile.[8] Limited pharmacological data are available for Roman chamomile, although many actions have been reported for German chamomile. In view of the similar chemical compositions, many of the activities described for German chamomile are thought to be applicable to Roman chamomile and thus support the traditional herbal uses[7]. Roman chamomile is stated to be of low toxicity, although allergic reactions (mainly contact dermatitis) have been reported.[G26]

References

See General References G1, G2, G3, G4, G9, G10, G11, G12, G14, G19, G21, G22, G23, G24, G26 and G32

1. Mann C, Staba EJ. The chemistry, pharmacology, and commercial formulations of chamomile. In: Herbs, spices, and medicinal plants: Recent advances in botany, horticulture, and pharmacology; vol 1. Craker LE, Simon JE, editors. Arizona: Oryx Press, 1986:235–80.

2. Opdyke DLJ. Chamomile oil roman. *Food Cosmet Toxicol* 1974: **12**: 853.

3. Casterline CL. Allergy to chamomile tea. *JAMA* 1980; **4**: 330–1.

4. Hausen BM *et al*. The sensitizing capacity of Compositae plants. *Planta Med* 1984; **50**: 229–34.

5. Melegari M *et al*. Chemical characteristics and pharmacological properties of the essential oils of *Anthemis nobilis*. *Fitoterapia* 1988; **59**: 449–55.

6. Achterrath-Tuckermann U *et al*. Pharmacologisch Untersuchungen von Kamillen-Inhaltestoffen. *Planta Med* 1980; **39**: 38–50.

7. Harris B, Lewis R. Chamomile—Part 1. *Int J Alternative Complementary Medicine* 1994; September 12.

8. Berry M. The chamomiles. *Pharm J* 1995; **254**: 191–3.

CHAPARRAL

Species (Family)

Larrea tridentata (DC) Coville (Zygophyllaceae)

Synonym(s)

Creosote Bush. *L. tridentata* (South-west USA and Northern Mexico) is now regarded as a separate species to *Larrea divaricata* Gav. (North-west Argentina).[1]

Part(s) Used

Herb

Pharmacopoeial Monographs

None

Legal Category (Licensed Products)

Chaparral is not included on the GSL.[G14]

Constituents[G10]

Amino Acids Arginine, aspartine, cystine, glutamic acid, glycine, isoleucine, leucine, phenylalanine, tryptophan, tyrosine, valine

Flavonoids More than 20 different compounds reported, including isorhamnetin, kaempferol and quercetin and their glycosidic and ether derivatives; gossypetin, herbacetin, and their acetate derivatives;[1–7] 2 *C*-glucosyl flavones

Lignans Major constituent nordihydroguaiaretic acid (NDGA) (up to 1.84%), norisoguaiacin, dihydroguaiaretic acid, partially demethylated dihydroguaiaretic acid, 3'-demethoxyisoguaiacin[8–10]

Resins (20%). Phenolic constituents on external leaf surfaces of *L. divaricata* and *L. tridentata* are reported to be identical, containing a number of flavone and flavonol glycosides, and two lignans (including NDGA).[5]

Volatile oils Many identified terpene components include calamene, eudesmol, limonene, α- and β-pinene, and 2-rossalene.[11]

Other constituents Two pentacyclic triterpenes,[12] saponins

Other plant parts A cytotoxic naphthoquinone derivative, larreantin, has been isolated from the roots.[13]

Food Use

Chaparral is not used in foods, although a related species *Larrea mexicana* Moric., also termed creosote bush, is listed by the Council of Europe as a natural source of food flavouring (category N2). This category indicates that creosote bush can be added to foodstuffs in small quantities, with a possible limitation of an active principle (as yet unspecified) in the final product.[G9] In the USA, NDGA is no longer permitted to be used as an antioxidant in foods following the results of toxicity studies in animals (*see* Side-effects, Toxicity).

Herbal Use

Chaparral has been used for the treatment of arthritis, cancer, venereal disease, tuberculosis, bowel cramps, rheumatism, colds.[G30]

Dose

None documented.

Pharmacological Actions

Animal studies Amoebicidal action against *Entamoeba histolytica* has been reported for a chaparral extract (0.01%).[14] This action may be attributable to the lignan constituents, which are documented as both amoebicidal and fungicidal.[9] NDGA has been reported to have antimicrobial activity against a number of organisms including *Penicillium*, *Salmonella*, and *Streptococcus* species, *Staphylococcus aureus*, *Bacillus subtilis*, *Pseudomonas aeruginosa* and various other pathogens and moulds.[8,15]

NDGA is an antioxidant, and has been documented to cause inhibition of hepatic microsomal enzyme function.[15–17]

Human studies Medical interest in chaparral increased following claims that an aqueous infusion of the herb had caused the regression of a malignant melanoma in the cheek of an 85-year-old man.[18] However, results of a subsequent study that investigated the antitumour action of chaparral, as a tea, were inconclusive.[G30]

Side-effects, Toxicity

Acute hepatitis has been associated with chaparral ingestion.[19,20,21] Contact dermatitis to chaparral has been reported.[22,23] Chaparral-induced toxic hepatitis has been reported for two patients in differnt parts of the USA. The adverse effects were attributed to ingestion of a herbal nutritional supplement derived from the leaves of chaparral. Five cases of serious posoning in the USA and another three in Canada have been linked to chaparral-containing products.[25] Some patients have developed irreversible renohepatic failure. Early investigations into the toxicity of NDGA concluded it to be low.[15] NDGA has been administered to humans, by intramuscular injection, in doses of up to 400 mg/kg body-weight for 5 to 6 months, with little or no toxicity reported.[15] Documented oral LD_{50} values for NDGA include 4 g/kg (mouse), 5.5 g/kg (rat), and 830 mg/kg (guinea-pig).[15] Results of chronic feeding studies (2 year, 0.25–1.0% of diet) in rats and mice reported no abnormalities in histological tests of the liver, spleen, and kidney. Inflammatory caecal lesions and slight cystic enlargement of lymph nodes near the caecum were observed in rats at the 0.5% feeding level. At this point NDGA was considered to be safe for food use. However, two later studies in rats (using NDGA at up to 3% of the diet) reported the development of cortical and medullary cysts in the kidney.[15] On the basis of these findings, NDGA was removed from GRAS (Generally Regarded As Safe) status in the USA and is no longer permitted to be used as an antoxidant in foods.[15]

Contra-indications, Warnings

In view of the reports of acute hepatitis associated with chaparral ingestion, and the uncertainty regarding NDGA toxicity, consumption should be avoided. Excessive doses may interfere with monoamine oxidase inhibitor (MAOI) therapy, because of the documented amino acid constituents.

Pregnancy and lactation In-vitro uteroactivity has been documented for chaparral.[G12] In view of the concerns regarding toxicity, chaparral should not be ingested during pregnancy or lactation.

Pharmaceutical Comment

The chemistry of chaparral is well studied and extensive literature has been published on the principal lignan component, NDGA. However, little documented evidence is available to justify the herbal uses of chaparral. In view of the concerns over the hepatic toxicity, the use of chaparral as a herbal remedy cannot be recommended.

References

See General References G9, G10, G12, G14, G30 and G34.

1.   Bernhard HO, Thiele K. Additional flavonoids from the leaves of *Larrea tridentata. Planta Med* 1981; **41**: 100–103.

2.   Sakakibara M *et al.* 6,8-Di-*C*-glucosylflavones from *Larrea tridentata* (Zygophyllaceae). *Phytochemistry* 1977; **16**: 1113–14.

3.   Sakakibara M *et al.* A new 8-hydroxyflavonol from *Larrea tridentata. Phytochemistry* 1975; **14**: 2097–8.

4.   Sakakibara M *et al.* New 8-hydroxyflavonols from *Larrea tridenta. Phytochemistry* 1975; **14**: 849–51.

5.   Sakakibara M *et al.* Flavonoid methyl ethers on the external leaf surface of *Larrea tridentata* and *L. divaricata. Phytochemistry* 1976; **15**: 727–31.

6.   Chirikdjian JJ. Isolation of kumatakenin and 4',5-dihydroxy-3, 3',7-trimethoxyflavone from *Larrea tridentata. Pharmazie* 1974; **29**: 292–3.

7.   Chirikdjian JJ. Flavonoids of *Larrea tridentata. Z Naturforsch* 1973; **28**: 32–5.

8.   Gisvold O, Thaker E. Lignans from *Larrea divaricata. J Pharm Sci* 1974; **63**: 1905–7.

9.   Fronczek FR *et al.* The molecular structure of 3'-demethoxynorisoguaiacin triacetate from creosote bush (*Larrea tridentata*). *J Nat Prod* 1987; **50**: 497–9.

10.   Page JO. Determination of nordihydroguaiaretic acid in creosote bush. *Analyt Chem* 1955; **27**: 1266–8.

11.   Bohnstedt CF, Mabry TJ. The volatile constituents of the genus *Larrea* (Zygophyllaceae). *Rev Latinoam Quim* 1979; **10**: 128–31.

12.   Xue H-Z *et al.* 3-β-(3,4-Dihydroxycinnamoyl)-erythrodiol and 3β-(4-hydroxycinnamoyl)-erythrodiol from *Larrea tridentata. Phytochemistry* 1988; **27**: 233–5.

13.   Luo, Z *et al.* Larreatin, a novel, cytotoxic naphthoquinone from Larrea tridentata. *J Org Chem* 1988; **53**: 2183–2185.

14.   Segura JJ *et al.* In-vitro amebicidal activity of Larrea tridentata. *Bol Estud Med Biol* 1979; **30**: 267–8.

15.   Oliveto EP. Nordihydroguaiaretic acid. A naturally occurring antioxidant. *Chem Ind* 1972: 677–9.

16.   Burk D, Woods M. Hydrogen peroxide, catalase, glutathione peroxidasequinones, nordihydroguaiaretic acid, and phosphopyridine in relation to X-ray action on cancer cells. *Radiation Res Suppl* 1963; **3**: 212–46.

17.   Pardini RS *et al.* Inhibition of mitochondrial electron transport by nor-dihydroguaiaretic acid (NDGA). *Biochem Pharmacol* 1970; **19**: 2695–9.

18.   Smart CR *et al.* An interesting observation on nordihydroguaiaretic acid (NSC-4291; NDGA) and a patient with malignant melanoma—a preliminary report. *Cancer Chemother Rep Part 1* 1969; **53**: 147.

19.   Katz M, Saibil F. Herbal hepatitis: subacute hepatic necrosis secondary to chaparral leaf. *J Clin Gastroenterol* 1990; **12**: 203–6.

20.   Anon. Chaparral-induced toxic hepatitis—California and Texas, 1992. *Morbidity Mortality Weekly Report* 1992; **41**: 812–4.

21.   Gordon DW *et al.* Chaparral ingestion—the broadening spectrum of liver injury caused by herbal medicines. *JAMA* 1995; **273**: 489–90.

22.   Leonforte JF. Contact dermatitis from *Larrea* (creosote bush). *J Am Acad Dermatol* 1986; **14**: 202–7.

23.   Shasky, D R. Contact dermatitis from *Larrea tridentata* (creosote bush). *J Am Acad Dermatol* 1986; **15**: 302.

24.   Clark F, Reed R. Chaparral-induced toxic hepatitis – California and Texas 1992. *Morb Mortal Weekly Report* 1992; **41**: 812–4.

25.   Anon. Toxic tea. *Pharm J* 1993; **250**: 366.

CINNAMON

Species (Family)
(i) *Cinnamomum zeylanicum* Blume (Lauraceae)
(ii) *Cinnamomum loureirii* Nees
(iii) *Cinnamomum burmanii* (Nees) Bl.

Synonym(s)
(i) *Cinnamomum verum* J. S. Presl, Ceylon Cinnamon, True Cinnamon
(ii) *Cinnamomum obtusifolium* Nees var. *loureirii* Perr. et Eb., Saigon Cinnamon, Saigon Cassia
(iii) Batavia Cassia, Batavia Cinnamon, Padang-Cassia, Panang Cinnamon

Part(s) Used
Inner bark

Pharmacopoeial Monographs
BHP 1983
BPC 1973
Martindale 30th edition
Pharmacopoeias—Aust., Br., Braz., Egypt., Eur., Fr., Gr., Mex., Neth., Port., Rom., and Swiss.

Legal Category (Licensed Products)
GSL[G14]

Constituents[G1,G19,G24,G29,G31,G32,G35]
Tannins Condensed
Volatile oils (Up to 4%). Cinnamaldehyde (60–75%), benzaldehyde and cuminaldehyde; phenols (4–10%) including eugenol, methyl eugenol and safrole, pinene, phellandrene, cymeme, and caryophyllene (hydrocarbons), eugenol acetate, cinnamyl acetate and benzyl benzoate (esters), linalool (an alcohol). Of the various types of cinnamon bark the oil of *C. zeylanicum* is stated to contain the highest amount of eugenol. Cinnamon oil differs from the closely related cassia oil in that the latter is reported to be devoid of eugenol, monoterpenoids, and sesquiterpenoids (*see* Cassia).
Other constituents Calcium oxalate, cinnzeylanin, cinnzeylanol, coumarin, gum, mucilage, resins, sugars
Other plant parts Cinnamon leaf oil contains much higher concentrations of eugenol, from 80–96% depending on the species. A cinnamon leaf oil of Chinese origin, *C. japonicum* Sieb., contains a high concentration of safrole (60%) and only about 3% eugenol.

Food Use
Cinnamon is listed by the Council of Europe as a natural source of food flavouring (category N2). This category indicates that cinnamon can be added to foodstuffs in small quantities, with a possible limitation of an active principle (as yet unspecified) in the final product.[G9] It is commonly used as a spice in cooking, although at levels much less than stated therapeutic doses. The acceptable daily intake of cinnamaldehyde has been temporarily estimated as 700 µg/kg body-weight.[G22] In the USA, cinnamon is listed as GRAS (Generally Regarded As Safe).[G19]

Herbal Use
Cinnamon is stated to possess antispasmodic, carminative, orexigenic, antidiarrhoeal, antimicrobial, refrigerant, and anthelmintic properties. It has been used for anorexia, intestinal colic, infantile diarrhoea, common cold, influenza, and specifically for flatulent colic, and dyspepsia with nausea.[G3] Cinnamon bark is also stated to be astringent, and cinnamon oil is reported to possess carminative and antiseptic properties.[G1,G19,G32]

Dose
Dried bark. 0.5–1.0 g as infusion three times daily[G3]
Liquid extract (1:1 in 70% alcohol) 0.5–1.0 mL three times daily[G3]
Tincture of Cinnamon (BPC 1949) 2–4 mL

Pharmacological Actions
Animal studies Cinnamon oil has antifungal, antiviral, bactericidal, and larvicidal properties.[G19] A carbon dioxide extract of cinnamon bark (0.1%) has been documented to suppress completely the growth of numerous micro-organisms including *Escherichia coli*, *Staphylococcus aureus*, and *Candida albicans*.[G19] *See* Cassia for details of the many pharmacological actions documented for cinnamaldehyde and Cinnamomi Cortex (Cinnamon Bark).

Antiseptic and anaesthetic properties have been documented for eugenol[1] and two insecticidal compounds, cinnzeylanin and cinnzeylanol, have been isolated.[G19] Tannins are known to possess astringent properties.

Weak tumour-promoting activity on the mouse skin and weak cytotoxic activity against HeLa cells has been documented for eugenol.[G19]

Side-effects, Toxicity
None documented for cinnamon bark. Cinnamon oil contains cinnamaldehyde, an irritant and sensitising principle.[G35] The dermal LD_{50} of the oil is reported to be 690 mg/kg body-weight. Refer to Cassia monograph. The accepted daily intake of eugenol is up to 2.5 mg/kg.[G22]

Contra-indications, Warnings
Contact with cinnamon bark or oil may cause an allergic reaction.[G26] Cinnamon oil is stated to be a dermal and mucous membrane irritant, and a dermal sensitiser.[G35] It is a hazardous oil and should not be used on the skin.[G35] The oil should not be taken internally.

Pregnancy and lactation There are no known problems with the use of cinnamon during pregnancy and lactation, provided that doses do not greatly exceed the amounts used in foods.

Pharmaceutical Comment

The reputed antimicrobial, antiseptic, anthelmintic, carminative, and antispasmodic properties of cinnamon are probably attributable to the volatile oil. The astringent properties of tannins may account for the claimed antidiarrhoeal action. Cinnamon should not be used in amounts greatly exceeding those used in foods.

References

See General References G1, G3, G7, G9, G14, G19, G22, G23, G24, G26, G29, G31, G32, G33 and G35.

1. Wagner H, Wolff P (eds). New natural products and plant drugs with pharmacological, biological or therapeutical activity. Berlin: Springer Verlag, 1977.

CLIVERS

Species (Family)
Galium aparine L. (Rubiaceae)

Synonym(s)
Cleavers, Galium, Goosegrass

Part(s) Used
Herb

Pharmacopoeial Monographs
BHP 1983
BHP 1990

Legal Category (Licensed Products)
GSL[G14]

Constituents[G2,G15,G18,G21,G24,G32]
Acids Caffeic acid, *p*-coumaric acid, gallic acid, *p*-hydroxy-benzoic acid, salicylic acid, citric acid.[1]
Coumarins Unspecified. Scopoletin and umbelliferone reported for related species *Galium cruciata* and *Galium tauricum*.[2]
Iridoids Asperuloside (rubichloric acid), monotropein[3,4]
Tannins Unspecified;[5] gallic acid is usually associated with hydrolysable tannins
Other constituents Alkanes (C_{19}-C_{31}),[4] flavonoids.
Other plant parts Anthraquinones have been documented for the roots, but not for the aerial parts.[1]

Food Use
Clivers is not used in foods.

Herbal Use
Clivers is stated to possess diuretic and mild astringent properties. It has been used for dysuria, lymphadenitis, psoriasis, and specifically for enlarged lymph nodes.[G2,G3,G4,G32]

Dose
Dried herb 2–4 g or by infusion three times daily[G2,G3]
Liquid extract (1:1 in 25% alcohol) 2–4 mL three times daily[G2,3]
Expressed juice 3–15 mL three times daily[G2,G3]

Pharmacological Actions
Animal studies None documented for clivers. Asperuloside and monotropein have been reported to elicit a mild laxative action in mice.[6] The action was stated to be approximately fifteen times less potent than senna, and of shorter duration.
Human studies None documented. Tannins are known to possess astringent activities.

Side-effects, Toxicity
None documented.

Contra-indications, Warnings
It has been stated that diabetics should only use the expressed juice with caution[G15] although no pharmacological data were located to support this statement.
Pregnancy and lactation In view of the lack of pharmacological and toxicological information, the use of clivers during pregnancy should be avoided.

Pharmaceutical Comment
Limited chemical information is available for clivers. No scientific evidence was found to support the herbal uses, although documented tannin constituents may account for the reputed mild astringent action. In view of the paucity of toxicity data, excessive use of clivers should be avoided.

References
See General References G2, G3, G4, G14, G15, G18, G21, G24, G25, G32 and G45.

1.   Hegnauer R. Chemotaxonomie der Pflanzen, vol.6. Basel and Stuttgart: Birhauser Verlag. 1973, pp. 158–9.

2.   Borisov MI. Coumarins of the genus Asperula and Galium. *Khim Prir Soedin* 1974; **10**: 82.

3.   Grimshaw J. Structure of asperuloside. *Chem Ind* 1961: 403–4.

4.   Corrigan D *et al*. Iridoids and alkanes in twelve species of *Galium* and *Asperula*. *Phytochemistry* 1978; **17**: 1131–3.

5.   Buckova A *et al*. Contents of tannins in some species of the Asperula and Galium genera. *Acta Fac Pharm Univ Comeniana* 1970; **19**: 7–28.

6.   Inouye H *et al*. Purgative activities of iridoid glucosides. *Planta Med* 1974; **25**: 285–8.

CLOVE

Species (Family)
Syzygium aromaticum (L.) Merr. & Perry (Myrtaceae)

Synonym(s)
Eugenia aromatica (L.) Baill., *Eugenia caryophyllata* Thunb., *Eugenia caryophyllus* (Spreng.) Bull. et Harr., *Caryophyllus aromaticus* L.

Part(s) Used
Clove (dried flowerbud), leaf, stem

Pharmacopoeial Monographs
BP 1993 (Clove, Powdered Clove, Clove Oil)
Martindale 30th edition (Clove, Clove Oil)
Pharmacopoeias—Aust., Br., Chin., Egypt., Eur., Fr., Gr., Hung., It., Jpn, Neth., and Swiss.

Legal Category (Licensed Products)
GSL[G14]

Constituents[G1,G10,G19,G24,G32,G35]
Volatile oils Clove bud oil (15–18%) containing eugenol (80–90%), eugenyl acetate (2–27%), β-caryophyllene (5–12%). Others include methyl salicylate, methyl eugenol, benzaldehyde, methyl amyl ketone, α-ylangene.
Leaf oil (2%) containing eugenol 82–88%
Stem oil (4–6%) with eugenol 90–95%. A more comprehensive listing is provided by reference.[G10]
Other constituents Campesterol, carbohydrates, kaempferol, lipids, oleanolic acid, rhamnetin, sitosterol, stigmasterol, vitamins

Food Use
Clove is listed by the Council of Europe as a natural source of food flavouring (category N2). This category indicates that clove can be added to foodstuffs in small quantities, with a possible limitation of an active principle (as yet unspecified) in the final product.[G9] Clove is commonly used in cooking, and as a flavouring agent in food products. In the USA, clove is listed as GRAS (Generally Regarded As Safe).[G19]

Herbal Use
Clove has been traditionally used as a carminative, antiemetic, toothache remedy, and counter-irritant.[G1,G19,G32]
Clove oil is stated to be a carminative occasionally used in the treatment of flatulent colic[G40] and is commonly used topically for symptomatic relief of toothache.[G22]

Dose
Clove 120–300 mg[G21]
Clove oil 0.05–0.2 mL[G21]

Pharmacological Actions
Animal studies The anodyne and mild antiseptic properties documented for clove oil have been attributed to eugenol.[G19] Clove oil is stated to possess antihistaminic and antispasmodic properties.[G19] Eugenol, eugenol acetate, and methyl acetate are reported to exhibit trypsin-potentiating activity.[G19]
Antibacterial, hypoglycaemic, and potent CNS depressant activities have been documented for *Syzygium cuminii* L., a related species cultivated in India.[1]
Human studies A tincture of cloves (15% in 70% alcohol) was effective in treating athlete's foot.[G19]

Side-effects, Toxicity
None documented for the bud, leaf, or stem of cloves. Clove oil is stated to be a dermal and mucous membrane irritant;[2] contact dermatitis, cheilitis, and stomatitis have been reported for clove oil.[G26] The irritant nature of the oil can be attributed to the eugenol content. Eugenol is also stated to have sensitising properties.[G26] An LD_{50} (rat, by mouth) value for clove oil is stated as 2.65 g/kg bodyweight.[G10]
In humans, the accepted daily intake of eugenol is up to 2.5 mg/kg body-weight.[G22]

Contra-indications, Warnings
None documented for the bud, leaf or stem. It is recommended that clove oil should be used with caution orally and should not be used on the skin.[G35] Repeated application of clove oil as a toothache remedy may result in damage to the gingival tissue.[G22] In view of the irritant nature of the volatile oil, concentrated clove oil is not suitable for internal use in large doses. Eugenol is a powerful inhibitor of platelet activity and it is recommended that caution be taken for patients taking anticoagulant therapy.[G35]
Pregnancy and lactation There are no known problems with the use of clove during pregnancy or lactation, provided that doses taken do not greatly exceed the amounts used in foods.

Pharmaceutical Comment
The pharmacological properties documented for cloves are associated with the volatile oil, in particular with eugenol which has local anaesthetic action. Cloves should not be taken in doses greatly exceeding those used in foods and caution exerted in patients taking anticoagulant or antiplatelet therapy.

References
See General References G1, G9, G10, G14, G19, G21, G22, G24, G26 and G32.

1. Chakraborty D *et al.* A new neuropsychopharmacological study of *Syzygium cuminii*. *Planta Med* 1986; **52**: 139–43.

COHOSH, BLACK

Species (Family)

Cimicifuga racemosa Nutt. (Ranunculaceae)

Synonym(s)

Actaeae Racemosae Radix, Black Snakeroot, Cimicifuga, Macrotys Actaeae

Part(s) Used

Rhizome, Root

Pharmacopoeial Monographs

BHP1983
BHP 1990
BPC 1934
Martindale 30th edition
Chin. includes the rhizome *C. heracleifolia*, *C. dahurica*, and *C. foetida*. Jpn includes the rhizome of *C. simplex* (=*foetida*).

Legal Category (Licensed Products)

GSL[G14]

Constituents[G2,G10,G14,G19,G32]

Alkaloids (quinolizidine-type) *N*-methylcytisine and other unidentified compounds
Tannins Type unspecified. Tannic and gallic acids are usually associated with hydrolysable tannins.
Terpenoids A mixture including actein, 12-acetylactein and cimigoside[1–7]
Other constituents Acetic acid, butyric acid, formic acid, isoferulic acid, oleic acid, palmitic acid, salicylic acid, racemosin, formononetin,[2] phytosterols, cimicifugin 15–20%, acteina (resinous mixture), volatile oil

Food Use

In the USA, black cohosh is listed by the FDA as a 'Herb of Undefined Safety'.[G10] Black cohosh is not used in foods.

Herbal Use

Black cohosh is stated to possess antirheumatic, antitussive, sedative, and emmenagogue properties. It has been used for intercostal myalgia, sciatica, whooping cough, chorea, tinnitus, dysmenorrhoea, uterine colic, and specifically for muscular rheumatism and rheumatoid arthritis.[G2,G3,G4,G32]

Dose

Dried rhizome/root 0.3–2.0 g or by decoction three times daily[G2,G3]
Liquid Extract (BP 1898) (1:1 in 90% alcohol) 0.3–2.0 mL
Tincture of Cimicifuga (BPC 1934) (1 in 10 in 60% alcohol) 2–4 mL

Pharmacological Actions

Animal studies A resinous component, termed acteina, has exhibited a hypotensive action in both unanaesthetised rabbits and anaesthetised cats. The effect in unanaesthetised dogs was found to be inconsistent.[8] An effective dose of acteina 1 mg/kg body-weight was recorded, with maximum hypotension attained using 10 mg/kg. It was stated that acteina may act by an action on the vasomotor centres. A methanolic rhizome extract reduced the serum concentration of luteinising hormone (LH) in the ovariectomised rat, and exhibited a binding affinity to oestrogen receptors in the isolated rat uterus.[1] *In vivo*, the activity of the methanolic extract was significantly reduced following enzymatic hydrolysis of glucosides present. Subsequent *in-vitro* studies isolated three compounds with endocrine activity, including an isoflavone, formononetin. Formononetin was found to exhibit competitive oestrogen receptor activity, but did not cause a reduction in serum concentrations of LH.[2]
Triterpene compounds in black cohosh have been shown to possess hypocholesterolaemic activity *in vivo* and an inhibitory effect on phytohaemagglutin-induced proliferative response *in vitro*. These activities were thought to be linked to molecular characteristics between the identified triterpenes and intermediates in cholesterol biosynthesis.[9]
The root of a related species, *Cimicifuga dahurica*, has been reported to exhibit antibacterial activity towards Gram-positive (*Bacillus subtilis*, *Mycobacterium smegmatis*, *Staphylococcus aureus*), and Gram-negative (*Escherichia coli*, *Shigella flexneri*, *Shigella sonnei*) organisms.[10]
Human studies Black cohosh has been reported to cause peripheral vasodilatation and an increase in peripheral blood flow, following the administration of a resinous constituent, acteina (500 µg/kg body-weight), to patients suffering from peripheral arterial disease.[8] The blood pressure of conscious individuals, both normotensive and hypertensive, was stated to be unaffected. The chemical composition of acteina is undefined.

Side-effects, Toxicity

Overdose may produce symptoms of nausea, vomiting, dizziness, visual and nervous disturbances, together with reduced pulse rate and increased perspiration.[G10,G20,G25] Pharmacological studies in animals have indicated that acteina does not provoke acute toxicity, stimulate any local effects, or affect the heart or spontaneous movement.

Contra-indications, Warnings

It has been recommended that black cohosh should only be used in therapeutic doses, and that high doses are potentially dangerous.[G20,G25]
Pregnancy and lactation In-vitro studies using the rat uterus have indicated that black cohosh binds to uterine oestrogen receptors. Black cohosh is contra-indicated in pregnancy;[G25] an overdose may cause premature birth.[G10]

Pharmaceutical Comment

The chemistry of black cohosh is well studied, although most of the documented information concerns the triterpene constituents. Pharmacological actions have been observed in both animals and humans, although none support the reputed traditional uses of the root. Little is known about the toxicity of black cohosh and excessive use should be avoided.

References

See General References G2, G3, G4, G5, G10, G14, G17, G19, G20, G22, G23, G25, and G32)

1.   Jarry H and Harnischfeger G. Untersuchungen zur endokrinen wirksamkeit von inhaltsstoffen aus *Cimicifuga racemosa* 1. Einfluss auf die serumspiegel von hypophysenhormonen ovariektomierter ratten. *Planta Med* 1985; **51**: 46–9.

2.   Jarry H *et al*. Untersuchungen zur endokrinen wirksamkeit von inhaltsstoffen aus *Cimicifuga racemosa* 2. *In vitro*-bindung von inhaltsstoffen an östrogenrezeptoren. *Planta Med* 1985; **51**: 316–319.

3.   Linde H. Die inhaltsstoffe von Cimicifuga racemosa 2. Mitt.: zur struktur des acteins. *Archiv der pharmazie* 1967; **300**: 885–92.

4.   Linde H. Die inhaltsstoffe von Cimicifuga racemosa 3. Mitt.: über die konstitution der ringe A, B und C des acteins. *Archiv der Pharmazie* 1967; **300**: 982–92.

5.   Linde H. Die inhaltsstoffe von Cimicifuga racemosa 4. Mitt.: actein: der ring D und seitenkette. *Archiv der Pharmazie* 1968; **301**: 120–38.

6.   Linde H. Die inhaltsstoffe von Cimicifuga racemosa 5. Mitt.: 27-desoxyacetylacteol. *Archiv der Pharmazie* 1968; **301**: 335–341.

7.   Radics L *et al*. Carbon-13 NMR spectra of some polycyclic triterpenoids. *Tetrahedron Lett* 1975; 4287–4290.

8.   Genazzani E and Sorrentino L. Vascular action of acteina: active constituent of *Actaea racemosa* L. *Nature* 1962; **194**: 544–5.

9.   Resing K and Fitzgerald A. Crystal data for 15-*o*-acetylacerinol and two related triterpenes isolated from Japanese *Cimicifuga* plants. *J Appl Cryst* 1978; **11**: 58.

10.   Moskalenko SA. Preliminary screening of Far-Eastern ethnomedicinal plants for antibacterial activity. *J Ethnopharmacol* 1986; **15**: 231–59.

COHOSH, BLUE

Species (Family)
Caulophyllum thalictroides (L.) Mich. (Berberidaceae)

Synonym(s)
Caulophyllum, Papoose Root, Squaw Root

Part(s) Used
Rhizome, Root

Pharmacopoeial Monographs
BHP 1983
BPC 1934

Legal Category (Licensed Products)
GSL[G14]

Constituents[G10,G19,G24,G32]
Alkaloids (quinolizidine and isoquinoline-types). Anagyrine, baptifoline, magnoflorine, methylcytisine (caulophylline). Other unidentified minor tertiary alkaloids [1]
Saponins Caulosaponin and cauloside D yielding hederagenin on hydrolysis [2]
Other constituents Citrullol, gum, resins, phosphoric acid, phytosterol, starch
Other Caulophyllum species A related species, *C. robustum.* Maxim., is rich in triterpene glycosides (caulosides A-G), most of which possess hederagenin as their aglycone.

Food Use
Blue cohosh is not used in foods.

Herbal Use
Blue cohosh is stated to possess antispasmodic, emmenagogue, uterine tonic, and antirheumatic properties. Traditionally, it has been used for amenorrhoea, threatened miscarriage, false labour pains, dysmenorrhoea, rheumatic pains, and specifically for conditions associated with uterine atony.[G3,G32]

Dose
Dried rhizome/root 0.3–1.0 g or by decoction three times daily[G3]
Liquid extract (1:1 in 70% alcohol) 0.5–1.0 mL three times daily[G3]

Pharmacological Actions
Animal studies A blue cohosh extract exhibited stimulant properties on the isolated guinea-pig uterus, although subsequent *in-vivo* studies in cats, dogs, and rabbits demonstrated no uterine activity.[3] Antifertility actions documented in rats were reported to be caused by inhibition of ovulation[4] and by interruption of implantation.[5]

Smooth muscle stimulation has been documented for a crystalline glycoside constituent on the uterus (*in vitro*), the small intestine (*in vitro*), and the coronary blood vessels (*in vivo*) of various small mammals.[6] The glycoside was also reported to cause erythrolysis and to be of an irritant nature. An earlier study that used a crystalline glycoside identified as caulosaponin, reported a variety of actions including an oxytocic effect on the isolated rat uterus, constriction of coronary and carotid blood vessels, a toxic action on cardiac muscle, and a spasmogenic action on the isolated intestine.[6]

Methylcytisine is stated to have a nicotinic-like action, causing an elevation in blood pressure and stimulating both respiration and intestinal motility.[G30]

An alcoholic extract of the aerial parts of blue cohosh produced up to 55% inhibition of inflammation in the carrageenan rat paw test[7].

Side-effects, Toxicity
Powdered blue cohosh is stated to be irritant, especially to mucous membranes.[G26] The leaves and seeds are reported to contain methylcytisine and some glycosides that can cause severe stomach pains. Children have been poisoned by eating the bright blue bitter-tasting seeds.[G10] Caulosaponin is reported to be cardiotoxic causing constriction of coronary blood vessels, produce intestinal spasms, and possess oxytocic properties.[G30]

Contra-indications, Warnings
Blue cohosh may interfere with existing therapy for angina and irritate gastrointestinal conditions. Excessive doses may cause a rise in blood pressure, because of the methylcytisine constituent and give rise to other symptoms of nicotine poisoning.
Pregnancy and lactation Blue cohosh should not be taken in pregnancy; it is reputed to be an abortifacient and to affect the menstrual cycle.[G12] It has been documented that blue cohosh should be avoided by pregnant women,[G10] only be taken once labour has commenced,[G25] only taken in small doses during the first trimester of pregnancy,[G3] or only be used under expert supervision.[G20]

Pharmaceutical Comment
Limited data are available on the chemistry of blue cohosh. Documented pharmacological actions support some of the reputed traditional uses, although many of these are not suitable indications for self-medication. No evidence regarding antirheumatic properties was located, although anti-inflammatory action has been documented for the aerial plant parts. In view of the potential toxicity associated with blue cohosh, it should be used with caution.

References

See General References G3, G5, G10, G12, G14, G19, G20, G21, G24, G25, G26, G30, G32 and G34.

1.   Flom MS *et al.*   Isolation and characterization of alkaloids from *Caulophyllum thalictroides*.   *J Pharm Sci* 1967; **56:** 1515–7.

2.   Strigina LI *et al.* Cauloside D a new triterpenoid glycoside from *Caulophyllum robustum*. Maxim. Identification of cauloside A. *Phytochemistry* 1976; **15:** 1583–6.

3.   Pilcher JD *et al.* The action of various female remedies on the excised uterus of the guinea-pig. *Arch Int Med* 1916; **18:** 557–83.

4.   Chaudrasekhar K and Sarma GHR. Observations on the effect of low and high doses of Caulophyllum on the ovaries and the consequential changes in the uterus and thyroid in rats. *J Reprod Fertil* 1974; **38:** 236–7.

5.   Chaudrasekkhar K and Raa Vishwanath C. Studies on the effect of Caulophyllum on implantation in rats. *J Reprod Fertil* 1974; **38:** 245–6.

6.   Ferguson HC, Edwards LD. A pharmacological study of a crystalline glycoside of *Caulophyllum thalictroides*. *J Amer Pharm Assoc* 1954; **43:** 16–21.

7.   Benoit PS *et al.* Biological and phytochemical evaluation of plants XIV. Anti-inflammatory evaluation of 163 species of plants. *Lloydia* 1976; **393** 160–171.

COLA

Species (Family)
(i) *Cola nitida* A. Chev. (Sterculiaceae)
(ii) *Cola acuminata* Schott & Endl. and related species

Synonym(s)
Cola Seed, Kola Nut, Guru Nut
(ii) *Sterculia acuminata* Beauv.

Part(s) Used
Cotyledon

Pharmacopoeial Monographs
BHP 1983
BHP 1990
BPC 1949
Martindale 30th edition (Xanthine-containing beverages)

Legal Category (Licensed Products)
GSL[G14]

Constituents[G2,G10,G19,G24,G31,G32]
Alkaloids (xanthine-types) Caffeine (0.6–3.0%), theobromine (up to 0.1%)
Tannins Condensed type, catechins
Other constituents Betaine, cellulose, enzyme, fats, a glucoside, protein, red pigment, sugars

Food Use
Cola is listed by the Council of Europe as a natural source of food flavouring (category N2). This category indicates that cola can be added to foodstuffs in small quantities, with a possible limitation of an active principle (as yet unspecified) in the final product.[G9] Cola is commonly used in foods. In the USA, cola is listed as GRAS (Generally Regarded As Safe).[G19]

Herbal Use
Cola is stated to possess CNS stimulant, thymoleptic, antidepressant, diuretic, cardioactive, and antidiarrhoeal properties. It has been used for depressive states, melancholy, atony, exhaustion, dysentery, atonic diarrhoea, anorexia, migraine, and specifically for depressive states associated with general muscular weakness.[G2,G3,G4, G32]

Dose
Powdered cotyledons 1–3 g or by decoction three times daily[G2,G3]
Liquid Extract of Kola (BPC 1949) (1:1 in 60% alcohol) 0.6–1.2 mL
Tincture of Kola (BPC 1934) (1:5 in 60% alcohol) 1–4 mL

Pharmacological Actions
The xanthine constituents, caffeine and theobromine, are the active principles in cola. The pharmacological properties of caffeine are well documented and include stimulation of the CNS, respiratory system and skeletal muscle, cardiac stimulation, coronary dilatation, smooth muscle relaxation, and diuresis.[G19] Cola-containing beverages are stated to provide active doses of caffeine.[G22]

Side-effects, Toxicity
Side-effects commonly associated with xanthine-containing beverages include sleeplessness, anxiety, tremor, palpitations, and withdrawal headache.[G40]

Contra-indications, Warnings
Consumption of cola should be restricted in individuals with hypertension or cardiac disorders, because of the caffeine content.
Pregnancy and lactation It is generally recommended that caffeine consumption should be restricted during pregnancy, although conflicting reports have been documented regarding the association between birth defects and caffeine consumption. In view of this, excessive consumption of cola during pregnancy should be avoided. Caffeine is excreted in breast milk, but at concentrations too low to represent a hazard to breast-fed infants.[G22] As with all xanthine-containing beverages, excessive consumption of cola by lactating mothers should be avoided.

Pharmaceutical Comment
The principal active constituent in cola is caffeine. The reputed herbal uses of cola can be attributed to the actions of caffeine, and precautions associated with other xanthine-containing beverages are applicable to cola.

References
See General References G2, G3, G4, G6, G9, G10, G14, G19, G22, G24, G31 and G32.

COLTSFOOT

Species (Family)
Tussilago farfara L. (Asteraceae/Compositae)

Synonym(s)
Farfara

Part(s) Used
Flower, Leaf

Pharmacopoeial Monographs
BHP 1983
BPC 1949
Martindale 28th edition
Pharmacopoeias—Port. Swiss describes the flowers. Aust., Ger., Pol. describe the leaf.

Legal Category (Licensed Products)
GSL[G14]

Constituents[G1,G10,G24,G32]

Acids Caffeic acid, caffeoyltartaric acid, ferulic acid, gallic acid, *p*-hydroxybenzoic acid, and tannic acid (phenolic); malic acid, tartaric acid (aliphatic)[1]

Alkaloids (pyrrolizidine-type). Senkirkine 0.015% and senecionine (minor) (unsaturated)[2,3] and tussilagine (saturated)[4]

Carbohydrates Mucilage (water-soluble polysaccharides) 7–8% yielding various sugars following hydrolysis (e.g. arabinose, fructose, galactose, glucose, uronic acid, and xylose); inulin (polysaccharide)[5]

Flavonoids Flavonols (e.g. kaempferol, quercetin) and their glycosides[1]

Tannins Up to 17% (type unspecified)

Other constituents Bitter (glycoside), choline, paraffin (fatty acid), phytosterols (sitosterol, stigmasterol, taraxasterol), triterpene (amyrin), tussilagone (sesquiterpene),[6] and volatile oil.

Food Use

Coltsfoot is not commonly used as a food but it is listed by the Council of Europe as a source of natural food flavouring (category N4). This category indicates that although coltsfoot is permitted for use as a food flavouring, there is insufficient data available for an assessment of toxicity to be made.[G9]

Herbal Use

Coltsfoot is stated to possess expectorant, antitussive, demulcent, and anticatarrhal properties. It has been used for asthma, bronchitis, laryngitis, and pertussis.[G1,G3,G25,G32]

Dose
Dried herb 0.6–2.0 g by decoction three times daily[G2]
Liquid extract (1:1 in 25% alcohol) 0.6–2.0 mL three times daily[G3]
Tincture (1:5 in 45% alcohol) 2–8 mL three times daily[G3]
Syrup (liquid extract 1:4 in syrup) 2–8 mL three times daily[G3]

Pharmacological Actions

Animal studies Antibacterial activity has been documented against various Gram-negative bacteria including *Staphylococcus aureus*, *Proteus hauseri*, *Bordetella pertussis*, *Pseudomonas aeruginosa*, and *Proteus vulgaris*.[7–9]

Anti-inflammatory activity comparable to that of indomethacin, determined in Selye's experimental chronic inflammation test, has been attributed to water-soluble polysaccharides in coltsfoot.[10] Weak acute anti-inflammatory activity has been reported for coltsfoot when tested against carrageenan-induced rat paw oedema.[11,12]

Platelet-activating factor (PAF) is known to be involved in various inflammatory, respiratory, and cardiovascular disorders. The aggregating action of PAF is known to be weaker if intracellular concentrations of calcium are low. A sesquiterpene, L-652,469, isolated from coltsfoot buds has been reported to be a weak inhibitor of both PAF-receptor binding and calcium entry blocker binding to membrane vesicles.[13] This combination of actions was found to effectively block PAF-induced platelet aggregation. L-652,469 was also found to be active orally, inhibiting PAF-induced rat paw oedema.[13] Interestingly, L-652,469 was reported to interact with the cardiac calcium-channel blocker receptor complex (dihydropyridine receptor), but was also found to be a calcium-channel blocker.[13]

Tussilagone has been reported to be a potent cardiovascular and respiratory stimulant.[6,14] Dose-dependent pressor activity following intravenous injection has been observed in the cat, rat, and dog.[14] The pressor effect is stated to be similar to that of dopamine, but without tachyphylaxis. A significant stimulation of respiration was also observed.[6] Cardiovascular and respiratory effects are thought to be mediated by peripheral and central mechanisms, respectively.[6]

Side-effects, Toxicity

Coltsfoot has been reported to be phototoxic in guinea-pig skin.[15]

Pyrrolizidine alkaloids with an unsaturated pyrrolizidine nucleus are known to be hepatotoxic in both animals and man (*see* Comfrey). Of the pyrrolizidine alkaloids documented for coltsfoot, senecionine and senkirkine are unsaturated. Chronic hepatotoxicity has been described in rats following the incorporation of coltsfoot into their diet at concentrations ranging from 4–33%.[16] After 600 days, it was found that rats fed more than 4% coltsfoot had developed hepatic tumours (haemangioendothelial sarcoma) while none were observed in the control group. Furthermore, histological changes associated with pyrrolizidine alkaloid toxicity such as centrilobular necrosis of the liver and cirrhosis were observed in many of the rats who had ingested coltsfoot but who had not developed tumours.[16] The hepatotoxicity of coltsfoot was attributed to senkirkine, which is present at a concentration of only 0.015%, thus highlighting the dangers associated with chronic exposure to low concentrations of pyrrolizidine alkaloids.

Newborn rats have been found to be more susceptible than weanlings to the hepatotoxic effects of senkirkine despite lacking the hepatic microsomal enzymes required for the formation of the toxic pyrrolic metabolites.[17] Fatal hepatic veno-occlusive disease has been documented in a newborn infant whose mother had regularly consumed a herbal tea during pregnancy.[18] Analysis of the herbal tea revealed the presence of 10 different plants including coltsfoot and a *Senecio* species (known source of pyrrolizidine alkaloids, *see* Liferoot). The mother exhibited no signs of hepatic damage, suggesting an increased sensitivity of the foetal liver to pyrrolizidine alkaloid toxicity.

Pre-blooming coltsfoot flowers are reported to contain the highest concentration of alkaloids.[3] Considerable loss of both senkirkine and senecionine has been observed upon prolonged storage of the dried plant material.[3] Senkirkine and senecionine are both easily extracted into hot water and, therefore, would presumably be ingested in a herbal tea prepared from the fresh plant.[3] A cup of tea prepared from 10 g pre-blooming flowers has been estimated to contain a maximum of 70 µg senecionine and 1.4 mg senkirkine. Tea from the young leaves or mature plant would presumably contain considerably less alkaloids.[3] These concentrations are not considered to represent a health hazard compared to the known hepatotoxicity of senecionine (intravenous LD_{50} 64 mg/kg body-weight, mice).[3] However, prolonged exposure to low concentrations of pyrrolizidine alkaloids have resulted in hepatotoxicity (*see* Comfrey).

Tussilagine LD_{50} (mice, intravenous injection) has been determined as 28.9 mg/kg.[14]

Contra-indications, Warnings

Excessive doses of coltsfoot may interfere with existing antihypertensive or cardiovascular therapy. In view of the known pyrrolizidine alkaloid content, excessive or prolonged ingestion should be avoided. In particular, herbal teas containing coltsfoot should be avoided.

Pregnancy and lactation Coltsfoot should not be taken during pregnancy or lactation in view of the toxicity associated with the pyrrolizidine alkaloid constituents. Coltsfoot is reputed to be an abortifacient.[G12]

Pharmaceutical Comment

The majority of the traditional uses associated with coltsfoot can be attributed to the mucilage content. However, coltsfoot also contains toxic pyrrolizidine alkaloids albeit at a low concentration. The risk of exposure to low concentrations of pyrrolizidine alkaloids is unclear although hepatotoxicity following prolonged exposure has been documented (*see* Comfrey). The regular or excessive consumption of coltsfoot, especially in the form of herbal teas, should therefore be avoided.

References

See General References G2, G3, G6, G9, G10, G12, G14, G21, G24, G25, G32 and G33.

1.   Didry N *et al.* Phenolic compounds from *Tussilago farfara*. *Ann Pharm Fr* 1980; **38:** 237–241.

2.   Culvenor CCJ *et al.* The occurrence of senkirkine in *Tussilago farfara*. *Aust J Chem* 1976; **29:** 229–30.

3.   Rosberger, D F *et al.* The occurrence of senecione in *Tussilago farfara*. *Mitt Geb Lebensm Hyg* 1981; **72:** 432–6.

4.   Röder E *et al.* Tussilagine—a new pyrrolizidine alkaloid from *Tussilago farfara*. *Planta Med* 1981; **41:** 99–102.

5.   Haaland E. Water-soluble polysaccharides from the leaves of *Tussilago farfara* L. *Acta Chem Scand* 1969; **23:** 2546–8.

6.   Yi-Ping L, Wang Y-M. Evaluation of tussilagone: a cardiovascular-respiratory stimulant isolated from Chinese herbal medicine. *Gen Pharmacol* 1988; **19:** 261–3.

7.   Didry N *et al.* Components and activity of *Tussilago farfara*. *Ann Pharm Fr* 1982; **40:** 75–80.

8.   Didry N, Pinkas M. Antibacterial activity of fresh leaves of *Tussilago* spp. *Bull Soc Pharm (Lille)* 1982; **38:** 51–2.

9.   Ieven M *et al.* Screening of higher plants for biological activities I. Antimicrobial activity. *Planta Med* 1979; **36:** 311–21.

10.   Engalycheva E-I *et al.* Anti-inflammatory activity of polysaccharides obtained from *Tussilago farfara* L. *Farmatsiya* 1982; **31:**37–40.

11.   Benoit PS *et al.* Biological and phytochemical evaluation of plants. XIV. Antiinflammatory evaluation of 163 species of plants. *Lloydia* 1976; **39:** 160–71.

12.   Mascolo N *et al.* Biological screening of Italian medicinal plants for anti-inflammatory activity. *Phytotherapy Res* 1987; **1:** 28–31.

13.   Hwang S-B *et al.* L-652,469—a dual receptor antagonist of platelet activating factor and dihydropyridines from *Tussilago farfara* L. *Eur J Pharmacol* 1987; **141:** 269–81.

14.   Wang Y-M. Pharmacological studies of extracts of *Tussilago farfara* L. II Effects on the cardiovascular system. *Acta Pharm Sinica* 1979; **5:** 268–76.

15.   Masaki H *et al.* Primary skin irritation and phototoxicity of plants extracts for cosmetic ingredients. *J Soc Cosmet Chem Japan* 1984; **18:** 47–9.

16.   Hirono I *et al.* Carcinogenic activity of coltsfoot, *Tussilago farfara* L. *Gann* 1976; **67:** 125–9.

17.   Schoental R. Hepatotoxic activity of retrorsine, senkirkine and hydroxysenkirkine in newborn rats, and the role of epoxides in carcinogenesis by pyrrolizidine alkaloids and aflatoxins. *Nature* 1970; **227:** 401–2.

18.   Roulet M *et al* Hepatic veno-occlusive disease in newborn infant of a woman drinking herbal tea. *J Pediatr* 1988; **112:**433–6.

COMFREY

Species (Family)
Symphytum officinale L. (Boraginaceae)

Synonym(s)
Consolidae Radix, Symphytum Radix, *Symphytum peregrinum* Ledeb.
Related species include Prickly Comfrey (*Symphytum asperum*), Quaker and Russian Comfrey (*Symphytum uplandicum*, hybrid of *S. officinale* × *S. asperum*)

Part(s) Used
Leaf, Rhizome, Root

Pharmacopoeial Monographs
BHP 1983 (leaf, root); BHP 1990 (root)
BPC 1934
Martindale 30th edition

Legal Category (Licensed Products)
GSL (external use only)[G14]

Constituents[G1,G2,G10,G19,G24,G32]
Alkaloids (pyrrolizidine-type) 0.3%. Symphytine, symlandine, echimidine, intermidine, lycopsamine, myoscorpine, acetyllycopsamine, acetylintermidine, lasiocarpine, heliosupine, viridiflorine, echiumine[1–5]
Carbohydrates Gum (arabinose, glucuronic acid, mannose, rhamnose, xylose); mucilage (glucose, fructose)
Tannins (pyrocatechol-type) 2.4%.
Triterpenes Sitosterol and stigmasterol (phytosterols), steroidal saponins, isobauerenol
Other constituents Allantoin 0.75–2.55%, caffeic acid, carotene 0.63%, chlorogenic acid, choline, lithospermic acid, rosmarinic acid, silicic acid

Food Use
Comfrey is occasionally used as an ingredient of soups and salads. It is listed by the Council of Europe as natural source of food flavouring (category N4). This category indicates that although comfrey is permitted for use as a food flavouring, insufficient data are available to assess toxicity.[G9]

Herbal Use
Comfrey is stated to possess vulnerary, cell-proliferant, astringent, antihaemorrhagic, and demulcent properties. It has been used for colitis, gastric and duodenal ulcers, haematemesis, and has been applied topically for ulcers, wounds and fractures.[G1,G2,G3,G4,G25,G32]

Dose
Dried root/rhizome 2–4 g in a decoction three times daily[G3]

Root, liquid extract (1:1 in 25% alcohol) 2–4 mL three times daily[G3]
Ointment Symphytum root 10–15% root extractive in usual type ointment basis three times daily[G3]
Dried leaf 2–8 g or by infusion three times daily[G3]
Leaf, liquid extract (1:1 in 25% alcohol) 2–8 mL three times daily[G3]

Pharmacological Actions
The classical pharmacology of pyrrolizidine alkaloids is overshadowed by the well recognised toxicity of this class of compounds. Consequently, the majority of data documented for comfrey involve toxicity. Many useful reviews have been published on the toxicity of pyrrolizidine alkaloids in man (*see below*).[5–11]
Animal studies Wound healing and analgesic activities have been documented in rats administered comfrey extract orally.[12] Percutaneous absorption of pyrrolizidine alkaloids obtained from comfrey is reported to be low in rats, with minimal conversion of the pyrrolizidine alkaloid N-oxides to the free pyrrolizidine alkaloids in the urine (reduction of the N-oxides is required before they can be metabolised into the reactive pyrrolic esters).[13,14]
Rosmarinic acid has been isolated from comfrey (*S. officinale*) as the main constituent with *in-vitro* anti-inflammatory activity.[15] Biological activity was determined by inhibition of malonic dialdehyde formation in human platelets. Minor components, chlorogenic and caffeic acids, were not found to exhibit any significant activity. The pyrrolic esters have been reported to possess mild antimuscarinic activity, which is more pronounced in the non-hepatotoxic esters of saturated aminoalcohols.[16] Conversely, the free aminoalcohols are reported to exert indirect cholinomimetic action involving the release of acetylcholine from post-ganglionic sites in the guinea-pig ileum.[16]
Comfrey has been reported to stimulate the activity of the hepatic drug-metabolising enzyme aminopyrine N-demethylase in rats.[17]
A comfrey extract has been reported to enhance uterine tone *in vitro*.[18] The action of comfrey was reported to be weaker than that exhibited by German chamomile, calendula, and plantain, but stronger than that shown by shepherd's purse, St. John's wort, and uva-ursi.
Human studies The antimuscarinic properties of certain pyrrolic esters has been utilised. Two non-hepatotoxic pyrrolizidine alkaloids, sarracine and platyphylline, have been used for the treatment of gastro-intestinal hypermotility and peptic ulceration.[16]

Side-effects, Toxicity
Two reports of human hepatotoxicity associated with the ingestion of comfrey have been documented.[19,20] One case involved a 13-year-old boy who had been given a comfrey root preparation to treat Crohn's disease in conjunction with

acupuncture.[19] The boy was diagnosed with veno-occlusive disease of the liver and the authors concluded comfrey to be the only possible causal factor of the liver disease. The second case involved a 49-year-old woman diagnosed with veno-occlusive disease.[20] She had been taking various food supplements including a herbal tea and comfrey-pepsin pills. Pyrrolizidine alkaloids were identified in both the tea (stated to contain ginseng) and the comfrey-pepsin pills. The authors estimated that over a period of six months the woman had ingested 85 mg of pyrrolizidine alkaloids, equivalent to 15 µg/kg body-weight per day. This report highlighted the potential toxicity associated with chronic ingestion of relatively small amounts of pyrrolizidine alkaloids.

The toxicity of pyrrolizidine alkaloids is well recognised. Pyrrolizidine alkaloids with an unsaturated pyrrolizidine nucleus are metabolised in the liver to toxic pyrrole metabolites.[8] Acute toxicity results in hepatic necrosis whereas chronic toxicity typically results in veno-occlusive disease characterised by the presence of greatly enlarged liver cells.[8,10]

Reports of human hepatotoxicity associated with pyrrolizidine alkaloid ingestion have been documented.[5,8–10,21–30] Many of these reports have resulted from crop (and subsequently flour and bread) contamination with Crotalaria, Heliotropium, and Senecio species and from the use of pyrrolizidine-containing plants in medicinal 'bush' teas. In addition, pyrrolizidine alkaloid poisoning has been associated with the use of herbal teas in Europe and the United States.[20,25–27] The diagnosis of veno-occlusive disease in a newborn infant who subsequently died highlights the susceptibility of the foetus to pyrrolizidine alkaloid toxicity.[30] In this case, the mother had consumed a herbal tea as an expectorant during pregnancy. The tea, which was purchased from a pharmacy in Switzerland, was analysed and found to contain pyrrolizidine alkaloids. The mother did not exhibit any signs of hepatotoxicity.

Interestingly, liver function tests in 29 chronic comfrey users have been reported to show no abnormalities.[31]

The hepatotoxicity of pyrrolizidine alkaloids is well documented in animals.[5] In addition, carcinogenicity has been described in rats fed a diet supplemented with comfrey.[32] The mutagenicity of comfrey has been attributed to lasiocarpine, [23] which is known to be mutagenic and carcinogenic. However, other workers have reported a lack of mutagenic activity for comfrey following assessment using direct bacterial test systems (Ames), host mediated assay (Legator), liver microsomal assay, and the micronucleus technique.[33,34]

Contra-indications, Warnings

In view of the hepatotoxic properties documented for the pyrrolizidine alkaloid constituents, comfrey should not be taken internally. The topical application of comfrey-containing preparations to broken skin should be avoided.

Pregnancy and lactation The safety of comfrey has not been established. In view of the toxicity associated with the alkaloid constituents, comfrey should not be taken during pregnancy or lactation.

Pharmaceutical Comment

Comfrey is characterised by its pyrrolizidine alkaloid constituents. The hepatotoxicity of these compounds is well known and cases of human poisoning involving comfrey have been documented. Human hepatotoxicity with pyrrolizidine-containing plants is well documented, particularly following the ingestion of Crotalaria, Heliotropium, and Senecio species. Comfrey has traditionally been used topically for treating wounds. Percutaneous absorption of pyrrolizidine alkaloids present in comfrey is reported to be low, although application of comfrey preparations to the broken skin should be avoided.

Licensed herbal products intended for internal use are not permitted to contain comfrey.

The inclusion of comfrey in products intended for topical application is permitted, provided the preparation is only applied to the unbroken skin and that its use is restricted to ten days or less at any one time.

As a result of a report by the Committee on Toxicity of Chemicals in Food to the Food Advisory Committee and the Ministry of Agriculture, Fisheries and Food, the health food trade voluntarily withdrew all products, such as tablets and capsules, and advice was issued that the root and leaves should be labelled with warnings against ingestion. It was considered that comfrey teas contained relatively low levels of pyrrolizidine alkaloids and did not need any warning labels.[36]

References

See General ReferencesG1, G2, G3, G4, G5, G9, G10, G14, G19, G22, G23, G24, G25, G32 and G33.

1.   Culvenor CCJ *et al*. Structure and toxicity of the alkaloids of Russian comfrey (*Symphytum* × *uplandicum* Nyman), a medicinal herb and item of human diet. *Experientia* 1980; **36:** 377–9.

2.   Smith LW, Culvenor CCJ. Hepatotoxic pyrrolizidine alkaloids. *J Nat Prod* 1981; **44:** 129–52.

3.   Huizing HJ. Phytochemistry, systematics and biogenesis of pyrrolizidine akaloids of *Symphytum* taxa. *Pharm Weekbl (Sci)* 1987; **9:** 185–7.

4.   Mattocks AR. Toxic pyrrolizidine alkaloids in comfrey. *Lancet* 1980; **ii:** 1136–7.

5.   Pyrrolizidine alkaloids. *Environmental Health Criteria 80* Geneva: WHO, 1988.

6.   Abbott PJ. Comfrey: assessing the low-dose health risk. *Med J Aust* 1988; **149:** 678–82.

7.   Awang DVC. Comfrey. *Canad Pharm J* 1987; **120:** 101–4.

8.   McLean EK. The toxic actions of pyrrolizidine (Senecio) alkaloids. *Pharmacol Rev* 1970; **22:** 429–83.

9.   Huxtable RJ. Herbal teas and toxins: novel aspects of pyrrolizidine poisoning in the United States. *Perspect Biol Med* 1980; **24:** 1–14.

10.   Mattocks AR. Chemistry and toxicology of pyrrolizidine alkaloids. London: Academic Press, 1986.

11.   Jadhav SJ *et al*. Pyrrolizidine alkaloids: A review. *J Food Sci Tech* 1982; **19:** 87–93.

12. Goldman RS *et al*. Wound healing and analgesic effect of crude extracts of *Symphytum officinale*. *Fitoterapia* 1985; **6**: 323–9.

13. Brauchli J *et al*. Pyrrolizidine alkaloids from *Symphytum officinale* L. and their percutaneous absorption in rats. *Experientia* 1982; **38**: 1085–7.

14. Brauchli J *et al*. Pyrrolizidine alkaloids in *Symphytum officinale* L. and their dermal absorption in rats. *Experientia* 1981; **37**: 667.

15. Gracza L *et al*. Biochemical-pharmacological investigations of medicinal agents of plant origin, I: Isolation of rosmarinic acid from *Symphytum officinale* L. and its anti-inflammatory activity in an *in-vitro* model. *Arch Pharm (Weinheim)* 1985; **318**: 1090–5.

16. Culvenor CCJ. Pyrrolizidine alkaloids: some aspects of the Australian involvement. *Trends Pharmacol Sci* 1985; **6**: 18–22.

17. Garrett BJ *et al*. Consumption of poisonous plants (*Senecio jacobaea*, *Symphytum officinale*, *Pteridium aquilinum*, *Hypericum perforatum*) by rats: Chronic toxicity, mineral metabolism, and hepatic drug-metabolizing enzymes. *Toxicol Lett* 1982; **10**: 183–8.

18. Shipochliev T. Extracts from a group of medicinal plants enhancing the uterine tonus. *Vet Med Nauki* 1981; **18**: 94–8.

19. Weston CFM *et al*. Veno-occlusive disease of the liver secondary to ingestion of comfrey. *Br Med J* 1987; **295**: 183.

20. Ridker PM *et al*. Hepatic venocclusive disease associated with the consumption of pyrrolizidine-containing dietary supplements. *Gastroenterology* 1985; **88**: 1050–54.

21. Anderson C. Comfrey toxicity in perspective. *Lancet* 1981; **i**: 944.

22. Huxtable RJ *et al*. Toxicity of comfrey-pepsin preparations. *New Engl J Med* 1986; **315**: 1095.

23. Furmanowa M *et al*. Mutagenic effects of aqueous extracts of *Symphytum officinale* L. and of its alkaloidal fractions. *J Appl Toxicol* 1983; **3**: 127–30.

24. Ridker PM, McDermott WV. Comfrey herb tea and hepatic veno-occlusive disease. *Lancet* 1989; **i**: 657–8.

25. Lyford CL *et al*. Hepatic veno-occlusive disease originating in Ecuador. *Gastroenterology* 1976; **70**: 105–8.

26. Kumana CR *et al*. Herbal tea induced hepatic veno-occlusive disease: quantification of toxic alkaloid exposure in adults. *Gut* 1985; **26**: 101–4.

27. Stillman AE *et al*. Hepatic veno-occlusive disease due to pyrrolizidine (Senecio) poisoning in Arizona. *Gastroenterology* 1977; **73**: 349–52.

28. McGee JO'D *et al*. A case of veno-occlusive disease of the liver in Britain associated with herbal tea consumption. *J Clin Path* 1976; **29**: 788–94.

29. Datta DV *et al*. Herbal medicines and veno-occlusive disease in India. *Postgrad Med J* 1978; **54**: 511–15.

30. Roulet M *et al*. Hepatic veno-occlusive disease in newborn infant of a woman drinking herbal tea. *J Pediatr* 1988; **112**: 433–6.

31. Anderson PC, McLean AEM. Comfrey and liver damage. *Hum Toxicol* 1989; **8**: 55–74.

32. Hirono I *et al*. Carcinogenic activity of *Symphytum officinale*. *J Natl Cancer Inst* 1978; **61**: 865–9.

33. Lim-Sylianco CY *et al*. Mutagenicity studies of aqueous extracts from leaves of comfrey (*Symphytum officinale* Linn). *NRCP Res Bull* 1977; **32**: 178–91.

34. White RD *et al*. An evaluation of acetone extracts from six plants in the Ames mutagenicity test. *Toxicol Lett* 1983; **15**: 23–31.

35. Food Safety Directive. FSD Information Bulletin May 1993; 2, and Food Sense Factsheet No. 14, May 1993.

CORN SILK

Species (Family)
Zea mays L. (Gramineae)

Synonym(s)
Stigma Maydis, Zea

Part(s) Used
Stigma, Style

Pharmacopoeial Monographs
BHP 1983
BHP 1990
BPC 1934

Legal Category (Licensed Products)
Cornsilk is not included on the GSL[G14]

Constituents[G1,G2,G18,G19,G21,G25,G32]
Amines 0.05%. Type not specified, although hordenine is listed for the genus *Zea*.
Fixed oils (1.85–2.25%). Contain glycerides of linoleic, oleic, palmitic and stearic acids.
Saponins 3% (unspecified)
Tannins Up to 11.5–13% (unspecified)
Other constituents Allantoin, bitter glycosides (1%), cryptoxanthin, cyanogenetic compound (unidentified),[1] flavone, gum, phytosterols (e.g. sitosterol, stigmasterol), pigments, resin, vitamins (C and K)

Food Use
Corn silk is listed as a natural source of food flavouring (category N2). This category indicates that corn silk can be added to foodstuffs in small quantities, with a possible limitation of an active principle (as yet unspecified) in the final product. In the USA, corn silk is listed as GRAS (Generally Regarded As Safe).[G19] The fruits are classified as category N1 with no restriction on their use.[G9] Corn (maize) oil and flour are commonly used in cooking.

Herbal Use
Corn silk is stated to possess diuretic and stone-reducing properties. It has been used for cystitis, urethritis, nocturnal enuresis, prostatitis, and specifically for acute or chronic inflammation of the urinary system.[G1,G2,G3,G4,G32]

Dose
Dried style/stigma 4–8 g or infusion three times daily[G2,G3]
Liquid Extract of Maize Stigmas (BPC 1923) 4–8 mL.
Tincture (1:5 in 25% alcohol) 5–15 mL thrice daily[G2,G3]
Syrup of Maize Stigmas (BPC 1923) 8–15 mL

Pharmacological Actions
Animal studies Corn silk is stated to possess cholagogue, diuretic, hypoglycaemic, and hypotensive activities in laboratory animals.[2,G19] Utilising aqueous extracts, a methanol-insoluble fraction has been reported to exhibit diuretic activity in rabbits,[G19] and an isolated crystalline component has been documented to have a hypotensive action and to stimulate uterine contraction in rabbits.[3] The latter two actions were thought to involve a cholinergic mechanism. The action of corn silk extract on experimental periodontolysis in hamsters has been documented.[4]

Cryptoxanthin is stated to possess vitamin A activity,[G24] and tannins are known to possess astringent properties.
Human studies It has been stated that an aqueous extract is strongly diuretic in humans,[G19] and that clinical studies have indicated corn silk to be effective in kidney and other diseases.[G19] No further information on human studies was located to support these statements.

Side-effects, Toxicity
Allergic reactions including contact dermatitis and urticaria have been documented for corn silk, its pollen, and for starch derived from corn silk.[G26] Cornstarch is considered to be a known allergen.[G26] The toxicity of a methanol-insoluble fraction of an aqueous corn silk extract has been reported to be low in rabbits. The effective intravenous dose for a diuretic action was documented as 1.5 mg/kg body-weight compared to the lethal intravenous dose of 250 mg/kg.[G19] Corn silk contains an unidentified toxic principle,[1,2] and is listed as being capable of producing a cyanogenetic compound.[1]

Contra-indications, Warnings
Corn silk may cause an allergic reaction in susceptible individuals. Excessive doses may interfere with hypoglycaemic drug therapy (*in-vivo* hypoglycaemic activity has been documented) or with hypertensive or hypotensive therapy (*in-vivo* hypotensive activity reported), and prolonged use may result in hypokalaemia because of the diuretic action.
Pregnancy and lactation Corn silk has been documented to stimulate uterine contractions in rabbits. In view of this, doses of corn silk greatly exceeding amounts used in foods should not be taken during pregnancy or lactation.

Pharmaceutical Comment
Limited information is available on the constituents of corn silk.Extracts have been reported to exhibit diuretic actions in both humans and animals, thus justifying the reputed herbal uses. However, no additional data were located to support these reported actions. In view of the lack of toxicity data, excessive use of corn silk should be avoided.

References
See General References G1, G2, G3, G4, G5, G9, G14, G18, G19, G21, G24, G25, G26 and G32
1. Seigler DS. Plants of the northeastern United States that produce cyanogenic compounds. *Economic Bot* 1976; **30:** 395–407.
2. Bever BO and Zahnd GR. Plants with oral hypoglycaemic action. *Quart J Crude Drug Res* 1979; **17:** 139–196.
3. Hahn SJ. Pharmacological action of Maydis stigma. *K'at'ollik Taehak Uihakpu Nonmunjip* 1973; **25:** 127–41.
4. Chaput A *et al.* Action of Zea Mays L. unsaponifiable titre extract on experimental periodontolysis in hamsters. *Med Hyg (Geneve)* 1972; **30:** 1470–1.

COUCHGRASS

Species (Family)
Agropyron repens (L.) Beauvais (Gramineae)

Synonym(s)
Agropyron, Dogs Grass, Quackgrass, Triticum, Twitchgrass, *Triticum repens* L.

Part(s) Used
Rhizome

Pharmacopoeial Monographs
BHP 1983
BPC 1934
Martindale 30th edition
Pharmacopoeias—Fr. and Hung.

Legal Category (Licensed Products)
GSL (Agropyron)[G14]

Constituents[G1,G3,G18,G19,G27,G32]
Carbohydrates Fructose, glucose, inositol, mannitol, mucilaginous substances (10%), pectin, triticin
Cyanogenetic glycosides Unspecified
Flavonoids Tricin and other unidentified flavonoids
Saponins No details documented
Volatile oils (0.05%). Agropyrene (95%). Presence of agropyrene has been disputed[1], with the oil reported to consist mainly of the monoterpenes carvacrol, *trans*-anethole, carvone, thymol, menthol, menthone, and *p*-cymene and three sesquiterpenes.
Other constituents Fixed oil, vanillin glucoside

Food Use
Couchgrass is listed by the Council of Europe as a natural source of food flavouring (category N2). This category indicates that couchgrass can be added to foodstuffs in small quantities, with a possible limitation of an active principle (as yet unspecified) in the final product.[G9] In the USA, couchgrass is listed as GRAS (Generally Regarded As Safe).[G19]

Herbal Use
Couchgrass is stated to possess diuretic properties. It has been used for cystitis, urethritis, prostatitis, benign prostatic hypertrophy, renal calculus, lithuria, and specifically for cystitis with irritation or inflammation of the urinary tract.[G1,G3,G32]

Dose
Dried rhizome 4–8 g or in decoction three times daily[G3]
Liquid extract (1:1 in 25% alcohol) 4–8 mL three times daily[G3]
Tincture (1:5 in 40% alcohol) 5–15 mL three times daily[G3]

Pharmacological Actions
Animal studies Couchgrass is stated to exhibit diuretic and sedative activities in rats and mice, respectively.[G19] Broad antibiotic activity has been documented for agropyrene and its oxidation product.[G19] An ethanolic extract was found to exhibit only weak inhibition (14%) of carrageenan-induced inflammation in the rat paw.[2]
Couchgrass has been reported to be phytotoxic with flavonoid components implicated as the active constituents.[3]

Side-effects, Toxicity
None documented for couchgrass. An unspecified cyanogenetic glycoside has been reported as a constituent of couchgrass, although no further details were located.[G3]

Contra-indications, Warnings
In view of its reputed diuretic action, excessive or prolonged use of couchgrass should be avoided since this may result in hypokalaemia.
Pregnancy and lactation In view of the limited pharmacological and toxicological data, the use of couchgrass during pregnancy and lactation should be avoided.

Pharmaceutical Comment
Limited chemical data are available for couchgrass and little scientific evidence was located to justify the traditional herbal uses. Agropyrene is regarded as the main active principle in couchgrass on account of its antibiotic effect, although the presence of agropyrene in the volatile oil has been disputed.[1] In view of the lack of toxicity data, excessive ingestion should be avoided.

References
See General References G1, G3, G5, G9, G14, G18, G19, G22, G23, G24, G27, and G32

1. Boesel R and Schilcher H. Composition of the essential oil of *Agropyrum repens* rhizome. *Planta Med* 1989; **55**: 399–400.

2. Mascolo N. Biological screening of Italian medicinal plants for anti-inflammatory activity. *Phytotherapy Res* 1987; **1**: 28–9.

3. Weston LA *et al.* Isolation, Characterization and Activity of Phytotoxic Compounds from Quackgrass [*Agropyron repens* (L.) Beauv.]. *J Chem Ecol* 1987; **13**: 403–21.

COWSLIP

Species (Family)
Primula veris L. (Primulaceae)

Synonym(s)
Paigle, Peagle, Primula, *Primula officinalis* (L.) Hill.

Part(s) Used
Flower

Pharmacopoeial Monographs
BHP 1983
Martindale 28th edition

Legal Category (Licensed Products)
GSL[G14]

Constituents[G1,G18,G25,G29,G31,G32]
Carbohydrates Arabinose, galactose, galacturonic acid, glucose, rhamnose, xylose, water soluble polysaccharide (6.2–6.6%)
Flavonoids Apigenin, isorhamnetin, kaempferol, luteolin, quercetin[1]
Phenols Glycosides primulaveroside (primulaverin) and primveroside
Quinones Primin and other quinone compounds
Saponins Primula acid in sepals but saponins absent from other parts of the flower.
Tannins Condensed (e.g. proanthocyanidin B2), pseudotannins (e.g. epicatechin, epigallocatechin)[1]
Other constituents Silicic acid, volatile oil (0.1–0.25%)
Other plant parts Saponins have been documented for the underground parts.[1] 'Primulic acid' is a collective term for the saponin mixture.[2] Primulic acid A glycoside (5–10%) yields primulagenin A as aglycone together with arabinose, galactose, glucose, glucuronic acid, rhamnose, and xylose.[3,4] The saponin content of the roots is stated to peak at two years.[5] After five years of storage the saponin content was reported to have decreased by 45%.

Food Use
Cowslip is not commonly used in foods. A related species *Primula eliator* is listed by the Council of Europe as a natural source of food flavouring (category N2). This category indicates that *Primula eliator* can be added to foodstuffs, provided that the concentration of coumarin does not exceed 2 mg/kg.[G9] Coumarins, however, are not documented as constituents of *Primula veris*, the subject of this monograph.

Herbal Use
Cowslip is stated to possess sedative, antispasmodic, hypnotic, mild diuretic, expectorant, and mild aperient properties. It has been used for insomnia, nervous excitability, hysteria, and specifically for anxiety states associated with restlessness and irritability.[G1,G3,G32]

Dose
Dried flowers 1–2 g as an infusion three times daily[G3]
Liquid extract (1:1 in 25% alcohol) 1–2 mL three times daily[G3]

Pharmacological Actions
Animal studies The saponin fraction has been reported to cause an initial hypotension followed by a long-lasting hypertension in anaesthetised animals. [6]
In vitro, the saponins have been documented to inhibit prostaglandin (PG)-synthetase, but to a lesser extent than aspirin because of insignificant protein binding; to exhibit a slight anti-inflammatory effect against carrageenan rat paw oedema; to contract isolated rabbit ileum; and to possess analgesic and antigranulation activity.[6]
Flavonoid and tannin constituents have been documented for cowslip. A variety of activities have been reported for flavonoids including anti-inflammatory and antispasmodic effects. The tannins are known to be astringent.

Side-effects, Toxicity
Allergic contact reactions to related *Primula* species have been documented; quinone compounds are stated to be the allergenic principles with primin described as a strong contact allergen.[7] Two positive patch test reactions to cowslip have been recorded, although allergenicity was not proven.[G26] An LD_{50} value (mice, intraperitoneal injection) for the saponin fraction is documented as 24.5 mg/kg body-weight compared to a value of 9.5 mg/kg for reparil (aescin). Haemolytic activity has been reported for the saponins, and an aqueous extract of cowslip is stated to contain saponins that are toxic to fish. Saponins are stated to be irritant to the gastro-intestinal tract.
The toxicity of cowslip seems to be associated with the saponin constituents. However, these compounds have only been documented for the underground plant parts, and not for the flowers which are the main plant parts used in the UK.

Contra-indications, Warnings
Cowslip may cause an allergic reaction in sensitive individuals. Excessive doses may interfere with hypo-/hypertensive therapy or cause gastrointestinal irritation.
Pregnancy and lactation The safety of cowslip has not been established. In view of the lack of toxicity data, use of cowslip during pregnancy and lactation should be avoided.

Pharmaceutical Comment
The chemistry of cowslip is not well documented and it is unclear whether saponins reported as constituents of the

underground plant parts are also present in the flowers. Little pharmacological information has been documented to justify the herbal uses of cowslip. In view of the lack of toxicity data, excessive use of cowslip should be avoided.

References

See General References G1, G3, G9, G14, G18, G21, G25, G26, G29, G31 and G32.

1.   Karl C *et al*. Die flavonoide in den blüten von Primula officinalis. *Planta Med* 1981; **41:** 96–9.

2.   Grecu L and Cucu V. Saponine aus *Primula officinalis* und *Primula elatior. Planta Med* 1975; **27:** 247–53.

3.   Kartnig T and Ri CY. Dünnschichtchromatographische untersuchungen an den zuckerkomponenten der saponine aus den wurzeln von *Primula veris* und *P. elatior. Planta Med* 1973; **23:** 379–80.

4.   Grecu L and Cucu V. Primulic acid aglycone from the roots of *Primula officinalis. Farmacia (Bucharest)* 1975; **23:** 167–170.

5.   Jentzsch K. *et al*. Saponin level in the radix of Primula veris. *Sci Pharm* 1973; **41:** 162–5. 162–5.

6.   Cebo B *et al*. Pharmacological properties of saponin fractions from Polish crude drugs. *Herb Pol* 1976; **22:** 154–162.

7.   Hausen BM. On the occurrence of the contact allergen primin and other quinoid compounds in species of the family of Primulaceae. *Arch Dermatol Res* 1978; **261:** 311–21.

DAMIANA

Species (Family)
Turnera diffusa Willd. var. *aphrodisiaca* Urb. (Bignoniaceae/Turneraceae) and related species indigenous to Texas and Mexico.

Synonym(s)
Damiana aphrodisiaca, *Turnera aphrodisiaca* L.F. Ward, *Turnera microphyllia* Desv., Turnera

Part(s) Used
Leaf, Stem

Pharmacopoeial Monographs
BHP 1983
BHP 1990
BPC 1934
Martindale 25th edition

Legal Category (Licensed Products)
GSL[G14]

Constituents[G2,G10,G18,G19,G32]
Carbohydrates Gum 13.5%, starch 6%, sugars
Cyanogenetic glycosides Tetraphyllin B[1]
Phenolic glycoside. Arbutin (up to 0.7%)[2]
Tannins (3.5%). Type unspecified
Volatile oils (0.5–1.0%). At least 20 components including 1,8-cineole 11%, *p*-cymene 2%, α- and β-pinene 2%, thymol, α-copaene, δ-cadinene, and calamene. The presence of 1,8-cineole and *p*-cymene has been disputed.[2]
Other constituents Acids (fatty, plant), alkanes (e.g. hexacosanol-1 and triacontane), damianin 7% (a bitter principle), flavone, β-sitosterol, resin 6.5%.[3]

Food Use
Damiana is used in foods and is listed by the Council of Europe as a natural source of food flavouring (category N2). This category indicates that damiana can be added to foodstuffs in small quantities with a possible limitation of an active principle (as yet unspecified) in the final product.[G9]

Herbal Use
Damiana is stated to possess antidepressant, thymoleptic, mild purgative, stomachic, and reputedly aphrodisiac properties.[4] It has been used for depression, nervous dyspepsia, atonic constipation, coital inadequacy, and specifically for anxiety neurosis with a predominant sexual factor.[G2,G3,G4, G32]

Dose
Dried leaf 2–4 g or by infusion three times daily[G2,G3]
Liquid Extract of Damiana (BPC 1934) 2–4 mL

Pharmacological Actions
Animal studies Hypoglycaemic activity has been reported in mice following both oral and intraperitoneal administration of damiana.[5] An ethanolic extract was stated to exhibit CNS-depressant activity although no other experimental details were available.[6]
Antibacterial activity against *Escherichia coli*, *Proteus mirabilis*, *Pseudomonas aeruginosa*, and *Staphylococcus aureus* has been documented for a mixed herbal preparation, with some of the activity attributed to damiana.[7] The same herbal preparation was also reported to inhibit acetylcholine-induced spasm of the isolated guinea-pig ileum, although none of the antispasmodic activity was attributed to damiana.[7]
Arbutin is stated to be responsible for the urinary antiseptic properties (*see* Uva-ursi). However, the arbutin content of damiana is much less than that quoted for uva-ursi (0.7% and 5 to 18%, respectively).
The roots of various *Turnera* species have exhibited uteroactivity.[G12]
Human studies A herbal preparation containing damiana as one of the ingredients was reported to have a favourable effect on the symptoms of irritable bladder associated with functional and neurohormonal disorders, and on bacterial bladder infections.[7]

Side-effects, Toxicity
Tetanus-like convulsions and paroxysms resulting in symptoms similar to those of rabies or strychnine poisoning have been described in one individual following the ingestion of approximately 200 g damiana extract; cyanide poisoning was considered to be a possible cause. No other reported side-effects for damiana were located.
High doses of arbutin (e.g. 1 g) are considered to be toxic, although the concentration of arbutin documented for damiana (1 g arbutin is equivalent to more than 100 g plant material) is probably too low to warrant concerns over safety.

Contra-indications, Warnings
Excessive use should be avoided because of the presence of cyanogenetic glycosides and arbutin; damiana may interfere with existing hypoglycaemic therapy.
Pregnancy and lactation The safety of damiana has not been established. In view of the lack of toxicity data and possible cyanogenetic constituents, doses greatly exceeding amounts used in foods should not be taken during pregnancy or lactation.

Pharmaceutical Comment
There is limited chemical information available on damiana. There has been little documented evidence to justify the herbal uses, and the reputation of damiana as an aphrodisiac is unproven.[7,8] In view of the lack of toxicity data

and reported cyanogenetic and arbutin constituents, excessive use of damiana should be avoided.

References

See General References G2, G3, G4, G5, G9, G10, G12, G14, G18, G19 and G32

1.   Spencer KC and Siegler DS. Tetraphyllin B from Turnera diffusa. *Planta Med* 1981; **43:** 175–8.

2.   Auterhoff H and Häufel H-P. Inhaltsstoffe der damiana-droge. *Archiv der Pharmazie* 1968; **301:** 537–544.

3.   Domínguez XA and Hinojosa M. Mexican medicinal plants. XXVIII Isolation of 5-hydroxy-7,3',4'-trimethoxy-flavone from *Turnera diffusa. Planta Med* 1976; **30:** 68–71.

4.   Braun JK and Malone MH. Legal highs. *Clin Toxicol* 1978; **12:** 1–31.

5.   Pérez RM *et al.* A study of the hypoglycemic effect of some Mexican plants. *J Ethnopharmacol* 1984; **12:** 253–62.

6.   Jiu J. A survey of some medical plants of Mexico for selected biological activity. *Lloydia* 1966; **29:** 250–259.

7.   Westendorf J. Carito-In-vitro-Untersuchungen zum Nachweis spasmolytischer und kontraktiler Einflüsse. *Therapiewoche* 1982; **32:** 6291–7.

8.   Lowry TP. Damiana. *J Psychoactive Drugs* 1984; **16:** 267–268.

DANDELION

Species (Family)

Taraxacum officinale Weber (Asteraceae/
Compositae)

Synonym(s)

Lion's Tooth, *Taraxacum palustre* (Lyons) Lam & DC.,
Leontodon taraxacum L., Taraxacum

Part(s) Used

Leaf, Root

Pharmacopoeial Monographs

BHP 1983
BHP 1990
BPC 1949
Martindale 30th edition
Pharmacopoeias—Aust., Chin., and Cz. specify Taraxacum
Herb from other species of *Taraxacum*.

Legal Category (Licensed Products)

GSL[G14]

Constituents[G1,G2,G4,G10,G19,G24,G28,G32]

Acids Caffeic acid, *p*-hydroxyphenylacetic acid, chlorogenic acid,[1] linoleic acid, linolenic acid, oleic acid, palmitic acid
Minerals Potassium 297 mg/100 g leaf
Resin Undefined bitter complex, taraxacin
Terpenoids Sesquiterpene lactones taraxinic acid (germac-
ranolide) esterified with glucose,[2] and eudesmanolides[3]
Vitamins Vitamin A 14 000 iu/100 g leaf (compared to
11 000 iu/100 g carrots)
Other constituents Carotenoids, choline, inulin, pectin, phytosterols (e.g. sitosterol, stigmasterol, taraxasterol, homo-
taraxasterol), sugars (e.g. fructose, glucose, sucrose),
triterpenes (e.g. β-amyrin, taraxol, taraxerol)

Food Use

Dandelion is used as a food, mainly in salads and soups.
The roasted root and its extract have been used as a coffee
substitute.[G19] Dandelion is listed by the Council of Europe
as a natural source of food flavouring (category N2). This
category indicates that dandelion can be added to foodstuffs
in small quantities, with a possible limitation of an active
principle (as yet unspecified) in the final product.[G9]

Herbal Use

Dandelion is stated to possess diuretic, laxative, cholagogue, and antirheumatic properties. It has been used for
cholecystitis, gallstones, jaundice, atonic dyspepsia with
constipation, muscular rheumatism, oliguria, and specifically for cholecystitis and dyspepsia.[G1,G2,G3,G4,G30,G32]

Dose

Dried leaf 4–10 g or by infusion three times daily[G2,G3]
Leaf, liquid extract (1:1 in 25% alcohol) 4–10 mL three
times daily[G2,G3]
Dried root 2–8 g or by infusion or decoction three times
daily[G2,G3]
Root, tincture (1:5 in 45% alcohol) 5–10 mL three times
daily[G2,G3]
Liquid Extract of Taraxacum (BPC 1949) 2–8 mL
Juice of Taraxacum (BPC 1949) 4–8 mL

Pharmacological Actions

Animal studies A diuretic effect in rats and mice has been
documented for dandelion extracts, following oral administration.[4] Herb extracts were found to produce greater diuresis than root extracts; a dose of 50 mL (equivalent to 2 g
dried herb)/kg body-weight produced an effect comparable
to that of frusemide 80 mg/kg.
Moderate anti-inflammatory activity against carrageenan
rat paw oedema has been documented for a dandelion root
extract.[5] Hypoglycaemic activity has been described in
normal, but not in diabetic alloxan-treated rabbits following
oesophageal administration.[6] Doses greater than 500 mg/
kg produced a significant blood-glucose concentration
which had returned to normal after 24 hours. The maximum
decrease produced by a dose of 2 g/kg was reported to be
65% of the effect produced by tolbutamide 500 mg/kg. Sul-
ponylureas (e.g. tolbutamide) act by stimulating pancreatic
beta-cells and a similar mechanism was proposed for dandelion.
In-vitro antitumour activity has been documented for an
aqueous extract of dandelion, given by intraperitoneal
injection in the tumour systems ddY-Ehrlich and C3H/He-
MM46.[7] The mechanism of action was thought to be similar to that of tumour polysaccharides such as lentinan.
Human studies Dandelion is one of nine herbal ingredients
of a proprietary preparation that has been used to treat viral
hepatitis.[8]

Side-effects, Toxicity

Contact allergic reactions to dandelion have been documented[9,G26] and animal studies have reported dandelion to
have a weak sensitising capacity.[10] Sesquiterpene lactones
are thought to be the allergenic principles in dandelion.[2]
These compounds contain an exocyclic α-methylene β-lac-
tone moiety, which is thought to be a prerequisite for allergenic activity of sesquiterpene lactones.
The acute toxicity of dandelion would appear to be low,
with LD_{50} values (mice, intraperitoneal injection) estimated
at 36.8 g/kg and 28.8 g/kg for the root and herb, respectively.[4] No visible signs of toxicity were observed in rabbits administered dandelion 3, 4, 5 and 6 g/kg body-weight
by mouth for up to seven days.[6] In addition, no behavioural
changes were recorded.

In-vitro antitumour activity has been documented for an aqueous extract of dandelion (*see* Animal studies).

Contra-indications, Warnings

Dandelion may precipitate an allergic reaction in susceptible individuals, although no reports following the ingestion of dandelion have been documented. Dandelion may potentiate the action of other diuretics and may interfere with existing hypoglycaemic activity.

Pregnancy and lactation There are no known problems with the use of dandelion during pregnancy, provided that doses do not greatly exceed the amounts used in foods.

Pharmaceutical Comment

Dandelion is a well known traditional herbal remedy, although limited scientific information is available to justify the reputed uses. Dandelion has also been used in foods for many years. The chemistry of dandelion has been investigated and animal studies indicate it to be of low toxicity. However, excessive ingestion of dandelion, particularly in amounts exceeding those normally consumed in foods, should be avoided.

References

See General References G1, G2, G3, G4, G6, G9, G10, G14, G19, G21, G22, G23, G24, G26, G28, G30, G32, G33 and G34.

1.   Clifford MN *et al*. The chlorogenic acids content of coffee substitutes. *Food Chem* 1987; **24:** 99–107.

2.   Hausen BM. Taraxinsäure-1'-O-β-D-glucopyranosid, das kontaktallergen des löwenzahns (Taraxacum officinale Wiggers). *Dermatosen* 1982; **30**:51–53.

3.   Hänsel R *et al*. Sequiterpenlacton-β-D-glucopyranoside sowie ein neues eudesmanolid aus *Taraxacum officinale*. *Phyotochemistry* 1980; 19: 857–61.

4.   Rácz-Kotilla *et al*. The action of Taraxacum officinale extracts on the body weight and diuresis of laboratory animals. *Planta Med* 1974; **26:** 212–17.

5.   Mascolo N *et al*. Biological screening of Italian medicinal plants for anti-inflammatory activity. *Phytotherapy Res* 1987; **1:** 28–29.

6.   Akhtar MS *et al*. Effects of Portulaca oleracae (kulfa) and Taraxacum officinale (dhudhal) in normoglycaemic and alloxan-treated hyperglycaemic rabbits. *JPMA* 1985; **35:** 207–210.

7.   Baba K *et al*. Antitumor activity of hot water extract of dandelion, *Taraxacum officinale*—correlation between antitumor activity and timing of administration. *Yagugaku Zasshi* 1981; **101:** 538–43.

8.   Sankaran JK. Livr-Doks in Viral Hepatitis. *The Antiseptic* 1977; **74:** 621–626.

9.   Hausen BM and Schulz KH. Allergische kontaktdermatitis durch löwenzahn (Taraxacum officinale Wiggers). *Dermatosen* 1978; **26:** 198.

10.   Davies MG and Kersey PJW. Contact allergy to yarrow and dandelion. *Contact Dermatitis* 1986; **14:** 256–257.

DEVIL'S CLAW

Species (Family)
Harpagophytum procumbens DC (Pedaliaceae)

Synonym(s)
Harpagophytum

Part(s) Used
Root

Pharmacopoeial Monographs
BHP 1983
BHP 1990

Legal Category (Licensed Products)
Devil's claw is not included on the GSL[G14]

Constituents[G1,G2,G4,G10,G17,G25,G30,G31,G32]

Carbohydrates Fructose, galactose, glucose and *myo*-inositol (monosaccharides), raffinose, stachyose (46%), and sucrose (oligosaccharides).[1]
Iridoids Harpagide, 8-*O*-(*p*-coumaroyl)-harpagide, harpagoside, procumide, 6'-*O*-(*p*-coumaroyl)-procumbide, and procumboside (glucosides).[2]
Phenols Acetoside and isoacetoside (glycosides), and a bioside.[3]
Other constituents Amino acids, flavonoids (kaempferol, luteolin)
Other plant parts The flower, stem, and ripe fruit are reported to be devoid of harpagoside; the leaf contains traces of iridoids.[4]

Food Use
Devil's claw is not used in foods.

Herbal Use
Devil's claw is stated to possess anti-inflammatory, antirheumatic, analgesic, sedative, and diuretic properties. It has been used for arthritis, gout, myalgia, fibrositis, lumbago, pleurodynia, and specifically for rheumatic disease.[G1,G2,G3,G4,G32]

Dose
Dried tuber 0.1–0.25 g three times daily[G2,G3]
Liquid extract (1:1 in 25% alcohol) 0.1–0.25 mL three times daily[G2,G3]
Tincture (1:5 in 25% alcohol) 0.5–1.0 mL three times daily[G2,G3]

Pharmacological Actions
Animal studies Conflicting reports have been documented on the anti-inflammatory activity of devil's claw. Following the administration of alcoholic extracts by mouth or aqueous extracts by intravenous injection, analgesic and anti-inflammatory activity have been described in guinea-pigs, mice, and rats.[5,6] Greatest activity was seen in semi-chronic, rather than acute, models. However, other studies have reported devil's claw to be ineffective as an anti-inflammatory agent in rats, when compared to indomethacin and aspirin.[7,8] *In vitro*, devil's claw (100 mg/mL) was reported to show no significant alteration to prostaglandin (PG) synthetase activity, whereas indomethacin (316 ng/mL) and aspirin (437 µg/mL) caused a 50% inhibition.[9] Results of studies investigating the antiphlogistic, analgesic, and antispasmodic effects of harpagoside, its aglycone, and an aqueous extract of devil's claw, reported activity comparable to that of phenylbutazone.[10] None of the above three fractions, however, gave positive results in the same test systems, demonstrating the difficulty in identifying the active principle in devil's claw.

Crude methanolic extracts of devil's claw have been shown to be cardioactive in *in-vitro* and *in-vivo* studies in rats. A protective action against ventricular arrhythmias induced by aconitine, calcium chloride, adrenaline/chloroform, or reperfusion has been reported.[11,12] The crude extract was found to exhibit greater activity than pure harpagoside, suggesting that the extract contains other constituents that show synergy with harpagoside.[12] Low doses of the extract have been reported to exhibit mild negative chronotropic and positive inotropic effects,[13] whereas high doses have caused a marked negative inotropic effect with reduction in coronary blood flow.[12] The change in inotropic response of the cardiac muscle to high and low doses of devil's claw was attributed to the harpagide component.

In vitro, harpagoside has been shown to decrease the contractile response of smooth muscle to acetylcholine and barium chloride on guinea-pig ileum and rabbit jejunum.[13] Harpagide was found to increase this response at lower doses, but antagonised it at higher concentrations.[13]

Methanolic extracts have also exhibited hypotensive properties in normotensive rats, causing a decrease in arterial blood pressure following oral doses of 300 mg/kg and 400 mg/kg body-weight.[11]

Devil's claw extracts possess weak antifungal activity against *Penicillium digitatum* and *Botrytis cinerea*.[14]

It has been stated that the therapeutic activity exhibited by devil's claw may be associated with the in-vivo formation of harpagogenin, by acid or enzymatic hydrolysis from harpagoside or harpagide.[15]

Human studies Devil's claw tablets (410 mg aqueous extract) were reported to be ineffective, in comparison with indomethacin, when given to 13 arthritic patients at a dose of 1.23 g daily, for six weeks.[8]

Side-effects, Toxicity
One arthritic patient withdrew from a study using devil's claw, after four days of treatment (*see* Human studies).[8] Symptoms documented including a throbbing frontal head-

ache in the morning, tinnitus, severe anorexia, and a loss of taste. No side-effects were reported by other patients in the study.

The toxicity of devil's claw is stated to be minimal, with oral LD_0 and LD_{50} values in mice reported to be greater than 13.5 g/kg body-weight. Clinical, haematological, and gross pathological findings have been described as unremarkable in rats given 7.5 g/kg by mouth for seven days. Hepatic changes could not be demonstrated. No chronic toxicity studies were located. Harpagoside is reported to be highly toxic following intravenous administration.

Contra-indications, Warnings

Devil's claw is stated to be contra-indicated in diabetics (hypoglycaemic action) and is recommended only to be taken under medical supervision. However, no scientific data were located to support this statement. Excessive doses may interfere with existing treatment for cardiac disorders and with hypo-/hypertensive therapy.

Pregnancy and lactation Devil's claw has been stated to be oxytoxic in animals. It should not be taken during pregnancy.[G20]

Pharmaceutical Comment

The chemistry of devil's claw has been well studied and iridoid constituents are thought to be responsible for the reputed anti-inflammatory activity. However, results of clinical and animal studies are conflicting. Further research is required with standardised iridoid preparations to assess the true therapeutic benefit of devil's claw. Excessive use of devil's claw should be avoided in view of the lack of chronic toxicity studies and possible cardioactivity.

References

See General References G1, G2, G3, G4, G10, G17, G20, G23, G25, G30, G31 and G32

1.   Ziller KH and Franz G. Analysis of the water-soluble fraction from the roots of Harpagophytum procumbens. *Planta Med* 1979; **37**: 340–8.

2.   Kikuchi T *et al*. New iridoid glucosides from *Harpagophytum procumbens* DC. *Chem Pharm Bull* 1983; **31**: 2296–2301.

3.   Burger JFW *et al*. Iridoid and phenolic glycosides from *Harpagophytum procumbens*. *Phytochemistry* 1987; **26**: 1453–7.

4.   Czygan FC and Krueger A. Pharmaceutical biological studies of the genus harpagophytum. Part 3 Distribution of the iridoid glycoside harpagoside in the different organs of Harpagophytum-Procumbens and Harpagophytum Zeyheri. *Planta Med* 1977; **31**: 305–7.

5.   Erdös A *et al*. Beitrag zur pharmakologie und toxikologie verschiedener extrakte, sowie des harpagosids aus Harpagophytum procumbens DC. *Planta Med* 1978; **34**: 97—108.

6.   Lanhers M-C *et al*. Anti-inflammatory and analgesic effects of an aqueous extract of *Harpagophytum procumbens*. *Planta Med* 1992; **58**: 117–123.

7.   McLeod DW *et al*. Investigations of *Harpagophytum procumbens* (Devil's Claw) in the treatment of experimental inflammation and arthritis in the rat. *Brit J Pharmacol* 1979; **66**: 140P.

8.   Grahame R and Robinson BV. Devil's Claw (Harpagophytum procumbens): pharmacological and clinical studies. *Ann Rheum Dis* 1981; **40**: 632.

9.   Whitehouse LW *et al*. Devil's Claw (*Harpagophytum procumbens*): no evidence for anti-inflammatory activity in the treatment of arthritic disease. *Can Med Assoc J* 1983; **129**: 249–251.

10.   Sticher O. Plant mono-, di- and sesquiterpenoids with pharmacological and therapeutical activity. In: New natural products with pharmacological, biological or therapeutical activity. H Wagner and P Wolff eds. Berlin: Springer Verlag, pp.137–176, 1977.

11.   Circosta C *et al*. A drug used in traditional medicine: *Harpagophytum procumbens* DC. II. Cardiovascular activity. *J Ethnopharmacol* 1984; **11**: 259–74.

12.   Costa de Pasquale R *et al*. A drug used in traditional medicine: *Harpagophytum procumbens* DC. III. Effects on hyperkinetic ventricular arrhythmias by reperfusion. *J Ethnopharmacol* 1985; **13**: 193–9.

13.   Occhiuto F *et al*. A drug used in traditional medicine: *Harpagophytum procumbens* DC. IV. Effects on some isolated muscle preparations. *J Ethnopharmacol* 1985; **13**: 201–8.

14.   Guérin J-C and Réveillère H-P. Activité antifongique d'extraits végétaux à usage thérapeutique. II. Étude de 40 extraits sur 9 souches fongiques. *Ann Pharmaceut Françaises* 1985; **43**: 77–81.

15.   Vanhaelen M *et al*. Biological Activity of Harpagophytum-Procumbens 1. Preparation and structure of Harpagogenin. *J Pharm Belg* 1981 **36**: 38–42.

DROSERA

Species (Family)
Drosera rotundifolia L. (Droseraeae)

Synonym(s)
Sundew

Part(s) Used
Herb

Pharmacopoeial Monographs
BHP 1983
Martindale 30th edition

Legal Category (Licensed Products)
Drosera is not included in the GSL[G14]

Constituents[G1,G18,G24,G27,G32]
Flavonoids Kaempferol, myricetin, quercetin, hyperoside.[1]
Quinones Plumbagin,[2] hydroplumbagin glucoside,[3] rossoliside (7-methyl-hydrojuglone-4-glucoside)[4]
Other constituents Carotenoids, plant acids, (e.g. butyric acid, citric acid, formic acid, gallic acid, malic acid, propionic acid), resin, tannins (unspecified), ascorbic acid (vitamin C)

Food Use
Drosera is not used in foods.

Herbal Use
Drosera is stated to possess antispasmodic, demulcent, and expectorant properties. It has been used for bronchitis, asthma, pertussis, tracheitis, gastric ulceration, and specifically for asthma and chronic bronchitis with peptic ulceration or gastritis.[G1,G3,G32]

Dose
Dried plant 1–2 g or by infusion three times daily[G3]
Liquid extract (1:1 in 25% alcohol) 0.5–2.0 mL three times daily[G3]
Tincture (1:5 in 60% alcohol) 0.5–1.0 mL three times daily[G3]

Pharmacological Actions
Animal studies Drosera is reported to prevent acetylcholine- or histamine-induced bronchospasm, and to relax acetylcholine- or barium chloride-induced spasm of the isolated intestine.[5] Drosera is stated to possess antitussive properties and has been reported to prevent coughing induced by excitation of the larynx nerve in the rabbit.[5] These antispasmodic actions have been attributed to the naphthoquinone constituents.[G27]
Antimicrobial properties have also been documented for the naphthoquinones.[6] *In vivo*, plumbagin is reported to exert a broad spectrum of activity against Gram-positive and Gram-negative bacteria, influenza viruses, pathogenic fungi, and parasitic protozoa. *In vitro*, a plumbagin solution (1:50 000) was reported to exhibit activity against *Staphylococci*, *Streptococci*, and *Pneumococci* (Gram-positive bacteria), but to lack activity against *Haemophilus pertussis* (Gram-negative bacteria).[5] Plumbagin administered orally to mice for five days, was found to be ineffective against *Lamblia muris* and tuberculosis infection. *Microsporum* infections in guinea-pigs were treated successfully by local applications of 0.25–0.5% solutions (in 40% alcohol) or of 1% emulsions.[6]
An aqueous drosera extract was reported to possess pepsin-like activity.[G27]
In vitro, drosera extracts and plumbagin, in concentrations of 0.01–1.0 mg/mL, have been documented to exert a cytotoxic or immunosuppressive effect in human granulocytes and lymphocytes.[2] Lower concentrations were reported to exhibit immunostimulating properties. Plumbagin possesses chemotherapeutic properties, but is irritant when administered at therapeutic doses.[6]

Side-effects, Toxicity
None documented for drosera. Plumbagin is stated to be an irritant principle[G26] and an LD_{50} (mice, intraperitoneal injection) has been reported to be 15 mg/kg body- weight.[G24] Cytotoxic properties have been documented for drosera and plumbagin (*see* Animal studies).

Contra-indications, Warnings
None documented.
Pregnancy and Lactation The safety of drosera has not been established. In view of the lack of toxicity data, the use of drosera during pregnancy and lactation should be avoided.

Pharmaceutical Comment
Limited chemical information is available for drosera. Documented animal studies support some of the herbal uses. Reported immunostimulant and immunosuppressant activities may warrant further research into the pharmacological activities of drosera. In view of the lack of chemical and toxicity data, excessive use of drosera should be avoided.

References
See General References G1, G3, G14, G18, G22, G23, G24, G26, G27, G32)

1. Ayuga C *et al*. Contribución al estudio de flavonoides en *D. rotundifolia* L. *An R Acad Farm* 1985; **51**: 321–326.

2. Wagner H *et al*. Immunological investigations of naphthoquinone-containing plant extracts, isolated quinones and other cytostatic compounds in cellular immunosystems. Phytochem Soc Europe Symposium. p.43, 1986.

3. Vinkenborg J *et al*. De aanwezigheid van hydroplumbagin-glucoside in Drosera rotundifolia. *Pharm Weekbl* 1969; **104**: 45–9.

4. Sampara-Rumantir N. Rossoliside. *Pharm Weekbl* 1971; **106**: 653–64.

5. Oliver-Bever B. Plants in tropical West Africa. Cambridge University Press: Cambridge, p. 129, 1986.

6. Vichkanova SA *et al*. Chemotherapeutic properties of plumbagin. In: ess. Aizenman BE, *Fitontsidy Mater Soveshch, 6th 1969*. Kiev: Naukova Dumka. p.183–5, 1972.

ECHINACEA

Species (Family)
(i) *Echinacea angustifolia* (DC) Heller. (Asteraceae/Compositae)
(ii) *Echinacea pallida* (Nutt.) Britt.
(iii) *Echinacea purpurea* Moensch.

Synonym(s)
Black Sampson, Coneflower
(i) *Brauneria angustifolia*
(ii) *Brauneria pallida* (Nutt.) Britt.

Part(s) Used
Rhizome, Root

Pharmacopoeial Monographs
BHP 1983
BHP 1990

Legal Category (Licensed Products)
GSL[G14]

Constituents[1–5,G1,G2,G17,G18,G24,G27,G32]
Alkaloids (saturated pyrrolizidine-type). Isotussilagine and tussilagine 0.006% in *Echinacea angustifolia* and *Echinacea purpurea*[6]
Amides Alkylamides, at least 20, especially isobutylamides of C_{11}–C_{16} straight-chain fatty acids;[7–11] echinacein, an unsaturated amide reported to be identical with neoherculin and α-sanshool
Carbohydrates High molecular-weight polysaccharides, echinacin (polysaccharide component), inulin, sugars (fructose, glucose, pentose)[12–14]
Glycosides Caffeic acid derivatives (e.g. echinacoside 0.5–1.0%).[9,15,16] Cynarin (quinic acid derivative) is reported to be specific to *E. angustifolia* and is stated to be the first documented isolation of cynarin from the genus *Echinacea*.
Polyenes Polyacetylenes are reported to be specific to *E. pallida*. However, polyacetylenes have also been documented for both *E. angustifolia* and *E. purpurea*.[9,17,18]
Terpenoids Sesquiterpene lactone esters (germacrane- or guaiane-type skeleton) isolated from *E. purpurea*[19] have subsequently been attributed to *Parthenium integrifolium*,[20] a known adulterant of *E. purpurea*.
Other constituents Betaine (carotenoid), fatty acids, phytosterol, resin, volatile oil (alkylketones main constituents in *E. pallida*).
Other plant parts The aerial parts of *E. purpurea* have been reported to contain amides (highly unsaturated), germacrene (a sesquiterpene) alcohol, a labdane derivative, methyl *p*-hydroxycinnamate, vanillin

Food Use
Echinacea is not used in foods.

Herbal Use
Echinacea is stated to possess antiseptic, antiviral, and peripheral vasodilator properties.Traditionally, it has been used for furunculosis, septicaemia, nasopharangeal catarrh, pyorrhoea, tonsillitis, and specifically for boils, carbuncles, and abscesses.[G1,G2,G3,G4,G32,1] It is under investigation for its immunostimulant action.

Dose
Dried root/rhizome 1 g or by infusion or decoction three times daily[G2,G3]
Liquid extract (1:1 in 45% alcohol) 0.25–1.0 mL three times daily[G2,G3]
Tincture (1:5 in 45% alcohol) 1–2 mL three times daily[G2,G3]

Pharmacological Actions[1–5]
Animal studies In-vivo immunostimulant activity in mice has been documented for echinacea, indicated by phagocytosis enhancement and by an increase in the serum elimination of carbon particles (carbon clearance test).[12,21] Documented *in-vitro* immunostimulant activity, indicated by phagocytosis enhancement and by TNF (tumour necrosis factor)-secretion stimulation in human macrophages and lymphocytes, is stated to be indicative of non-specific T-cell activation.[12,22]

Immunostimulant activity has been associated with polysaccharide and polyacetylene fractions (PSF and PCF, respectively) in both *in-vivo* and *in-vitro* studies.[23] However, no direct infuence on T-lymphocytes and only a moderate induction of B-lymphocyte proliferation were reported for a PSF, from *E. purpurea*, that was found to selectively induce macrophage cytotoxicity against tumour targets *in vitro*.

Phagocytosis enhancement *in vitro* has also been reported for non-volatile sesquiterpene esters isolated from *E. purpurea*,[19] and tissue culture experiments have yielded immunologically active polysaccharides.[24]

In-vitro antiviral activity has been described for alcoholic and aqueous echinacea extracts.[25] Incubation of mouse cells with the extracts was stated to result in 24 hour resistance to *Influenza*, *Herpes*, and *Vesicular* [pox] viruses.[25] Documented immunostimulant and antiviral properties are thought to be partly mediated via the binding of the PSF to carbohydrate receptors on the cell surface of T-cell lymphocytes, resulting in non-specific T-cell activation (e.g. interferon production, lymphokine (TNF) secretion).[26,27]

In-vivo anti-inflammatory activity has been reported for the PSF in the carrageenan rat paw oedema test and in the croton oil mouse ear test, with the PSF administered intravenously and topically, respectively.[13] The isolated PSF was stated to be twice as active as the total aqueous extract in the carrageenan test, and to be about half as active as indomethacin in the croton oil test.

In addition, an aqueous echinacea extract was reported to be more effective in the croton oil test than benzydamine, a topical non-steroidal anti-inflammatory drug. When an echinacea leaf extract was administered orally to rats, it was stated to be devoid of anti-inflammatory activity in the carageenan test.[28]

A long-chain alkene from *E. angustifolia* is stated to possess significant antitumour *in vivo*, inhibiting the growth of Walker tumours in rats and lymphocytic leukaemia (P388) in mice.[29]

Antibacterial activity against *Escherichia coli*, *Proteus mirabilis*, *Pseudomonas aeruginosa*, and *Staphylococcus aureus* has been demonstrated for a multi-herbal preparation containing echinacea and other herbal ingredients, with slight activity against *Staphylococcus aureus* and *Proteus mirabilis* attributed to echinacea.[30]

The same preparation exhibited *in-vitro* antispasmodic activity against acetylcholine-induced spasm of the isolated guinea-pig ileum. Echinacea was one of two components to which the main antispasmodic activity was attributed.[30]

Echinacin, a polysaccharide extract, has been used experimentally as an antagonist of hyaluronidase.[31] The wound healing properties documented for echinacea have been attributed to echinacin (polysaccharide extract), which is said to inhibit the action of hyaluronidase via formation of a stable hyaluronic acid polysaccharide complex and to stimulate fibroblast cell growth.[G1]

Echinacea is stated to have some cortisone-like activity.[31]

Human studies Echinacea has been used for its non-specific action on cell-mediated immunity. A single 2 mL subcutaneous injection (stated as equivalent to 0.1 g of press sap) followed by a free interval of one week was reported to stimulate cell-mediated immunity, whereas daily administration of the injection was stated to have a depressant effect on cell-mediated immunity.[30]

A multi-herbal preparation containing echinacea as one of the ingredients was reported to have a favourable effect on the symptoms of irritable bladder associated with functional and neurohormonal disorders, and on bacterial bladder infections. Contributions of the individual ingredients to the overall efficacy of the preparations were assessed in animal experiments (*see* Animal studies).[30]

Numerous trials have been undertaken with the commercial preparations Echinacin® (fresh juice of the aerial parts) and Esberitox® (a mixture of *Echinacea purpurea*, *Echinacea angustifolia*, *Baptista tinctoria* and *Thuja occidentalis*). The majority of these trials, which utilised i.v. injections and small groups of patients, were not randomised and controlled double-blind trials. The clinical conditions studied have included infections and wound healing, polyarthritis, influenza, colds, upper respiratory tract infections, eczema, psoriasis, urogenital infections, allergies, candidiasis, gynaecological infections, chronic osteomyelitis and chronic skin ulcers.[3]

Side-effects, Toxicity

Echinacea is stated to have produced positive patch test reactions in four patients with a previous history of plant dermatitis.[G26] Trace amounts of echinacin (polysaccharide extract) placed on the tongue are stated to produce excessive salivation and an intense burning paralytic effect on the tongue and on the mucous membranes of the lips and mouth. The roots are stated to produce a similar but milder effect.[G17]

Pyrrolizidine alkaloids with an unsaturated pyrrolizidine nucleus are reported to be hepatotoxic in both animals and humans (*see* Comfrey). The alkaloids isotussilagine and tussilagine have been documented for echinacea; they possess a saturated pyrrolizidine nucleus and are not thought to be toxic.

In-vivo antitumour activity and *in-vitro* stimulation of TNF secretion have been reported for echinacea. TNF is one of a group of polypeptide inflammatory mediators which have been collectively termed cytokines (produced by various cell types) or lymphokines (produced by lymphocytes).[G22] TNF is stated to be produced mainly by lymphocytes and macrophages. In addition to its antitumour effects, TNF is stated to be a mediator of cachexia and the manifestations of endotoxic shock. Concern has been expressed over the possible toxicity of TNF.[G22]

Contra-indications, Warnings

None documented. Echinacea may interfere with immunosuppressive therapy.

Pregnancy and lactation The safety of echinacea has not been established. In view of the lack of toxicity data, excessive use of echinacea during pregnancy should be avoided.

Pharmaceutical Comment

The chemistry of echinacea is well documented.[1–20] *E. angustifolia* and *E. pallida* are described under the same monograph heading in the BHP 1983, although it has been proposed that the two species are in fact chemically dissimilar. *E. purpurea* and *E. angustifolia* both contain amides as their major lipophilic constituents, but of differing structural types.[9,10] By contrast, the lipophilic fraction of *E. pallida* is characterised by polyacetylenes and contains only very low concentrations, if any, of amides.[9,10]

Commercial echinacea samples may contain one or more of the three *Echinacea* species mentioned above, and the reported presence of polyenes in commercial samples of *E. angustifolia* is thought to result from sample contamination with *E. pallida*.[9]

The polyene components are stated to be susceptible to auto-oxidation resulting in the formation of artefacts during storage. It has therefore been recommended that the roots should be stored full-size and that extracts should be kept in solution.[G1,9]

Documented scientific evidence from animal studies supports some of the uses for echinacea as well as the more recent interest in immunostimulant properties.[1–5] Reported pharmacological activities seem to be mainly associated with polyene and high-molecular-weight polysaccharide constituents. Further well designed clinical studies using standardised preparations and larger numbers of patients are required in order to verify the efficacy of echinacea.

In view of the lack of toxicity data, excessive use of echinacea should be avoided.

References

See General References G1, G2, G3, G4, G12, G14, G15, G17, G18, G22, G24, G27 and G32

1. Bauer R and Wagner H. *Echinacea. Ein Handbuch für Ärzte, Apotheker und andere Naturwissenschaftler*. Stuttgart: Wissenschaftliche Verlagsgesellschaft, 1990. pp. 182.

2. Bauer R and Wagner H. Echinacea - Der Sonnenhut – Stand der Forschung. *Z Phytotherapie* 1988; **9**: 151-9.

3. Hobbs C. *The Echinacea Handbook*, Miovich M, ed. Portland, Oregon: Eclectic Medical Publications 1989, pp. 118.

4. Hobbs C. Echinacea - a literature review. *Herbalgram* 1994; **No.30**: 33-47.

5. Houghton PJ. Echinacea. *Pharm J* 1994; **253**: 342-3.

6. Röder E *et al*. Pyrrolizidine in *Echinacea angustifolia* DC und *Echinacea purpurea* M. *Arzneim-Forsch* 1984; **124**: 2316-7.

7. Jacobson M. The structure of echinacein, the insecticidal component of American coneflower roots. *J Org Chem* 1967; **32**: 1646-7.

8. Bohlman F and Hoffmann M. Further amides from *Echinacea purpurea*. *Phytochemistry* 1983; **22**: 1173-5.

9. Bauer R *et al*. Analysis of *Echinacea pallida* and *E. angustifolia* roots. *Planta Med* 1988; **54**: 426-30.

10. Bauer R and Remiger P. TLC and HPLC analysis of alkamides in *Echinacea* drugs. *Planta Med* 1989; **55**: 367-71.

11. Bauer R *et al*. Alkamides from the roots of *Echinacea angustifolia*. *Phytochemistry* 1989; **28**: 505-8.

12. Wagner H *et al*. Immunostimulating polysaccharides (heteroglycans) of higher plants. *Arzneim-Forsch* 1985; **35**: 1069-75.

13. Tubaro A *et al*. Anti-inflammatory activity of a polysaccharide fraction of *Echinacea angustifolia*. *J Pharm Pharmacol* 1987; **39**: 567-9.

14. Protsch A and Wagner H. Structural analysis of a 4-*O*-methylgluconoarabinoxylan with immunostimulating activity from *Echinacea purpurea*. *Phytochemistry* 1987; **26**: 1989-93.

15. Becker H *et al*. Structure of echinoside. *Z Naturforsch* 1982; **37c**: 351-3.

16. Becker H and Hsieh WC. Cichoric acid and its derivatives from Echinacea species. *Z Naturforsch* 1985; **40c**: 585-7.

17. Schulte KE *et al*. Das Vorkommen von Polyacetylen-Verbindungen in *Echinacea purpurea* Mnch. und *Echinacea angustifolia* DC. *Arzneim-Forsch* 1967; **17**: 825-9.

18. Bauer R *et al*. Two acetylenic compounds from *Echinacea pallida* roots. *Phytochemistry* 1987; **26**: 1198-200.

19. Bauer R *et al*. Structure and stereochemistry of new sesquiterpene esters from *Echinacea purpurea*. *Helv Chim Acta* 1985; **68**: 2355-8.

20. Bauer R *et al*. Nachweis einer Verfälschung von *Echinacea purpurea* (L.) Moench mit *Parthenium integrifolium* L. *Dtsch Apoth Ztg* 1987; **127**: 1325.

21. Bauer R *et al*. Immunologische *in-vivo* und *in-vitro* Untersuchungen mit *Echinacea* Extracten. *Arzneim-Forsch* 1988; **38**: 276-81.

22. Vömel T. Der einfluss eines pflanzelischen Immunostimulans auf die Phagozytose von Erythozyten durch das retikulohistozytäre System der isoliert perfundierten Rattenleber. *Arzneim-Forsch* 1985; **35**: 1437-9.

23. Stimpel M *et al*. Macrophage activation and induction of macrophage cytotoxicity by purified polysaccharide fractions from the plant *Echinacea purpurea*. *Infection Immunity* 1984; **46**: 845-9.

24. Wagner H *et al*. Immunologically active polysaccharides of *Echinacea purpurea* cell cultures. *Phytochemistry* 1988; **27**: 119-26.

25. Wacker A and Hilbig W. Virus inhibition by *Echinacea purpurea*. *Planta Med* 1978; **33**: 89-102.

26. Mose J. Effect of echinacin on phagocytosis and natural killer cells. *Med Welt* 1983; **34**: 1463-7.

27. Wagner H *et al*. Immunostimulating polysaccharides (heteroglycans) of higher plants – preliminary communications. *Arzneim-Forsch* 1984; **34**: 659-60.

28. Tragni E *et al*. Evidence from two classical irritation tests for an anti-inflammatory action of a natural extract, echinacea B. *Fd Chem Toxic* 1985; **23**: 317-9.

29. Voaden DJ and Jacobson M. Tumour inhibitors. 3. Identification and synthesis of an oncolytic hydrocarbon from American coneflower roots. *J Med Chem* 1972; **15**: 619-23.

30. Westendorf J. Carito® – *in-vitro* Untersuchungen zum Nachweiss spasmolytischer und kontraktiler Einflüsse. *Therapiewoche* 1982; **32**: 6291-7.

31. Busing K. Hyaluronidasehemmung durch echinacin. *Arzneim-Forsch* 1952; **2**: 467-9.

ELDER

Species (Family)
Sambucus nigra L. (Caprifoliaceae)

Synonym(s)
Black Elder, European Elder, Sambucus
Sambucus canadensis L. refers to American Elder

Part(s) Used
Flower

Pharmacopoeial Monographs
BHP 1983
BHP 1990
BPC 1949
Martindale 30th edition
National pharmacopoeias—Aust., Cz., Fr., Hung., Rom., and Swiss.

Legal Category (Licensed Products)
GSL[G14]

Constituents[G1,G2,G19,G31,G32]
Flavonoids Flavonols (kaempferol, quercetin), quercetin glycosides (1.5–3.0%) including hyperoside, isoquercitrin, and rutin.
Triterpenes α- and β-amyrin, oleanolic and ursolic acids.
Volatile oils (0.3%). 66% fatty acids (primarily linoleic, linolenic, and palmitic) and 7% alkanes (C_{19}, C_{21}, C_{23}, and C_{25}). Numerous other constituent types have been identified including ethers and oxides, ketones, aldehydes, alcohols, and esters.[1]
Other constituents Chlorogenic acid, tannin, mucilage, plastocynin (protein),[2] pectin, and sugar.
Other plant parts. *Leaf* Sambunigrin (0.042%), prunasin, zierin, and holocalin (cyanogenetic glycosides),[3] choline, flavonoids (rutin, quercetin), sterols (sitosterol, stigmasterol, campesterol), triterpenes (α- and β-amyrin palmitates, oleanolic and ursolic acids), alkanes, fatty acids, tannins, and others.[G19]
Bark Lectin (mol. wt 140 000) rich in asparagine/aspartic acid, glutamine/glutamic acid, valine, and leucine,[4] phytohaemagglutinin,[5] triterpenoids (α-amyrenone, α-amyrin, betulin, oleanolic acid, β-sitosterol).[6]

Food Use
Elder is listed by the Council of Europe as a source of natural food flavouring (categories N1 and N2). Category N1 refers to the fruit and indicates that there are no restrictions on quantities used. Category N2 refers to the restrictions on the concentrations of hydrocyanic acid that are permitted, namely 1 mg/kg in beverages and foods, 1 mg/kg for every per cent proof of alcoholic beverages, 5 mg/kg in stone fruit juices, 25 mg/kg in confectionery, and 50 mg/kg in marzi-

pan.[G9] In the USA, the flowers have a regulatory status of GRAS (Generally Regarded As Safe).[G19]

Herbal Use
Elder is stated to possess diaphoretic and anticatarrhal properties. Traditionally, it has been used for influenza colds, chronic nasal catarrh with deafness, and sinusitis.[G4] Elder is also stated to act as a diuretic, laxative, and local anti-inflammatory agent.[G1,G2,G3,G4,G19,G25,G32]

Dose
Dried flower 2–4 g by infusion three times daily[G2,G3]
Liquid extract (1:1 in 25% alcohol) 2–4 mL three times daily[G2,G3]

Pharmacological Actions
Animal studies Elder is stated to possess diuretic and laxative properties.[G19]
Moderate (27%) anti-inflammatory action in carrageenan rat paw oedema has been documented for an elder preparation given one hour before carrageenan (100 mg/kg, by mouth).[7] Indomethacin as a control exhibited 45% inhibition at a dose of 5 mg/kg.[7]
An infusion made from the flowers of elder, St. John's wort herb, and root of soapwort (*Saponaria officinalis*) has exhibited antiviral activity versus influenza types A and B (*in-vivo* and *in-vitro*) and herpes simplex virus type 1 (*in-vitro*).[8]
A diuretic effect in rats exceeding that exerted by theophylline has been reported for elder.[9] An infusion and extracts rich in potassium and in flavonoids all caused diuresis. Greatest activity was exerted by the combined potassium- and flavonoid-rich extracts.
In-vitro antispasmodic activity (rat ileum, rabbit/guinea-pig intestine) and spasmogenic activity (rat uterus) have been reported for lectins isolated from elder.[10]
A lectin isolated from elder bark was found to be a lactose-specific haemagglutinin with a slightly higher affinity for erythrocytes from blood group A.[4] Unlike many other plant lectins, the lectin did not inhibit protein synthesis.[4] The carbohydrate binding properties of a lectin isolated from elder bark have been studied.[11]
Phytohaemagglutinins are biologically active extracts isolated from various plants and represent a class of lectin. They are associated with haemagglutination and mitogenic, antigenic, and immunosuppressant properties.[5] *In-vitro*, phytohaemagglutinin has been found to stimulate production of an interferon-like substance in human leucocytes.[G22]
Hepatoprotective activity against CCl_4-induced toxicity has been reported for triterpenes isolated from *Sambucus formosana* Nakai.[12]
Human studies None documented for elder. Phytohaemagglutinin extracts have been used clinically to treat drug-

induced leucopenia and some types of anaemia.[5] The blastogenic response of lymphocytes to phytohaemagglutinin has been used extensively as a measure of immunocompetence.[G22]

Side-effects, Toxicity

No reported side-effects specifically for elder were located. Human poisoning has occurred with *Sambucus* species.[13] The roots, stems, and leaves, and much less the flowers and unripe berries, are stated to contain a poisonous alkaloid and cyanogenic glycoside causing nausea, vomiting, and diarrhoea.[13] The flowers and ripe fruit are stated to be edible without harm.[13]

The effects of a lectin isolated from elder bark on mammalian embryonic and foetal development has been studied.[5] The lectin exerted mainly a toxic effect and, to a lesser degree, a teratogenic effect when administered subcutaneously to pregnant mice. In view of the high doses administered, the authors stated that the results did not indicate a potential hazard to human foetuses exposed to lectins.[5]

Contra-indications, Warnings

Excessive or prolonged use may result in hypokalaemia in view of the documented diuretic effect. Plant parts other than the flowers are reported to be poisonous and should not be ingested.

Pregnancy and lactation The safety of elder taken during pregnancy has not been established. In view of the lack of toxicity data, the use of elder during pregnancy and lactation should be avoided.

Pharmaceutical Comment

Phytochemical details have been documented for elder, with flavonoids and triterpenes representing the main biologically active constituents. Anti-inflammatory, antiviral, and diuretic effects have been observed in *in-vivo* studies thus supporting the herbal uses of elder. No documented studies in humans were found. Potentially toxic compounds have been reported for the bark (lectins) and the leaves (cyanogenetic glycosides); the flowers are suitable for use as a herbal remedy.

References

See General References G1, G2, G3, G4, G6, G9, G14, G19, G22, G23, G24, G25, G31 and G32.

1.   Toulemonde B, Richard HMJ. Volatile constituents of dry elder (*Sambucus nigra* L.) flowers. *J Agric Food Chem* 1983; **31:** 365–70.

2.   Scawen MD *et al.* The amino-acid sequence of plastocyanin from *Sambucus nigra* L. (elder). *Eur J Biochem* 1974; **44:** 299–303.

3.   Jensen SR, Nielsen BJ. Cyanogenic glucosides in *Sambucus nigra* L. *Acta Chem Scand* 1973; **27:** 2661–85.

4.   Broekaert WF *et al.* A lectin from elder (*Sambucus nigra* L.) bark. *Biochem J* 1984; **221**; 163–9.

5.   Paulo E. Effect of phytohaemagglutinin (PHA) from the bark of *Sambucus nigra* on embryonic and foetal development in mice. *Folia Biol (Kraków)* 1976; **24:**213–22.

6.   Lawrie W *et al.* Triterpenoids in the bark of elder (*Sambucus nigra*). *Phytochemistry* 1964; **3:** 267–8.

7.   Mascolo N *et al.* Biological screening of Italian medicinal plants for anti-inflammatory activity. *Phytotherapy Res* 1987; **1:** 28.

8.   Serkedjieva J *et al.* Antiviral activity of the infusion (SHS-174) from flowers of *Sambucus nigra* L., aerial parts of *Hypericum perforatum* L., and roots of *Saponaria officinalis* L. against influenza and herpes simplex viruses. *Phytotherapy Res* 1990; **4:** 97.

9.   Rebuelta M *et al.* Étude de l'effet diurétique de différentes préparations des fleurs du *Sambucus nigra* L. *Plant Méd Phytothér* 1983; **17:** 173–81.

10.   Richter A. Changes in the motor activity of smooth muscles of the rat uterus *in vitro* as the effect of phytohaemagglutinins from *Sambucus nigra*. *Folia Biol* 1973; **21:** 33–48.

11.   Shibuya N *et al.* The elderberry (*Sambucus nigra* L.) bark lectin recognizes the Neu5Ac(α2-6)Gal/GalNAc sequence. *J Biol Chem* 1987; **262:** 1596–1601.

12.   Lin C-N, Tome W-P. Antihepatotoxic principles of *Sambucus formosana*. *Planta Med* 1988; **54:** 223–4.

13.   Hardin JW, Arena JM, editors. Human poisoning from native and cultivated plants. 2nd edn. North Carolina: Duke University Press, 1974.

ELECAMPANE

Species (Family)
Inula helenium L. (Asteraceae/Compositae)

Synonym(s)
Alant, Horseheal, Inula, Scabwort, Yellow Starwort, *Helenium grandiflorum* Gilib., *Aster officinalis* All., *Aster helenium* (L.) Scop.
An elecampane extract has been referred to as helenin. Alantolactone is also known as elecampane camphor, alant camphor, helenin, and inula camphor.[G22]

Part(s) Use
Rhizome, Root

Pharmacopoeial Monographs
BHP 1983
BHP 1990
Martindale 28th edition

Legal Category (Licensed Products)
GSL[G14]

Constituents[G1,G2,G19,G32]
Carbohydrates Inulin (up to 44%), mucilage
Terpenoids β- and γ-sitosterols, stigmasterol, and damaradienol (sterols), friedelin
Volatile oils (1–4%). Mainly contains sesquiterpene lactones including alantolactone, isoalantolactone, and dihydroalantolactone (eudesmanolides), alantic acid, azulene
Other constituents Resin

Food Use
Elecampane is listed by the Council of Europe as a natural source of food flavouring (category N2). This category indicates that elecampane can be added to foodstuffs in small quantities, with a possible limitation of an active principle (as yet unspecified) in the final product.[G9]
In the USA, elecampane is only approved for use in alcoholic beverages.[G19]

Herbal Use
Elecampane is stated to possess expectorant, antitussive, diaphoretic, and bactericidal properties. Traditionally, it has been used for bronchial/tracheal catarrh, cough associated with pulmonary tuberculosis, and dry irritating cough in children.[G1,G2,G3,G4,G32]
Alantolactone has been used as an anthelmintic in the treatment of roundworm, threadworm, hookworm, and whipworm infection.[G21,G22]

Dose
Rhizome/Root 1.5–4.0 g or by decoction three times daily[G2,G3]

Liquid extract 1.5–4.0 mL (1:1 in 25% alcohol) three times daily[G2,G3]

Alantolactone 300 mg daily for two courses of 5 days, with an interval of 10 days. *Children*, 50–200 mg daily[G21]

Pharmacological Actions
Animal studies Elecampane infusion has exhibited a pronounced sedative effect in mice.[G19] Alantolactone has been reported to exhibit hypotensive, hyperglycaemic (large doses), and hypoglycaemic (smaller doses) actions in animals.[G19] Antibacterial properties have also been documented. Alantolactone and isoalantolactone have been reported to exhibit high bactericidal and fungicidal properties *in vitro*.[G19]

The volatile oil has been reported to exert a potent smooth muscle relaxant effect *in vitro* on guinea-pig ileal and tracheal muscle.[1]

Various activities have been documented for *Inula racemosa*: an extract lowered plasma insulin and glucose concentrations in rats 75 minutes after oral administration,[2] counteracted adrenaline-induced hyperglycaemia in rats,[2] exhibited negative inotropic and chronotropic effects on the frog heart,[2] and provided a preventative and curative action against experimentally induced myocardial infarction in rats.[3] Pretreatment was found to be most effective.[3]

Sesquiterpene lactones with antitumour activity have been isolated from *Helenium microcephalum*.[4,5]

Human studies Alantolactone has been used as an anthelmintic in the treatment of roundworm, threadworm, hookworm, and whipworm infection.[G21,G22]

Inula racemosa has been reported to prevent ST-segment depression and T-wave inversion in patients with proven ischaemic heart disease,[2] and to have a beneficial effect on angina pectoris.[6]

Side-effects, Toxicity
Elecampane has been reported to cause allergic contact dermatitis.[G26] Sensitising properties have been documented for the volatile oil,[G26,G35] and for alantolactone and isoalantolactone.[7] *In-vitro* cytotoxicty has been reported for alanto-lactone and isoalantolactone.[8]

Contraindications, Warnings
Elecampane may cause an allergic reaction, particularly in individuals with an existing allergy or sensitivity to other plants in the Asteraceae family. Elecampane may interfere with existing hypoglycaemic and antihypertensive treatment.

Pregnancy and lactation The safety of elecampane taken during pregnancy has not been established. In view of the lack of toxicity data, the use of elecampane during pregnancy and lactation should be avoided.

Pharmaceutical Comment

The pharmacological actions documented for elecampane seem to be attributable to the sesquiterpene lactone constituents, in particular alantolactone and isoalantolactone. The demulcent action of mucilage and reported *in-vivo* antispasmodic activity of the volatile oil support the traditional uses of this remedy in coughs. In addition, alantolactone has been utilised as an anthelmintic. A number of interesting cardiovascular activities have been documented for a related species, *I. racemosa*. Whether the constituents responsible for these actions are also present in elecampane is unclear. In view of the paucity of toxicity data for elecampane, excessive or prolonged use should be avoided.

References

See General References G1, G2, G3, G4, G9, G14, G19, G21, G22, G24, G26, G32 and G35

1.   Reiter M, Brandt W. Relaxant effects on tracheal and ileal smooth muscles of the guinea pig. *Arzneimittelforschung* 1985; **35**: 408–14.

2.   Tripathi YB *et al*. Assessment of the adrenergic beta-blocking activity of *Inula racemosa*. *J Ethnopharmacol* 1988; **23**: 3–9.

3.   Patel V *et al*. Effect of indigenous drug (puskarmula) on experimentally induced myocardial infarction in rats. *Act Nerv Super (Praha)* 1982; (Suppl 3): 387–94.

4.   Sims D *et al*. Antitumor agents 37. The isolation and structural elucidation of isohelenol, a new antileukemic sesquiterpene lactone, and isohelenalin from *Helenium microcephalum*. *J Nat Prod* 1979; **42**: 282–6.

5.   Imakura Y *et al*. Antitumor agents XXXVI: Structural elucidation of sesquiterpene lactones microhelenins-A, B, and C, microlenin acetate, and plenolin from *Helenium microcephalum*. *J Pharm Sci* 1980; **69**: 1044–9.

6.   Tripathi SN *et al*. Beneficial effect of *Inula racemosa* (pushkarmoola) in angina pectoris: A preliminary report. *Indian J Physiol Pharmacol* 1984; **28**: 73–5.

7.   Stampf JL *et al*. The sensitising capacity of helenin and two of its main constituents the sesquiterpene lactones alantolactone and isoalantolactone: a comparison of epicutaneous and intradermal sensitising methods in different strains of guinea pig. *Contact Dermatitis* 1982; **8**: 16–24.

8.   Woerdenbag HJ. In vitro cytotoxicity of sesquiterpene lactones from *Eupatorium cannabinum* L. and semi-synthetic derivatives from eupatoriopicrin. *Phytotherapy Res* 1988; **2**: 109–14

EUCALYPTUS

Species (Family)
Eucalyptus globulus Labill. (Myrtaceae)

Synonym(s)
Fevertree, Gum Tree, Tasmanian Bluegum

Part(s) Used
Leaf

Pharmacopoeial Monographs
Martindale 30th edition (Eucalyptus oil)
National pharmacopoeias—Aust., Belg., Br., Chin., Cz., Egypt., Eur., Fr., Ger., Gr., Hung., Ind., It., Jpn, Mex., Neth., Port., Rom., Rus., and Swiss include Eucalyptus oil.

Legal Category (Licensed Products)
GSL[G14]

Constituents[G1,G10,G19,G24,G32]
Flavonoids Eucalyptrin, hyperoside, quercetin, quercitrin, rutin
Volatile oils (0.5–3.5%). Eucalyptol (cineole) 70–85%. Others include monoterpenes (e.g. α-pinene, β-pinene, *d*-limonene, *p*-cymene, α-phellandrene, camphene, γ-terpinene) and sesquiterpenes (e.g. aromadendrene, alloaromadendrene, globulol, epiglobulol, ledol, viridiflorol), aldehydes (e.g. myrtenal) and ketones (e.g. carvone, pinocarvone)
Other constituents Tannins and associated acids (e.g. gallic acid, protocatechuic acid), caffeic acid, ferulic acids, gentisic acid, resins, waxes

Food Use
Eucalyptus is listed by the Council of Europe as a natural source of food flavouring (category N2). This category indicates that eucalyptus can be added to foodstuffs in small quantities, with a possible limitation of an active principle (as yet unspecified) in the final product.[G9] Both eucalyptus and eucalyptol (cineole) are used as flavouring agents in many food products.[G19] In the USA, eucalyptus is approved for food use and eucalyptol is listed as a synthetic flavouring agent.[G19]

Herbal Use
Eucalyptus leaves and oil have been used as an antiseptic, febrifuge, and expectorant.[G1,G19,G32]

Dose
Eucalyptol (cineole BPC 1973) 0.05–0.2 mL
Eucalyptus Oil (BPC 1973) 0.05–0.2 mL
Fluid extract 2–4 g
Oil for local application 30 mL oil to 500 mL lukewarm water

Pharmacological Actions
Animal studies Hypoglycaemic activity in rabbits has been documented for a crude leaf extract rich in phenolic glycosides. Purification of the extract resulted in a loss of activity.[G19] Expectorant and antibacterial activities have been reported for eucalyptus oil and for eucalyptol.[G19] Various *Eucalyptus* species have been shown to possess antibacterial activity against both Gram-positive and Gram-negative organisms. Gram-positive organisms were found to be the most sensitive, particularly *Bacillus subtilis* and *Micrococcus glutamious*.[1]

In-vitro antiviral activity against influenza type A has been documented for quercitrin and hyperoside.[G19]

Human studies Eucalyptus oil has been taken orally for catarrh, used as an inhalation, and applied as a rubefacient.[G22] A plant preparation containing tinctures of various herbs including eucalyptus has been used successfully in the treatment of chronic suppurative otitis.[2] The efficacy of the preparation was attributed to the antibacterial and anti-inflammatory actions of the herbs included.

Side-effects, Toxicity
Externally, eucalyptus oil is stated to be generally non-toxic, non-sensitising, and non-phototoxic.[G35] Undiluted eucalyptus oil is toxic and should not be taken internally unless suitably diluted. A dose of 3.5 mL has proved fatal.[G22] Symptoms of poisoning with eucalyptus oil include epigastric burning, nausea and vomiting, dizziness, muscular weakness, miosis, a feeling of suffocation, cyanosis, delirium, and convulsions.

Contra-indications, Warnings
Eucalyptus may interfere with existing hypoglycaemic therapy. Eucalyptus oil should be diluted before internal or external use.
Pregnancy and lactation Eucalyptus oil should not be taken internally during pregnancy.

Pharmaceutical Comment
Eucalyptus is characterised by its volatile oil components. Antiseptic and expectorant properties have been attributed to the oil, in particular to the principal component eucalyptol. The undiluted oil is toxic if taken internally. Essential oils should not be applied to the skin unless they are diluted with a carrier vegetable oil.

References
See General References G1, G9, G10, G14, G19, G22, G23, G24 , G32, G33 and G35.

1. Kumar A *et al*. Antibacterial properties of some *Eucalpytus* oils. *Fitoterapia* 1988; **59**: 141–4.

2. Shaparenko *et al*. On use of medicinal plants for treatment of patients with chronic suppurative otitis. *Zh Ushn Gorl Bolezn* 1979; **39**: 48–51.

EUPHORBIA

Species (Family)
Euphorbia hirta L. (Euphorbiaceae)

Synonym(s)
Pillbearing spurge, Snakeweed, *Euphorbia pilulifera* L., *Euphorbia capitata* Lam.

Part(s) Use
Herb

Pharmacopoeial Monographs
BHP 1983
BPC 1934
Martindale 28th edition

Legal Category (Licensed Products)
GSL[G14]

Constituents[G19,G24,G32]
Flavonoids Leucocyanidin, quercetin, quercitrin, xanthorhamnin
Terpenoids α- and β-Amyrin, taraxerol and esters, friedelin; campesterol, sitosterol, stigmasterol (sterols)
Other constituents Choline, alkanes, inositol, phenolic acids (eg. ellagic, gallic, shikimic), sugars, resins

Food Use
Euphorbia is not used in foods

Herbal Use
Euphorbia is stated to be used for respiratory disorders, such as asthma, bronchitis, catarrh, and laryngeal spasm. It has also been used for intestinal amoebiasis.
[G3,G32]

Dose
Herb 120–300 mg or as infusion[G3]
Liquid Extract of Euphorbia (BPC 1949) 0.12–0.3 mL
Euphorbia Tincture (BPC 1923) 0.6–2.0 mL

Pharmacological Actions
Animal studies Euphorbia has been reported to have antispasmodic and histamine-potentiating properties.[G19] Smooth muscle relaxing and contracting activities have been exhibited by euphorbia *in vitro* (guinea-pig ileum) and have been attributed to shikimic acid and to choline, respectively.[1]

In-vivo antitumour activities have been documented for euphorbia.[G19]

Antibacterial activity *in-vitro* versus both Gram-positive and Gram-negative bacteria has been documented for euphorbia.[2] Stem extracts were slightly more active than leaf extracts. *In-vitro* amoebicidal activity versus *Entamoeba histolytica* has been reported for a euphorbia decoction.[3]

Side-effects, Toxicity
None documented for euphorbia. Carcinogenic properties in mice have been reported for shikimic acid, although no mutagenic activity was observed in the Ames assay.[G19]

Contra-indications, Warnings
None documented.

Pregnancy and lactation The safety of euphorbia has not been established. Euphorbia has been reported to cause both contraction and relaxation of smooth muscle. In view of the lack of pharmacological and toxicity data, the use of euphorbia during pregnancy and lactation should be avoided.

Pharmaceutical Comment
There is little published information concerning euphorbia, although documented actions observed in animals do support the traditional herbal uses. There is a lack of information concerning toxicity, although the documented constituents of euphorbia do not indicate any obvious toxic component. Nevertheless, excessive or prolonged ingestion should be avoided.

References
See General References G3, G5, G14, G19, G21, G24 and G32

1.   El-Naggar L *et al*. A note on the isolation and identification of two pharmacologically active constituents of *Euphorbia pilulifera*. *Lloydia* 1978; **41**: 73–75.

2.   Ajao AO *et al*. Antibacterial activity of *Euphorbia hirta*. *Fitoterapia* 1985; **56**: 165–7.

3.   Basit N *et al*. In vitro effect of extracts of *Euphorbia hirta* Linn. on *Entamoeba histolytica*. *Riv Parasitol* 1977; **38**: 259–62.

EVENING PRIMROSE

Species (Family)
Oenothera species including *Oenothera biennis* L. (Onagraceae)

Synonym
King's Cureall

Part(s) Used
Seed oil

Pharmacopoeial Monographs
Martindale 30th edition

Legal Category (Licensed Products)
Evening primrose is not included on the GSL.[G14] Gamolenic acid is a Prescription Only Medicine

Constituents
Fixed oils (14%). *cis*-Linoleic acid (LA) 72% (65–80%), *cis*-gammalinolenic acid (gamolenic acid, GLA) 2–16%, oleic acid 9%, palmitic acid 7%, stearic acid (3%) [1–5]

Food Use
Evening primrose root has been used as a vegetable with a peppery flavour.[5] The seed oil has been used as a food supplement for many years. LA and gamolenic acid are both essential fatty acids (EFA), with LA representing the main EFA in the diet, whilst gamolenic acid is found in human milk, in oats and barley, and in small amounts in a wide variety of common foods.[4,5]

Herbal Use
An infusion of the whole plant is reputed to have sedative and astringent properties, and has traditionally been used for asthmatic coughs, gastro-intestinal disorders, whooping cough, and as a sedative pain killer.[5] Externally, poultices were reputed to ease bruises and to speed wound healing.[5] Evening primrose oil (EPO) is licensed for the treatment of atopic eczema, and cyclical and non-cyclical mastalgia. Other conditions in which evening primrose oil is used include premenstrual syndrome, psoriasis, multiple sclerosis, hypercholesterolaemia, rheumatoid arthritis, Raynaud's phenomenon, Sjögren's syndrome, post-viral fatigue syndrome, asthma, and diabetic neuropathy. [1–3,5]

Dose
Recommended doses for evening primrose oil are specific to the condition being treated.
Daily doses for a licensed evening primrose oil product are 6 to 8 g (adults) and 2 to 4 g (children) in atopic eczema.[6] In cyclical and non-cyclical mastalgia, a daily dose of 3 to 4 g is recommended. These doses are based on a standardised gamolenic acid content of 8%. No special precautions are noted for the elderly. The oil may be swallowed directly, mixed with milk or another liquid, or taken with food.
A patient may need to receive evening primrose oil for a period of three months before a clinical response is observed.[3,6]

Pharmacological Actions
The pharmacological actions of evening primrose oil have been reviewed.[1–3,5]
The actions of evening primrose oil are attributable to the essential fatty acid content of the oil and to the involvement of these compounds in prostaglandin biosynthetic pathways.
Gamolenic acid and its metabolite dihomogamma-linolenic acid (DGLA) are precursors of both the inflammatory prostaglandin E_2 series (PGE_2) via arachidonic acid (AA), and of the less inflammatory PGE_1 series. Actions attributed to PGE_1 include anti-inflammatory, immunoregulatory, and vasodilatory properties, inhibition of platelet aggregation and cholesterol biosynthesis, hypotension, and elevation of cyclic AMP (inhibits phospholipase A2, *see below*).[1–3]
Dietary supplementation with gamolenic acid has been noted to have a favourable effect on the DGLA:AA ratio. Although an increase in arachidonic acid concentrations is also seen, this is much smaller and less consistent compared to the increase seen for DGLA.[3] Contributory factors to this negative effect on arachidonic acid are PGE_1 and 15-hydroxy-DGLA. The latter inhibits conversion of arachidonic acid to inflammatory lipoxygenase metabolites including leukotrienes, whilst PGE_1 inhibits the enzyme phospholipase A_2 which is required for the mobilisation of arachidonic acid from phospholipid membrane stores.[3] In addition, DGLA desaturation to arachidonic acid is a rate-limiting step in humans and proceeds very slowly.[3]
gamolenic acid is not normally obtained directly from dietary sources and the body relies on metabolic conversion from dietary LA. This conversion is readily saturable and is considered to be the rate-limiting step in the production of gamolenic acid. A reduced rate of LA conversion to gamolenic acid has been observed in a number of clinical situations including ageing, diabetes, cardiovascular disorders and high cholesterol concentrations, high alcohol intake, viral infections, cancer, nutritional deficits, atopic eczema, and premenstrual syndrome.[1–3] Direct dietary supplementation with gamolenic acid effectively by-passes this rate-limiting conversion step and has a beneficial effect on the ratio of inflammatory:non-inflammatory prostaglandin compounds.
Evening primrose oil represents a good source of both LA and, more importantly, of gamolenic acid. Numerous papers have been published on the biochemical rationale for the therapeutic uses of evening primrose oil, and on its efficacy in various disease states associated with low concentrations of gamolenic acid. Horrobin[3] reviewed the use of evening

primrose oil in various disease states which include atopic eczema, premenstrual syndrome including mastalgia, diabetic neuropathy, rheumatoid arthritis, Sjögrens Syndrome, cardiovascular, renal, hepatic and gastro-intestinal disorders, viral infections, endometriosis, schizophrenia, alcoholism, Alzheimer's disease, and cancers.

Atopic eczema An inherited slow rate of 6-desaturation (LA to gamolenic acid conversion) has been documented in this condition. Normal or elevated concentrations of LA are associated with reduced concentrations of their metabolites. Randomised, double-blind, placebo-controlled trials have shown gamolenic acid to produce a highly significant improvement in all features of atopic eczema, especially in itch.[1–3,7,8] The requirement for topical and oral steroids, histamines, and antibiotics was also reduced.[3] However, attention has been drawn to the conflicting evidence of clinical trials on evening primrose oil. Two large trials have not shown evidence of benefit[10,11] whereas other trials have resulted in benefits, particularly for patients with moderate or severe eczema.[12,13] Adequate doses of evening primrose oil for treatment of atopic eczema are 160–320 mg of gamolenic acid daily in children aged 1–12 years and 320–480 mg in adults for 3 months.[9]

Cyclical/Non-cyclical mastalgia PGE$_1$ is thought to modulate the action of prolactin. Abnormal concentrations may result in an excessive peripheral action of prolactin.[3]

Several placebo-controlled studies have demonstrated that gamolenic acid is superior compared to placebo in the treatment of both premenstrual syndrome and breast pain.[1–3,14] Overall, cyclical mastalgia responds better than non-cyclical to all treatments (danazol, bromocriptine, evening primrose oil).

Premenstrual syndrome The use of evening primrose oil for the treatment of premenstrual syndrome has been rationalised on the grounds that hypersensitivity to prolactin is due to low levels of PGE$_1$.[15] High levels of linoleic acid and low levels of gamma-linolenic acid have been observed for patients with premenstrual syndrome. Several clinical studies have been reported and the conclusions vary from no beneficial effects being observed to marked improvements.[1–3,16]

Diabetic neuropathy Diabetes has been associated with reduced ability to desaturate EFAs, with deficits resulting in abnormal neuronal membrane structure. Animal studies have shown that diabetic neuropathy can be either prevented or reversed by the provision of gamolenic acid as evening primrose oil. In humans, a double-blind, placebo-controlled trial has demonstrated reversal of diabetic neuropathy by gamolenic acid.[17]

Multiple sclerosis The results of clinical trials on the use of evening primrose oil for the treatment of multiple sclerosis are contradictory.[1,2] Patients with recent onset or less severe forms of the disease are more likely to respond. Linoleic acid may have a beneficial effect on the severity and duration of relapses and on the progression of the disease.[1] It is suggested that linoleic acid is involved in the immunosuppressive effect at the cellular level and may be of use when combined with a low animal fat/high polyunsaturated fat diet.[2]

Rheumatoid arthritis A double-blind, randomly assigned trial has demonstrated a significant improvement in subjective symptoms of RA (indicated by a reduction in required NSAID treatment) in the active group receiving evening primrose oil compared to the placebo group. However, no objective changes were observed in any of the biochemical indicators of RA.[1–3]

Sjögren's syndrome This disease is associated with the loss of secretions from exocrine glands throughout the body, but especially from the salivary and lacrimal glands. One of the features of EFA deficiency is exocrine gland atrophy. Placebo-controlled trials have shown a modest improvement in tear flow together with relief of lethargy, a prominent feature of the syndrome.[1,3]

Coronary heart disease Abnormal intake and metabolism of EFAs (both *n*-3 and *n*-6) are thought to be important risk factors for CHD, resulting in enhanced cholesterol and triglyceride biosynthesis, enhanced platelet aggregation, and elevated blood pressure. Dietary supplementation with foods or oils rich in LA (*n*-6) or in marine (*n*-3) EFAs have been found to decrease significantly the risk of CHD, although it is considered that an optimum balance between *n*-3 and *n*-6 EFAs may well be important.[1–3,18] gamolenic acid has been reported to decrease blood pressure and platelet aggregation in both animal and human studies[3].

Renal disease Renal tissue is especially rich in EFAs, and prostaglandins of the E series are believed to be important in maintaining adequate renal blood flow. Administration of gamolenic acid to animals has been reported to prevent or attenuate renal damage. A single placebo-controlled trial involving post-renal transplant patients demonstrated better graft survival rate for the group receiving evening primrose oil (45 patients) compared to the placebo group (44 patients).[3]

Liver disease PGE$_1$ has been administered to patients with liver failure, and has been observed to exert some cytoprotective effect and to maintain the normal function of the liver. There is little experience of gamolenic acid supplementation in liver disease.[17]

Gastro-intestinal disorders A double-blind placebo-controlled crossover trial has indicated a beneficial effect of evening primrose oil on irritable bowel syndrome exacerbated by premenstrual syndrome. A beneficial effect superior to that of fish oil or placebo has been reported for evening primrose oil in ulcerative colitis. A protective effect of gamolenic acid against gastric ulceration has yet to be shown in humans.[3]

Viral infections/Post viral fatigue A single placebo-controlled study has demonstrated significant beneficial effects in patients with well-defined PVF receiving evening primrose oil compared to those on placebo. Symptoms arrested were muscle weakness, aches and pains, lack of concentration, exhaustion, memory loss, depression, dizziness, and vertigo.[1,3]

Endometriosis A placebo-controlled trial has shown that gamolenic acid in combination with eicosapentaenoic acid (*n*-3 EFA metabolite) reduced symptoms in 90% women, whereas 90% of the placebo group reported no relief from symptoms.[3]

Schizophrenia It is believed that EFAs, in particular PGE_1, antagonise the excessive central dopaminergic activity that is thought to be a possible cause of schizophrenia. Low concentrations of LA in plasma phospholipids have been observed in populations of schizophrenics from Ireland, England, Scotland, Japan, and the USA. It is thought that a poor recovery rate from the disease is associated with the presence of saturated fats in the diet, but not with unsaturated fats. Various open and placebo-controlled trials of gamolenic acid and DGLA supplementation have reportedly produced mixed results. Administration of evening primrose oil with co-factors known to be important in EFA metabolism (zinc, pyridoxine, niacin, and vitamin C) enhanced the improvements in memory loss, schizophrenic symptoms, and tardive dyskinesia that were observed in evening primrose oil-treated compared to placebo-treated patients.[1–3]

Alcoholism Evening primrose oil has been documented to reduce symptoms in the first three weeks of withdrawal, indicated by a reduced requirement for tranquillisers, and to significantly improve the rate of return to normal liver function. However, in the longer term, evening primrose did not affect the relapse rate.[3]

Dementia Alzheimer's disease and other forms of dementia are associated with low serum concentrations of EFAs. A single placebo-controlled trial in patients with Alzheimer's disease reported improvements in cerebral function in the evening primrose oil group compared to the placebo group.

Hyperactivity in children Hyperactive children tend to have abnormal levels of essential fatty acids. No improvements in behavioural patterns and no changes in blood fatty acids were observed in one trial with evening primrose oil.[2]

Cancer In-vitro studies have observed that malignant cells die following exposure to gamolenic acid and related fatty acids at concentrations that are non-lethal to normal cells. *In-vitro* studies have shown gamolenic acid to inhibit the growth of various human cancer cell lines, and *in-vivo* studies have described an inhibitory effect of gamolenic acid on tumour growth. Human studies are currently ongoing to assess the impact of gamolenic acid supplementation in various human cancers.[3]

Side-effects, Toxicity

Evening primrose oil appears to be well tolerated with very few side-effects reported, despite it being available for many years in a number of countries as a food supplement.[3] Mild gastro-intestinal effects, indigestion, nausea and softening of stools, and headache have occasionally occurred.[3,5] It has been noted that there may be an increased risk of temporal lobe epilepsy in schizophrenic patients being treated with epileptogenic drugs such as phenothiazines.[6] In cases of overdosage, symptoms of loose stools and abdominal pain have been noted. No special treatment is required.[6]

Toxicity studies have indicated evening primrose oil to be non-toxic.[3] The two principal components in evening primrose oil are LA and gamolenic acid. LA is commonly ingested as part of the diet. It has been estimated that the concentration of gamolenic acid provided by evening prim-rose oil is comparable to that metabolised in the body from normal dietary LA.[4] In addition, it has been calculated that a breastfed infant receives a higher proportion (mg/kg) of LA and gamolenic acid from human milk compared to that received from evening primrose oil.[4]

Contra-indications, Warnings

Evening primrose oil may have the potential to make manifest undiagnosed temporal lobe epilepsy, especially in schizophrenic patients and/or those who are already receiving known epileptogenic drugs such as phenothiazines.[6] No epileptic events have been reported in patients not being treated with phenothiazines.[6]

Pregnancy and lactation Animal studies have indicated evening primrose oil to be non-teratogenic.[6] However, data on the safety of evening primrose oil during human pregnancy are not available and therefore the risk of taking evening primrose oil during pregnancy should be carefully considered against the perceived benefit to the patient. Both LA and gamolenic acid are normally present in breast milk (see Side-effects, Toxicity) and therefore it is reasonable to assume that evening primrose oil may be taken while breast feeding.

Pharmaceutical Comment

Interest in the seed oil of the evening primrose plant lies in its essential fatty acid content, in particular in the linoleic acid (LA) and gamolenic acid (GLA) content. Both of these compounds are prostaglandin precursors and dietary gamolenic acid supplementation has been shown to increase the ratio of non-inflammatory:inflammatory prostaglandin compounds.

The use of evening primrose oil in various disease states associated with low gamolenic acid concentrations has been extensively investigated and a vast body of published literature is available. The beneficial effects of evening primrose oil in treating atopic eczema and and mastalgia (cyclical/non-cyclical) have been recognised with product licences granted to evening primrose oil-containing preparations for these indications.[6] However, doubt has also been expressed over the effectiveness of evening primrose oil in eczema.[2,9,10,11,19] Alternative natural oil sources such as blackcurrant or borage (but see monograph) that offer a higher gamolenic acid yield compared to evening primrose oil have been identified, although these oils have not been found to exhibit the same biological effects as those observed for evening primrose oil.[3]

Evening primrose oil is reported to be virtually non-toxic with only minor adverse effects such as headache and nausea occasionally associated with its use. The range of potential uses for evening primrose oil is extensive and results of further human studies are awaited to establish its efficacy in various therapeutic conditions.

References

See General References G32

1.   Li Wan Po A. Evening primrose oil. *Pharm J* 1991; **246:** 670–676

2.   Barber HJ. Evening primrose oil: a panacea? *Pharm J* 1988; **240:** 723–5.

3.   Horrobin DF. Gammalinolenic acid: an intermediate in essential fatty acid metabolism with potential as an ethical pharmaceutical and as a food. *Rev Contemp Pharmacother* 1990; **1:** 1–45.

4.   Carter JP. Gamma-linolenic acid as a nutrient. *Food Technology* 1988; 72.

5.   Briggs CJ. Evening primrose. *Rev Pharm Canad* 1986; **119:** 249–54.

6.   Anon. Data Sheet Compendium 1994–95, 1520-1. Efamast, Epogam, Epogam Paediatric (Searle).

7.   Lovell CR *et al*. Treatment of atopic eczema with evening primrose oil. *Lancet* 1981; **1:** 278.

8.   Schalin-Karrila M *et al*. Evening primrose oil in the treatment of atopic eczema : effect on clinical status, plasma phospholipid fatty acids and circulating blood prostaglandins. *Br J Dermatol* 1987; **117:** 11–19.

9.   McHenry PM *et al*. Management of atopic eczema. *Br Med J* 1995; **310:** 843–7.

10.   Bamford JTM *et al*. Atopic eczema unresponsive to evening primrose oil (linolenic and gamma-linolenic acids). *J Am Acad Dermatol* 1985; **13:** 959–65

11.   Berth-Jones J and Graham-Brown RAC. Placebo-controlled trial of essential fatty acid supplementation in atopic dermatitis. *Lancet* 1993; **341:** 1557–60.

12.   Wright S, Burton JL. Oral evening primrose seed oil improves atopic eczema. *Lancet* 1982; **ii:** 1120–2.

13.   Stewart JCM *et al*. Treatment of severe and moderately severe atopic dermatitis with evening primrose oil (Epogam); a multicentre study. *J Nutr Med* 1991; **2:** 9–15.

14.   Pye JK *et al*. Clinical experience of drug treatments for mastalgia. *Lancet* 1985; **ii:** 373–7.

15.   Brush MG. Efamol (evening primrose oil) in the treatment of the premenstrual syndrome. In: Clinical uses for essential fatty acids. Horrobin DF ed. Buffalo, New York: Eden Press, 1982, p.155.

16.   Horrobin DF.The role of essential fatty acids and prostaglandins in the premenstrual syndrome. *J Reprod Med* 1983; **28:** 465–8.

17.   Jamal GA *et al*. Gamma–linolenic acid in diabetic neuropathy. *Lancet* 1986; **i:** 1098.

18.   Horrobin DF and Manku MS. How do polyunsaturated fatty acids lower plasma cholesterol levels? *Lipids* 1983; **18:** 558–62.

19.   Anon. Gamolenic acid in atopic eczema: Epogam. *Drug Ther Bull* 1990; **28:** 69–70.

EYEBRIGHT

Species (Family)
Euphrasia species including
(i) *Euphrasia brevipila* Burnat & Gremli
(ii) *Euphrasia officinalis* L.
(iii) *Euphrasia rostkoviana* Hayne (Scrophulariaceae)

Synonym(s)
Euphrasia

Part(s) Used
Herb

Pharmacopoeial Monographs
BHP 1983
Martindale 28th edition

Legal Category (Licensed Products)
Not included on the GSL[G14]

Constituents[G1,G10,G18,G32]
Unless otherwise stated, constituents listed are for *E. officinalis*.
Acids Caffeic acid, ferulic acid.[1]
Alkaloids Unidentified tertiary alkaloids, choline, steam volatile bases[1]
Amino acids Glycine, leucine, valine
Flavonoids Four compounds (unidentified). Quercetin and rutin stated to be absent.[1] Quercetin, quercitrin, and rutin have been documented for *E. rostkoviana*.
Iridoids Aucubin 0.05%. Additional glycosides have been reported for related *Euphrasia* species including catalpol, euphroside, eurostoside, geniposide, ixoroside, and mussaenoside for *E. rostkoviana*.[2–5]
Phenethyl glycosides Dehydroconiferyl alcohol-4-β-D-glucoside[3] and eukovoside (3,4-dihydroxy-4-phenethyl-*O*-α-L-rhamnoside(1→3)-4-*O*-isoferuoyl-β-D-glucoside)[4] from *L. rostkoviana*
Tannins (about 12%). Condensed and hydrolysable; gallic acid is among the hydrolysis products.[1]
Volatile oils (about 0.2%). Seven major and numerous minor components, mainly unidentified; four of the major compounds are thought to be aldehydes or ketones.[1]
Other constituents Bitter principle, β-carotene, phytosterols (e.g. β-sitosterol, stigmasterol),[1] resin, carbohydrates (e.g. arabinose, glucose, galactose), vitamin C

Food Use
Eyebright is listed by the Council of Europe as a natural source of food flavouring (category N3). This category indicates that eyebright can be added to foodstuffs in the traditionally accepted manner, although there is insufficient information available for an adequate assessment of potential toxicity.[G9]

Herbal Use
Eyebright is stated to possess anticatarrhal, astringent, and anti-inflammatory properties. Traditionally it has been used for nasal catarrh, sinusitis, and specifically for conjunctivitis when applied locally as an eye lotion.[G1,G3,G32]

Dose
Dried herb 2–4 g or by infusion three times daily[G3]
Liquid extract (1:1 in 25% alcohol) 2–4 mL three times daily[G3]
Tincture (1:5 in 45% alcohol) 2–6 mL three times daily[G3]

Pharmacological Actions
Animal studies None documented for eyebright. Caffeic acid is bacteriostatic,[1] and a purgative action in mice has been documented for iridoid glycosides.[6] The purgative action of aucubin is approximately 0.05 times the potency of sennosides, with onset of diarrhoea stated to occur more than six hours after aucubin administration.[6] Tannins are known to possess astringent properties.

Side-effects, Toxicity
It has been stated that 10 to 60 drops of eyebright tincture could induce toxic symptoms including mental confusion and cephalalgia, raised pressure in the eyes with lachrymation, pruritus, redness, swelling of the eyelid margins, dim vision, photophobia, weakness, sneezing, nausea, toothache, constipation, cough, dyspnoea, insomnia, polyuria, and diaphoresis.[G10]

Contra-indications, Warnings
The use of eyebright for ophthalmic application has been discouraged.[G30]
Pregnancy and lactation The safety of eyebright has not been established. In view of the lack of pharmacological and toxicity data, the use of eyebright during pregnancy and lactation should be avoided.

Pharmaceutical Comment
Limited information is available regarding the constituents of eyebright, and it is unclear which *Euphrasia* species is most commonly utilised. In addition, eyebright is also used as a common name for plants other than *Euphrasia* species. Little scientific information was found to justify the reputed herbal uses, although tannin constituents would provide an astringent effect. The use of home-made preparations for ophthalmic purposes should be avoided. Little is known regarding the toxicity of eyebright and, in view of the reported presence of unidentified alkaloids, it should be used with caution avoiding excessive doses.

References
See General References G1, G3, G9, G10, G14, G18, G21, G30 and G32.

1.   Harkiss KJ, Timmins P. Studies in the Scrophulariaceae Part VIII. Phytochemical investigation of *Euphrasia officinalis*. *Planta Med* 1973; **23:** 342–7.

2.   Sticher O, Salama O. Iridoid glucosides from *Euphrasia rostkoviana*. *Planta Med* 1981; **42:** 122–3.

3.   Salama O *et al*. A lignan glucoside from *Euphrasia rostkoviana*. *Phytochemistry* 1981; **20:** 2003–4.

4.   Sticher O *et al*. Structure analysis of eukovoside, a new phenylpropanoid glycoside from *Euphrasia rostkoviana*. *Planta Med* 1982; **45:** 159.

5.   Salama O, Sticher O. Iridoidglucoside von *Euphrasia rostkoviana* 4. Mitteilung über Euphrasia-Glykoside. *Planta Med* 1983; **47:** 90–4.

6.   Inouye H *et al*. Purgative activities of iridoid glycosides. *Planta Med* 1974; **25:** 285–8.

FALSE UNICORN

Species (Family)
Chamaelirium luteum (L.) A. Gray (Liliaceae)

Synonym(s)
Blazing Star, Helonias, Starwort, *Chamaelirium carolianum* Wild., *Helonias dioica* Pursh., *Helonias lutea* Ker-Gawl., *Veratrum luteum* L.

Part(s) Used
Rhizome, Root

Pharmacopoeial Monographs
BHP 1983
BHP 1990

Legal Category (Licensed Products)
GSL[G14]

Constituents[G18,G24,G32]
Limited chemical information is available on false unicorn. It is stated to contain a steroidal saponin glycoside, chamaelirin, and another glycoside helonin.

Food Use
False unicorn is not used in foods.

Herbal Use
False unicorn is stated to possess an action on the uterus. Traditionally it has been used for ovarian dysmenorrhoea, leucorrhoea, and specifically for amenorrhoea. It is reported to be useful for vomiting of pregnancy and threatened miscarriage.[G3,G4,G32]

Dose
Dried rhizome/root 1–2g or by infusion three times daily[G3]

Liquid extract (1:1 in 45% alcohol) 1–2 mL three times daily[G3]

Tincture (1:5 in 45% alcohol) 2–5 mL three times daily[G3]

Pharmacological Actions
None documented.

Side-effects, Toxicity
No reported side-effects or documented toxicity studies were located. It is stated that large doses of false unicorn may cause nausea and vomiting.[G3]

Contra-indications, Warnings
None documented.

Pregnancy and lactation The safety of false unicorn has not been established. In view of the lack of phytochemical, pharmacological, and toxicity data, and its reputed action as a uterine tonic, the use of false unicorn during pregnancy and lactation should be avoided.

Pharmaceutical Comment
The chemistry of false unicorn is poorly documented and no scientific evidence was located to justify the herbal uses. In view of this and the lack of toxicity data, the use of false unicorn should be avoided.

References
See General References G3, G4, G14, G18, G24 and G32.

FENUGREEK

Species (Family)
Trigonella foenum-graecum L. (Leguminosae)

Synonym(s)
Bockshornsame

Part(s) Used
Seed

Pharmacopoeial Monographs
BHP 1983
BPC 1949
Martindale 30th edition
National pharmacopoeias—Aust. and Chin.

Legal Category (Licensed Products)
GSL[G14]

Constituents[G1,G19,G24,G32]
Alkaloids (pyridine-type) Gentianine, trigonelline (up to 0.13%), choline (0.05%)
Proteins and amino acids Protein (23–25%) containing high quantities of lysine and tryptophan. Free amino acids include 4-hydroxyisoleucine (0.09%), histidine, lysine, arginine
Flavonoids Flavone (apigenin, luteolin) glycosides including orientin and vitexin, quercetin (flavonol)
Saponins (0.6–1.7%). Glycosides yielding steroidal sapogenins diosgenin and yamogenin (major), with tigogenin, neotigogenin, gitogenin, neogitogenin, smilagenin, sarsasapogenin, yuccagenin;[1] fenugreekine, a sapogenin-peptide ester involving diosgenin and yamogenin;[2] trigofoenosides A-G (furostanol glycosides).[3–6]
Other constituents Coumarin,[7] lipids (5–8%),[10] mucilaginous fibre (50%),[10] vitamins (including nicotinic acid), minerals

Food Use
Fenugreek is listed by the Council of Europe as a natural source of food flavouring (category N2). This category indicates that fenugreek can be added to foodstuffs in small quantities, with a possible limitation of an active principle (as yet unspecified) in the final product.[G9] In the USA, fenugreek extracts are permitted in foods at concentrations usually below 0.05%. In addition, fenugreek is listed as GRAS (Generally Regarded As Safe) in the USA.

Herbal Use
Fenugreek is stated to possess mucilaginous demulcent, laxative, nutritive, expectorant and orexigenic properties, and has been used topically as an emollient and vulnerary. Traditionally, it has been used in the treatment of anorexia, dyspepsia, gastritis, and convalescence, and topically for furunculosis, myalgia, lymphadenitis, gout, wounds, and leg ulcers.[G1,G3,G10,G32]

Dose
Seed 1–6 g or equivalent three times daily[G25]

Pharmacological Actions
Animal studies Hypocholesterolaemic activity has been reported for fenugreek in rats[8,G19] and alloxan-diabetic dogs.[9] Activity has been attributed to the fibre and saponin fractions, and not to lipid or amino acid fractions.[8,9] Studies have reported a reduction in cholesterol but not triglyceride concentrations,[8] or in both cholesterol and triglyceride concentrations but without significant alterations in HDL and LDL concentrations.[9]

Hypoglycaemic activity has been observed in rabbits, rats, and dogs, and attributed to the defatted seed fraction (DSF),[10] trigonelline, nicotinic acid, and coumarin.[7,11] Oral administration of DSF reduced hyperglycaemia in four alloxan-diabetic dogs, and reduced the response to an oral glucose tolerance test in eight normal dogs, whereas the lipid fraction had no effect on serum glucose and insulin concentrations.[10] The high fibre content (50%) of DSF was thought to contribute to its antidiabetic effect although the initial rate of glucose absorption was not affected.[10] Nicotinic acid and coumarin were reported to be the major hypoglycaemic components of fenugreek seeds, following administration to normal and alloxan-diabetic rats.[7] The hypoglycaemic action exhibited by coumarin was still significant 24 hours post-administration.[7] In addition, a slight antidiuretic action was noted for coumarin.[7] Trigonelline inhibited cortisone-induced hyperglycaemia in rabbits if administered (250 mg/kg) concomitantly or two hours before, but not 2 hours after, cortisone.[11] In addition, trigonelline exhibited significant hypoglycaemic activity in alloxan-diabetic rats (50 mg/kg), lasting 24 hours.[11]

A stimulant action on the isolated uterus (guinea-pig), especially during late pregnancy, has been noted for both aqueous and alcoholic extracts.[G19] An aqueous extract is stated to increase the number of heart beats in the isolated mammalian heart.[G19]

In-vitro antiviral activity against vaccinia virus has been reported for fenugreekine, which also possesses cardiotonic, hypoglycaemic, diuretic, antiphlogistic, and antihypertensive properties.[2]

Human studies A transient hypoglycaemic effect was observed in 5 of 10 diabetic patients who received 500 mg oral trigonelline whilst fasting.[11] Increasing the dose did not increase this effect, and 500 mg ingested three times a day for 5 days did not alter the diurnal blood-glucose concentration.[11] Hypoglycaemic activity in healthy individuals has been reported for whole seed extracts, with slightly lesser activity exhibited by gum isolate, extracted seeds, and cooked seeds.[12] The addition of fenugreek to an oral glucose tolerance test reduced serum glucose and insulin concentrations. Chronic ingestion (21 days) of extracted seeds (25 g seeds daily incorporated into two meals) by non-insulin-dependent diabetics improved plasma glucose and insulin responses (no control group), and reduced 24-hour urinary glucose concentrations.[12] Furthermore, in two diabetic insulin-dependent subjects, daily administration of 25 g fenugreek seed powder reduced fasting plasma-glucose profile, glycosuria, and daily insulin requirements (56 to 20 units) after 8 weeks. A significant reduction in serum-cholesterol concentrations in diabetic patients was also noted.[12]

Side-effects, Toxicity

No reported side-effects were located for fenugreek. Acute toxicity values (LD_{50}) documented for fenugreek alcoholic seed extract are 5 g/kg (rat, oral), and 2 g/kg (rabbit, dermal).[13] The alcoholic seed extract is reported to be non-irritating and non-sensitising to human skin, and non-phototoxic (mice, pigs).[13] Coumarin is a toxic seed component.[7] Acute LD_{50} (rat, oral) values per kg documented for various seed constituents are 5 g (trigonelline), 8.8 g (nicotinic acid), 7.4 g (nicotinamide), and 0.72 g (coumarin).[7]

Contra-indications, Warnings

Hypoglycaemic activity has been reported for fenugreek, which may therefore interfere with existing hypoglycaemic therapy. Caution is advisable in patients receiving MAOI, hormonal or anticoagulant therapies in view of amine, steroidal saponin and coumarin constituents respectively, although their clinical significance is unclear. Cardioactivity has been documented *in vitro*. The absorption of drugs taken concomitantly with fenugreek may be affected (high mucilaginous fibre content).

Pregnancy and lactation Fenugreek is reputed to be oxytocic[G10] and *in-vitro* uterine stimulant activity has been documented. In view of this, and the documented pharmacologically active components, the use of fenugreek during pregnancy and lactation in doses greatly exceeding those normally encountered in foods is not advisable.

Pharmaceutical Comment

Fenugreek seeds contain a high proportion of mucilaginous fibre, together with various other pharmacologically active compounds including steroidal and amine components. The majority of the traditional uses of fenugreek are probably attributable to the mucilage content. In addition, hypocholesterolaemic and hypoglycaemic actions have been documented for fenugreek in both laboratory animals and humans. The mechanism by which fenugreek exerts these

actions is unclear. Proposed theories include a reduction in carbohydrate absorption by the mucilaginous fibre,[12] and an effect on cholesterol metabolism, cholesterol absorption and bile acid excretion by the saponin components.[8] Toxicity studies indicate fenugreek seeds to be relatively non-toxic, although the presence of pharmacologically active constituents would suggest that excessive ingestion is inadvisable.

References

See General References G1, G3, G6, G9, G10, G14, G18, G19, G22, G23, G24, G25, and G32.

1. Gupta RK *et al*. Minor steroidal sapogenins from fenugreek seeds, *Trigonella foenum-graecum*. *J Nat Prod* 1986; **49:** 1153.

2. Ghosal S *et al*. Fenugreekine, a new steroidal sapogenin-peptide ester of *Trigonella foenum-graecum*. *Phytochemistry* 1974; **13:** 2247–51.

3. Gupta RK *et al*. Two furostanol saponins from *Trigonella feonum-graecum*. *Phytochemistry* 1986; **25:** 2205–7.

4. Varshney IP *et al*. Saponins from *Trigonella foenum-graucum* leaves. *J Nat Prod* 1984; **47:** 44–6.

5. Gupta RK *et al*. Furostanol glycosides from *Trigonella foenum-graecum* seeds. *Phytochemistry* 1984; **23:** 2605–7.

6. Gupta RK *et al*. Furostanol glycosides from *Trigonella foenum-graecum* seeds. *Phytochemistry* 1985; **24:** 2399–2401.

7. Shani J *et al*. Hypoglycaemic effect of *Trigonella foenum graecum* and *Lupinus termis* (Leguminosae) seeds and their major alkaloids in alloxan-diabetic and normal rats. *Arch Int Pharmacodyn Ther* 1974; **210:** 27–37.

8. Sharma RD. An evaluation of hypocholesterolemic factor of fenugreek seeds (*T. foenum graecum*) in rats. *Nutr Rep Int* 1986; **33:** 669–77.

9. Ribes G *et al*. Hypocholesterolaemic and hypotriglyceridaemic effects of subfractions from fenugreek seeds in alloxan diabetic dogs. *Phytotherapy Res* 1987; **1:** 38–42.

10. Ribes G *et al*. Effects of fenugreek seeds on endocrine pancreatic secretions in dogs. *Ann Nutr Metab* 1984; **28:** 37–43.

11. Mishkinsky J *et al*. Hypoglycaemic effect of trigonelline. *Lancet* 1967; **2:** 1311–12.

12. Sharma RD. Effect of fenugreek seeds and leaves on blood glucose and serum insulin responses in human subjects. *Nutr Res* 1986; **6:** 1353–64.

13. Opdyke DLJ. Fenugreek absolute. *Food Cosmet Toxicol* 1978; **16**(Suppl): 755–6.

FEVERFEW

Species (Family)

Tanacetum parthenium (L.) Schultz Bip. (Asteraceae/Compositae)

Synonym(s)

Altamisa, *Chrysanthemum parthenium* (L.) Bernh., *Leucanthemum parthenium* (L.) Gren & Godron, *Pyrethrum parthenium* (L.) Sm.[28]

Part(s) Used

Leaf, Aerial parts

Pharmacopoeial Monographs

BHP 1990
Martindale 30th edition

Legal Category (Licensed Products)

Feverfew is not included on the GSL[G14]

Constituents[G2,G10,G25,G32]

Terpenoids Sesquiterpene lactones: germacranolides(GE), guaianolides(GU) and eudesmanolides(EU). The structural feature common to all three types is an α-unsaturated γ-lactone moiety, and examples of each type include parthenolide, 3-β-hydroxy-parthenolide, costunolide, 3-β-hydroxycostunolide, artemorin, 8-α-hydroxyestafiatin and chrysanthemonin (novel dimeric nucleus) (GE); artecanin, chrysanthemin A (canin) and B (stereoisomers), chrysanthemolide, partholide, 2 chlorine-containing sesquiterpene lactones (GU); magnolialide, reynosin, santamarine, 1-β-hydroxyarbusculin and 5-β-hydroxyreynosin (EU)[1–5]
Volatile oils (0.02–0.07%). Various monoterpene and sesquiterpene components (e.g. camphor, borneol, α-pinene derivatives, germacrene, farnesene and their esters)
Other constituents Pyrethrin, flavonoids, tannins (type unspecified)

Food Use

Feverfew is not generally used in foods.

Herbal Use

Feverfew has traditionally been used in the treatment of migraine, tinnitus, vertigo, arthritis, fever, menstrual disorders, difficulty during labour, stomach ache, toothache, and insect bites.[G2,G4,G25,G32]

Dose

Limited information is available regarding the traditional dose of feverfew. The dose that has been recommended for migraine prophylaxis is:
Leaf (fresh) 2.5 leaves daily with or after food
Leaf (freeze-dried) 50 mg daily with or after food[5]
Aerial parts (dried) 50–200 mg daily [G2]

Pharmacological Actions

Animal studies Feverfew extracts have been documented to inhibit platelet aggregation and prostaglandin, thromboxane, and leukotriene production, although feverfew has also been reported to have no effect on cyclo-oxygenase (the mechanism by which non-steroidal anti-inflammatory drugs inhibit prostaglandin production).[6–8] Instead, feverfew is thought to act by inhibiting the enzyme phospholipase A_2, which facilitates the release of arachidonic acid from the phospholipid cellular membrane.[7–9] The clinical significance of this action has been questioned.[10] In addition, *in-vitro* experiments have shown that feverfew extracts inhibit the interaction of human platelets with collagen substrates.[11,12] Feverfew has been shown to inhibit granule secretion in blood platelets and neutrophils, which has been associated with the aetiology of migraine and rheumatoid arthritis, respectively.[13] Feverfew was also found to inhibit the release of vitamin B_{12}-binding protein from polymorphonuclear leucocytes, but to be ineffective against platelet and polymorphonucleocyte secretion induced by calcium ionophore A2318.[13] Sesquiterpene lactone constituents of feverfew containing an α-methylene butyrolactone unit are thought to be responsible for the antisecretory activity.[14] Their inhibitory effect on platelet aggregation is thought to involve neutralisation of sulphydryl groups on specific enzymes of proteins that are necessary for platelet aggregation and secretion.[15] A similar mode of action has been proposed for the inhibitory action of feverfew on polymorphonuclocyte secretion.[16] In addition, feverfew extracts have been reported to produce a dose-dependent inhibition of anti-IgE-induced histamine release from mast cells.[17] The authors concluded that the mechanism of action of the feverfew extract was different to that of both cromoglycate and quercetin.

The presence of high numbers of lymphocytes and monocytes in the synovium is considered to be of significance in rheumatoid arthritis.[18] Feverfew extract and parthenolide have been documented to inhibit mitogen-induced proliferation of human peripheral blood mononuclear cells and mitogen-induced PGE_2 production by synovial cells.[18] The feverfew extract and parthenolide also proved to be cytotoxic to mitogen treated peripheral blood mononuclear cells and the authors considered that this cytotoxicity was responsible for the actions observed.[18]

Parthenolide has been documented to have cytotoxic activity in Eagle's 9KB carcinoma of the nasopharynx cell culture system, the activity being associated with the presence of an α-methylene-γ-lactone moiety in the molecule.[19]

Antimicrobial properties against Gram-positive bacteria, yeasts, and filamentous fungi *in vitro* have been documented for parthenolide.[20] Gram-negative bacteria were not affected.

Human studies Two documented clinical trials have investigated the use of feverfew to treat migraine.[21,22] Johnson *et* al[21] recruited 17 patients who had been successfully controlling their migraine by eating raw feverfew leaves for at least 3 months into a double-blind placebo-controlled trial. Patients either continued to receive feverfew (50 mg daily) or were given a placebo for six periods of 4 weeks. The authors reported that the placebo group experienced a significant increase in the frequency and severity of headache. Those given the feverfew showed no change. It was suggested that the placebo group were in fact suffering withdrawal symptoms from feverfew and a 'Post-Feverfew Syndrome' was described (see Side-effects, Toxicity). Murphy et al[22] carried out a randomised double-blind, placebo-controlled cross-over study with 72 volunteers. Adults who had suffered from migraine for more than 2 years and who had at least one attack per month were eligible for the study. The only concurrent medication allowed was the oral contraceptive. Patients completed a 1 month single-blind placebo run-in followed by 4 months placebo/active and 4 months crossover. The authors reported that patients experienced a 24% reduction in the number of attacks during feverfew treatment (one capsule daily; 70 to 114 mg feverfew equivalent to 2.19 µg parthenolide) although the duration of each individual attack was not significantly affected. Interestingly, patients allocated to the active and then placebo group did not experience the withdrawal symptoms documented by Johnson et al,[21] although feverfew use had been over a longer period of time in these latter patients. A double-blind, placebo-controlled non-crossover trial studying the use of feverfew in rheumatoid arthritis has also been documented.[23] Forty-one female patients with inflammatory joint symptoms inadequately controlled by non-steroidal anti-inflammatory drugs were given either one feverfew capsule (70 to 86 mg equivalent to 2 to 3 µmol parthenolide) daily or one placebo capsule for 6 weeks. Current non-steroidal therapy was maintained. It was concluded that patients in the trial had experienced no additional benefit from feverfew.[22] The authors commented that while concomitant non-steroidal anti-inflammatory drug therapy has been stated to reduce the effectiveness of feverfew, the majority of rheumatoid arthritis sufferers will use feverfew to supplement existing therapy.

Side-effects, Toxicity

The following side-effects were documented in a double-blind placebo-controlled trial[21]: mouth ulcers, dry and sore tongue, swollen lips and mouth with loss of taste, unpleasant and bitter taste, abdominal pain and indigestion, diarrhoea, flatulence, nausea and vomiting, and hypersensitivity reactions. No significant side-effects were reported in another study, which produced a higher occurrence of mouth ulcers in the placebo group.[22] A 'Post-Feverfew Syndrome' has been described[21] (see Human Studies) with

symptoms such as nervousness, tension headaches, insomnia, stiffness/pain in joints and tiredness.

The onset of side-effects with feverfew is reported to vary, with symptoms becoming apparent within the first week of treatment, or appearing gradually over the first two months. Sesquiterpene lactones that contain an α-methylene butyrolactone ring are known to cause allergic reactions.[24,G26] Compounds with this structure are present in feverfew and reports of contact dermatitis have been documented.[25–28] No documented allergic reactions following oral ingestion were located.

An LD_{50} value for feverfew has not been estimated. No adverse effects were reported for rats and guinea-pigs receiving feverfew at doses 100 and 150 times the human daily dose, respectively.[29] No chronic toxicity studies have been reported. However, detailed haematological analysis of 60 feverfew users, some of whom had used feverfew for more than one year, did not show any significant differences when compared to that of controls.[29] A human toxicity study has investigated whether the sesquiterpene lactones in feverfew induce chromosomal or other changes in normal human cells of individuals who have taken the herb.[30] The study compared 30 chronic female feverfew users (leaves, tablets or capsules taken daily for more than 11 consecutive months) with matched non-users. The results of lymphocyte cultures established from blood samples taken over a period of several months were stated to indicate that feverfew affects neither the frequency of chromosomal aberrations nor the frequency of sister chromatid exchanges in the circulating peripheral lymphocytes.

Contra-indications, Warnings

Feverfew is contra-indicated in individuals with a known hypersensitivity to other members of the family Compositae (Asteraceae), such as chamomile, ragweed, and yarrow. Feverfew should not be ingested by individuals who develop a rash on contact with the plant.

Feverfew should only be considered as a treatment for migraine that has proved unresponsive to conventional forms of medication. Although traditionally recommended as a remedy for rheumatic conditions, self-medication with feverfew should not be undertaken without first consulting a doctor.

Pregnancy and lactation Feverfew is contra-indicated during pregnancy. It is reputed to be an abortifacient and to affect the menstrual cycle. It is documented to modify menstural flow, cause abortion in cattle, and induce uterine-contraction in full-term women.[G10,12]

Pharmaceutical Comment

Feverfew is characterised by the sesquiterpene lactone constituents, in particular by parthenolide which is thought to be the main active component. Numerous *in-vitro* studies have supported the reputation of feverfew as a herb used to treat migraine and arthritis. Studies with human volunteers have indicated that feverfew may be a useful prophylactic remedy against migraine,[31,32] although it has been recommended that feverfew should only be used by sufferers who have proved unresponsive to conventional forms of migraine treatment. Those using feverfew as a remedy for migraine should preferably do so under medical supervision. Results of a study that investigated the usefulness of feverfew in treating rheumatoid arthritis were less encouraging: feverfew provided no additional benefit when added to existing non-steroidal anti-inflammatory treatment. Feverfew products currently available are unlicensed and vary in their recommended daily doses.[29-] Furthermore, variation between the stated and actual amount of feverfew in commercial products (based on their ability to inhibit platelet secretion) has been reported.[12]

References

See General References G2, G4, G9, G10, G12, G14, G23, G25, G26, G32 and G33.

1. Stefanovic M *et al*. Sesquiterpene lactones from the domestic plant species Tanacetum parthenium L. (Compositae). *J Serb Chem Soc* 1985; **50:** 435–41.

2. Bohlmann F, Zdero C. Sesquiterpene lactones and other constituents from *Tanacetum parthenium. Phytochemistry* 1982: **21:** 2543–9.

3. Osawa T, Taylor D. Revised structure and stereochemistry of chrysartemin B. *Tetrahedron Lett* 1977; **13:** 1169–72.

4. Hylands DM, Hylands PJ. New sesquiterpene lactones from feverfew. *Phytochemical Society of Europe Symposium*, 1986; P17.

5. Wagner H *et al*. New chlorine-containing sesquiterpene lactones from *Chrysanthemum parthenium. Planta Med* 1988; **54:** 171–2.

6. Collier HOJ *et al*. Extract of feverfew inhibits prostaglandin biosynthesis. *Lancet* 1980; **ii:** 922–73.

7. Makheja AM, Bailey JM. The active principle in feverfew. *Lancet* 1981; **ii,** 1054.

8. Capasso F. The effect of an aqueous extract of *Tanacetum parthenium* L. on arachidonic acid metabolism by rat peritoneal leucocytes. *J Pharm Pharmacol* 1986; **38:** 71–2.

9. Makheja AM, Bailey JM. A platelet phospholipase inhibitor from the medicinal herb feverfew (*Tanacetum parthenium*). *Prostaglandins Leukot Med* 1982; **8:** 653–60.

10. Biggs MJ *et al*. Platelet aggregation in patients using feverfew for migraine. *Lancet* 1982; **ii:** 776.

11. Loesche W *et al*. Feverfew — an antithrombotic drug? *Folia Haematol* 1988; **115:** 181–4.

12. Groenewegen WA, Heptinstall S. Amounts of feverfew in commercial preparations of the herb. *Lancet* 1986; **i:** 44–5.

13. Heptinstall S *et al*. Extracts of feverfew inhibit granule secretion in blood platelets and polymorphonuclear leucocytes. *Lancet* 1985; **i:** 1071–3.

14. Groenewegen WA *et al*. Compounds extracted from feverfew that have anti-secretory activity contain an α-methylene butyrolactone unit. *J Pharm Pharmacol* 1986; **38:** 709–12.

15. Heptinstall S *et al*. Extracts of feverfew may inhibit platelet behaviour via neutralization of sulphydryl groups. *J Pharm Pharmacol* 1987; **39:** 459–65.

16. Lösche W *et al*. Inhibition of the behaviour of human polynuclear leukocytes by an extract of *Chrysanthemum parthenium. Planta Med* 1988; **54:** 381–384.

17. Hayes NA, Foreman JC. The activity of compounds extracted from feverfew on histamine release from rat mast cells. *J Pharm Pharmacol* 1987; **39:** 466–70.

18. O'Neill LAJ *et al*. Extracts of feverfew inhibit mitogen-induced human peripheral blood mononuclear cell proliferation and cytokine mediated responses: a cytotoxic effect. *Br J Clin Pharmac* 1987; **23:** 81–3.

19. Berry MI. Feverfew faces the future. *Pharm J* 1984; **232:** 611–14.

20. Blakeman JP, Atkinson P. Antimicrobial properties and possible role in host-pathogen interactions of parthenolide, a sesquiterpene lactone isolated from glands of *Chrysanthemum parthenium. Physiol Plant Pathol* 1979; **15:** 183–92.

21. Johnson ES *et al*. Efficacy of feverfew as prophylactic treatment of migraine. *Br med J* 1985; **291:** 569–73.

22. Murphy JJ *et al*. Randomised double-blind placebo-controlled trial of feverfew in migraine prevention. *Lancet* 1988; **ii:** 189–92.

23. Pattrick M *et al*. Feverfew in rheumatoid arthritis: a double blind, placebo controlled study. *Ann Rheum Dis* 1989; **48:** 547–9.

24. Rodríguez E *et al*. The role of sesquiterpene lactones in contact hypersensitivity to some North and South American species of feverfew (*Parthenium* – Compositae). *Contact Dermatitis* 1977; **3:** 155–162.

25. Burry J. Compositae dermatitis in South Australia: Contact dermatitis from *Chrysanthemum parthenium. Contact Dermatitis* 1980; **6:** 445.

26. Mitchell JC *et al*. Allergic contact dermatitis caused by *Artemisia* and *Chrysanthemum* species. The role of sesquiterpene lactones. *J Invest Dermatol* 1971; **56:** 98–101.

27. Schmidt RJ, Kingston T. Chrysanethemum dermatitis in South Wales; diagnosis by patch testing with feverfew (*Tanacetum parthenium*) extract. *Contact Dermatitis* 1985; **13:** 120–7.

28. Mensing H *et al*. Airborne contact dermatitis. *Der Hautarzt* 1985; **36:** 398–402.

29. Baldwin CA *et al*. What pharmacists should know about feverfew. *Pharm J* 1987; **239:** 237–8

30. Johnson ES *et al*. Investigation of possible genetoxic effects of feverfew in migraine patients. *Hum Toxicol* 1987; **6:** 533–4.

31. Awang DVC. Feverfew fever—a headache for the consumer. *Herbalgram* 1993; No.29: 34–36,66.

32. Berry M. Feverfew. *Pharm J* 1994; **253:** 806–8.

FIGWORT

Species (Family)

Scrophularia nodosa L. (Scrophulariaceae)

Synonym(s)

Common Figwort, Scrophularia

Part(s) Used

Herb

Pharmacopoeial Monographs

BHP 1983

Legal Category (Licensed Products)

Figwort is not included on the GSL[G14]

Constituents[G31,32]

Amino acids Alanine, isoleucine, leucine, lysine, phenylalanine, threonine, tyrosine, valine[1]

Flavonoids Diosmetin, diosmin, acacetin rhamnoside[2]

Iridoids Aucubin, acetylharpagide, harpagide, harpagoside, isoharpagoside, procumbid, and a catalpol glycoside.[3-5] Figwort is stated to have the same qualitative iridoid composition as devil's claw, but about half the content of harpagoside.

Acids Various acids including caffeic acid, cinnamic acid, ferulic acid, sinapic acid and vanillic acid, present as both esters and glycosides[6,7]

Food Use

Figwort is not used in foods.

Herbal Use

Figwort is stated to act as a dermatological agent and a mild diuretic, and to increase myocardial contraction. Traditionally, it has been used for chronic skin disease, and specifically for eczema, psoriasis, and pruritus.[G3,G32]

Dose

Dried herb 2–8 g by infusion[G3]

Liquid extract (1:1 in 25% alcohol) 2–8 mL[G3]

Tincture (1:10 in 45% alcohol) 2–4 mL[G3]

Pharmacological Actions

Animal studies The iridoid glycosides aucubin and catalpol have been documented to exert a purgative action in mice.[8] Cardioactive properties and anti-inflammatory activity have been claimed for harpagide and the other iridoid constituents (*see* Devil's claw).[G31]

Human studies None documented. The iridoids are stated to be bitter principles.[G31]

Side-effects, Toxicity

None documented.

Contra-indications, Warnings

Figwort should be avoided in ventricular tachycardia.[G3] The recommendation that devil's claw should not be taken by diabetics may also apply to figwort, in view of their similar constituents.

Pregnancy and lactation The safety of figwort has not been established. In view of the lack of pharmacological and toxicity data, use of figwort during pregnancy and lactation should be avoided.

Pharmaceutical Comment

The chemistry of figwort is well studied and it is stated to be an acceptable substitute for devil's claw (*Harpagophytum procumbens*) with the same qualitative composition of bitter principles but half the content of harpagoside.[G31] Little scientific evidence was located to justify the herbal uses. In view of the lack of toxicity data and possible cardioactive properties, excessive use of figwort should be avoided.

References

See General References G3, G14, G31 and G32.

1. Toth L *et al*. Amino acids in Scrophulariaceae species. *Bot Kozl* 1977; **64**: 43–52.

2. Marczal G *et al*. Flavonoids as biologically active agents and their occurrence in the Scrophulariaceae family. *Acta Pharm Hung* 1974; **44**(Suppl): 83–90.

3. Swann K, Melville C. Iridoid content of some *Scrophularia* species. *J Pharm Pharmacol* 1972; **24**: 170P.

4. Swiatek L. Iridoid glycosides in the Scrophulariaceae family. *Acta Pol Pharm* 1973; **30**: 203–12.

5. Weinges K, Von der Eltz H. Natural products from medicinal plants. XXIII. Iridoid glycosides from Scrophularia nodosa L. *Justus Liebigs Ann Chem* 1978; **12**: 1968–73.

6. Swiatek L. Phenolic acids of underground parts of Scrophularia nodosa. *Pol J Pharmacol Pharm* 1973; **25**: 461–4.

7. Swiatek L. Pharmacobotanical investigations of some Scrophulariaceae species. *Diss Pharm Pharmacol* 1970; **22**: 321–8.

8. Inouye H *et al*. Purgative activities of iridoid glucosides. *Planta Med* 1974; **25**:285–288.

FRANGULA

Species (Family)
Rhamnus frangula L. (Rhamnaceae)

Synonym(s)
Alder Buckthorn, *Frangula alnus* Mill.

Part(s) Used
Bark

Pharmacopoeial Monographs
BHP 1983
BHP 1990
BPC 1949
Martindale 30th edition
National pharmacopoeias—Aust., Belg., Br., Cz., Eur., Fr., Ger., Gr., Hung., It., Neth., Nord., Pol., Rom., Rus., Swiss, and Yug. Br. also describes Powdered Frangula Bark.

Legal Category (Licensed Products)
GSL[G14]

Constituents[G1,G2,G10,G19,G24,G29,G31,G32]
Anthraquinones (3–7%). Frangulosides as major components including frangulin A and B (emodin glycosides) and glucofrangulin A and B (emodin diglycosides); emodin derivatives including emodin dianthrone and its monorhamnoside, palmidin C (*see* Rhubarb) and its monorhamnoside, emodin glycoside; also glycosides of chrysophanol and physcione, and various free aglycones.
Other constituents Flavonoids, tannins

Food Use
Frangula is listed by the Council of Europe as a natural source of food flavouring (category N4). While this category recognises the use of frangula as a flavouring agent, it indicates that there is insufficient information available to classify it further into categories N1, N2, or N3.[G9]

Herbal Use
Frangula is stated to possess mild purgative properties and has been used traditionally for constipation.[G1,G2,G3,G4,G32]

Dose
Dried Bark 0.5–2.5 g [G2]
Liquid extract (1:1 in 25% alcohol) 2–5 mL three times daily[G3]

Pharmacological Actions
The pharmacological activity of frangula can be attributed to the anthraquinone glycoside constituents. The laxative action of these compounds is well recognised (*see* Senna).

Side-effects, Toxicity[G34]
None documented specifically for frangula or frangulosides. *See* Senna for side-effects and toxicity associated with anthraquinones.

Contra-indications, Warnings
See Senna for contra-indications and warnings associated with anthraquinones.
Pregnancy and lactation The use of stimulant laxatives, particularly unstandardised preparations, is not generally recommended during pregnancy (*see* Senna).

Pharmaceutical Comment
The chemistry of frangula is characterised by the anthraquinone glycoside constituents. The laxative action of these compounds is well recognised and supports the herbal use of frangula as a laxative. The use of non-standardised anthraquinone-containing preparations should be avoided, since their pharmacological effect will be variable and unpredictable. In particular, the use of products containing combinations of anthraquinone laxatives should be avoided.

References
See General References G1, G2, G3, G4, G6, G9, G10, G14, G19, G22, G24, G29, G31, G32 and G34.

FUCUS

Species (Family)
Fucus vesiculosus L. and other *Fucus* species (Fucaceae)

Synonym(s)
Black Tang, Bladderwrack, Kelp, Kelpware, Rockweed, Seawrack

Brown seaweeds refer to species of *Fucus*, *Ascophyllum*, *Laminaria*, and *Macrocystis*. 'Kelps' refer to species of *Laminaria* and *Macrocystis*, although kelp is often used in reference to species of *Fucus*.

Part(s) Used
Thallus (whole plant)

Pharmacopoeial Monographs
BHP 1983
BHP 1990
BPC 1949
Martindale 28th edition

Legal Category (Licensed Products)
GSL[G14]

Constituents[G1,G2,G32]
Carbohydrates Polysaccharides: alginic acid (algin) as the major component; fucoidan and laminarin (sulphated polysaccharide esters).[1]

Iodine Content of various *Laminaria* species has been reported as 0.07–0.76% of dry weight.[2]

Other constituents Various vitamins and minerals, particularly ascorbic acid (vitamin C) (0.013–0.077% of fresh material).[2]

Food Use
Seaweeds are commonly included in the diet of certain populations. The gelling properties of alginic acid, the major polysaccharide in brown seaweeds including fucus, are extensively utilised in the dairy and baking industries to improve texture, body and smoothness of products.[1] Fucus is listed by the Council of Europe as a natural source of food flavouring (category N2). This category indicates that fucus can be added to foodstuffs in small quantities, with a possible limitation of an active principle (as yet unspecified) in the final product.[G9]

Herbal Use
Fucus is stated to possess antihypothyroid, anti-obesic and antirheumatic properties. Traditionally, it has been used for lymphadenoid goitre, myxoedema, obesity, arthritis, and rheumatism.[G1,G2,G3,G4,G32]

Dose
Dried thallus 5–10 g or infusion three times daily[G2,G3]

Liquid extract (1:1 in 25% alcohol) 4–8 mL three times daily[G2,G3]

Pharmacological Actions
There is a paucity of information documented specifically for *Fucus vesiculosus*, although pharmacological activities are recognised for individual constituents and other brown seaweed species.

Alginic acid is a hydrophilic colloidal substance that swells to approximately 25–35 times its original bulk in an alkaline environment and as such exerts a bulk laxative action.[3] It is stated to compare favourably with the carboxylic type of cation exchange resins. The colloidal properties of alginates have been utilised in wound dressings and skin grafts.[3]

Anticoagulant properties have been documented for brown seaweeds.[3] The glucose polymer laminarin has been identified as the anticoagulant principle in a Laminaria species.[4] A fucoidan fraction has been isolated from *Fucus vesiculosus* with 40–50% blood anticoagulant activity of heparin.[5]

The iodine content of seaweeds is well recognised. The low incidence of goitre amongst maritime people has been attributed to the inclusion of seaweeds in their diet.[3,4] Similarly, the traditional use of *Fucus vesiculosus* in 'slimming teas' is thought to be attributable to the effect of iodine on hypothyroidism.[4]

Extracts of various brown seaweeds including *Ascophyllum nodosum* and *Fucus vesiculosus* have been reported to exhibit a high *in-vitro* inhibitory activity towards mammalian digestive enzymes (α-amylase, trypsin, and lipase) isolated from the porcine pancreas.[6] Activity was attributed to high molecular weight (30 000–100 000) polyphenols.[6]

Inhibitory effects of laminarin sulphate on lipidaemia and atherosclerosis (*in-vivo*, rabbit) have been partially attributed to the *in-vitro* inhibition of lipid synthesis observed in cultured chick aortic cells.[7]

Hypotensive activity observed in rats intravenously administered extracts of commercial seaweed (*Laminaria* species) preparations has been attributed to their histamine content.[8] However, histamine concentrations varied considerably between preparations, and authentic specimens of the *Laminaria* species were devoid of histamine.

Kelp extracts have antiviral activity [9] and laminarin is reported to have exhibited some tumour-inhibiting actions.[1]

Side-effects, Toxicity
Hyperthyroidism has been associated with the ingestion of kelp and is attributable to the iodine content in the plant.[10, 11] Typical symptoms of hyperthyroidism (weight loss, sweating, fatigue, frequent soft stools) were exhibited by a 72-year-old woman following 6 months ingestion of a commercial kelp product.[10] Laboratory tests confirmed the hyperthyroidism although no pre-existing evidence of thy-

roid disease was found and the condition resolved in 6 months following discontinuation of the tablets. Analysis of the kelp tablets reported an iodine content of 0.7 mg/tablet representing a daily intake of 2.8–4.2 mg iodine.[10] Clinically evident hyperthyroidism developed in an otherwise healthy woman following the daily ingestion of six 200 mg kelp tablets.[11] Symptoms gradually resolved on cessation of therapy.

The association between halogen salts and acneiform eruptions is well established.[12] Ingestion of kelp products has been associated with the worsening of pre-existing acne and the development of acneiform eruptions, which improved following withdrawal of the tablets.[12]

The ability of marine plants to accumulate heavy metals and other toxic elements is recognised, and the uptake of various radioactive compounds by seaweeds has been reported.[3,13,14] Fifteen samples of kelp-containing dietary supplements have been analysed for their iodine and arsenic contents.[19] The levels of arsenic were low in all but one product. The iodine levels varied widely, even between different samples of the same product, and in some products the iodine levels were high in relation to safe daily intake.

Brown algae (*Ascophyllum nodosum* and *Fucus vesiculosus*) have been found to be capable of synthesising volatile halogenated organic compounds (VHOCs).[15] VHOCs are considered to be troublesome pollutants because land plants and animals have difficulty in degrading the compounds which consequently persist in terrestrial ecosystems.[15] VHOCs released into the seawater predominantly contain bromine with iodine-containing compounds showing a slower rate of turnover.[15] Concentration of iron by brown seaweeds has been attributed to fucoidan, and alginic acid exhibits a high specificity for the binding of strontium.[13] Elevated urinary arsenic concentrations (138 and 293 µg/24 hour) in two female patients have been associated with the ingestion of kelp tablets. Subsequent analysis of the arsenic content of various kelp preparations revealed concentrations ranging from 16 to 58 µg/g product.[16,17] The botanical source of the kelp in the products was not stated.[17]

Ascophyllum nodosum is commonly added to animal foodstuffs as a source of vitamin and minerals, with beneficial results reported for dairy cattle, sheep, pigs and poultry.[13] Feeding studies using *A. nodosum* have highlighted an atypical toxic response of rabbits compared to that of rats and pigs.[13,18] Addition of *A. nodosum* to the diet of rabbits (at 5–10%) caused a severe drop in haemoglobin content, serum iron concentrations and packed cell volume, leading to weight loss and death in two-thirds of the animals.[13] No differences in renal and liver function, and in lipid metabolism were found between test and control animals.[13] Similar, but much milder, toxicity has also been observed in rabbits fed *Fucus serratus*.[18] Subsequent studies incorporating *A. nodosum* into the feed of rats and pigs failed to demonstrate the toxic effects observed in rabbits.[18] The toxic components in *A. nodosum* have been reported to be non-extractable with chloroform, ethanol, water and 20% sodium carbonate solution, remaining in the insoluble residue.[18]

Contra-indications, Warnings

The iodine content in kelp may cause hyper- or hypothyroidism and may interfere with existing treatment for abnormal thyroid function. In view of this, ingestion of kelp preparations by children is inadvisable. The iodine content in kelp has also been associated with acneiform eruptions and aggravation of pre-existing acne. In general, brown seaweeds are known to concentrate various heavy metals and other toxic elements. Elevated urinary arsenic concentrations have been traced to the ingestion of kelp tablets. Prolonged ingestion of kelp may reduce gastrointestinal iron absorption (binding properties of fucoidan), resulting in a slow reduction in haemoglobin, packed cell volume and serum iron concentrations. Prolonged ingestion may also affect absorption of sodium and potassium ions (alginic acid) and cause diarrhoea.

Pregnancy and lactation The safe use of kelp products during pregnancy and lactation has not been established. In view of the potential actions on the thyroid gland and possible contamination with toxic elements, the use of kelp should be avoided.

Pharmaceutical Comment

Kelp is a generic term that strictly speaking refers to *Laminaria* and *Macrocystis* species of brown seaweeds, although in practice it may be used in reference to other species of brown algae including *Nereocystis* and *Fucus*. The species *Fucus vesiculosus* is reported to be commonly used in the preparation of kelp products.[G30] The principal constituents of seaweeds are polysaccharides. For brown seaweeds the major polysaccharide is alginic acid (algin). Fucoidan, present in all brown algae, is thought to refer to a number of related polysaccharide esters whose main sugar component is fucose. The traditional uses of kelp in obesity and goitre are presumably attributable to the iodine content, although the self-diagnosis and treatment of these conditions with a herbal remedy is not suitable. There have been no documented studies supporting the traditional use of kelp in rheumatic conditions. In view of the iodine and potential accumulation of toxic elements, excessive ingestion of kelp is inadvisable. Doubt over the quality of commercial seaweed preparations has been reported.[10]

References

See General References G1, G2, G3, G4, G6, G9, G14, G21, G24, G30 and G32.

1. Wood CG. Seaweed extracts. A unique ocean resource. *J Chem Ed* 1974;**51**:449–52.

2. Algae as food for man. In: Chapman VJ, editor. Seaweeds and their uses. London: Methuen, 1970: 115.

3. Whistler RL, editor. Industrial gums. 2nd edn. New York: Academic Press, 1973: 13.

4. Burkholder PR. Drugs from the sea. *Armed Forces Chem J* 1963; **17**:6,8,10,12–16.

5. Doner LW. Fucoidan. In: Whistler RL, editor. Industrial gums. 2nd edn. New York: Academic Press, 1973: 115–21.

6.   Barwell CJ et al. Inhibitors of mammalian digestive enzymes in some species of marine brown algae. Br Phycol J 1983; 18: 200.

7.   Murata K. Supression of lipid synthesis in cultured aortic cells by laminaran sulfate. J Atheroscl Res 1969; 10: 371–8.

8.   Funayama S, Hikino H. Hypotensive principle of Laminaria and allied seaweeds. Planta Med 1981; 41: 29–33.

9.   Kathan RH. Kelp extracts as antiviral substances. Ann NY Acad Sci 1965; 130: 390–7.

10.   Shilo S, Hirsch HJ. Iodine-induced hyperthyroidism in a patient with a normal thyroid gland. Postgrad Med J 1986; 62: 661–2.

11.   Smet PAGM de et al. Kelp in herbal medicines: hyperthyroidism. Nederlands Tijdschrift voor Geneeskunde 1990; 134: 1058–9.

12.   Harrell BL, Rudolph AH. Kelp diet: A cause of acneiform eruption. Arch Dermatol 1976; 112: 560.

13.   Blunden G, Jones RT. Toxic effects of Ascophyllum nodosum as a rabbit food additive. In: Food — Drugs from the Sea Proceedings 1972. Washington: Marine Technology Society, 1972: 267–293.

14.   Hodge VF et al. Rapid accumulation of plutonium and polonium on giant brown algae. Health Physics 1974; 27: 29–35.

15.   Halocarbons. Natural pollution by algal seaweeds. Chem Br 1985: 513–14.

16.   Walkiw O, Douglas DE. Health food supplements prepared from kelp — a source of elevated urinary arsenic. Can Med Assoc J 1974; 111: 1301–2.

17.   Walkiw O, Douglas DE. Health food supplements prepared form kelp — a source of elevated urinary arsenic. Clin Toxicol 1975; 8: 325–31.

18.   Jones RT et al. Effects of dietary Ascophyllum nodosum on blood parameters of rats and pigs. Botanica Marina 1979; 22: 393–4.

19.   Norman JA et al. Human intake of arsenic and iodine from seaweed-based food supplements and health foods available in the UK. Food Additives Contaminants 1987; 5: 103–9.

FUMITORY

Species (Family)
Fumaria officinalis L. (Fumariaceae)

Synonym(s)
Fumitory

Part(s) Used
Herb

Pharmacopoeial Monographs
BHP 1983
BHP 1990

Legal Category (Licensed Products)
GSL[G14]

Constituents[G1,G2,G18,G32]
Alkaloids (Isoquinoline-type). Protopines including protopine (fumarine) as the major alkaloid and cryptopine,[1,2] protoberberines including aurotensine, stylopine, sinactine and *N*-methylsinactine,[3] spirobenzylisoquinolines including fumariline, fumaricine and fumariline,[4,5] benzophenanthridines including sanguinarine,[6] and indenobenzazepines including fumaritridine and fumaritrine.[6,7]
Flavonoids Glycosides of quercetin including isoquercitrin, rutin and quercetrin-3,7-diglucoside-3-arabinoglucoside.[8,9]
Acids Chlorogenic, caffeic and fumaric acids.[8]
Other constituents Bitter principles, mucilage, resin.

Food Use
Fumitory is listed by the Council of Europe as a natural source of food flavouring (category N3). This category indicates that fumitory can be added to foodstuffs in the traditionally accepted manner, although there is insufficient information available for an adequate assesment of potential toxicity.[G9]

Herbal Use
Fumitory is stated to possess weak diuretic and laxative properties and to act as a cholagogue. Traditionally, it has been used to treat cutaneous eruptions, conjunctivitis (as an eye lotion) and, specifically, chronic eczema.[G1,G2,G3,G4,G32]

Dose
Herb 2–4 g or by infusion three times daily[G2,G3]
Liquid extract (1:1 in 25% alcohol) 2–4 mL three times daily[G2,G3]
Tincture (1:5 in 45% alcohol) 1–4 mL three times daily[G2,3]

Pharmacological Actions
Animal studies The herb had no effect on normal choloresis but it modified bile flow which was artificially increased or decreased.[10] Antispasmodic activity on smooth muscle has been reported.[11] Extracts inhibited formation of gall-bladder calculi in animals.[12] The major alkaloid protopine has antihistaminic,[13] hypotensive, bradycardic and sedative activities in small doses,[14] whereas larger doses cause excitation and convulsions.[14] Bactericidal activity against Gram-positive organisms *Bacillus anthracis* and *Staphylococcus* have been reported.[14]
Human studies Clinical studies on 105 patients with biliary disorders claimed favourable results.[15]

Side-effects, Toxicity
No reported side-effects or documented toxicity studies were located, although possible adverse effects include raised intraocular pressure and oedema.[16]

Contra-indications, Warnings
Hypotensive actions have been documented in animal studies.
Pregnancy and lactation The safety of fumitory during pregnancy and lactation has not been established. In view of lack of pharmacological and toxicty data, the use of fumitory during pregnancy and lactation should be avoided.

Pharmaceutical Comment
Fumitory is characterised by isoquinoline alkaloids which represent the principal active ingredients. Animal studies support some of the traditional uses, but it should not be used in home-made ophthalmic preparations. In view of the active constituents and the lack of safety data, excessive ingestion of fumitory should be avoided.

References
See General References G1, G2, G3, G4, G9, G14 and G32.

1. Sener B. Turkish species of *Fumaria* L. and their alkaloids. VII Alkaloids from *Fumaria officinalis* L. and *F. cilicica* Hansskn. *Gazi Univ Eczacilik Fak Derg* 1985; **2**: 45-49.

2. Hermansson J, Sandberg F. Alkaloids of *Fumaria officinalis*. *Acta Pharm Suec* 1973; **10**: 520-2.

3. Mardirossian ZH et al. Alkaloids of *Fumaria officinalis*. *Phytochemistry* 1983; **22**: 759-61.

4. MacLean DB *et al.* Structure of three minor alkaloids of *Fumaria officinalis*. *Can J Chem* 1969; **47**: 3593-9.

5. Murav'eva DA et al. Isolation of fumaritine from *Fumaria officinalis*. *Khim Farm Zh* 1974; **8**: 32-4.

6. Forgacs P et al. Alcaloides des Papavéracées II: Composition chimique de dix-sept espèces de *Fumaria*. *Plantes med phytother* 1986; **20**: 64-81.

7. Forgacs P et al. Composition chimique des Fumariacées. Alcaloides de quatorze espèces de *Fumaria*. *Plantes med phytother* 1982; **16**: 99-115.

8. Massa V et al. Sur les pigments phenoliques du *Fumaria officinalis* L. *Trav Soc Pharm Montpellier* 1971; **31:** 233-6.

9. Torck M *et al.* Flavonoids of *Fumaria officinalis* L. *Ann Pharm Fr* 1971; **29:** 591-6.

10. Boucard M, Laubenheimer B. Action du nébulisat de fumeterre sur le débit bilaire du rat. *Therapie* 1966; **21:** 903-11.

11. Reynier M *et al.* Action du nébulisat de fumeterre officinal sur la musculature lisse. Contribution à l'étude du mécanisme de son activité thérapeutique. *Trav Soc Pharm Montpellier* 1977; **37:** 85-102.

12. Lagrange E, Aurousseau M. Effect of spray-dried product of *Fumaria officinalis* on experimental gall bladder lithiasis in mice. *Ann Pharm Fr* 1973; **31:** 357-62.

13. Abdul Habib Dil. Activité anti-histaminique de la fumarine. *Therapie* 1973; **28:** 767-74.

14. Preininger V. The pharmacology and toxicology of the papaveraceae alkaloids. In: RHF Manske (ed). *The Alkaloids XV.* London Academic Press, 1975, pp. 207-61.

15. Fiegel G. Die amphocholoretische Wirkung der *Fumaria officinalis.* *Z Allgemeinmed Landarzt* 1971; **34:** 1819-20.

16. Anderson LA, Phillipson JD. Herbal medicine, education and the pharmacist. *Pharm J* 1986; **236:** 303-5.

GARLIC

Species (Family)
Allium sativum L. (Amaryllidaceae/Liliaceae)

Synonym(s)
Ajo, Allium

Part(s) Used
Bulb (clove)

Pharmacopoeial Monographs
BHP 1983
BHP 1990
BPC 1949
Martindale 30th edition

Legal Category (Licensed Products)
GSL[G14]

Constituents[G2,G19,G32,35]

Enzymes Allinase, peroxidases, myrosinase
Volatile oils (0.1–0.36%). Sulphur-containing compounds including alliin, compounds produced enzymatically from alliin including allicin (diallyl thiosulphinate), allylpropyl disulphide, diallyl disulphide, diallyl trisulphide; ajoene and vinyldithiines (secondary products of alliin produced non-enzymatically from allicin); *S*-allylmercaptocysteine (ASSC) and *S*-methylmercaptocysteine (MSSC); terpenes include citral, geraniol, linalool, α- and β-phellandrene
Other constituents Protein, minerals, vitamins, lipids, amino acids, prostaglandins (A_2 and $F_{1\alpha}$)[1]

Food Use

Garlic is used extensively in foods. It is listed by the Council of Europe as a natural source of food flavouring (category N1). This category indicates that there are no restrictions on the use of garlic in foods.[G9]

Herbal Use

Garlic is stated to possess diaphoretic, expectorant, antispasmodic, antiseptic, bacteriostatic, antiviral, promoter of leucocytosis, hypotensive, and anthelmintic properties. Traditionally, it has been used to treat chronic bronchitis, respiratory catarrh, recurrent colds, whooping cough, bronchitic asthma, influenza, and chronic bronchitis.[G1,G2,G3,G4,G32]

Dose

Dried bulb 2–4 g three times daily[G2,G3]
Tincture (1:5 in 45% alcohol) 2–4 mL three times daily[G2, G3]
Oil 0.03–0.12 mL three times daily[G2,G3]
Juice of Garlic (BPC 1949) 2–4 mL
Syrup of Garlic (BPC 1949) 2–8 mL

Pharmacological Actions

Many reviews have been published on the pharmacological activities of garlic.[2–9]

Details of a symposium on the chemistry, pharmacology, and medical applications of garlic, held in Germany in 1989 have also been published.[10]

Animal studies The hypocholesterolaemic activity of garlic is well documented in animal studies and has been attributed to diallyl disulphide, a decomposition product of allicin.[11] A reduction in both blood and tissue lipid concentrations in animals fed a diet supplemented with dried garlic powder, garlic oil, or allicin has been documented.[3,12]

Garlic has been noted to reduce serum cholesterol, serum triglyceride, and low density lipoprotein (LDL) concentrations, and increase high density lipoprotein (HDL) concentrations. It has been suggested that an increase in HDL may enhance the removal of cholesterol from arterial tissue.[3] The cholesterol lowering effect of garlic is reported to be dose-related and proposed mechanisms of action include inhibition of lipid synthesis and increased excretion of neutral and acidic sterols.[3,5] The hypolipidaemic effect of garlic is thought to involve reduction in triacylglycerol biosynthesis via a reduction in tissue concentrations of NADPH, increase in hydrolysis of triacylglycerols via increased lipase activity and inactivation of enzymes involved in lipid synthesis via an interaction with enzyme thiol groups.[3,5,11] Garlic has also been reported to reduce hepatic triglyceride and cholesterol concentrations in rats, and to reduce aortic lipid deposition and atheromatous lesions in rabbits fed a high fat diet.[3]

Antithrombotic activity is well documented for garlic in both *in-vitro* and *in-vivo* animal studies. Increased serum-fibrinogen concentrations together with a decrease in blood coagulation time and fibrinolytic activity are associated with a high fat diet and enhance thrombosis.[3] Garlic has been shown to have a beneficial effect on all of these parameters. Garlic has been shown to inhibit platelet aggregation[13,14] caused by a number of inducers such as ADP, collagen, arachidonic acid, adrenaline, and calcium ionophore A23187.[15] A number of mechanisms have been proposed by which garlic is thought to exert an anti-aggregatory action. These include inhibition of thromboxane synthesis via cyclo-oxygenase and lipoxygenase inhibition[5], inhibition of membrane phospholipase activity and incorporation of arachidonic acid into platelet membrane phospholipids[16], intraplatelet mobilisation of calcium uptake, and inhibition of calcium uptake into platelets.[15] Garlic oil has been reported to reduce artificial surface adhesion of platelets *in vitro*.[17] Garlic is thought to contain more than one inhibitor of platelet aggregation and release; allicin is considered to be the major inhibitor.[18]

Many studies have investigated the role of ajoene (a secondary degradation product of alliin) as an inhibitor of platelet aggregation and release.[10] Ajoene inhibits platelet aggregation caused by various inducers. Its action is noted to be dose dependent and reversible both *in vitro* and *in vivo*.[10] It has been suggested that this latter feature may be of clinical significance in instances where a rapid inhibition of platelet aggregation is required with subsequent reversal, such as chronic haemodialysis and coronary bypass surgery.[10] It has been proposed that ajoene exerts its anti-aggregatory effect by altering the platelet membrane via an interaction with sulphydryl groups.[19] The inhibitory action of ajoene on granule release from platelets is thought to involve alteration of the microviscosity in the inner part of the plasma membrane.[20] Ajoene is reported to synergistically potentiate the anti-aggregatory action of prostacyclin, forskolin, indomethacin, and dipyridamole,[21] and to potentiate the inhibitory action of prostaglandin PGI_2 on platelet aggregation.[21] Approximately 96% inhibition of prostaglandin synthetase and 100% inhibition of lipoxygenase has been described for ajoene *in vitro*.[16] Structure-activity investigations suggested that an allylic structure in the open disulphide ring is required for activity.[16]

A hypotensive effect in dogs administered garlic extract has been documented; prior administration of antagonists to known endogenous hypotensive substances such as histamine, acetylcholine, serotonin, and kinins did not affect the hypotensive effect.[23]

Antimicrobial activity is well documented for garlic.[4] Bacterial species sensitive to garlic include *Staphylococcus*, *Escherichia*, *Proteus*, *Salmonella*, *Providencia*, *Citrobacter*, *Klebsiella*, *Hafnia*, *Aeromonas*, *Vibrio*, and *Bacillus* genera.[4] *Pseudomonas aeruginosa* is not sensitive to garlic.[4] Garlic has also been documented to inhibit growth in 30 strains of mycobacteria, consisting of 17 species, including *Mycobacterium tuberculosis*.[23] It has been proposed that garlic inhibits bacterial cell growth by primarily inhibiting RNA synthesis.[24] Broad spectrum activity against fungi has been documented for garlic including the genera *Microsporum*, *Epidermophyton*, *Trichophyton*, *Rhodotorula*, *Torulopsis*, *Trichosporon*, *Cryptococcus neoformans*, and *Candida* including *Candida albicans*.[4] Garlic extract has been reported as more effective than nystatin against pathogenic yeasts, especially *Candida albicans*.[4] Inhibition of lipid synthesis is thought to be an important factor in the anticandidal activity of garlic, with a disulphide-containing component such as allicin thought to be the main active component.[25] Garlic has been found to inhibit the growth and toxin production of *Aspergillus parasiticus*.[26]

In-vitro antiviral activity against parainfluenza type 3, *Herpes simplex* type 1, and *Influenza* B has been documented.[27,28] Activity was attributed to allicin or an allicin derivative. Garlic was reported to be ineffective towards coxsackie B1 virus.[29]

Garlic has been documented to cause both smooth-muscle relaxation and contraction.[14,22,29] Garlic oil has been reported to depress gastro-intestinal movements in mice, induced by charcoal meal and castor oil.[29] Garlic has also inhibited acetylcholine- and PGE_2-induced contraction of the rat gastric fundus, with the most active components exhibiting the weakest antiplatelet aggregatory activity.[14]

Garlic has also elicited contractions on the rat uterus and the guinea-pig ileum *in vitro*.[22] Both actions were blocked by flufenamic acid but not by atropine or cyproheptadine, indicating a prostaglandin-like mode of action.

Antihepatotoxic activity *in vitro* and *in vivo* has been reported for garlic oil[30] and some of its constituents, namely alliin, *S*-allylmercapto-cysteine (ASSC), and *S*-methylmercapto-cysteine (MSSC) in carbon tetrachloride- and galactosamine-induced hepatotoxicity.[30] Inhibition of benzo[*a*]pyrene-induced neoplasia of the forestomach and lung in female mice has been documented for four allyl group-containing derivatives in garlic.[31] Structure-activity requirements underlined the importance of the unsaturated allyl groups for activity. Saturated analogues containing propyl groups instead of allyl were devoid of activity.

Immunostimulant activity has been described for a high-molecular-weight protein fraction obtained from an aged garlic extract.[32] The fraction was found to strongly stimulate mice peritoneal macrophages *in vitro*, and to stimulate carbon clearance in mice *in vivo*. The authors commented that garlic may suppress tumour cell growth by the stimulation of immunoresponder cells.

Garlic oil and juice have been reported to protect against isoprenaline-induced myocardial necrosis in rats.[33]

Hypoglycaemic activity has been documented for an alcoholic garlic extract following oral administration to rabbits (dose equivalent to 50 g dry garlic powder). 59% activity compared to that of 500 mg tolbutamide was observed.[34]

Human studies Documented studies have shown garlic to have a beneficial effect on serum lipids, reducing serum cholesterol (CH), serum triglycerides (TG) and LDL, and improving the LDL/HDL ratio.[2,3,5,10,35,36] An initial rise in CH, TG, and LDL following garlic administration has also been noted.[35] Supplementation of a fatty meal with garlic is reported to prevent the subsequent rise in serum lipids.[3] Epidemiological studies in India have associated low total serum TG with regular consumption of both garlic and onion.[3] Decreases in LDL and very low density lipoprotein (VLDL) and a progressive rise of HDL have been observed in coronary heart disease patients given garlic oil 0.25 mg/kg body-weight for 10 months.[3] However, garlic has also been reported to be ineffective in lowering serum lipids.[3,37] Treatment of post-myocardial infarction patients with garlic has been reported to reduce reinfarction and mortality rate, as well as lowering systolic and diastolic blood pressure and serum-cholesterol concentrations.[10]

Few controlled studies concerning the hypotensive effect of garlic have been documented.[10] Studies using a proprietary preparation containing powdered garlic have reported a reduction in both systolic and diastolic blood pressure.[10] The daily dose of 600 to 900 mg was equivalent to 1.8 to 2.7 g fresh garlic. An average reduction of 12 to 30 mmHg systolic blood pressure and 7 to 20 mmHg diastolic blood pressure has been described for patients with essential hypertension who regularly ingested garlic.[2]

Antithrombotic activity has been noted for garlic in humans. A decrease in serum fibrinogen concentrations and an increase in fibrinolytic activity has been documented.[5,10]

A 72 to 85% increase in fibrinolytic activity was recorded in patients with ischaemic heart disease who had received garlic daily for one month.[2] An epidemiological study has shown a positive correlation between fibrinolysis activity and the recorded garlic consumption.[2] Garlic has also been found to inhibit serotonin-induced platelet aggregation.[5] Antiplatelet activity has been documented for garlic in *in-vitro* studies using human platelets.[2,38] Garlic consumption has been noted to abolish the normal post-prandial increase in thrombocyte aggregation.[2] Garlic consumption has also been associated with a reduction in the mean plasma viscosity and in haematocrit values.[10]

A reduction in blood-sugar concentrations and an increase in insulin have been observed following allyl propyl disulphide administration to normal volunteers, whereas other workers have stated that garlic exhibits hypoglycaemic actions in diabetic patients but not in controls.[2] It is also reported that garlic can prevent tolbutamide- and adrenaline-induced hyperglycaemia.[2]

Side-effects, Toxicity[G33,G35]

Garlic is generally considered to be non-toxic.[5,39] Adverse effects that have been documented in humans include a burning sensation in the mouth and gastro-intestinal tract, nausea, diarrhoea, and vomiting.[5] A potential interaction between garlic and warfarin has been documented.[40] Cases of contact dermatitis resulting from occupational exposure to garlic have been reported. [G26,10,41]. The allergenic property of garlic is well recognised and allergens have been identified as diallyldisulphide, allylpropylsulphide, and allicin (latter may be an irritant).[42] A garlic antigen in the serum of affected patients has also been identified.[10] There have not been any documented cases of asthma or contact dermatitis following the medicinal use of garlic oil or extract.[10]

Erratic pulse rates, abnormal ECGs, weight loss, lethargy and weakness, soft faeces, dehydration, and tender skin on fore and hindlimbs have been observed in spontaneously hypertensive rats administered garlic extract at 0.25 and 0.5 mL/kg every 6 hours for 28 days.[43] The effects were most pronounced in animals receiving doses two or three times a day. Conversely, acute toxicity studies for garlic extract in mice and rats have reported LD_{50} values for various routes of administration (by mouth, intraperitoneal injection, intravenous injection) as all greater than 30 mL/kg.[39] Early studies, in 1944, reported LD_{50} values for allicin in mice as 120 mg/kg (subcutaneous injection) and 60 mg/kg (intravenous injection).[10] Results of chronic toxicity studies are stated to be conflicting.[10] High doses are reported to cause anaemia due to both decreased haemoglobin synthesis and haemolysis.[10] A chronic toxicity study in rats given a garlic extract (2 g/kg) five times a week for 6 months, reported no toxic symptoms.[44] High doses were found to decrease food consumption slightly, but did not inhibit weight gain. There were no significant differences in urinary, haematological, or serological examinations, and no toxic symptoms in histopathological examinations. Genotoxicity studies using the micronucleus test have reported both positive[45] and negative[46] findings. No evidence of mutagenicity has been reported when assessed using the Ames and Ree assay.[45]

Slight cytotoxic signs have been observed at high doses in HEp2 and chinese hamster embryo primary cultured cells.[45]

Contra-indications, Warnings

In view of the pharmacological actions documented for garlic, therapeutic doses of garlic may interfere with existing hypoglycaemic and anticoagulant therapies. Garlic may potentiate the antithrombotic effects of anti-inflammatory drugs such as aspirin, and is likely to be synergistic with eicosapentaenoic acid (EPA) in fish oils.[5] Gastro-intestinal irritation may occur particularly if the clove is eaten raw by individuals not accustomed to ingesting garlic.

Pregnancy and lactation Garlic is reputed to act as an abortifacient and to affect the menstrual cycle, and is also reported to be uteroactive.[G12] *In-vitro* uterine contraction has been documented.[29] There are no experimental or clinical reports on adverse effects during pregnancy or lactation.[G33] In view of this, doses of garlic greatly exceeding amounts used in foods should not be taken during pregnancy and lactation.

Pharmaceutical Comment

Considerable literature exists for garlic, with reseach primarily focussing on antimicrobial and cardiovascular properties. Garlic is characterised by the odiferous sulphur-containing principles in the volatile oil. Pharmacological activities documented for garlic are also associated with these principles. It is recognised that allicin, the unstable compound formed by enzymatic action of allinase on alliin when the garlic clove is crushed, is required for the antimicrobial activity that has been demonstrated by garlic. However, serum concentrations of allicin achieved in humans following oral ingestion of garlic are unclear. The hypolipidaemic and antithrombotic actions documented for garlic have been attributed to many of the degradation products of alliin.

One of the difficulties in comparing studies that have investigated the efficacy of garlic, is establishing the concentration of active principles present in the garlic preparations used. It has been reported that the percentage of active constituents in fresh garlic may vary by a factor of ten.[10] It has been suggested that one way of standardising garlic preparations is by estimating the allicin-releasing potential.[10] Dried garlic powder contains both alliin and allinase and therefore has an allicin-releasing potential. Garlic preparations produced by heat or solvent extraction processes are stated to contain alliin but to be devoid of allinase and therefore have no allicin releasing potential.[10] Garlic oil macerates and steam distillation products are rich in secondary alliin metabolites, such as ajoene. However, it is unclear to what extent these secondary compounds are formed in the body following the ingestion of garlic and whether, therefore, these products exhibit the pharmacological actions of fresh garlic.[10]

Fermented garlic preparations are considered to be practically devoid of the active sulphur-containing compounds.[10]

Many 'odourless' garlic preparations are available: obviously one should establish if these products are odourless due to the formulation of the product or because they are devoid of the odoriferous, active principles. Further controlled human studies with standardised preparations are required to establish the true usefulness of garlic in reducing serum lipids, blood pressure, platelet aggregation, and exerting an antimicrobial effect. Therapeutic doses of garlic should not be given to those whose blood clots slowly and caution is recommended for patients on anticoagulant therapy.[G35]

References

See General References G1, G2, G3, G4, G6, G9, G12, G14, G19, G22, G23, G26, G32, G33 and G35.

1.   Al-Nagdy SA *et al*. Evidence for some prostaglandins in *Allium sativum* extracts. *Phytotherapy Res* 1988; **2**: 196–7.

2.   Ernst E. Cardiovascular effects of garlic (*Allium sativum*): a review. *Pharmatherapeutica* 1987; **5**: 83–9.

3.   Lau BHS *et al*. *Allium sativum* (garlic) and atherosclerosis: a review. *Nutr Res* 1983; **3**: 119–28.

4.   Adetumbi M, Lau BHS. *Allium sativum* (garlic) — a natural antibiotic. *Med Hypoth* 1983; **12**: 227–37.

5.   Fulder S. Garlic and the prevention of cardiovascular disease. *Cardiology In Practice* 1989; **7**: 30–5.–

6.   Pizzorno JE, Murray MT. A textbook of natural medicine. Seattle, WA: John Bastyr College Publications. 1985 (looseleaf).

7.   Hamon NW. Garlic and the genus Allium. *Canad Pharm J* 1987; **120**: 493–8.

8.   Fenwick GR, Hanley AB. The genus *Allium*. In: CRC Critical Reviews in Food Science and Nutrition; **22**: 199–376; **23**: 1–73.

9.   McElnay, JC and Li Wan Po, A. Garlic. *Pharm J* 1991; **246**: 324–6.

10.   Symposium on the chemistry, pharmacology and medical applications of garlic. *Cardiology In Practice* 1989; **7**: 1–15.

11.   Adoga GI. The mechanism of the hypolipidemic effect of garlic oil extract in rats fed on high sucrose and alcohol diets. *Biochem Biophys Res Comm* 1987; **142**: 1046–52.

12.   Kamanna VS and Chandrasekhara N. Effect of garlic (*Allium sativum* Linn.) on serum lipoproteins and lipoprotein cholesterol levels in Albino rats rendered hypercholesteremic by feeding cholesterol. *Lipids* 1982; **17**: 483–8.

13.   Boullin DJ. Garlic as a platelet inhibitor. *Lancet* 1981; **i**: 776–7.

14.   Gaffen JD *et al*. The effect of garlic extracts on contractions of rat gastric fundus and human platelet aggregation. *J Pharm Pharmacol* 1984; **36**: 272–4.

15.   Srivastava KC, Winslows JB. Evidence for the mechanism by which garlic inhibits platelet aggregation. *Prostaglandins Leukot Med* 1986; **22**: 313–21.

16.   Wagner H *et al*. Effects of garlic constituents on arachidonate metabolism. *Planta Med* 1987; **53**: 305–6.

17.   Sharma CP, Nirmala NV. Effects of garlic extract and of three pure components isolated from it on human platelet aggregation, arachidonate metabolism, release reaction and platelet ultrastructure — comments. *Thromb Res* 1985; **37**: 489–90.

18.   Mohammad SF, Woodward SC. Characterization of a potent inhibitor of platelet aggregation and release reaction isolated from *Allium sativum* (garlic). *Thromb Res* 1986; **44**: 793–806.

19.   Block E *et al*. Antithrombotic organosulfur compounds from garlic: Structural, mechanistic, and synthtic studies. *J Am Chem Soc* 1986; **108**: 7045–55.

20.   Rendu F *et al*. Ajoene, the antiplatelet compound derived from garlic, specifically inhibits platelet release reaction by affecting the plasma membrane internal microviscosity. *Biochem Pharmacol* 1989; **38**: 1321–28.

21.   Apitz-Castro R *et al*. Ajoene. The antiplatelet principle of garlic, synergistically potentiates the antiaggregatory action of prostacyclin, forskolin, indomethacin and dypiridamole on human platelets. *Thromb Res* 1986; **42**: 303–11.

22.   Rashid A, Khan HH. The mechanism of hypotensive effect of garlic extract. *JPMA* 1974; **35**: 357–62.

23.   Delaha ED, Garagusi VF. Inhibition of mycobacteria by garlic extract (*Allium sativum*). *Antimicrob Agents Chemother* 1985; **27**: 485–6.

24.   Feldberg RS *et al*. In vitro mechanism of inhibition of bacterial cell growth by allicin. *Antimicrob Agents Chemother* 1988; **32**: 1763–8.

25.   Adetumbi M *et al*. *Allium sativum* (garlic) inhibits lipid synthesis by *Candida albicans*. *Antimicrob Agents Chemother* 1986; **30**: 499–501.

26.   Graham HD, Graham EJF. Inhibition of *Aspergillus parasiticus* growth and toxin production by garlic. *J Food Safety* 1987; **8**: 101–8.

27.   Hughes BG *et al*. Antiviral constituents from *Allium sativum*. *Planta Med* 1989; **55**: 114.

28.   Tsai Y *et al*. Antiviral properties of garlic: *In vitro* effects on influenza B, Herpes simplex and Coxsackie viruses. *Planta Med* 1985; **51**: 460–1.

29.   Joshi DJ *et al*. Gastrointestinal actions of garlic oil. *Phytotherapy Res* 1987; **1**: 140–1.

30.   Hikino H *et al*. Antihepatotoxic actions of *Allium sativum* bulbs. *Planta Med* 1986; **52**: 163–8.

31.Sparnins VL *et al*. Effects of organosulfur compounds from garlic and onions on benzo[a]pyrene-induced neoplasia and glutathione S-transferase activity in the mouse. *Carcinogenesis* 1988; **9**: 131–4.

32.   Hirao Y *et al*. Activation of immunoresponder cells by the protein fraction from aged garlic extract. *Phytotherapy Res* 1987; **1**: 161–4.

33.   Saxena KK *et al*. Effect of garlic pretreatment on isoprenaline–induced myocardial necrosis in albino rats. *Indian J Physiol Pharmacol* 1980; **24**: 233–6.

34.   Brahmachari HD, Augusti KT. Orally effective hypoglycaemic agents from plants. *J Pharm Pharmacol* 1962; **14**: 254–5.

35. Lau BHS *et al*. Effect of an odor-modified garlic preparation on blood lipids. *Nutr Res* 1987; **7:** 139–49.

36. Ernst E *et al*. Garlic and blood lipids. *Br Med J* 1985; **291:** 139.

37. Luley C *et al*. Lack of efficacy of dried garlic in patients with hyperlipoproteinemia. *Arzneimittelforschung* 1986; **36:** 766–8.

38. Apitz-Castro A *et al*. Effects of garlic extract and of three pure components isolated from it on human platelet aggregation, arachidonate metabolism, release reaction and platelet ultrastructure. *Thromb Res* 1983; **32:** 155–69.

39. Nakagawa S *et al*. Acute toxicity test of garlic extract. *J Toxicol Sci* 1984; **9:** 57–60.

40. Sunter W. Warfarin and garlic. *Pharm J* 1991; **246:** 722.

41. Lautier R, Wendt V. Contact Allergy to Alliaceae/Case-report and literature survey. *Dermatosen* 1985; **33:** 213–15.

42. Papageorgiou C *et al*. Allergic contact dermatitis to garlic (*Allium sativum* L.) Identification of the allergens: The role of mono-, di-, and trisulfides present in garlic. *Arch Dermatol Res* 1983; **275:** 229–34.

43. Ruffin J, Hunter SA. An evaluation of the side effects of garlic as an antihypertensive agent. *Cytobios* 1983; **37:** 85–9.

44. Sumiyoshi H *et al*. Chronic toxicity test of garlic extract in rats. *J Toxicol Sci* 1984; **9:** 61–75.

45. Yoshida S *et al*. Mutagenicity and cytotoxicity tests of garlic. *J Toxicol Sci* 1984; **9:** 77–86.

46. Abraham SK, Kesavan PC. Genotoxicity of garlic, turmeric and asafoetida in mice. *Mutat Res* 1984; **136:** 85–8.

GENTIAN

Species (Family)
Gentiana lutea L. (Gentianaceae)

Synonym(s)
Bitter Root, Gentiana, Yellow Gentian

Part(s) Used
Rhizome, Root

Pharmacopoeial Monographs
BHP 1990
BPC 1973
Martindale 30th edition
Pharmacopoeias—Aust., Br., Cz., Egypt., Fr., Ger., Gr., Hung., It., Jpn, Neth., Nord., Port., Rom., Swiss, and Yug. Br. also includes Powdered Gentian.
Aust., Cz., and Hung. also allow other species of *Gentiana*. Jpn also includes Japanese Gentian from *Gentiana scabra*. Chin. specifies *G. scabra* and other species.

Legal Category (Licensed Products)
GSL[G14]

Constituents[G1,G2,G10,G14,G19,G30,G31,G32]
Alkaloids (pyridine-type) Gentianine 0.6–0.8%, gentialutine
Bitters Major component is secoiridoid glycoside gentiopicroside (also known as gentiamarin and gentiopicrin) 2%, with lesser amounts of amarogentin (0.01–0.04%) and swertiamarine.[1] The glycosides amaropanin and amaroswerin are reported to be present in related species *Gentiana pannonica*, *Gentiana punctata*, and *Gentiana purpurea*, but are absent from *Gentiana lutea*. Gentianose (a trisaccharide bitter principle).
Xanthones Gentisein, gentisin (gentianin), isogentisin, 1,3,7-trimethoxyxanthone
Other constituents Carbohydrates (e.g. gentiobiose, sucrose and other common sugars), pectin, tannin (unspecified), triterpenes (e.g. β-amyrin, lupeol), volatile oil (trace)

Food Use
Gentian is listed by the Council of Europe as a natural source of food flavouring (category N2). This category indicates that gentian can be added to foodstuffs in small quantities, with a possible limitation of an active principle (as yet unspecified) in the final product.[G9]

Herbal Use
Gentian is stated to possess bitter, gastric stimulant, sialogogue, and cholagogue properties. Traditionally, it has been used for anorexia, atonic dyspepsia, gastro-intestinal atony, and specifically for dyspepsia with anorexia.[G1,G2,G4,G30,G32]

Dose
Dried rhizome/root 0.6–2 g or by infusion or decoction three times daily[G2]
Tincture (1:5 in 45% alcohol) 1–4 mL three times daily[G2]

Pharmacological Actions
Animal studies Choleretic properties have been documented for gentian,[G19] and gentianine has been reported to possess anti-inflammatory activity.[G10] In general, bitter principles are known to stimulate gastric secretions.

Mutagenic activity in the Ames test (*Salmonella typhimurium* TA100 with S9 mix) has been documented for gentian, with gentisin and isogentisin identified as mutagenic components.[2] Gentian root 100 g was reported to yield approximately 100 mg total mutagenic compounds, of which gentisin and isogentisin comprised approximately 76 mg.[2]

Side-effects, Toxicity
Mutagenic activity has been documented for gentian (*see* Animal studies).

Contra-indications, Warnings
Gentian is stated to be contra-indicated in individuals with high blood pressure,[G30] although no rationale is given to this statement.

Pregnancy and lactation Gentian is reputed to affect the menstrual cycle,[G10,G30] and it has been stated that gentian should not be used in pregnancy.[G30] In view of this and the documented mutagenic activity, gentian is best avoided in pregnancy and lactation.

Pharmaceutical Comment
The major constituents of pharmacological importance in gentian are the bitter principles; limited information is available on the other compounds present. The herbal uses of gentian are supported by the known properties of the bitter principles present in the root. Excessive doses should be avoided in view of the lack of toxicity data.

References
See General References G1, G2, G3, G4, G7, G8, G9, G10, G11, G14, G19, G22, G23, G29, G30, G31 and G32.

1. Verotta L. Isolation and HPLC determination of the active principles of *Rosmarinus officinalis* and *Gentiana lutea*. *Fitoterapia* 1985; **56:** 25–9.

2. Morimoto I *et al*. Mutagenic activities of gentisin and isogentisin from Gentianae radix (Gentianaceae). *Mutat Res* 1983; **116:** 103–17.

GINGER

Species (Family)

Zingiber officinale Roscoe (Zingiberaceae)

Synonym(s)

Zingiber

Part(s) Used

Rhizome

Pharmacopoeial Monographs

BHP 1983
BHP 1990
BPC 1973
Martindale 30th edition
Pharmacopoeias—Aust., Br., Chin., Egypt., Jpn and Swiss.

Legal Category (Licensed Products)

GSL[G14]

Constituents[G1,G2,G14,G19,G32]

Carbohydrates Starch (major constituent, up to 50%)

Lipids (6–8%). Free fatty acids (e.g. palmitic acid, oleic acid, linoleic acid, caprylic acid, capric acid, lauric acid, myristic acid, pentadecanoic acid, heptadecanoic acid, stearic acid, linolenic acid, arachidic acid);[1] triglycerides, phosphatidic acid, lecithins

Oleo-resin Gingerol homologues (major, about 33%) including derivatives with a methyl side-chain,[2] shogaol homologues (dehydration products of gingerols), zingerone (degradation product of gingerols), volatile oils

Volatile oils (1–3%). Complex, predominately hydrocarbons. β-Bisabolene and zingiberene (major); other sesquiterpenes include zingiberol, zingiberenol, *ar*-curcumene, β-sesquiphellandrene, β-sesquiphellandrol (*cis* and *trans*); numerous monoterpene hydrocarbons, alcohols, and aldehydes (e.g. phellandrene, camphene, geraniol, neral, linalool, *d*-nerol). See reference 1 for a detailed analysis of the volatile oil.

Other constituents Amino acids (e.g. arginine, aspartic acid, cysteine, glycine, isoleucine, leucine, serine, threonine, valine), protein (about 9%), resins, vitamins (especially nicotinic acid (niacin) and vitamin A), minerals.[1]

Food Use

Ginger is listed by the Council of Europe as a natural source of food flavouring (category N2). This category indicates that ginger can be added to foodstuffs in small quantities, with a possible limitation of an active principle (as yet unspecified) in the final product.[G9] It is used widely in foods as a spice.

Herbal Use

Ginger is stated to possess carminative, diaphoretic, and antispasmodic properties. Traditionally, it has been used for colic, flatulent dyspepsia, and specifically for flatulent intestinalcolic.[G1,G2,G3,G4,G32]. Ginger has also been investigated for the prevention of motion sickness.

Dose

Dried rhizome 0.25–1.0 g or by infusion or decoction three times daily[G2,G3]
Weak Ginger Tincture (BP) 1.5–3.0 mL
Strong Ginger Tincture (BP) 0.25–0.5 mL

Pharmacological Actions

Animal studies Ginger has been reported to have hypoglycaemic, hypo- and hypertensive, cardiac, prostaglandin and platelet aggregation inhibition, antihypercholesterolaemic, cholagogic and stomachic properties.

A hypoglycaemic effect in both non-diabetic and alloxan-induced diabetic rabbits and rats has been documented for fresh ginger juice administered orally. The effect was stated to be significant in the diabetic animals.[3]

The pharmacological actions of (6)-shogaol and capsaicin have been compared.[4] Both compounds caused rapid hypotension followed by a marked pressor response, bradycardia, and apnoea in rats after intravenous administration. The pressor response was thought to be a centrally acting mechanism. Contractile responses in isolated guinea-pig trachea with both compounds, and positive inotropic and chronotropic responses in isolated rat atria with (6)-shogaol were thought to involve the release of an unknown active substance from nerve endings.[4] A potent, positive inotropic action on isolated guinea-pig atria has been documented and gingerols were identified as the cardiotonic principles.[5]

(6)-Gingerol, (6)- and (10)-dehydrogingerdione, (6)- and (10)-gingerdione have been reported to be potent inhibitors of prostaglandin biosynthesis (PG synthetase) *in vitro*, with the latter four compounds stated to be more potent than indomethacin.[6] Dose-dependent inhibition of platelet aggregation, *in vitro*, induced by ADP, adrenaline, collagen, and arachidonic acid has been described for an aqueous ginger extract.[7] Ginger was also found to reduce platelet synthesis of prostaglandin-endoperoxides, thromboxane, and prostaglandins. A good correlation was reported between concentrations of the extract required to inhibit platelet aggregation and concentrations necessary to inhibit platelet-thromboxane synthesis.[7]

Ginger oleo-resin, by intragastric administration, has been reported to inhibit elevation in serum and hepatic cholesterol concentrations in rats by impairing cholesterol absorption.[8] Antihypercholesterolaemic activity has also been documented for dried ginger rhizome when given to both rats fed a cholesterol-rich diet and those with existing hypercholesterolaemia.[9] Fresh ginger juice was not found to have an effect on serum-cholesterol concentrations within four hours of administration. In addition, serum-cholesterol concentrations were not greatly increased within four hours of cholesterol administration. The authors concluded that ginger should be taken daily for several days for any hypocholesterolaemic benefits to be observed.

A cholagogic action in rats has been described for an acetone extract of ginger administered intraduodenally.[10] (6)-Gingerol and (10)-gingerol were reported to be the active components, the former more potent with a significant increase in bile secretion still apparent four hours after administration.

The effect of ginger (acetone extract) and zingiberene on hydrochloric acid/ethanol-induced gastric lesions in rats has been examined.[11] (6)-Gingerol and zingiberene, both 100 mg/kg body-weight by mouth, significantly inhibited gastric lesions by 54.5% and 53.6%, respectively. The total extract inhibited lesions by 97.5% at 1 g/kg. Oral administration of both aqueous and methanol ginger extracts to rabbits has been reported to reduce gastric secretions (gastric juice volume, acid and pepsin output).[12] Both extracts were found to be comparable with cimetidine (50 mg/kg) with respect to gastric juice volume; the aqueous extract was comparable with cimetidine and superior to the methanol extract for pepsin output, and the methanol extract superior to both the aqueous extract and comparable to cimetidine for acid output.

In-vitro anthelmintic activity against *Ascaridia galli* Schrank has been documented for the volatile oil of *Zingiber purpureum* Roxb.[13] Activity exceeding that of piperazine citrate was exhibited by the oxygenated compounds fractionated from the volatile oil.

Uteroactivity has been described for a phenolic compound isolated from *Zingiber cassumunar* Roxb.[14] The compound was found to exhibit a dose-related relaxant effect on the non-pregnant rat uterus *in situ*; the uterine response from pregnant rats was stated to vary with the stage of pregnancy, the post-implantation period being the most sensitive. The compound was thought to act by a similar mechanism to papaverine.[14]

Human studies In a study of seven women, raw ginger 5 g by mouth reduced thromboxane B$_2$ concentrations in serum collected after clotting,[15] thus indicating a reduction in eicosanoid synthesis (associated with platelet aggregation).

A reduction in joint pain and improvement in joint movement in seven rheumatoid arthritis sufferers has been documented for ginger, with a dual inhibition of cyclo-oxygenase and lipoxygenase pathways reported as a suggested mechanism of action.[15,16] Patients took either fresh ginger in amounts ranging from 5 to 50 g or powdered ginger 0.1 to 1.0 g daily.

Ginger has been reported to be effective as a prophylactic against seasickness.[17,18] Ingestion of powdered ginger root 1 g was found to significantly reduce the tendency to vomit and cold sweating in 40 naval cadets compared to 39 receiving placebo.[17] Powdered ginger root 1.88 g has been reported to be superior to dimenhydrate 100 mg in preventing the gastro-intestinal symptoms of motion sickness

induced by a rotating chair.[18] However, a second study reported ginger (500 mg powdered, 1 g powdered/fresh) to be ineffective in the prevention of motion sickness induced by a rotating chair.[19] The study concluded hyoscine 600 µg and dexamphetamine 10 mg to be the most effective combination, with dimenhydrinate 50 mg as the over-the-counter motion sickness medication of choice.[19] Two more controlled trials have investigated the effect of ginger root on symptoms of motion sickness, collectively known as kinetosis (e.g. vertigo, cold sweating, vomiting).[17] In one of these trials, ginger reduced symptoms of vertigo, while in the second it was ineffective when compared to hyoscine hydrobromide and cinnarizine.[17]

Side-effects, Toxicity

None documented for ginger. Ginger oil is stated to be non-irritating and non-sensitising although dermatitis may be precipitated in hypersensitive individuals. Phototoxicity is not considered to be of significance.[20] Ginger oil is stated to be of low toxicity[G35] with acute LD$_{50}$ values (rat, by mouth; rabbit, dermal) reported to exceed 5 g/kg.[20]

Mutagenic activity has been documented for an ethanolic ginger extract, gingerol, and shogaol in *Salmonella typhimurium* strains TA 100 and TA 1535 in the presence of metabolic activation (S9 mix) but not in TA 98 or TA 1538 with or without S9 mix.[21] Zingerone was found to be non-mutagenic in all four strains with or without S9 mix, and was reported to suppress mutagenic activity of gingerol and shogaol. Ginger juice has been reported to exhibit antimutagenic activity whereas mutagenic activity has been described for (6)-gingerol in the presence of known chemical mutagens.[22] It was suggested that certain mutagens may activate the mutagenic activity of (6)-gingerol so that it is not suppressed by antimutagenic components present in the juice.[22]

Contra-indications, Warnings

Ginger has been reported to possess both cardiotonic and antiplatelet activity *in vitro* and hypoglycaemic activity in *in-vivo* studies. Excessive doses may therefore interfere with existing cardiac, antidiabetic, or anticoagulant therapy. An oleo-resin component, (6)-shogaol has been reported to affect blood pressure (initially decrease then increase) *in vivo*.

Pregnancy and lactation Ginger is reputed to be an abortifacient[G12] and uteroactivity has been documented for a related species. Doses of ginger that greatly exceed the amounts used in foods should not be taken during pregnancy or lactation.

Pharmaceutical Comment

The chemistry of ginger is well documented with respect to the oleo-resin and volatile oil. Oleo-resin components are considered to be the main active principles in ginger and documented pharmacological actions generally support the traditional uses. In addition, a number of other pharmacological activities have been documented, including hypoglycaemic, antihypercholesterolaemic, anti-ulcer, and inhibition of prostaglandin synthesis, all which require further investigation. The use of ginger as a prophylactic remedy against motion sickness is contentious. It seems likely that ginger may act by a local action on the gastro-intestinal tract, rather than by a centrally mediated mechanism.

References

See General References G1, G2, G3, G4, G7, G8, G9, G12, G14, G19, G22, G23, G32 and G35.

1.   Lawrence BM, Reynolds RJ. Major tropical spices — ginger (*Zingiber officinale* Rosc.). *Perf Flav* 1984; **9**: 1–40.

2.   Chen C-C *et al*. Chromatographic analyses of gingerol compounds in ginger (*Zingiber officinale* Roscoe) extracted by liquid carbon dioxide. *J Chromatogr* 1986; **360**: 163–74.

3.   Sharma M, Shukla S. Hypoglycaemic effect of ginger. *J Res Ind Med Yoga Homoeopath* 1977; **12**: 127–30.

4.   Suekawa M *et al*. Pharmacological studies on ginger. V. Pharmacological comparison between (6)-shogaol and capsaicin. *Folia Pharmac Japonica* 1986; **88**: 339–47.

5.   Shoji N *et al*. Cardiotonic principles of ginger (*Zingiber officinale* Roscoe). *J Pharm Sci* 1982; **71**: 1174–5.

6.   Kiuchi F *et al*. Inhibitors of prostaglandin biosynthesis from ginger. *Chem Pharm Bull* 1982; **30**: 754–7.

7.   Srivastava KC. Effects of aqueous extracts of onion, garlic and ginger on platelet aggregation and metabolism of arachidonic acid in the blood vascular system: in vitro study. *Prostaglandins Leukot Med* 1984; **13**: 227–35.

8.   Gujral S *et al*. Effect of ginger (*Zingiber officinale* Roscoe) oleorosin on serum and hepatic cholesterol levels in cholesterol fed rats. *Nutr Rep Int* 1974; **17**: 183–9.

9.   Giri J *et al*. Effect of ginger on serum cholesterol levels. *Indian J Nutr Dietet* 1984; **21**: 433–6.

10.   Yamahara J *et al*. Cholagogic effect of ginger and its active constituents. *J Ethnopharmacol* 1985; **13**: 217–25.

11.   Yamahara J *et al*. The anti-ulcer effect in rats of ginger constituents. *J Ethnopharmacol* 1988; **23**: 299–304.

12.   Sakai K *et al*. Effect of extracts of Zingiberaceae herbs on gastric secretion in rabbits. *Chem Pharm Bull* 1989; **37**: 215–17.

13.   Taroeno *et al*. Anthelmintic activities of some hydrocarbons and oxygenated compounds in the essential oil of *Zingiber purpureum*. *Planta Med* 1989; **55**: 105.

14.   Kanjanapothi D *et al*. A uterine relaxant compound from *Zingiber cassumunar*. *Planta Med* 1987; **53**: 329–32.

15.   Srivastava KC. Effect of onion and ginger consumption on platelet thromboxane production in humans. *Prostaglandins Leukot Essent Fatty Acids* 1989; **35**: 183–5.

16.   Srivastava K *et al*. Ginger and rheumatic disorders. *Med Hypoth* 1989; **29**: 25–8

17.   Grontved A *et al*. Ginger root against seasickness. A controlled trial on the open sea. *Acta Otolaryngol* 1988; **105**: 45–9.

18.   Mowrey DB, Clayson DE. Motion sickness, ginger, and psychophysics. *Lancet* 1982; **i**: 655–7.

19.   Wood CD *et al*. Comparison of efficacy of ginger with various antimotion sickness drugs. *Clin Res Pract Drug Reg Affairs* 1988; **6**: 129–36.

20.   Opdyke DLJ. Ginger oil. *Food Cosmet Toxicol* 1974; **12**: 901–2.

21.   Nagabhushan M *et al*. Mutagenicity of ginergol and shogaol and antimutagenicity of zingerone in salmonella/microsome assay. *Cancer Lett* 1987; **36**: 221–33.

22.   Nakamura H, Yamamoto T. Mutagen and anti-mutagen in ginger, *Zingiber officinale*. *Mutat Res* 1982; **103**: 119–26.

GINKGO

Species (Family)
Ginkgo biloba L. (Ginkgoaceae)

Synonym(s)
Maidenhair Tree, Kew Tree, Fossil Tree

Part(s) Used
Leaf, Seed

Pharmacopoeial Monographs
Martindale 30th edition
Pharmacopoeias—Chin. and Fr.

Legal Category (Licensed Products)
Not included on GSL[G14]

Constituents[G24,G32]
Leaf *Amino acids* 6-Hydroxykynurenic acid (2-carboxy-4-one-6-hydroxyquinoline), a metabolite of tryptophan[1-3]
Flavonoids Dimeric flavones (e.g. bilobetin, ginkgetin, isoginkgetin, sciadopitysin);[4] flavonols (e.g. quercetin, kaempferol) and their glycosides[1,5]
Proanthocyanidins [6]
Terpenoids (diterpenes) Bilobalide.[6] Ginkgolides A, B, C, J, M which are unique cage molecules[6-9,G24]

Seeds *Alkaloids* Ginkgotoxin (4-O-methylpyridoxine)[10]
Amino acids [6]
Cyanogenetic glycosides [6]
Phenols A series of long-chain phenols including anacaric acid, bilobol and cardanol have been isolated from the seeds[11]

Food Use
The seed is edible and is sold in the Far East.[6,G24]

Herbal Use
The medicinal use of the leaves was recorded by the Chinese in 'Chen Houng Pen T'sao' published in 2800 BC and a monograph exists in the modern Chinese pharmacopoeia.[7,8] The leaves are recommended as being beneficial to the heart and lungs; inhalation of a decoction of leaves is used for the treatment of asthma; boiled leaves are used against chilblains.[8] Standardised concentrated extracts of *G. biloba* leaves are marketed in several European countries (e.g. as Tanakan™ in France, and as Tebonin™ and Rokan™ in Germany).[6] The seed is used as an antitussive and expectorant in Japan and China.[10]

Dose
Leaf extract 80–120 mg daily[6,8]
Solid extract 40 mg three times daily[6]
Fluid extract (1:1) 0.5 mL three times daily[6]

Pharmacological Actions
The pharmacological activities of ginkgo have been reviewed.[6-9,12]

Animal studies Ginkgolides competitively inhibit the binding of platelet-activating factor (PAF) to its membrane receptor.[6-9]

Ginkgolide B antagonises thrombus formation induced by PAF and in the guinea-pig it also induces a rapid curative thromblysis. A protective effect is exerted by ginkgolides on PAF-induced bronchoconstriction and airway hyperactivity in immuno-anaphylaxis and in antigen-induced bronchial provocation tests. Oral or intravenous injection of ginkgolide B antagonises cardiovascular impairments and bronchoconstriction induced by PAF. Ginkgolide B does not appear to interfere with cyclo-oxygenase, but at an earlier step involving PAF receptors and phospholipase activation. Eosinophil infiltration occurs in asthma and in allergic reactions, the number of eosinophils increasing during late phase. Since PAF is a potent activator of eosinophil function it is argued that ginkgolide B may interfere with the late phase response.[7] Antigen-induced pulmonary impairment is inhibited by ginkgolides in guinea-pigs. The protective effect of ginkgolides on immune bronchoconstriction is associated with values of blood pH, PO_2, and thromboxane B_2 concentrations returning to normal.

Decrease in myocardial contractility and coronary flow, induced by PAF in perfused guinea-pig heart, are antagonised by ginkgolides. Ginkgolide B inhibits the suppressive effects of PAF on T-lymphocyte profiliferation and cytokine production. Cardiac allograft survival in rats is increased by ginkgolide A, which acts synergistically with azathioprine and cyclosporin A. Ginkgolide A also prevents cyclosporin A-induced nephrotoxicity. PAF is released from mesangial cells of isolated perfused rat kidneys and glomeruli, and ginkgolides are able to inhibit the resulting release of thromboxane B_2, prostaglandins, and reactive oxygen species. Significant protection from endotoxic shock has been observed in animals injected with ginkgolide B. Endotoxin-induced ulceration of the gastro-intestinal tract in animals is inhibited by ginkgolide B. When ginkgolide B is injected intravenously into rats or guinea-pigs it inhibits inflammation and vascular permeability induced by PAF and it is also liable to antagonise skin damage produced by low doses of lymphokine. Ginkgolides are able to antagonise the adverse effects of PAF on retinas of rabbits and rats. *G. biloba* leaf extract reduces superoxide release in polymorphonuclear cells taken from whole body gamma irradiated rabbits.[10]

PAF is implicated in panic disorders and although ginkgolides do not modify behavioural patterns in animals, they do reduce immobility in despair tests. *G. biloba* leaf extract improves cerebral metabolism and protects brain tissue against hypoxic damage in various animal models of cerebral ischemia by PAF antagonism. Although ginkgolide

B is not a direct free radical scavenger it does inhibit lipid peroxidation occurring in animal post-ischemic lesions.[6-9]

Three long chain phenols, anacardic acid, bilobol, and cardanol isolated from seeds of *G. biloba* are active against Sarcoma 180 ascites in mice.[11]

Human studies Double-blind clinical trials with matched patient groups with peripheral arterial insufficiency of the lower limbs have demonstrated that a standardised extract *G. biloba* leaf is clinically effective.[6] Significant improvements in pain-free walking time and in maximum walking distance were achieved.[6] Intradermal injections of PAF induce a biphasic inflammatory response similar to that observed in sensitised individuals subjected to moderate doses of allergen. A single dose of a mixture of ginkgolides antagonises this response.[6] Oral administration of ginkgolides resulted in a reduction of eosinophil infiltration in atopic patients given intracutaneous injections of PAF [6]

In a double-blind, randomised cross-over study, 80 and 120 mg capsules containing a standardised mixture of ginkgolides A, B, and C (ratio of 40:40:20) were given as a single oral dose two hours before challenge by intradermal PAF/histamine. Both dose ranges inhibited flare which was maximal after 5 minutes. Within 15 to 30 minutes wheal volume was reduced, greatest effect being observed for the higher dose treatments. The protection was still present eight hours after oral dosing.[8] Similar inhibition of PAF was observed for platelet aggregation with single oral doses of 80 and 120 mg extract which were given two hours before blood withdrawal. The ginkgolide mixture given orally also blocked PAF-induced airway hyper-responsiveness.

Antagonism of the effects of PAF by a standarised mixture of ginkgolides was assessed in a double-blind, placebo-controlled cross-study in six normal subjects aged 25 to 35 years.[13] Wheal and flare responses to PAF examined two hours after ingestion of 80 mg and 120 mg of ginkgolide mixture were inhibited in a dose-related manner. Both doses significantly inhibited PAF-induced platelet aggregation in platelet-rich plasma.[13]

A double-blind, randomised cross-over study was undertaken with atopic asthmatic patients who were challenged with their specific dust or pollen antigen. Some 6.5 hours later they were subjected to a new provocation test with acetylcholine so that the treatment of later stages of an asthma attack could be assessed. Mixed ginkgolide standardised extract, 40 mg three times daily, or placebo, were given during the three days before the test and a final single dose of 120 mg of extract was given 2 hours before the challenge. The trial demonstrated that ginkgolides were effective in both the early phase and the late phase of airway hyperactivity.[8]

Some 112 patients with a mean age of 70.5 years suffering with chronic cerebral insufficiency were treated as outpatients with *G. biloba* leaf standardised extract at 120 mg per day in an open one-year trial.[14] The results showed that there was a statistically significant regression of major symptoms including vertigo, headache, tinnitus, short term memory, vigilance and mood disturbance. During the period of the trial no changes were noted for heat rate or blood pressure and the blood concentrations of cholesterol and of triglycerides remained unchanged.[14]

Eight healthy female volunteers with a mean age of 32 years were given a standardised extract of *G. biloba* leaf at dose ranges of 120, 240, and 600 mg and a placebo according to nine randomised, double-blind cross-over design.[15] One hour following treatment the subjects were given a series of psychological tests. Memory was found to be significantly improved with the 600 mg dose as compared with placebo. The author concluded that there was a potential use of *G. biloba* leaf extract for the treatment of individuals suffering from senile or presenile dementia in which impaired memory function is a prevailing characteristic.[15]

A review of *G. biloba* published in 1986 details clinical investigations into its use for the treatment of cerebral disorders due to ageing, memory impairment, acute cochlear deafness, tinnitus, and oedema.[9]

Side-effects, Toxicity

No significant side-effects or interactions with existing medication, including cardiac glycosides and antidiabetic preparations, were noted in one trial involving 112 patients treated with 120 mg/day of *G. biloba* leaf extract.[14] No significant adverse reactions have been reported in patients ingesting as much as 600 mg of leaf extract in single doses.[6] Mild adverse reactions including gastro-intestinal upset and headache have been reported.[6]

Contact or ingestion of the fruit pulp has produced severe allergic reactions including erythema, oedema, blisters, and itching.[6] The seed contains the toxin 4-*O*-methylpyridoxine which is reported to be responsible for 'gin-nan' food poisoning in Japan and China.[10] The main symptoms are convulsion and loss of consciousness and lethality is estimated in about 27% of cases in Japan, infants being particularly vulnerable.

Contra-indications, Warnings

The fruit pulp has produced severe allergic reactions and should not be handled or ingested. The seed causes severe adverse effects when ingested.

Pregnancy and lactation No studies appear to have been reported on the effects of *G. biloba* leaf extracts or ginkgolides in pregnant or lactating women. In view of the many pharmacological actions documented and the lack of toxicity data, use of ginkgo during pregnancy and lactation should be avoided.

Pharmaceutical Comment

G. biloba leaf, its extract, or purified mixtures of ginkgolides are present in some herbal preparations. There is considerable literature evidence to show that the ginkgolides present in *G. biloba* leaf are able to alleviate the adverse effects of platelet-activating factor in a number of tissues and organs both in animals and in humans.[16-18] Clinical data based on trials with small numbers of patients indicate that *Ginkgo* preparations are effective in the treatment of arterial insufficiency in the limbs and in the brain. Improvements in allergic responses (e.g. in asthma) have been observed in humans and inflammation due to PAF is reduced. The claims that *Ginkgo* preparations are beneficial in the treatment of geriatric illness, including impairment of memory is of considerable interest and further clinical trials are being undertaken. The intended uses of ginkgo are not suitable for self-medication.

References

See General References G24 and G32.

1.   Victoire C, *et al*. Isolation of flavonoid glycosides from *Ginkgo biloba* leaves. *Planta Med* 1988; **54:** 245–7.

2.   Schenne A, Holzl J. 6-Hydroxykynurensaure, die erste N-haltige Verbindung aus den Blattern von *Ginkgo biloba*. *Planta Med* 1986; **52:** 235–6.

3.   Nasr C, *et al*. 2-Quinoline carboxylic acid-4,6-dihydroxy from *Ginkgo biloba*. Phytochemical Society of Europe Symposium: Biologically active natural products, Lausanne (1986), p. 9.

4.   Briancon-Scheid F, *et al*. HPLC separation and quantitative determination of biflavones in leaves from *Ginkgo biloba*. *Planta Med* 1983; **49:** 204–20.

5.   Vanhaelen M, Vanhaelen-Fastre R. Kaempferol-3-*O*-β-glucoside (astragalin) from *Ginkgo biloba*. *Fitoterapia* 1988; **59**: 511.

6   Pizzorno JE and Murray MT. A textbook of natural medicine. Seattle, WA: John Bastyr College Publications 1985 (looseleaf).

7.   Hosford D, *et al*. Natural antagonists of platelet-activating factor. *Phytotherapy Res* 1988; **2**: 1–17.

8   Braquet P. The ginkgolides: potent platelet-activating factor antagonists isolated from *Ginkgo biloba* L.: Chemistry, pharmacology and clinical applications. *Drugs of the Future* 1987; **12**: 643–99.

9.   Anonymous. Extract of *Ginkgo biloba* (EGb 761). *Presse Med* 1986; **15:** (31) 1438–1598.

10.   Wada K, *et al*. Studies on the constitution of edible medicinal plants. 1. Isolation and identification of 4-*O*-methylpyridoxine, toxic principle from the seed of *Ginkgo biloba* L. *Chem Pharm Bull* 1988; **36**: 1779–82.

11.   Itokawa H, *et al*. Antitumour principles from *Ginkgo biloba* L. *Chem Pharm Bull* 1987; **35:** 3016–20.

12.   Clostre F and De Fendis (editors). Cardiovascular effects of *Ginkgo biloba* extract (EGb761). Advances in *Ginkgo biloba* extract research, vol.3. Paris: Elsevier, 1994. pp.1–162.

13.   Chung KF. Effect of a ginkgolide mixture (BN 52063) in antagonising skin and platelet responses to platelet activating factor in man. *Lancet* 1987; **i**: 248–51.

14.   Vorberg G. *Ginkgo biloba* extract (GBE): A long term study on chronic cerebral insufficiency in geriatric patients. *Clin Trials J* 1985; **22**: 149–57.

15.   Hindmarsh SZ. The psychopharmacological effects of *Ginkgo biloba* extract in normal healthy volunteers. *Int J Clin Pharmacol Res* 1984; **4**: 89–93.

16.   Houghton PJ. Ginkgo. *Pharm J* 1994; **253**: 122–3.

17.   Braquet P (ed.). Ginkgolides — chemistry, biology, pharmacology and clinical perspectives, vol.1. Barcelona: JR Prous, 1988.

18.   Braquet, P (ed.). Ginkgolides — chemistry, biology, pharmacology and clinical perspectives, vol.2. Barcelona: JR Prous, 1989.

GINSENG, ELEUTHEROCOCCUS

Species (Family)
Eleutherococcus senticosus (Rupr. & Maxim.) Maxim (Araliaceae)

Synonym
Devil's Shrub, Eleuthero and Siberian Ginseng, Touch-Me-Not, Wild Pepper, *Acanthopanax senticosus*, *Hedera senticosa*

Part(s) Used
Root

Pharmacopoeial Monographs
BHP 1990

Legal Category (Licensed Products)
Not included on the GSL[G14]

Constituents[1,2,G2]
Eleutherosides A–M Heterogenous group of compounds including sterol(A), phenylpropanoid(B), coumarin (B1, B3), monosaccharide(C), and lignan(B_4,D,E) structural types, many present as glycosides. Characterised eleutherosides include daucosterol(A), syringin(B), isofraxidin glucoside(B_1), (–)-sesamin(B_4), methyl-α-D-galactoside(C), (–)-syringaresinol glucoside(D), acanthoside D(E) and hedera-saponin B(M).
Carbohydrates Polysaccharides (glycans); some have been referred to as eleutherans.[10] Galactose, glucose, maltose, sucrose
Some of the additional documented constituents represent aglycones of the eleutherosides, namely β-sitosterol, isofraxidin, (–)-syringaresinol and sinapyl alcohol.
Phenylpropanoids Caffeic acid and ester, coniferyl aldehyde
Terpenoids Oleanolic acid
Volatile oils (0.8%). Individual components not documented

Food Use
Eleutherococcus ginseng is not used in foods

Herbal Use
Eleutherococcus ginseng does not have a traditional herbal use in the UK, although it has been used for many years in the former Soviet Union. Like Panax ginseng, Eleutherococcus ginseng is claimed to be an adaptogen in that it increases the body's resistance to stress and builds up general vitality.[G2,G4,G25]

Dose
Dry root 0.6–3 g daily for up to one month has been recommended.[G2,G25] Russian studies in healthy human subjects have involved the administration of an ethanolic extract in doses ranging from 2–16 mL one to three times daily, for up to 60 consecutive days.
Doses in non-healthy individuals ranged from 0.5–6.0 mL one to three times daily for up to 35 days. In both groups, multiple dosing regimens were separated by an extract free period of 2 to 3 weeks.[1]

Pharmacological Actions
The adaptogenic properties of Eleutherococcus ginseng have been extensively investigated in the USSR. Pharmacological studies on extracts of Eleutherococcus ginseng started in the 1950s and have been primarily reported by two groups of Russian scientists. In 1962, a 33% ethanolic extract of *Eleutherococcus senticosus* was approved for human use by the Pharmacological Committee of USSR Ministry of Health, and in 1976 it was estimated that some 3 million people were regularly using this extract.[1]
A review by Farnsworth *et al*[1] describes the chemistry and toxicity of Eleutherococcus ginseng and documents results of *in-vitro*, *in-vivo*, and human studies involving the oral administration of an ethanolic extract.
The majority of literature on Eleutherococcus ginseng has been published in the Russian language and therefore great difficulty is encountered in obtaining translations.[1] This monograph will draw mainly on data included in the Farnsworth review as well as on more recent papers that have been published in English. When used in this monograph , 'ginseng' will refer to Eleutherococcus ginseng unless indicated otherwise.

Animal studies
Hypo/Hyperglycaemic activity has been documented in both normal animals and in those with induced hyperglycaemia (rabbit, mouse), but with little effect on alloxan-induced hyperglycaemia (rat).[1,3] Hypoglycaemic activity (mice, intraperitoneal injection) of an aqueous ginseng extract has been attributed to polysaccharide components termed Eleutherans A–G.[4]

Central nervous system effects Sedative actions (rat, mouse), CNS stimulant effects (intravenous/subcutaneous injection, rabbit), and a decrease/increase in barbiturate sleeping time has been reported.[1,5]

Immunostimulant, antitoxic actions Increased resistance to induced listeriosis infection (mouse, rabbit) with prophylactic ginseng administration and reduced resistance with simultaneous administration, stimulation of specific antiviral immunity (guinea-pig, mouse), regulation of complement titre and lysozyme activity post immunisation have been documented.[1] In addition, protection against cardiac glycoside (intravenous injection, frog), diethylglycolic acid (mouse) and alloxan (rat) toxicity has also been described.[1]

Immune stimulant effects have been reported for polysaccharide components, together with an ability to lessen thioacetamide, phytohaemagglutinin and X-ray toxicity, and to exhibit antitumour effects.[4] Immunostimulant activity *in vitro* (using granulocyte, carbon clearance, and lymphocyte-transformation tests) has been documented for high molecular weight polysaccharide components.[6,7]

Effects on overall performance   A beneficial action on parameters indicative of stress (rat) and on overall work capacity (mouse) has been reported,[1] although a lack of adaptogenic response has also been reported in mice receiving various ginseng infusions (Siberian, Korean and American).[8,9] In one study, mice receiving a commercial concentrated extract of Eleutherococcus ginseng were noted to exhibit significantly more aggressive behaviour.[8] Ginseng is claimed to result in a more economical utilisation of glycogen and high energy phosphorus compounds, and in a more intense metabolism of lactic and pyruvic acids during stress.[1] It has been claimed that the adaptogenic effect of ginseng involves regulation of energy, nucleic acid, and protein metabolism in tissues.[1]

Steroidal activity   Gonadotrophic activity in immature male mice (intraperitoneal injection), oestrogenic activity in immature female mice, and an anabolic effect in immature rats (intraperitoneal injection) has been reported.[1] *In-vitro* studies have reported that ginseng extracts bind to progestin, mineralocorticoid, glucocorticoid and oestrogen receptors.[1]

Cardiovascular activity   3,4-Dihydroxybenzoic acid (DBA) has been identified as an anti-aggregatory component in Eleutherococcus ginseng.[10] Compared to aspirin, activity of DBA was comparable versus collagen- and ADP-induced platelet aggregation, but less potent versus arachidonic acid-induced platelet aggregation.[10] Anti-oedema and anti-inflammatory actions (intravenous injection, mouse, have also been described.[1]

Effect on reproductive capacity   Ginseng has been reported to improve the reproductive capacity of bulls and cows, and to have no adverse effects on the various blood parameters (haemoglobin, total plasma protein, albumin and globulin, protein coefficient) measured.[1]

Other actions documented for ginseng include the stimulation of liver regeneration in partially hepatectomised mice,[1] an increase in catecholamine concentrations in the brain, adrenal gland, and urine,[1] a variable effect on induced hypothermia (rabbit, rat, mouse),[1] and *in-vitro* inhibition (66%) of hexobarbitone metabolism.[5]

Human studies

In Russia, ginseng extract has been administered orally to more than 4300 human subjects in studies involving either healthy or non-healthy individuals.[1]

Administration to healthy subjects   These studies were designed to investigate the adaptogenic effects of ginseng and measured parameters such as the ability of humans to withstand adverse conditions (heat, noise, motion, workload increase, exercise, decompression), improvement in auditory disturbances, quality of work under stress conditions and in athletic performance, and increase in mental alertness and work output.[1] The studies involved more than 2100 subjects and included both male and female subjects ranging in age from 19 to 72 years. Doses ranged from 2 to 16 mL of an ethanolic extract (33%), administered orally one to three times a day, for periods of up to 60 consecutive days. Multiple dosing regimens usually involved a 2 to 3 week interval between courses.[1] For many of the studies, it is unclear whether ginseng had a beneficial effect because this is not stated in the Farnsworth review. However, ginseng was found to exert favourable effects in a number of situations including ability to perform physical labour, quality of proofreading, adaptation to a high temperature environment, speed and quality of work by radiotelegraphers in noisy conditions, resistance to hypoxemia and physical burdens in skiers, ability to withstand conditions designed to induce motion sickness, capillary resistance, haematological parameters in blood donors, and number of days lost to sickness amongst factory workers. Ginseng was also reported to increase excretion of vitamins B_1, B_2 and C given concurrently with the ginseng. On its own, ginseng did not affect the excretion of water-soluble vitamins.

Administration to non-healthy subjects   These studies involved more than 2200 subjects with various ailments and included both males and females ranging in age from 19 to 60 years. Ginseng doses ranging from 0.5 to 6 mL were administered orally between one to three times daily for up to 35 days, with as many as eight courses employed. Multiple dosing regimens involved a 2 to 3 week ginseng-free interval in between courses.[1] A favourable effect was noted in atherosclerosis (although treatment was stated to be less effective in patients with high blood pressure), acute pyelonephritis, various forms of diabetes mellitus (although no marked effect was noted in another study), hypertension and hypotension (tendancy to normalisation), acute craniocerebral trauma, various types of neuroses, rheumatic heart disease (reduced blood coagulation properties), chronic bronchitis, and in children with abating forms of pulmonary tuberculosis.[1] An increase in the working capacity of six males, in a single blind crossover study using placebo and no treatment as comparators, has been reported for a 33% ethanolic ginseng extract.[13] The observed increase in working capacity was partially attributed to an improvement in bodily oxygen metabolism, reflected by the increase in all four measured parameters (oxygen uptake, oxygen pulse, total work and exhaustion time).[11]

Immunostimulant activity   A strong immunomodulatory effect has been documented for an ethanolic extract of ginseng, in a placebo-controlled double-blind study using healthy volunteers.[12] A significant increase in the total lymphocyte count, especially in the T-lymphocyte cells, was noted in the ginseng-treated group who received a daily dose of 30–40 mL extract (eleutheroside B 0.2%w/v). Specificity of action on the lymphocytes was confirmed by the fact that neither granulocyte or monocyte levels were significantly altered.[12]

Side-effects, Toxicity

No side-effects were documented from Russian studies involving more than 2100 healthy subjects.[1] Studies involving patients with various ailments have reported a few side-effects: insomnia, shifts in heart rhythm, tachycardia, extrasystole and hypertonia in some athersclerotic patients; headaches, pericardial pain, palpitations, and elevated blood pressure in 2 of 55 patients (at high dose level) with rheumatic heart disease; insomnia, irritability, melancholy and anxiety in hypochondriac patients receiving higher doses of extract; hypersensitivity reaction (symptoms unspecified) in stressed individuals.[1] Hypertension and mastalgia have been documented as side-effects of ginseng (species unknown).[13]

Results of various animal toxicity studies have indicated ginseng to be non-toxic.[1] Many species have been exposed to extracts including mice, rats, rabbits, dogs, minks, deer, lambs, and piglets.[1] Documented acute oral LD_{50} values for various preparations include: 23 mL/kg and 14.5 g/kg (mice), and greater than 20 mL/kg (dogs) for a 33% ethanolic extract[1,3]; 31 g/kg (mice) for the powdered root; greater than 3 g/kg (mice) for an aqueous aqueous (equivalent to 25 g dried roots/kg).[3] No deaths occurred in mice administered single 3 g/kg doses of a freeze-dried aqueous extract.[11] Symptoms observed in dogs receiving 7.1 mL/kg doses of the ethanolic extract (sedation, ataxia, loss of righting reflex, hypopnoea, tremors, increased salivation and vomiting) were attributed to the ethanol content of the extract.[1] A chronic toxicity study reported no toxic manifestations or deaths in rats fed 5 mL/kg ethanolic extract for 320 days.[1]

Teratogenicity studies in male and female rats, pregnant minks, rabbits and lambs have reported no abnormalities in the off-spring and no adverse effects in the animals administered the extracts. Premature death in parent female rabbits fed 13.5 mL/kg ethanolic extract daily was attributed to ethanol intoxication.[1]

Mutagenicity studies using Salmonella typhimurium TA100 and TA98, and the micronucleus test in mice have reported no activity for ginseng.[14] Differences in various serum biochemical parameters have been reported between test (ginseng) and control groups.[14] Parameters affected included ALP and gamma-GT enzymes (increased), serum triglycerides (decreased), and creatinine and BUN (increased).[14] No pathological changes were found in rats receiving a ginseng extract.[14]

Contra-indications, Warnings

It has been stated that ginseng should be avoided by individuals who are highly energetic, nervous, tense, hysteric, manic or schizophrenic, and that it should not be taken with stimulants, including coffee, antipsychotic drugs or during treatment with hormones.[13] In view of documented pharmacological actions ginseng may interfere with a number of therapies including cardiac, anticoagulant, hypoglycaemic, and hypo/hypertensive. Ginseng is stated to be unsuitable for individuals with high blood pressure (180/90 mmHg or greater)[1] and has been advised to be avoided by premenopausal women.[13]

Russian recommendations advise that healthy people under the age of 40 should not use ginseng and that middle-aged people can be treated with small doses of ginseng on a daily basis.[13] Individuals considered suitable to use ginseng are recommended to abstain from alcoholic beverages, sexual activity, bitter substances, and spicy foods.[13]

In general, long-term use of ginseng is not recommended and one author has documented that the main side-effect of prolonged use manifests as an inflamed nerve, frequently the sciatic, which then causes muscle spasm in the affected area.[13] Human studies involving long-term administration of ginseng have involved ginseng-free periods of 2–3 weeks every 30–60 days.

Pregnancy and lactation Teratogenicity studies in various animal species have not reported any teratogenic effects for ginseng. However, in view of the many pharmacological actions documented for ginseng, and the general recommendation that it should not be used by premenopausal women, the use of ginseng during both pregnancy and lactation should be avoided. It is unknown whether the pharmacologically active constituents in ginseng are secreted in the breast milk.

Pharmaceutical Comment

Phytochemical studies have revealed that there is no one constituent type that is characteristic of Eleutherococcus ginseng. Studies have shown that components thought to represent the main active constituents ('eleutherosides') consist of a heterogenous mixture of common plant constituents. Since the 1950s, many studies (animal and human) have been carried out in Russia, and more recently in Western countries, to investigate the reputed adaptogen properties of Eleutherococcus ginseng. An adaptogen is a substance that is defined as having three characteristics, namely lack of toxicity, non-specific action, and a normalising action.[1] Results of numerous studies in animals and humans seem to support these three criteria for Eleutherococcus ginseng, although pharmacological explanations for the observed actions are less well understood.[1] As with Panax ginseng, Eleutherococcus ginseng has been shown to possess a wide range of pharmacological activities. Consequently, it should be used with appropriate regard to traditional guidelines that have been drawn up in China and Russia.

References
See General References G2, G4, G14, G25.

1. Farnsworth NR *et al.* Siberian ginseng (*Eleutherococcus senticosus*): Current status as an adaptogen. In: Economics and Medicinal Plant Research, vol 1, Wagner H et al, eds. London: Academic Press, 1985: 155–209

2.   Phillipson JD, Anderson LA. Ginseng — quality, safety and efficacy? *Pharm J* 1984; **232:** 161–5.

3.   Medon PJ *et al.* Hypoglycaemic effect and toxicity of *Eleutherococcus senticosus* following acute and chronic administration in mice. *Acta Pharmacol Sinica* 1981; **2:** 281–5.

4.   Hikino H *et al.* Isolation and hypoglycaemic activity of eleutherans A, B, C, D, E, F, and G: Glycans of *Eleutherococcus senticosus* roots. *J Nat Prod* 1986; **49:** 293–7.

5.   Medon PJ *et al.* Effects of *Eleutherococcus senticosus* extracts on hexobarbital metabolism *in vivo* and *in vitro*. *J Ethnopharmacol* 1984; **10:** 235–41.

6.   Wagner H *et al.* Immunstimulierend wirkende Polysaccharide (heteroglykane) aus höheren Pflanzen. *Arzneimittelforschung* 1985; **35:** 1069.

7.   Wagner H. Immunostimulants from medicinal plants. In: Chang HM *et al*, editors. Advancesin Chinese Medicinal Materials Research. Singapore: World Scientific, 1985: 159. 159.

8.   Lewis WH *et al.* No adaptogen response of mice to ginseng and *Eleutherococcus* infusions. *J Ethnopharmacol* 1983; **8:** 209–14.

9.   Martinez B, Staba EJ. The physiological effects of *Aralia, Panax* and *Eleutherococcus* on exercised rats. *Jpn J Pharmacol* 1984; **35:** 79–85.

10.   Yun-Choi HS *et al.* Potential inhibitors of platelet aggregation from plant sources, III. *J Nat Prod* 1987; **50:** 1059–64.

11.   Asano K *et al.* Effect of *Eleutherococcus senticosus* extract on human physical working capacity. *Planta Med* 1986; **52:** 175.

12.   Bohn B *et al.* Flow-cytometric studies with *Eleutherococcus senticosus* extract as an immunomodulatory agent. *Arzneimittelforschung* 1987; **37:** 1193–6.

13.   Baldwin CA *et al.* What pharmacists should know about ginseng. *Pharm J* 1986; **237:** 583.

14.   Hirosue T *et al.* Mutagenicity and subacute toxicity of *Acanthopanax senticosus* extracts in rats. *J Food Hyg Soc Jpn* 1986; **27:** 380–6.

GINSENG, PANAX

Species (Family)
Various *Panax* species (Araliaceae) including:
(i) *Panax ginseng* Meyer
(ii) *Panax quinquefolius* L.
(iii) *Panax notoginseng* (Burkhill) Hoo & Tseng

Synonym(s)
(i) *Panax pseudoginseng* Wallich, *Panax schinseng* Nees, Jintsam, Ninjin, Schinsent; Asiatic, Chinese, Korean, Japanese, and Oriental ginseng.
(ii) American, Sanchi, and Tienchi ginseng
(iii) American and Western ginseng, Five-Fingers, Sang

Part(s) Used
Root
White ginseng represents the peeled and sun-dried root whilst red ginseng is unpeeled, steamed and dried.

Pharmacopoeial Monographs
BHP 1990
Martindale 30th edition
Pharmacopoeias—Aust., Chin., Cz., Fr., Jpn, Rus., and Swiss. Chin. also includes Radix Notoginseng from *Panax notoginseng*, Rhizoma Panacis from *Panax japonicus*, and Rhizoma Panacis Majoris from *Panax japonicus* var. *major* and *Panax japonicus* var. *bipinnatifidus*. Red Ginseng (Jpn P.) is the dried root of *Panax ginseng* that has been steamed.

Legal Category (Licensed Products)
GSL[G14]

Constituents[G1,G2,G19,G32]
Terpenoids Complex mixture of compounds (ginsenosides or panaxosides) involves three aglycone structural types — two tetracyclic dammarane-type sapogenins (protopanaxadiol and protopanaxatriol) and a pentacyclic triterpene oleanolic acid-type. Different naming conventions have been used for these compounds. In Japan, they are known as ginsenosides and are represented by R_x where 'x' indicates a particular saponin. For example, R_a, R_{b-1}, R_c, R_d, R_{g-1}. In Russia, the saponins are referred to as panaxosides and are represented as panaxoside X where 'X' can be A–F. The suffixes in the two systems are not equivalent and thus panaxoside A does not equal R_a but R_{g-1}.[1]
The saponin content varies between different *Panax* species. For example, in *P. ginseng* the major ginsenosides are R_{b-1}, R_c and R_{g-1} whereas in *P. quinquefolis* R_{b-1} is the only major ginsenoside.[1]
Other constituents Volatile oil (trace) mainly consisting of sesquiterpenes including panacene, limonene, terpineol, eucalyptol, α-phellandrene, and citral,[2] sesquiterpene alcohols including the panasinsanols A and B, and ginsenol,[3,4] polyacetylenes,[5,6] sterols, polysaccharides (mainly pectins and glucans),[7] starch (8–32%), β-amylase,[8] free sugars, vitamins (B_1, B_2, B_{12}, panthotenic acid, biotin), choline (0.1–0.2%), fats, minerals.
The sesquiterpene alcohols are stated to be characteristic components of *Panax ginseng* in that they are absent from the volatile oils of other *Panax* species.[4]

Food Use
Ginseng is listed by the Council of Europe as a natural source of food flavouring (category N2). This category indicates that ginseng can be added to foodstuffs in small quantities, with a possible limitation of an active principle (as yet unspecified) in the final product.[G9]

Herbal Use
Ginseng is stated to possess thymoleptic, sedative, demulcent, and stomachic properties, and is reputed to be an aphrodisiac. Traditionally, it has been used for neurasthenia, neuralgia, insomnia, hypotonia, and specifically for depressive states associated with sexual inadequacy.[G1,G2,G4,G32]
Ginseng has been used traditionally in Chinese medicine for many thousands of years as a stimulant, tonic, diuretic and stomachic.[9] Traditionally, ginseng use has been divided into two categories: *short-term*—to improve stamina, concentration, healing process, stress resistance, vigilance and work efficiency in healthy individuals and *long-term*—to improve well-being in debilitated and degenerative conditions especially those associated with old age.

Dose
Traditionally, dosage recommendations differ between the short term use in healthy individuals and the long term use in elderly or debilitated persons.

Short-term (For the young and healthy)
0.5–1.0 g root daily, as two divided doses, for a course generally lasting 15–20 days and with a root-free period of approximately two weeks between consecutive courses. Doses are recommended to be taken in the morning, two hours before a meal, and in the evening, not less than two hours after a meal.[9]

Long-term. (For the old and sick)
0.4–0.8 g root daily. Doses may be taken continuously.[1]

Pharmacological Actions
In the 1950s, early studies on ginseng reported its ability to improve both physical endurance and mental ability in animals and man.[10] In addition, the 'tonic' properties of ginseng were confirmed by the observation that doses taken for a prolonged period of time increased the overall well-being of an individual, measured by various qualitative parameters such as appetite, sleep and absence of moodiness, resulting in an increased work efficiency. Furthermore,

these effects were felt for sometime after cessation of ginseng treatment.[10] In addition, gonadotrophic activity, slight anti-inflammatory activity and an effect on carbohydrate metabolism were noted.[10] Since then, numerous studies have investigated the complex pharmacology of ginseng in both animals and man. The saponin glycosides (ginsenosides/panaxosides) are generally recognised as the main active constituents in ginseng, although pharmacological activities have also been associated with non-saponin components.

The following sections on animal and human studies are intended to give an indication of the type of research that has been published for ginseng rather than to provide a comprehensive bibliography of ginseng research papers.

Animal studies

Many of the activities exhibited by Panax ginseng have been compared to **corticosteroid-like actions** and results of endocrinological studies have suggested that the ginsenosides may primarily augment adrenal steroidogenesis via an indirect action on the pituitary gland.[11] Ginsenosides have increased adrenal cAMP in intact but not in hypophysectomised rats and dexamethasone, a synthetic glucocorticoid that provides positive feedback at the level of the pituitary gland, has blocked the effect of ginsenosides on pituitary corticotrophin and adrenal corticosterone secretion.[11] Hormones produced by the pituitary and adrenal glands are known to play a significant role in the adaptation capabilities of the body.[12] Working capacity is one of the indices used to measure adaptation ability and ginseng has been shown to increase the working capacity of rats following single (132%) and seven day (179%) administration (intraperitoneal). Furthermore, seven day administration of ginseng decreased the reduction seen in working capacity when the pituitary–adrenocortical system is blocked by prior administration of hydrocortisone.[12]

Hypoglycaemic activity has been documented for ginseng and attributed to both saponin and polysaccharide constituents. In-vitro studies using isolated rat pancreatic islets have shown that ginsenosides promote an insulin release which is independent of extracellular calcium and which utilises a different mechanism to that of glucose.[13] In addition, in-vivo studies in rats have reported that a ginseng extract increases the number of insulin receptors in bone marrow and reduces the number of glucocorticoid receptors in rat brain homogenate.[14] Both of these actions are thought to contribute to the antidiabetic action of ginseng, in view of the known diabetogenic action of adrenal corticoids and the knowledge that the number of insulin receptors generally decreases with ageing.[14]

Hypoglycaemic activity observed in both normal and alloxan-induced hyperglycaemic mice administered ginseng (ip) has also been attributed to non-saponin but uncharacterised principles[15–18] and to glycan (polysaccharide) components, Panaxans A–E and Q–U.[19–23] Glycans isolated from Korean or Chinese ginseng (A–E) were found to possess stronger hypoglycaemic activity than those isolated from Japanese ginseng (Q–U).[23] Proposed mechanisms of action have included elevated plasma-insulin concentration due to an increase of insulin secretion from pancreatic islets, and enhancement of insulin sensitivity.[21] However, these mechanisms do not explain the total hypoglycaemic activity that has been exhibited by the polysaccharides and further mechanisms are under investigation.[21]

The effect of panaxans A and B on the activities of key enzymes participating in carbohydrate metabolism has been studied.[18] DPG-3-2, a non-saponin component isolated from ginseng, has been shown to stimulate insulin biosynthesis in pancreatic preparations from various hyperglycaemic (but not normoglycaemic) animals; ginsenosides Rb_1 and Rg_1 were found to decrease islet insulin concentrations to an undetectable level.[16]

Cardiovascular activity Individual saponins have been reported to have different actions on cardiac haemodynamics.[25] For instance R_g, R_{g-1} and total flower saponins have increased cardiac performance whilst R_b and total leaf saponins have decreased it; calcium antagonist activity has been reported for R_b but not for R_g; R_b but not R_g has produced a protective effect on experimental myocardial infarction in rabbits.[25] Negative chronotropic and inotropic effects in vitro have been observed for ginseng saponins and a mechanism of action similar to that of verapamil has been suggested.[26] In-vitro studies on the isolated rabbit heart have reported an increase in coronary blood flow together with a positive inotropic effect.[27] Anti-arrhythmic action on aconitine and barium chloride (rat) and adrenaline (rabbit)-induced arrhythmias, and prolongation of RR, PR and QT_c intervals (rat), have been documented for saponins R_{c-1} and R_{d-1}. The mode of action was thought to be similar to that of amiodarone.[28] Ginsenosides (i.p.) have been reported to protect mice against metabolic disturbances and myocardial damage associated with conditions of severe anoxia.[29]

Ginseng has produced a marked hypotensive response together with bradycardia following intravenous administration to rats. The dose-related effect was blocked by many antagonists suggesting multi-site activity.[27] Higher doses of ginseng were found to cause vasoconstriction rather than vasodilation in renal, mesenteric and femoral arteries.[27]

The total ginseng saponin fraction has been reported to be devoid of haemolytic activity. However, individual ginsenosides have been found to exhibit either haemolytic or protective activities. Protective ginsenosides include R_c, R_{b-2} and R_e, whereas haemolytic saponins have included R_g, R_h and R_f.[30] The number and position of sugars attached to the sapogenin moiety was thought to determine activity.[30] Haemostatic activity has also been documented for ginseng.[31]

Oral administration of ginseng to rats fed a high cholesterol diet reduced serum cholesterol and triglycerides, increased HDL-cholesterol, decreased platelet adhesiveness, and decreased fatty changes to the liver.[32] Ginseng has also been reported to reduce blood coagulation and enhance fibrinolysis.[33] Panaxynol and the ginsenosides R_o, R_{g-1} and R_{g-2} have been documented as the main antiplatelet components in ginseng inhibiting aggregation, release reaction and thromboxane formation *in vitro*.[33] Anti-inflammatory activity and inhibition of 5-HPTE and thromboxane b_2 have previously been described for panaxydol.[33] Anticomplementary activity *in vitro* (human serum) has been documented for ginseng polysaccharides with highest activity observed in strongly acidic polysaccharide fractions.[7]

Effects on neurotransmitters Studies in rats have shown that a standardised ginseng extract (G115) inhibits the development of morphine tolerance and physical dependence, of a decrease in hepatic glutathione concentrations, and of dopamine receptor sensitivity without antagonising morphine analgesia, as previously documented for the individual saponins.[34] The inhibition of tolerance was thought to be asociated with a reduction in morphinone production, a toxic metabolite which irreversibly blocks the opiate receptor sites, and with the activation of morphinone–glutathione conjugation, a detoxication process. The mechanism of inhibition of physical dependence was unclear but thought to be associated with changed ratios of adrenaline, noradrenaline, dopamine and serotonin in the brain.[34]

A total ginsenoside fraction has been reported to inhibit the uptake of various neurotransmitters into rat brain synaptosomes in descending order of gamma-aminobutyrate and noradrenaline, dopamine, glutamate and serotonin.[35–37] The fraction containing ginsenoside R_d was most effective. Uptake of metabolic substrates 2-deoxy-D-glucose and leucine was only slightly affected and therefore it was proposed that the ginseng extracts were acting centrally rather than locally as surface active agents.

Studies in rats have indicated that the increase in dopaminergic receptors in the brain observed under conditions of stress is prevented by pretreatment with ginseng.[38]

Hepatoprotective activity Antioxidant and detoxifying activities have been documented for ginseng.[39] Protection against carbon tetrachloride- and galactosamine-induced hepatotoxicity has been observed in cultured rat hepatocytes for specific ginsenosides (oleanolic acid and dammarane series).[39,40] However, at higher doses certain ginsenosides from both series were found to exhibit simultaneous cytotoxic activity.[37]

Cytotoxic and antitumour activity Cytotoxic activity (ED_{50} 0.5μg/mL) versus L1210 has been documented for polyacetylenes isolated from the root.[5,6,41] The antitumour effect of ginseng polysaccharides in tumour-bearing mice has been associated with an immunological mechanism of action.[42] Ginseng polysaccharides have been reported to increase the lifespan of tumour-bearing mice and to inhibit the growth of tumour cells *in vivo*, although cytocidal action was not seen *in vitro*.[42] Antitumour activity *in vitro* versus several tumour cell lines has been documented for a polyacetylene, panaxytriol.[43]

Antiviral activity Antiviral activity (versus Semliki forest virus; 34–40% protection) has been documented for ginseng extract (G115, Pharmaton) administered orally to rats.[38] The ginseng extract also enhanced the level of protection afforded by 6-MFA, an interferon-inducing agent of fungal origin.[44] Ginseng has been found to induce *in-vitro* and *in-vivo* production of interferon and to augment the natural killer and antibody dependent cytotoxic activities in human peripheral lymphocytes.[44,45] In addition, ginseng enhances the antibody forming cell response to sheep red blood cells in mice and stimulates cell mediated immunity both *in-vitro* and *in-vivo*.[44,45] In view of these observations, it has been proposed that the antiviral activity of ginseng may be immunologically mediated.[44,45]

Human studies

Improvements in serum total cholesterol, HDL-cholesterol, triglycerides, non-essential fatty acids and lipoperoxides have been observed in 67 hyperlipidaemic patients administered 2.7 g/day red ginseng.[28] The addition of ginseng (3 g/65 kg body-weight) to alcohol consumption (72 g/65 kg body-weight of 25% ethanol) has been reported to enhance blood alcohol clearance by 32 to 51%.[46]

A preparation containing ginseng extract with multivitamins and trace elements has been shown to modify some indices of metabolic and liver function in elderly patients with chronic hepatotoxicity induced by alcohol and drugs.[47] Patients who received ginseng exhibited an increase in bromosulphthalein excretion (which is related to hepatic detoxification) and improved serum-zinc concentrations.[47]

A favourable effect on various tests of psychomotor performance (attention, processing, integrated sensory motor function and auditory reaction time) in healthy individuals receiving a ginseng extract (200 mg daily for 12 weeks) has been documented in a double-blind placebo-controlled study.[48] No difference was observed between ginseng and placebo groups in tests of pure motor function, recognition and visual reaction time.[48]

Ginseng has been reported to improve the overall control of status asthmaticus when added to conventional steroid, bronchodilator and antibiotic therapies.[49]

Ginseng has been shown to reduce blood-sugar concentrations in both diabetics and non-diabetics [1], such that in one study insulin therapy was no longer required in a proportion of the patients investigated.[1]

Ginseng has also been reported to normalise both high and low blood pressure states.[1]

Ginseng has been found to affect concentrations of corticosteroids such as ACTH and cortisol and noradrenaline.[1]

Ginseng has been reported to successfully treat cases of diabetic polyneuropathy, reactive depression, psychogenic impotence, enuresis, and various child psychiatric disorders.[53]

Side-effects, Toxicity

In Japan, ginseng (*Panax*) has been given to more than 500 individuals over the course of two studies with no side-effects experienced.[1] However, suspected adverse events associated with ginseng treatment have been documented although it is often difficult to assess individual cases due to a lack of information concerning dose, duration of treatment, species of ginseng used, and concurrent medication.[1]

Nevertheless, symptoms documented include hypertension[1] (ginseng species unspecified), diarrhoea[1], insomnia[1] (as a result of over stimulation), mastalgia[1], skin eruptions[1], and vaginal bleeding[1]. A case of vaginal bleeding in a post-menopausal woman has been associated with the use of a ginseng face cream.[51] In 1979, two studies referred to a Ginseng Abuse Syndrome (GAS) which emphasised that most side-effects documented for ginseng were associated with the ingestion of large doses of ginseng together with other psychomotor stimulants, including tea and coffee.[1] GAS was defined as diarrhoea, hypertension, nervousness, skin eruptions and sleeplessness. Other symptoms occasionally observed included amenorrhoea, decreased appetite, depression, euphoria, hypotension and oedema. However, these two studies have been widely criticised over the variety of ginseng and other preparations used, and over the lack of authentication of the ginseng species ingested[1]. Elsewhere, symptoms of overdose have been described as those exhibited by individuals allergic to ginseng, namely palpitations, insomnia and pruritus, together with heart pain, decrease in sexual potency, vomiting, haemorrhagic diathesis, headache and epistaxis; ingestion of very large doses have even been reported to be fatal.[9]

Two cases of a suspected interaction between ginseng and phenelzine have been documented.[52] Symptoms of headache and tremulousness in one 64 year old woman and of manic-like symptoms in a 42-year-old woman were described.[52]

Results documented for toxicity studies carried out in a number of animal species using standardised extracts (SE) indicate ginseng to be of low toxicity.[53–57]

Acute toxicity—single doses of up to 2 g SE have been administered to mice and rats with no toxic effects observed.[56] LD_{50} values (po) in mice and rats have been estimated at 2 g/kg and greater than 5 g/kg.[53] In addition, LD_{50} values (ip, mice) have been estimated for individual ginsenosides as 305 mg/kg (R_{b-2}), 324 mg/kg (R_d), 405 mg/kg (R_e), 410 mg/kg (R_c), 1110 mg/kg (R_{b-1}), 1250 mg/kg (R_{g-1}), and 1340 mg/kg (R_f); an LD_{50} (iv, mice) of 3806 mg/kg has been estimated for the saponins R_{c-1} and R_{d-1}.[53]

Sub-acute toxicity—doses of approximately 720 mg of a ginseng extract (G115) have been administered orally to rats for 20 days with no side-effects documented.[57]

Chronic toxicity—daily doses of up to 15 mg G115/kg body-weight have been administered orally to dogs for 90 days with no toxic effects documented. An initial increase in excitability which disappeared after 2 to 3 weeks was the only observation reported in rats fed 200 mg G115/kg body-weight for 25 weeks.[56]

P.quinquefolis has been reported to be devoid of mutagenic potential when investigated versus *Salmonella typhimurium* strain TM677.[58]

Contra-indications, Warnings

Ginseng may potentiate the action of MAOIs (inhibits uptake of various neurotransmitter substances)[35] and two cases of suspected ginseng interaction with phenelzine have been documented.[52] The use of ginseng has been contra-indicated during acute illness, any form of haemorrhage and during the acute period of coronary thrombosis[1]. It has been recommended that ginseng should be avoided by individuals who are highly energetic, nervous, tense, hysteric, manic or schizophrenic, and that it should not be taken with stimulants, including coffee, antipsychotic drugs or during treatment with hormones.[1,G25]

In view of documented pharmacological actions and side-effects, ginseng should also be used with caution in the following circumstances: cardiac disorders, diabetes, hyper- and hypotensive disorders, and with all steroid therapy. Women may experience oestrogenic side-effects.

In Russia, it is recommended that healthy people under the age of 40 should not use ginseng and that middle-aged people can be treated with small doses of ginseng on a daily basis. In general, long-term use of ginseng is not recommended and one author has documented that the main side-effect of prolonged use manifests as an inflamed nerve, frequently the sciatic, which then causes muscle spasm in the affected area.[1] In Russia, those individuals considered suitable to use ginseng are recommended to abstain from alcoholic beverages, sexual activity, bitter substances and spicy foods [9] Patients allergic to ginseng may exhibit symptoms of palpitation, insomnia, and pruritus.[9]

Pregnancy and lactation No foetal abnormalities have been observed in rats and rabbits administered a standardised extract (40 mg/kg, po) from day 1 to day 15 of pregnancy.[56] Ginseng has also been fed to two successive generations of rats in doses of up to 15 mg G115/kg body-weight/day (equivalent to approximately 2700 mg ginseng extract) with no teratogenic effects observed.[53] However, the safety of ginseng during pregnancy has not been established in humans and therefore its use should be avoided. Similarly, there are no published data concerning the secretion of pharmacologically active constituents from ginseng into the breast milk and use of ginseng during lactation is therefore best avoided.

Pharmaceutical Comment

Phytochemical studies on Panax ginseng are well documented and have initially concentrated on the saponin components (ginsenosides) which are generally considered to be the main active constituents. More recently, pharmacological actions documented for the non-saponin components, principally polysaccharides, have stimulated research into identifying non-saponin active constituents. Many of the pharmacological actions documented for ginseng directly oppose one another and this has been attributed to the actions of the individual ginsenosides. For example, ginsenoside R_{b1} exhibits CNS-depressant, hypotensive and tranquillising actions whilst ginsenoside R_{g1} exhibits CNS-stimulant, hypertensive, and anti-fatigue actions. These opposing actions are thought to explain the 'adaptogenic' reputation of ginseng, that is the ability to increase the overall resistance of the body to stress and to balance bodily functions.

In summary, ginseng has been shown to possess a wide range of pharmacological activities and it should consequently be used with appropriate regard to the traditional guidelines drawn up in China, Japan and Russia, to the health of the individual and to any concomitant therapies. When used appropriately, ginseng appears to be relatively non-toxic and most documented side-effects are associated with inappropriate use when compared with traditional warnings and guidelines.

References

See General References G1, G2, G4, G9, G14, G19, G23, G25 and G32.

1. Baldwin CA *et al*. What pharmacists should know about ginseng. *Pharm J* 1986; **237**: 583–6.

2. Chung BS. Studies on the components of Korean ginseng (II) On the composition of ginseng essential oils. *Kor J Pharmacog* 1976; **7**: 41–4.

3. Iwabuchi H *et al*. Studies on the sesquiterpenoids of *Panax ginseng* C.A. Meyer III. *Chem Pharm Bull* 1989; **37**: 509–10.

4. Iwabuchi H *et al*. Studies on the sesquiterpenoids of *Panax ginseng* C.A. Meyer II. Isolation and structure determination of ginsenol, a novel sesquiterpene alcohol. *Chem Pharm Bull* 1988; **36**: 2447–51.

5. Ahn B-Z *et al*. Acetylpanaxydol and panaxydolchlorohydrin, two new poly-ynes from Korean ginseng with cytotoxic activity against L1210 cells. *Arch Pharm (Weinheim)* 1989; **322**: 223–6.

6. Fujimoto Y, Satoh M. A new cytotoxic chlorine-containing polyacetylene from the callus of *Panax ginseng*. *Chem Pharm Bull* 1988; **36**: 4206–8.

7. Gao Q-P *et al*. Chemical properties and anti-complementary activities of polysaccharide fractions from roots and leaves of *Panax ginseng*. *Planta Med* 1989; **55**: 9–12.

8. Yamasaki K *et al*. Purification and characterization of β-amylase from ginseng. *Chem Pharm Bull* 1989; **37**: 973–8.

9. Baranov AI. Medicinal uses of ginseng and related plants in the Soviet Union: recent trends in the Soviet literature. *J Ethnopharmacol* 1982;**6**: 339–53.

10. Brekhman II. *Panax* ginseng-1. *Med Sci Service* 1967; **4**: 17–26.

11. Li TB *et al*. Effects of ginsenosides, lectins and *Momordica charantia* insulin-like peptide on corticosterone production by isolated rat adrenal cells. *J Ethnopharmacol* 1987; **21**: 21–9.

12. Filaretov AA *et al*. Role of pituitary-adrenocortical system in body adaptation abilities. *Exp Clin Endocrinol* 1988; **92**: 129–36.

13. Guodong L, Zhongqi L. Effects of ginseng saponins on insulin release from isolated pancreatic islets of rats. *Chinese J Integr Trad Western Med* 1987; **7**: 326.

14. Yushu H, Yuzhen C. The effect of *Panax ginseng* extract (GS) on insulin and corticosteroid receptors. *J Trad Chinese Med* 1988; **8**: 293–5.

15. Kimura M *et al*. Pharmacological sequential trials for the fractionation of components with hypoglycemic activitiy in alloxan diabetic mice from *Ginseng radix*. *J Pharm Dyn* 1981; **4**: 402–9.

16. Waki I *et al*. Effects of a hypoglycemic component of *Ginseng radix* on insulin biosynthesis in normal and diabetic animals. *J Pharm Dyn* 1982; **5**: 547–54.

17. Avakian EV *et al*. Effect of *Panax ginseng* extract on energy metabolism during exercise in rats. *Planta Med* 1984; **50**: 151–154.

18. Suzuki Y, Hikino H. Mechanisms of hypoglycemic activity of panaxans A and B, glycans of *Panax ginseng* roots: Effects on the key enzymes of glucose metabolism in the liver of mice. *Phytotherapy Res* 1989; **3**: 15–19.

19. Oshima Y *et al*. Isolation and hypoglycemic activity of quinquefolans A, B, and C, glycans of *Panax quinquefolium* roots. *J Nat Prod* 1987; **50**: 188–90.

20. Konno C, Hikino H. Isolation and hypoglycemic activity of panaxans M, N, O and P, glycans of *Panax ginseng* roots. *Int J Crude Drug Res* 1987; **25**: 53–6.

21. Suzuki Y, Hikino H. Mechanisms of hypoglycemic activity of panaxans A and B, glycans of *Panax ginseng* roots: effects of plasma level, secretion, sensitivity and binding of insulin in mice. *Phytotherapy Res* 1989; **3**: 20–4.

22. Konno C *et al*. Isolation and hypoglycaemic activity of panaxans A, B, C, D and E, glycans of *Panax ginseng* roots. *Planta Med* 1984; **50**: 434–6.

23. Konno C *et al*. Isolation and hypoglycaemic activity of panaxans Q,R,S,T and U, glycans of *Panax ginseng* roots. *J Ethnopharmacol* 1985; **14**: 69–74.

25. Manren R *et al*. Calcium antagonistic action of saponins from *Panax notoginseng* (sanqi-ginseng). *J Trad Chinese Med* 1987; **7**: 127–30.

26. Wu J-X, Chen J-X. Negative chronotropic and inotropic effects of *Panax saponins*. *Acta Pharmacol Sin* 1988; **9**: 409–12.

27. Lei X-L *et al*. Cardiovascular pharmacology of *Panax notoginseng* (Burk) F.H. Chen and *Salvia militiorrhiza*. *Am J Chinese Med* 1986; **14**: 145–52.

28. Li XJ, Zhang BH. Studies on the antiarrhythmic effects of panaxatriol saponins (PTS) isolated from *Panax notoginseng*. *Acta Pharm Sin* 1988; **23**: 168–73.

29. Yunxiang F, Xiu C. Effects of ginenosides on myocardial lactic acid, cyclic nucleotides and ultrastructural myocardial changes of anoxia on mice. *Chinese J Integr Trad Western Med* 1987; **7**: 326.

30. Namba T *et al*. Fundamental studies on the evaluation of the crude drugs. (I). Hemolytic and its protective activity of ginseng saponins. *Planta Med* 1974; **28**: 28–38.

31. Kosuge T *et al*. Studies on antihemorrhagic principles in the crude drugs for hemostatics. I. On hemostatic activities of the crude drugs for hemostatics. *Yakugaku Zasshi [J Pharm Soc Japan]* 1981; **101**: 501–3.

32. Yamamoto M, Kumagai M. Anti-atherogenic action of *Panax ginseng* in rats and in patients with hyperlipidemia. *Planta Med* 1982; **45**: 149–66.

33. Kuo S-C *et al*. Antiplatelet components in *Panax ginseng*. *Planta Med* 1990; **56**: 164–7.

34.   Kim H-S *et al*. Antinarcotic effects of the standardized ginseng extract G115 on morphine. *Planta Med* 1990; **56**: 158–63

35.   Tsang D *et al*. Ginseng saponins: Influence on neurotransmitter uptake in rat brain synaptosomes. *Planta Med* 1985; **51**: 221–4.

36.   Kobayashi S *et al*. Inhibitory actions of phospholipase A_2 and saponins including ginsenoside Rb_1 and glycyrrhizin on the formation of nicotinic acetylcholine receptor clusters on cultured mouse myotubes. *Phytotherapy Res* 1990; **4**: 106–11.

37.   Tsang D *et al*. Ginenoside modulates K^+ stimulated noradrenaline release from rat cerebral cortex slices. *Planta Med* 1986; **52**: 266–8.

38.   Saksena AK *et al*. Effect of *Withania somnifera* and *Panax ginseng* on dopaminergic receptors in rat brain during stress. *Planta Med* 1989 **55**: 95.

39.   Nakagawa S *et al*. Cytoprotective activity of components of garlic, ginseng and ciuwjia on hepatocyte injury induced by carbon tetrachloride *in vitro*. *Hiroshima J Med Sci* 1985; **34**: 303–9.

40.   Hikino H *et al*. Antihepatotoxic actions of ginsenosides from *Panax ginseng* roots. *Planta Med* 1985; **51**: 62–4.

41.   Ahn B-Z, Kim SI. Heptadeca-1,8*t*-dien-4,6-diin-3,10-diol, ein weiteres, gegen L1210—Zellen cytotoxisches Wirkprinzip aus der Koreanischen Ginsengwurzel. *Planta Med* 1988; **54**: 183.

42.   Qian B-C *et al*. Effects of ginseng polysaccharides on tumor and immunological function in tumor-bearing mice. *Acta Pharmacol Sin* 1987; **8**: 277–88.

43.   Matsunaga H *et al*. Studies on the panaxytriol of *Panax ginseng* C.A. Meyer. Isolation, determination and antitumor activity. *Chem Pharm Bull* 1989; **37**: 1279–81.

44.   Singh VK *et al*. Combined treatment of mice with *Panax ginseng* extract and interferon inducer. *Planta Med* 1983; **47**: 235–6.

45.   Singh VK *et al*. Immunomodulatory activity of *Panax ginseng* extract. *Planta Med* 1984; **50**: 462–5.

46.   Lee FC *et al*. Effects of *Panax ginseng* on blood alcohol clearance in man. *Clin Exp Pharmac Physiol* 1987; **14**: 543–6.

47.   Zuin M *et al*. Effects of a preparation containing a standardized ginseng extract combined with trace elements and multivitamins against hepatotoxin-induced chronic liver disease in the elderly. *J Int Med Res* 1987; **15**: 276–81.

48.   D'Angelo L *et al*. A double-blind, placebo-controlled clinical study on the effect of a standardized ginseng extract on psychomotor performance in healthy volunteers. *J Ethnopharmacol* 1986; **16**: 15–22.

49   Peigen X, Keji C. Recent advances in clinical studies of Chinese medicinal herbs. 2. Clinical trials of Chinese herbs in a number of chronic conditions. *Phytotherapy Res* 1988; **2**: 55–60.

50.   Chong SKF, Oberholzer VG. Ginseng — is there a use in clinical medicine? *Postgrad Med J* 1988; **64**: 841–6.

51.   Hopkins MP *et al*. Ginseng face cream and unexplained vaginal bleeding. *Am J Obstet Gynecol* 1988; **159**: 1121–2.

52.   Jones BD *et al*. Interaction of ginseng with phenelzine. *J Clin Psychopharmacol* 1987; **7**: 201–2.

53.   Berté F. Toxicological investigation of the standardized ginseng extract G115 after unique administration [LD_{50}]. Manufacturer's data, on file. 1982, pp. 1–12.

54.   Hess FG *et al*. Reproduction study in rats of ginseng extract G115. *Food Chem Toxicol* 1982; **20**: 189–92.

55.   Hess FG *et al*. Effects of subchronic feeding of ginseng extract G115 in beagle dogs. *Food Chem Toxicol* 1983; **21**: 95–7.

56.   Trabucchi E. Toxicological and pharmacological investigation of Geriatric Pharmaton. Manufacturer's data on fil., 1971, pp. 1–22.

57.   Savel J. Toxicological report on Geriatric Pharmaton. Manufacturer's data on file. 1971, pp. 1–31.

58.   Chang YS *et al*. Evaluation of the mutagenic potential of American ginseng (*Panax quinquefolius*). *Planta Med* 1986; **52**: 338.

GOLDEN SEAL

Species (Family)
Hydrastis canadensis L. (Ranunculaceae)

Synonym(s)
Yellow Root

Yellow root also refers to *Xanthorhiza simplicissima* Marsh, which is also a member of the Ranunculaceae family and contains berberine as the major alkaloid constituent.

Part(s) Used
Rhizome, Root

Pharmacopoeial Monographs
BHP 1983
BHP 1990
BPC 1934
Martindale 30th edition
Pharmacopoeias—Braz., Egypt., Fr., and Rom.

Legal Category (Licensed Products)
GSL[G14]

Constituents[G2,G10,G18,G19,G31,G32]
Alkaloids (isoquinoline-type) (2.5–6.0%). Hydrastine (major, 1.5–4.0%), berberine (0.5–6.0%), berberastine (2-3%), and canadine (1%), with lesser amounts of related alkaloids including candaline and canadaline.[1–3]
Other constituents Chlorogenic acid, carbohydrates, fatty acids (75% saturated, 25% unsaturated), volatile oil (trace), resin, meconin (meconinic acid lactone)

Food Use
Golden seal is not used in foods, although it is reported to be used in herbal teas.[G19] The concentration of berberine permitted in foods is limited to 0.1 mg/kg, and 10 mg/kg in alcoholic beverages.[G9]

Herbal Use
Golden seal is stated to be a stimulant to involuntary muscle, and to possess stomachic, oxytocic, antihaemorrhagic, and laxative properties. Traditionally it has been used for digestive disorders, gastritis, peptic ulceration, colitis, anorexia, upper respiratory catarrh, menorrhagia, post-partum haemorrhage, dysmenorrhoea, topically for eczema, pruritus, otorrhoea, catarrhal deafness, and tinnitus, conjunctivitis, and specifically for atonic dyspepsia with hepatic symptoms.[G2,G3,G4]

Dose
Dried rhizome 0.5–1.0 g or by decoction three times daily[G2,G3]
Liquid Extract of Hydrastis (BPC 1949) 0.3–1.0 mL
Tincture of Hydrastis (BPC 1949) 2–4 mL

Pharmacological Actions
The pharmacological activity of golden seal is attributed to the isoquinoline alkaloid constituents, primarily hydrastine and berberine,[3,4] which are reported to have similar properties.[G19] Antibiotic, immunostimulant, anticonvulsant, sedative, hypotensive, uterotonic, choleretic, and carminative activities have been described for berberine.[3]

Animal studies Limited work has been documented for golden seal, although the pharmacology of berberine and hydrastine is well studied.

The total alkaloid fraction of golden seal has been reported to exhibit anticonvulsant activity in smooth muscle preparations (e.g. mouse intestine, uterus).[5] However, *in vitro*, canadine is reported to exhibit uterine stimulation in guinea-pig and rabbit tissues.[4] Berberine, canadine, and hydrastine are all stated to exhibit uteroactivity.[G12]

Berberine and hydrastine have produced a hypotensive effect in laboratory animals following intravenous administration.[6,7,G19] High doses of hydrastine are documented to produce an increase in blood pressure.[7] *In vitro*, berberine has been reported to decrease the anticoagulant action of heparin in canine and human blood.[7]

Berberine is reported to exert a stimulant action on the heart and to increase coronary blood flow, although higher doses are stated to inhibit cardiac activity.[7]

Antimuscarinic and antihistamine actions have been documented for berberine.[7]

In rats, berberine has exhibited antipyretic activity three times as effective as aspirin.[3]

Berberine potentiated barbiturate sleeping time, but did not exhibit any analgesic or tranquillising effects.[7]

A broad spectrum of antimicrobial activity against bacteria, fungi, and protozoa has been reported for berberine. Sensitive organisms include *Staphylococcus* spp., *Streptococcus* spp., *Chlamydia aureus*, *Corynebacterium diphtheriae*, *Salmonella typhi*, *Diplococcus pneumoniae*, *Pseudomonas aeruginosa*, *Shigella dysenteriae*, *Trichomonas vaginalis*, *Neisseria gonorrhoeae*, *Neisseria meningitidis*, *Treponema pallidum*, *Giardia lamblia*, and *Leishmania donovani*.[3] Berberine is reported to be effective against diarrhoeas caused by enterotoxins such as *Vibrio cholerae* and *Escherichia coli*.[7] *In-vivo* and *in-vitro* studies in hamsters and rats have reported significant activity for berberine against *Entamoeba histolytica*.[3]

Anticancer activity has been reported for berberine in B1, KB, and PS tumour systems.[G10] In addition, berberine sulphate was found to inhibit the action of teleocidin, a known tumour promoter, on the formation of mouse skin tumours initiated with 7,12-dimethylbenz[a]anthracene.[5]

Human studies None documented for golden seal. Berberine is stated to have shown significant success in the treatment of acute diarrhoea in several clinical studies.[3] It has been found effective against diarrhoeas caused by *Escherichia coli*, *Shigella dysenteriae*, *Salmonella para-*

typhi B, *Klebsiella, Giardia lamblia* and *Vibrio cholerae*.[3] Berberine has been used to treat trachoma, an infectious ocular disease caused by *Chlamydia trachomatis* that is a major cause of blindness and impaired vision in underdeveloped countries.[3]

Clinical studies have shown berberine to stimulate bile and bilirubin secretion and to improve symptoms of chronic cholecystitis, and to correct raised levels of tyramine in patients with liver cirrhosis.[3]

Side-effects, Toxicity

Berberine and berberine-containing plants are considered to be non-toxic.[3] However, the alkaloid constituents are potentially toxic and symptoms of golden seal poisoning include stomach upset, nervous symptoms, and depression; large quantities may even be fatal.[8] High doses of hydrastine are reported to cause exaggerated reflexes, convulsions, paralysis, and death from respiratory failure.[4] The root may cause contact ulceration of mucosal surfaces.

Contra-indications, Warnings

Golden seal is contra-indicated in individuals with raised blood pressure.[G3,G10,G25] Prolonged use of golden seal may decrease vitamin B absorption.[G10] Coagulant activity opposing the action of heparin, and cardiac stimulant activity have been documented for berberine. The use of golden seal as a douche should be avoided because of the potential ulcerative side-effects.[G10] The alkaloid constituents of golden seal are potentially toxic and excessive use should be avoided.

Pregnancy and lactation Golden seal is contra-indicated for use during pregnancy.[3,G3,G25] Berberine, canadine, hydrastine, and hydrastinine have all been reported to produce uterine stimulant activity.[G12] It is not known whether the alkaloids are excreted in breast milk. The use of golden seal during lactation should be avoided.

Pharmaceutical Comment

Golden seal is characterised by the isoquinoline alkaloid constituents. These compounds, primarily hydrastine and berberine, represent the main active components of golden seal. Numerous activities have been documented many of which support the traditional herbal uses of the root. However, in view of the pharmacological properties of the alkaloid constituents, excessive use of golden seal should be avoided.

References

See General References G2, G3, G4, G5, G9, G10, G12, G14, G18, G19, G22, G23, G24, G31 and G32.

1. Gleye J *et al.* La canadaline: nouvel alcaloide d'*Hydrastis canadensis*. *Phytochemistry* 1974; **13**: 675–6.

2. El-Masry S *et al.* Colorimetric and spectrophotometric determination of *Hydrastis* alkaloids in pharmaceutical preparations. *J Pharm Sci* 1980; **69**: 597–8.

3. Pizzorno JE, Murray MT. *Hydrastis canadensis, Berberis vulgaris, Berberis aquitolium* and other berberine containing plants. In:Textbook of natural medicine. Seattle WR: John Bastyr College Publications, 1985 (looseleaf).

4. Genest K, Hughes DW. Natural products in Canadian pharmaceuticals iv. *Hydrastis canadensis. Can J Pharm Sci* 1969; **4**: 41–5.

5. Nishino H *et al.* Berberine sulphate inhibits tumour-promoting activity of teleocidin in two-stage carcinogenesis on mouse skin. *Oncology* 1986; **43**: 131–4.

6. Wisniewski W, Gorta T. Effect of temperature on the oxidation of hydrastine to hydrastinine in liquid extracts and rhizomes of *Hydrastis canadensis* in the presence of air and steam. *Acta Pol Pharm* 1969; **26**: 313–7.

7. Preininger V. The pharmacology and toxicology of the Papaveraceae alkaloids. In: The alkaloids Vol 15, Manske RHF, Holmes HL eds. New York: Academic Press 1975, p. 239.

8. Hardin JW, Arena JM. Human poisoning from native and cultivated plants, 2nd edn. Durham, North Carolina: Duke University Press 1974.

GRAVEL ROOT

Species (Family)
Eupatorium purpureum L. (Asteraceae/Compositae)

Synonym(s)
Kydney Root, Joe-Pye Weed, Purple Boneset, Queen of the Meadow.

Part(s) Used
Rhizome, Root

Pharmacopoeial Monographs
BHP 1983

Legal Category (Licensed Products)
GSL[G14]

Constituents[G18,G20,G24,G25,G32,G34]
Little information is available on the chemistry of gravel root. It is stated to contain euparin (a benzofuran compound), eupatorin (a flavonoid), resin, and volatile oil.

Other plant parts The herb is reported to contain echinatine, an unsaturated pyrrolizidine alkaloid.[1]

Food Use
Gravel root is not used in foods.

Herbal Use
Gravel root is stated to possess antilithic, diuretic, and antirheumatic properties. Traditionally, it has been used for urinary calculus, cystitis, dysuria, urethritis, prostatitis, rheumatism, gout, and specifically for renal or vesicular calculi.[G3,G32]

Dose
Dried rhizome/root 2–4 g or by decoction three times daily[G3]

Liquid extract (1:1 in 25% alcohol) 2–4 mL three times daily[G3]

Tincture (1:5 in 40% alcohol) 1–2 mL three times daily[G3]

Pharmacological Actions
None documented.

Side-effects, Toxicity[G34]
None documented for gravel root although pyrrolizidine alkaloids are constituents of many species of *Eupatorium*[1, G34]. Pyrrolizidine alkaloids with an unsaturated pyrrolizidine nucleus are reported to be hepatotoxic in both animals and humans (*see* Comfrey). An unsaturated pyrrolizidine alkaloid, echinatine, has been reported for the aerial parts of gravel root.

Contra-indications, Warnings
None documented.

Pregnancy and lactation The safety of gravel root has not been established. In view of the lack of phytochemical, pharmacological and toxicological information the use of gravel root during pregnancy and lactation should be avoided.

Pharmaceutical Comment
The chemistry of gravel root is poorly studied and no scientific evidence was located to justify the herbal uses. Excessive use of gravel root should be avoided.

References
See General References G3, G14, G18, G20, G24, G25, G32 and G34.

1. Pyrrolizidine Alkaloids. *Environmental Health Criteria 80* Geneva: WHO, 1988.

GROUND IVY

Species (Family)
Nepeta hederacea (L.) Trev. (Labiatae)

Synonyms
Glechoma hederacea L.

Part(s) Used
Herb

Pharmacopoeial Monographs
BHP 1983
BHP 1990

Legal Category (Licensed Products)
GSL[G14]

Constituents[G2,G10,G24,G32]

Amino acids Asparagic acid, glutamic acid, proline, tyrosine, valine

Flavonoids Flavonol glycosides (e.g. hyperoside, isoquercitrin, rutin) and flavone glycosides (e.g. luteolin diglucoside, cosmosyin)[1]

Steroids β-Sitosterol

Terpenoids Oleanolic acid, α-ursolic acid, β-ursolic acid[2]

Volatile oils (0.03–0.06%). Various terpenoid components including *p*-cymene, linalool, limonene, menthone, α-pinene, β-pinene, pinocamphone, pulegone, and terpineol; glechomafuran (a sesquiterpene).[3]

Other constituents Palmitic acid, rosmarinic acid, succinic acid, bitter principle (glechomin), choline, gum, diterpene lactone (marrubiin), saponin, tannin, wax

Food Use
Ground ivy is listed by the Council of Europe as a natural source of food flavouring (category N3). This category indicates that ground ivy can be added to foodstuffs in the traditionally accepted manner, although there is insufficient information available for an adequate assessment of potential toxicity.[G9]

Herbal Use
Ground ivy is stated to possess mild expectorant, anticatarrhal, astringent, vulnerary, diuretic, and stomachic properties. Traditionally, it has been used for bronchitis, tinnitus, diarrhoea, haemorrhoids, cystitis, gastritis, and specifically for chronic bronchial catarrh.[G2,G3,G4,G25,G32]

Dose
Dried herb 2–4 g or by infusion three times daily[G2,G3]
Liquid extract (1:1 in 25% alcohol) 2–4 mL three times daily[G2,G3]

Pharmacological Actions
Animal studies In-vivo anti-inflammatory activity has been reported for an ethanolic extract of ground ivy, which was stated to exhibit a moderate inhibition (27%) of carrageenan-induced rat paw oedema.[4]

Ursolic acid analogues, 2α- and 2β-hydroxyursolic acid, have been documented to provide significant ulcer-protective activity in mice.[5]

The astringent activity documented for ground ivy has been attributed to rosmarinic acid, a polyphenolic acid.[6]

Glechomin and marrubiin are stated to be bitter principles, and α-terpineol is known to be an antiseptic component of volatile oils.[G24,G25]

Anti-inflammatory and astringent properties are generally associated with flavonoids and tannins, respectively. Anti-inflammatory properties have been documented for rosmarinic acid (*see* Rosemary)

In-vitro antiviral activity against the Epstein-Barr virus has been documented for ursolic acid.[7] Both oleanolic and ursolic acids were found to inhibit tumour production by TPA in mouse skin, with activity comparable to that of retinoic acid, a known tumour-promoter inhibitor.[7]

Significant cytotoxic activity has also been reported for ursolic acid in lymphocytic leukaemia (P-388, L-1210) and human lung carcinoma (A-549), and marginal activity in KB cells, human colon (HCT-8), and mammary (MCF-7) tumour cells.[8]

Side-effects, Toxicity
Poisoning in cattle and horses has been documented in eastern Europe.[9] Symptoms include accelerated weak pulse, difficulty in breathing, conjunctival haemorrhage, elevated temperature, dizziness, spleen enlargement, dilation of the caecum, and gastro-enteritis revealed at post-mortem. Anti-tumour and cytotoxic activities have been reported for oleanolic and ursolic acids (*see* Animal studies).

Ground ivy volatile oil contains many terpenoids and terpene-rich volatile oils are irritant to the gastro-intestinal tract and kidneys. Pulegone is an irritant, hepatotoxic, and abortifacient principle of the volatile oil of Pennyroyal. However, in comparison with pennyroyal the overall yield of volatile oil is much less (0.03–0.06% in ground ivy and 1–2% in pennyroyal).

Contra-indications, Warnings
Ground ivy is contra-indicated in epilepsy,[G3] although no rationale for this statement has been found. Excessive doses may be irritant to the gastro-intestinal mucosa and should be avoided by individuals with existing renal disease.

Pregnancy and lactation The safety of ground ivy has not been established. In view of the lack of toxicity data and the possible irritant and abortifacient action of the volatile oil, the use of ground ivy during pregnancy and lactation should be avoided.

Pharmaceutical Comment

The chemistry of ground ivy is well studied. Documented pharmacological activities support some of the herbal uses, although no references to human studies were located. In view of the lack of toxicity data and the reported cytotoxic activity of ursolic acid, excessive use of ground ivy should be avoided.

References

See General References G2, G3, G4, G9, G10, G14, G24, G25, and G32.

1.   Zieba J. Isolation and identification of flavonoids from *Glechoma hederacea*. *Pol J Pharmacol Pharm* 1973; **25:** 593–7.

2.   Zieba J. Isolation and identification of nonheteroside triterpenoids from *Glechoma hederacea*. *Pol J Pharmacol Pharm* 1973; **25:** 587–92.

3.   Stahl E, Datta SN. New sesquiterpenoids of the ground ivy (*Glechoma hederacea*). *Justus Liebigs Ann Chem* 1972; **757:** 23–32.

4.   Mascolo N *et al*. Biological screening of Italian medicinal plants for anti-inflammatory activity. *Phytotherapy Res* 1987; **1:** 28–31.

5.   Okuyama E *et al* Isolation and identification of ursolic acid-related compounds as the principles of *Glechoma hederacea* having an antiulcerogenic activity. *Shoyakugaku Zasshi* 1983; **37:** 52–5.

6.   Okuda T *et al*. The components of tannic activities in Labiatae plants. I. Rosmarinic acid from Labiatae plants in Japan. *Yakugaku Zasshi* 1986; **106:** 1108–11.

7.   Tokuda H *et al*. Inhibitory effects of ursolic and oleanolic acid on skin tumor promotion by 12-*O*-tetradecanoylphorbol-13-acetate. *Cancer Lett* 1986; **33:** 279–85.

8.   Lee K-H *et al*. The cytotoxic principles of *Prunella vulgaris*, *Psychotria serpens*, and *Hyptis capitata*: Ursolic acid and related derivatives. *Planta Med* 1988; **54:** 308.

9.   MAFF. Poisonous plants in Britain. London: HMSO, 1984; 139.

GUAIACUM

Species (Family)
(i) *Guaiacum officinale* L. (Zygophyllaceae)
(ii) *Guaiacum sanctum* L.

Synonym(s)
Guaiac, Guajacum, Lignum Vitae

Part(s) Used
Resin obtained from the heartwood

Pharmacopoeial Monographs
BHP 1983
BHP 1990
BPC 1949
Martindale 30th edition

Legal Category (Licensed Products)
GSL[G14]

Constituents[G2,G24,G32]
Resins (15–20%). Guaiaretic acid, dehydroguaiaretic acid, guaiacin, isoguaiacin, α-guaiaconic acid (lignans), furoguaiacin and its monomethyl ether, furoguaiacidin, tetrahydrofuroguaiacin-A and tetrahydrofuroguaiacin-B (furanolignans), furoguaiaoxidin (enedione lignan)[1–4]
Steroids β-Sitosterol
Terpenoids Saponins, oleanolic acid[5,6]

Food Use
Guaiacum is listed by the Council of Europe as a natural source of food flavouring (category N2). This category indicates that guaiacum can be added to foodstuffs in small quantities, with a possible limitation of an active principle (as yet unspecified) in the final product.[G9]

Herbal Use
Guaiacum is stated to possess antirheumatic, anti-inflammatory, diuretic, mild laxative, and diaphoretic properties. Traditionally, it has been used for subacute rheumatism, prophylaxis against gout, and specifically for chronic rheumatism and rheumatoid arthritis.[G2,G3,G4,G32]

Dose
Dried wood 1–2 g or by decoction three times daily[G2,G3]
Liquid extract (1:1 in 80% alcohol) 1–2 mL three times daily[G2,G3]
Tincture of Guaiacum (BPC 1934) 2–4 mL

Pharmacological Actions
Animal studies None documented. Antimicrobial properties are associated with lignans and much has been documented for nordihydroguaiaretic acid, the principal lignan constituent in chaparral (*see* Chaparral monograph).

Side-effects, Toxicity
Guaiacum resin has been reported to cause contact dermatitis.[G26] The resin is documented to be of low toxicity; the oral LD_{50} in rats is greater than 5 g/kg body-weight.[G24]

Contra-indications, Warnings
It is recommended that guaiacum is avoided by individuals with hypersensitive, allergic, or acute inflammatory conditions.[G25]

Pregnancy and lactation The safety of guaiacum during pregnancy has not been established. In view of this, and the overall lack of pharmacological and toxicological data, the use of guaiacum during pregnancy and lactation should be avoided.

Pharmaceutical Comment
Guaiacum is characterised by the resin fraction of the heartwood and much has been documented on the constituents (principally lignans) of the resin, although little is known regarding other constituents. No scientific information was found to justify the herbal use of guaiacum as an antirheumatic or anti-inflammatory agent. In view of the lack of toxicity data, excessive use of guaiacum should be avoided.

References
See General References G2, G3, G4, G9, G14, G23, G24, G25, G26, and G32.

1. King FE and Wilson JG. The chemistry of extractives from hardwoods. Part XXXVI. The lignans of *Guaiacum officinale* L. *J Chem Soc* 1964; 4011–24.

2. Kratochvil JF *et al*. Isolation and characterization of α-guaiaconic acid and the nature of guaiacum blue. *Phytochemistry* 1971; **10**: 2529–31.

3. Majumder PL and Bhattacharyya M. Structure of furoguaiacidin: a new furanoid lignan of the heartwood of *Guaiacum officinale* L. *Chem Ind* 1974; 77–8.

4. Majumder P and Bhattacharyya M. Furoguaiaoxidin—a new enedione lignan of *Guaiacum officinale*: a novel method of sequential introduction of alkoxy functions in the 3- and 4-methyl groups of 2,5-diaryl-3,4-dimethylfurans. *JCS Chem Comm* 1975; 702–3.

5. Ahmad VU *et al*. Officigenin, a new sapogenin of *Guaiacum officinale*. *J Nat Prod* 1984; **47**: 977–82.

6. Ahmad VU *et al*. Guaianin, a new saponin from *Guaiacum officinale*. *J Nat Prod* 1986; **49**: 784–6.

HAWTHORN

Species (Family)

(i) *Crataegus oxyacanthoides* Thuill. (Rosaceae)

(ii) *Crataegus monogyna* Jacq.

Synonym(s)

Whitethorn

Part(s) Used

Fruit

Pharmacopoeial Monographs

BHP 1983

Martindale 30th edition

Pharmacopoeias—Braz., Chin., Cz., Fr., Ger., Hung., Rus., and Swiss.

Legal Category (Licensed Products)

Hawthorn is not included on the GSL.[G14]

Constituents[G1,G10,G31,G32]

Amines Phenylethylamine, *O*-methoxyphenethylamine, tyramine[1]

Flavonoids Flavonol (e.g. kaempferol, quercetin) and flavone (e.g. apigenin, luteolin) derivatives, rutin, hyperoside, vitexin glycosides, orientin glycosides,[2–5] procyanidins[6,7]

Tannins Condensed (proanthocyanidins)

Other constituents Cyanogenetic glycosides, saponins

Food Use

Hawthorn is not commonly used in foods. It is listed by the Council of Europe as a natural source of food flavouring (category N2). This category indicates that hawthorn can be added to foodstuffs in small quantities, with a possible limitation of an active principle (as yet unspecified) in the final product.[G9]

Herbal Use

Hawthorn is stated to possess cardiotonic, coronary vasodilator, and hypotensive properties. Traditionally, it has been used for cardiac failure, myocardial weakness, paroxysmal tachycardia, hypertension, arteriosclerosis, and Buerger's disease.[G1,G3]

Dose

Dried fruit 0.3–1.0 g or by infusion three times daily[G3]

Liquid extract (1:1 in 25% alcohol) 0.5–1.0 mL three times daily[G3]

Tincture (1:5 in 45% alcohol) 1–2 mL three times daily[G3]

Pharmacological Actions

Animal studies Cardiovascular activity has been documented for hawthorn and attributed to the flavonoid components, in particular the procyanidins. Hawthorn extracts have been documented to increase coronary blood flow both *in vitro* (in the guinea-pig heart) and *in vivo* (in the cat, dog, and rabbit), reduce blood pressure *in vivo* (in the cat, dog, rabbit, and rat), increase (head, skeletal muscle, and kidney) and reduce (skin, gastro-intestinal tract) peripheral blood flow *in vivo* (in the dog) and reduce peripheral resistance *in vivo* (in the dog).[6,8–13] The hypotensive activity of hawthorn has been attributed to a vasodilation action rather than via adrenergic, muscarinic, or histaminergic receptors.[12] Beta-adrenoceptor blocking activity (versus adrenaline-induced tachycardia) has been exhibited *in vivo* in the dog and *in vitro* in the frog heart using flower, leaf, and fruit extracts standardised on their procyanidin content.[6] The authors reported a direct relationship between the concentration of procyanidin and observed actions.

Negative chronotropic and positive inotropic actions have been observed *in vitro* using the guinea-pig heart and attributed to flavonoid and proanthocyanidin fractions.[14] A positive inotropic effect has also been exhibited by amine constituents *in vitro* using guinea-pig papillary muscle.[1]

In vivo Hawthorn extracts have also been reported to lack any effect on the heart rate and muscle contractility in studies that have observed an effect on blood pressure in the dog and rat.[11,12] Hawthorn extracts have exhibited some prophylactic anti-arrhythmic activity in rabbits administered intravenous aconitine.[15] Extracts infused after aconitine did not affect the induced arrhythmias. *In vitro*, vitexin rhamnoside has been reported to have no effect on the action of ouabain and aconitine.[15] A crude extract of *Crataegus pinnatifidia* Bge. var *major* N.E.Br. and the flavonoid vitexin rhamnoside have been reported to exert a protective action on experimental ischaemic myocardium in anaesthetised dogs.[17] The extracts were observed to decrease left ventricular work, decrease the consumption of oxygen index, and increase coronary sinus blood-oxygen concentrations resulting in a decrease in oxygen consumption and balance of oxygen metabolism. In contrast to other studies, an increase in coronary blood flow was not observed. The authors attributed these opposing results to the variation in concentrations of active constituents between the different plant parts. *In vitro*, vitexin rhamnoside has been reported to exert a protective action towards cardiac cells deprived of oxygen and glucose.[16]

A mild CNS depressant effect has been documented in mice that received oral administration of hawthorn flower extracts.[8] An increase in barbiturate sleeping time and a decrease in spontaneous basal motility were the most noticeable effects.

Free radicals have been linked with the ageing process. When fed to mice, a hawthorn fruit (*C. pinnatifidia*) extract has been reported to enhance the action of superoxide dismutase (SOD), which promotes the scavenging of free radicals.[19] An inhibition of lipid peroxidation, which can be caused by highly reactive free radicals was also documented.[19]

Human studies A commercial preparation containing 30 mg hawthorn extract standardised to 1 mg procyanidins has been used in a double-blind controlled study involving 80 patients (35 active, 45 placebo).[20] The active group was reported to exhibit greater overall improvement of cardiac function and of subjective symptoms such as dyspnoea and palpitations. Improvements in ECG recordings were not found to differ between the active and placebo groups.

A commercial product containing hawthorn, valerian, camphor, and cereus was given to 2243 patients with functional cardiovascular disorders and/or hypotension or meteorosensitivity in an open multicentre study.[21] An improvement in 84% of treated individuals was reported.

A commercial hawthorn preparation has been reported to be effective in treating 60 patients with a stable form of angina, increasing coronary perfusion and economising myocardial oxygen consumption.[22] The patients received the hawthorn preparation (60 mg three times daily) in a randomised controlled double-blind trial.

A commercial hawthorn/passionflower extract (standardised on flavone and proanthocyanidin content) has been used in a randomised, placebo-controlled double-blind trial involving 40 patients with chronic heart failure (20 active, 20 placebo).[23] Each group received 6 mL extract daily for 42 days. Significant improvements were noted in the active group for exercise capacity, heart rate at rest, diastolic blood pressure at rest, and total plasma cholesterol and low-density lipids. Non-significant improvements were noted in the active group for maximum exercise capacity, breathlessness, and physical performance. The authors commented that a higher dose of the extract administered over a longer period was necessary for further investigation of the observed improvements.[23]

Side-effects, Toxicity

Nausea[20] and fatigue, sweating, and rash on the hands[23] have been reported as side-effects in clinical trials using commercial preparations of hawthorn.[20]

General symptoms of acute toxicity observed in a number of animal models (e.g. guinea pig, frog, tortoise, cat, rabbit, rat) have been documented as bradycardia and respiratory depression leading to cardiac arrest and respiratory paralysis.[8–10] Acute toxicity (LD_{50}) of isolated constituents (mainly flavonoids) has been documented as 50–2600 mg/kg (by intravenous injection) and 6 g/kg (by mouth) in various animal preparations.[8–10] The documented acute toxicity of commercial hawthorn preparations has also been reviewed.[8–10]

Contra-indications, Warnings

Hawthorn has been reported to exhibit many cardiovascular activities and as such may affect the existing therapy of patients with various cardiovascular disorders such as hypertension, hypotension and cardiac disorders. These patient groups are likely to be most susceptible to the pharmacological actions of hawthorn.

Pregnancy and lactation In-vivo and *in-vitro* uteroactivity (reduction in tone and motility) has been documented for hawthorn extracts.[8–10] In view of the pharmacological activities described for hawthorn, it should not be taken during pregnancy and lactation.

Pharmaceutical Comment

Hawthorn is characterised by its phenolic constituents, in particular the flavonoid components to which many of the pharmacological properties associated with hawthorn have been attributed. Pharmacological actions documented in both animal and human studies support the traditional actions of hawthorn and include cardioactive, hypotensive and coronary vasodilator.[24] Further clinical studies are required to establish the true usefulness of hawthorn in treating various cardiovascular disorders. In view of the nature of the actions documented for hawthorn, it is not suitable for self-medication.

References

See General References G1, G3, G9, G10, G23, G31, and G32.

1. Wagner H, Grevel J. Cardioactive drugs IV. Cardiotonic amines from *Crataegus oxyacantha*. *Plant Med* 1982; **45:** 99–101.

2. Nikolov N *et al*. New flavonoid glycosides from *Crataegus monogyna* and *Crataegus pentagyna*. *Planta Med* 1982; **44:** 50–3.

3. Ficarra, P *et al*. High-performance liquid chromatography of flavonoids in *Crataegus oxyacantha* L. *Il Farmaco Ed Pr* 1984; **39:** 148–57.

4. Ficcara P *et al*. Analysis of 2-phenyl-chromon derivatives and chlorogenic acid. II — High-performance thin layer chromatography and high-performance liquid chromatography in flowers, leaves and buds extractives of *Crataegus oxyacantha* L. *Il Farmaco Ed Pr* 1984; **39:** 342–54.

5. Pietta P *et al*. Isocratic liquid chormatographic method for the simultaneous determination of *Passiflora incarnata* L. and *Crataegus monogyna* flavonoids in drugs. *J Chromatogr* 1986; **357:** 233–8.

6. Rácz-Kotilla E *et al*. Hypotensive and beta-blocking effect of procyanidins of *Crataegus monogyna*. *Planta Med* 1980; **39:** 239.

7. Vanhaelen M, Vanhaelen-Fastre R. TLC-densitometric determination of 2,3-*cis*-procyanidin monomer and oligo-mers from hawthorn (*Crataegus laevigata* and *C. monogyna*). *J Pharm Biomed Anal* 1989; **7:** 1871–5.

8. Ammon HPT, Händel M. Crataegus, toxicology and pharmacology. Part I: Toxicity. *Planta Med* 1981; **43:** 105–20.

9. Ammon HPT, Händel M. Crataegus, toxicology and pharmacology. Part II: Pharmacodynamics. *Planta Med* 1981; **43:** 209–39.

10. Ammon HPT, Händel M. Crataegus, toxicology and pharmacology. Part III: Pharmacodynamics and pharmacokinetics. *Planta Med* 1981; **43:** 313–22.

11. Lièvre M *et al*. Assessment in the anesthetized dog of the cardiovascular effects of a pure extract (hyperoside) from hawthorn. *Ann Pharm Fr* 1985; **43:** 471–7.

12.   Abdul-Ghani A-S *et al*. Hypotensive effect of *Crateagus oxyacantha*. *Int J Crude Drug Res* 1987; **25:** 216–20.

13.   Petkov V. Plants with hypotensive, antiatheromatous and coronarodilatating action. *Am J Chinese Med* 1979; **7:** 197–236.

14.   Leukel A *et al*. Studies on the activity of *Crataegus* compounds upon the isolated guinea pig heart. *Planta Med* 1986; **52:** 65.

15.   Thompson EB *et al*. Preliminary study of potential antiarrhythmic effects of *Crataegus monogyna*. *J Pharm Sci* 1974; **63:** 1936–7.

16.   Lianda L *et al*. Studies on hawthorn and its active principle. II. Effects on cultured rat heart cells deprived of oxygen and glucose. *J Trad Chinese Med* 1984; **4:** 289–92.

17.   Lianda L *et al*. Studies on hawthorn and its active principle. I. Effect on myocardial ischemia and hemodynamics in dogs. *J Trad Chinese Med* 1984; **4:** 283–8.

18.   Della Loggia R *et al*. Depressive effect of *Crataegus oxyacantha* L. on central nervous system in mice. *Sci Pharm* 1983; **51:** 319–24.

19.   Dai Y-R *et al*. Effect of extracts of some medicinal plants on superoxide dismutase activity in mice. *Planta Med* 1987; **53:** 309–10.

20.   Iwamoto M *et al*. Klinische Wirkung von Crataegutt bei Herzerkrankungen ischämischer und/oder hypertensiver Genese. *Planta Med* 1981; **42:** 1–16.

21.   Busanny-Caspari E *et al*. Indikationen Herzbeschwerden, Hypotonie und Wetterfühligkeit. *Therapiewoche* 1986; **36:** 2545–50.

22.   Hanak Th, Brückel M-H. Behandlung von leichten stabilen Formen der Angina pectoris mit Crataegutt novo. *Therapiewoche* 1983; **33:** 4331–3.

23.   von Eiff M *et al.*. Hawthorn/Passionflower extract and improvement in physical exercise capacity of patients with dyspnoea Class II of the NYHM functional classification. *Acta Ther* 1994; **20:** 47–66.

24.   Hobbs C, Foster S. Hawthorn — a literature review. *Herbalgram* 1990; No.22: 19–33.

HOLY THISTLE

Species (Family)
Cnicus benedictus L. (Asteraceae/Compositae)

Synonym(s)
Blessed Thistle, Carbenia Benedicta, Carduus Benedictus, Cnicus

Part(s) Used
Herb

Pharmacopoeial Monographs
BHP 1983
BHP 1990
Martindale 30th edition
Pharmacopoeias—Aust. and Hung.

Legal Category (Licensed Products)
GSL[G14]

Constituents[G1,G2,G12,G18,G31,G32]
Lignans Arctigenin, nortracheloside, 2-acetyl nortracheloside, trachelogenin[1]

Polyenes Several polyacetylenes[2]

Steroids Phytosterols (e.g. *n*-nonacosan, sitosterol, sitosteryl glycoside, stigmasterol)[3]

Tannins Type unspecified (8%)

Terpenoids Sesquiterpenes including cnicin 0.2–0.7%,[4] yielding salonitenolide as aglycone,[5] and artemisiifolin. Shoot and flowering head are reported to be devoid of cnicin.[4] Triterpenoids including α-amyrenone, α-amyrin acetate, α-amyrine, multiflorenol, multiflorenol acetate, oleanolic acid[3]

Volatile oils Many components, mainly hydrocarbons[6]

Other constituents Lithospermic acid, mucilage, nicotinic acid and nicotinamide complex, resin

Food Use
Holy thistle is listed by the Council of Europe as natural source of food flavouring (category N2). This category indicates that holy thistle can be added to foodstuffs in small quantities, with a possible limitation of an active principle (as yet unspecified) in the final product.[G9]

Herbal Use
Holy thistle is stated to possess bitter stomachic, antidiarrhoeal, antihaemorrhagic, febrifuge, expectorant, antibiotic, bacteriostatic, vulnerary, and antiseptic properties. Traditionally, it has been used for anorexia, flatulent dyspepsia, bronchial catarrh, topically for gangrenous and indolent ulcers, and specifically for atonic dyspepsia, and enteropathy with flatulent colic.[G1,G2,G3,G4,G32]

Dose
Dried flowering tops 1.5–3.0 g or by infusion three times daily[G2,G3]

Liquid extract (1:1 in 25% alcohol) 1.5–3.0 mL three times daily[G2,G3]

Pharmacological Actions
Animal studies Antibacterial activity has been reported for an aqueous extract of the herb, for cnicin, and for the volatile oil.[6–9] Activity has been documented against *Bacillus subtilis*, *Brucella abortus*, *Brucella bronchoseptica*, *Escherichia coli*, *Proteus* species, *Pseudomonas aeruginosa*, *Staphylococcus aureus*, and *Streptococcus faecalis*. The antimicrobial activity of holy thistle has been attributed to cnicin and to the polyacetylene constituents.[9] Cnicin has exhibited *in-vivo* anti-inflammatory activity (carrageenan rat paw oedema test) virtually equipotent to indomethacin.[4] Antitumour activity has been documented in mice against sarcoma 180 for the whole herb,[8] and against lymphoid leukaemia for cnicin;[8] cnicin has also been reported to exhibit *in-vitro* activity against KB cells.[8] An α-methylene-γ-lactone moiety is thought to be necessary for the antibacterial and antitumour activities of cnicin.[8]

Lithospermic acid is thought to be responsible for the antigonadotrophic activity documented for holy thistle.[G12] The sesquiterpene lactone constituents are stated to be bitter principles.[G31]

Tannins are generally known to possess astringent properties.

Side-effects, Toxicity
None documented for holy thistle. The toxicity of cnicin has been studied in mice: the acute oral LD_{50} was stated to be 1.6–3.2 mmol/kg body-weight and intraperitoneal administration was reported to cause irritation of tissue. In the writhing test, cnicin was found to cause abdominal pain with an ED_{50} estimated as 6.2 mmol/kg.[4]

Antitumour activity has been documented for the whole herb and for cnicin (*see* Animal studies).

Contra-indications, Warnings
None documented for holy thistle. Plants containing sesquiterpene lactones with an α- methylene-γ-lactone moiety are generally considered to be allergenic, although no documented hypersensitivity reactions to holy thistle were located. Holy thistle may cause an allergic reaction in individuals with a known hypersensitivity to other members of the Compositae (e.g. chamomile, ragwort, tansy).

Pregnancy and lactation The safety of holy thistle has not been established. In view of the lack of toxicity data, excessive use of holy thistle during pregnancy and lactation should be avoided.

Pharmaceutical Comment

The chemistry of holy thistle is well documented and the available pharmacological data support most of the stated herbal uses, although no references to human studies were located. In view of the lack of toxicity data, excessive use of holy thistle should be avoided.

References

See General References G1, G2, G3, G4, G9, G12, G14, G18, G22, G23, G31 and G32.

1.   Vanhaelen M, Vanhaelen-Fastré R. Lactonic lignans from *Cnicus benedictus*. *Phytochemistry* 1975; **14:** 2709.

2.   Vanhaelen-Fastré R. Constituents polyacetyleniques de *Cnicus benedictus* L. *Planta Med* 1974; **25:** 47–59.

3.   Ulubelen A, Berkan T. Triterpenic and steroidal compounds of *Cnicus benedictus*. *Planta Med* 1977; **31:** 375–7.

4.   Schneider G, Lachner I. A contribution to analytics and pharmacology of Cnicin. *Planta Med* 1987; **53:** 247–51.

5.   Vanhaelen-Fastré R, Vanhaelen M. Presence of saloniténolide in *Cnicus benedictus*. *Planta Med* 1974; **26:** 375–9.

6.   Vanhaelen-Fastré R. Constitution and antibiotical properties of the essential oil of *Cnicus benedictus*. *Planta Med* 1973; **24:** 165–75.

7.   Cobb E. Antineoplastic agent from *Cnicus benedictus*. *Brit Pat* 1,335,181 (Cl.A61k) 24 Oct 1973, Appl.54,800/69 (via Chemical Abstracts 1975; **83**: 48189j).

8.   Vanhaelen-Fastré R. Antibiotic and cytotoxic activities of cnicin isolated from *Cnicus benedictus*. *J Pharm Belg* 1972; **27:** 683–8.

9.   Vanhaelen-Fastré R. *Cnicus benedictus*: Separation of antimicrobial constituents. *Plant Med Phytother* 1968; **2:** 294–9.

HOPS

Species (Family)
Humulus lupulus L. (Cannabinaceae/Moraceae)

Synonym(s)
Humulus, Lupulus

Part(s) Used
Strobile

Pharmacopoeial Monographs
BHP 1983
BHP 1990
BPC 1949
Martindale 28th edition

Legal Category (Licensed Products)
GSL[G14]

Constituents[G1,G2,G10,G19,G24,G25,G32]
Flavonoids Astragalin, kaempferol, quercetin, quercitrin, rutin

Chalcones Isoxanthohumol, xanthohumol, 6-isopentenyl-naringenin, 3'-(isoprenyl)-2',4-dihydroxy-4',6'-dimethoxy-chalcone, 2',6'-dimethoxy-4,4'-dihydroxychalcone[9]

Oleo-resin (3–12%). Various phenolic compounds including α-bitter acids (e.g. humulone, cohumulone, adhumulone, prehumulone, posthumulone), β-bitter acids (e.g. lupulone, colupulone, adlupulone), and their oxidative degradation products including 2-methyl-3-buten-2-ol[2,3]

Tannins (2–4%). Condensed; gallocatechin identified.[4]

Volatile oils (0.3–1.0%). More than 100 terpenoid components identified; primarily (at least 90%) β-caryophyllene, farnescene, and humulene (sesquiterpenes), and myrcene (monoterpene)

Other constituents Amino acids, phenolic acids, gamma-linoleic acids, lipids, oestrogenic substances (disputed)[5]

Food Use
Hops are listed by the Council of Europe as a natural source of food flavouring (category N2). This category indicates that hops can be added to foodstuffs in small quantities, with a possible limitation of an active principle (as yet unspecified) in the final product.[G9]

Herbal Use
Hops are stated to possess sedative, hypnotic, and topical bactericidal properties. Traditionally, they have been used for neuralgia, insomnia, excitability, priapism, mucous colitis, topically for crural ulcers, and specifically for restlessness associated with nervous tension headache and/or indigestion.[G1,G2,G3,G4,G32]

Dose
Dried strobile 0.5–1.0 g or by infusion; 1–2 g as a hypnotic
Liquid extract (1:1 in 45% alcohol) 0.5–2.0 mL
Tincture (1:5 in 60% alcohol) 1–2 mL

Pharmacological Actions

Animal studies Antibacterial activity, mainly towards Gram-positive bacteria, has been documented for hops and attributed to the humulone and lupulone constituents.[6] The activity of the bitter acids towards Gram-positive bacteria is thought to involve primary membrane leakage. Resistance of Gram-negative bacteria to the resin acids is attributed to the presence of a phospholipid-containing outer membrane, as lupulone and humulone are inactivated by serum phospholipids.[6] Structure activity studies have indicated the requirement of a hydrophobic molecule and a six-membered central ring for such activity.[7]

The humulones and lupulones are thought to possess little activity towards fungi or yeasts. However, antifungal activity has been documented for the bitter acids towards *Trichophyton*, *Candida*, *Fusarium*, and *Mucor* species.[8] Flavonone constituents have also been documented to possess antifungal activity towards *Trichophyton* and *Mucor* species, and antibacterial activity towards *Staphylococcus aureus*.[9]

Antispasmodic activity has been documented for an alcoholic hop extract on various isolated smooth muscle preparations.[10] Hops have been reported to exhibit hypnotic and sedative properties.[G19] 2-Methyl-3-buten-2-ol, a bitter acid degradation product, has been identified as a sedative principle in hops.[2,3] 2-Methyl-3-buten-2-ol has been shown to possess narcotic properties in mice and motility depressant activity in rats, with the latter not attributable to a muscle-relaxant effect.[11] It has also been suggested that isovaleric acid residues present in hops may contribute towards the sedative action.

Hops have previously been reported to possess oestrogenic constituents.[5] However, when a number of purified components, including the volatile oil and the bitter acids, were examined using the uterine weight assay in immature female mice, no oestrogenic activity was found.[5]

Human studies The documented human studies generally refer to hops given in combination with one or more additional herbs. Hops have been reported to improve sleep disturbances when given in combination with valerian.[12] It has been stated that only low amounts of 2-methyl-3-buten-2-ol, the sedative principle identified in hops, are present in sedative tablets containing hops.[2] However, it is thought that 2-methyl-3-buten-2-ol is formed *in vivo* by metabolism of the α-bitter acids and, therefore, the low amount of 2-methyl-3-buten-2-ol in a preparation may not indicate low sedative activity.[13] Interestingly, relatively high concentrations of 2-methyl-3-buten-2-ol were found in bath preparations, suggesting that high concentrations of 2-methyl-3-buten-2-ol may be achieved in both tea and bath products containing hops.[2]

Hops, in combination with chicory and peppermint, have also been documented to relieve pain in patients with chronic cholecystitis (calculous and non-calculous).[14] A herbal product containing a mixture of plant extracts, including hops and uva-ursi, and alpha tocopherol acetate has improved irritable bladder and urinary incontinence.[15] Excellent results were reported for 772 out of 915 patients treated.

Side-effects, Toxicity

Respiratory allergy caused by the handling of hop cones have been documented;[16] a subsequent patch test using dried, crushed flowerheads proved negative. Positive patch test reactions have been documented for fresh hop oil, humulone, and lupulone. Myrcene, present in the fresh oil but readily oxidised, was concluded to be the sensitising agent in the hop oil.[G26] Contact dermatitis to hops has long been recognised[G26] and is attributed to the pollen.[G19] Small doses of hops are stated to be non-toxic.[G20] Large doses administered to animals by injection have resulted in a soporific effect followed by death, with chronic administration resulting in weight loss before death.[G17]

Contra-indications, Warnings

It has been stated that hops should not be taken by individuals suffering from depressive illness, as the sedative effect may accentuate symptoms.[G22,G25] The sedative action may potentiate the effects of existing sedative therapy and alcohol. Allergic reactions have been reported for hops, although only following external contact with the herb and oil.

Pregnancy and lactation In-vitro antispasmodic activity on the uterus has been documented. In view of this and the lack of toxicity data, the excessive use of hops during pregnancy and lactation should be avoided.

Pharmaceutical Comment

The chemistry of hops is well documented and is characterised by the bitter acid components of the oleo-resin. Documented pharmacological activities justify the herbal uses, although excessive use should be avoided in view of the limited toxicity data.

References

See General References G1, G2, G3, G4, G6, G9, G10, G14, G17, G19, G20, G21, G24, G25, G26 and G32.

1. Song-San S *et al.* Chalcones from *Humulus lupulus. Phytochemistry* 1989; **28:** 1776–7.

2. Hänsel R *et al.* The sedative-hypnotic principle of hops. 3. Communication: Contents of 2-methyl-3-buten-2-ol in hops and hop preparations. *Planta Med* 1982; **45:** 224–8.

3. Wohlfart R *et al.* Detection of sedative–hypnotic hop constituents, V: Degradation of humulones and lupulones to 2-methyl-3-buten-2-ol, a hop constituent possessing sedative-hypnotic activity. *Arch Pharm (Weinheim)* 1982; **315:** 132–7.

4. Gorissen H *et al.* Separation and identification of (+)-gallocatechin in hops. *Arch Int Physiol Biochem* 1968; **76:** 932–4.

5. Fenselau C, Talalay P. Is oestrogenic activity present in hops? *Food Cosmet Toxicol* 1973; **11:** 597–603.

6. Teuber M, Schmalreck AF. Membrane leakage in *Bacillus subtilis* 168 induced by the hop constituents lupulone, humulone, isohumulone and humulinic acid. *Arch Mikrobiol* 1973; **94:** 159–71.

7. Schmalreck AF *et al.* Structural features determining the antibiotic potencies of natural and synthetic hop bitter resins, their precursors and derivatives. *Can J Microbiol* 1975; **21:** 205–12.

8. Mizobuchi S, Sato Y. Antifungal activities of hop bitter resins and related compounds. *Agric Biol Chem* 1985; **49:** 399–405.

9. Mizobuchi S, Sato Y. A new flavanone with antifungal activity isolated from hops. *Agric Biol Chem* 1984; **48:** 2771–5.

10. Caujolle F *et al.* Spasmolytic action of hop (*Humulus lupulus*). *Agressologie* 1969; **10:** 405–10.

11. Wohlfart R *et al.* The Sedative-hypnotic principle of hops. 4. Communication: Pharmacology of 2-methyl-3-buten-2-ol. *Planta Med* 1983; 48: 120–3.

12. Müller-Limmroth W, Ehrenstein W. Untersuchungen über die Wirkung von Seda- Kneipp auf den Schlaf schlafgestörter Menschen. *Med Klin* 1977; **72:** 1119–25.

13. Hänsel R, Wohlfart R. Narcotic action of 2-methyl-3-butene-2-ol Contained in the exhalation of hops. *Z Naturforsch* 1980; **35:** 1096–7.

14. Chakarski I *et al.* Clinical study of a herb combination consisting of *Humulus lupulus, Cichorium intybus, Mentha piperita* in patients with chronic calculous and non-calculous cholecystitis. *Probl Vatr Med* 1982; **10:** 65–9.

15. Lenau H *et al.* Wirksamkeit und Verträglichkeit von Cysto Fink bei Patienten mit Reizblase und/oder Harninkontinenz. *Therapiewoche* 1984; **34:** 6054.

16. Newmark FM. Hops allergy and terpene sensitivity: An occupational disease. *Ann Allergy* 1978; **41:** 311–12.

HOREHOUND, BLACK

Species (Family)
Ballota nigra L. (Labiatae)

Synonym(s)
Ballota

Part(s) Used
Herb

Pharmacopoeial Monographs
BHP 1983

Legal Category (Licensed Products)
Not included on the GSL[G14]

Constituents[G25,G32]
Limited chemical information is available for black horehound. Documented constituents include diterpenes (e.g. ballotenol, ballotinone, preleosibirin),[1-3] flavonoids, and volatile oil.

Food Use
Black horehound is listed by the Council of Europe as a natural source of food flavouring (category N3). This category indicates that black horehound can be added to foodstuffs in the traditionally accepted manner, although insufficient information is available for an adequate assessment of potential toxicity.[G9]

Herbal Use
Black horehound is stated to possess anti-emetic, sedative, and mild astringent properties. Traditionally, it has been used for nausea, vomiting, nervous dyspepsia, and specifically for vomiting of central origin.[G3,G32]

Dose
Dried herb 2–4 g or by infusion three times daily[G3]

Liquid extract (1:1 in 25% alcohol) 1–3 mL three times daily[G3]

Tincture (1:10 in 45% alcohol) 1–2 mL three times daily[G3]

Pharmacological Actions
None documented.

Side-effects, Toxicity
None documented.

Contra-indications, Warnings
None documented.

Pregnancy and lactation Black horehound is reputed to affect the menstrual cycle.[G12] In view of the lack of phytochemical, pharmacological, and toxicity data, the use of black horehound during pregnancy and lactation should be avoided.

Pharmaceutical Comment
Limited phytochemical or pharmacological information is available for black horehound to justify its use as a herbal remedy. In view of the lack of toxicity data, excessive use should be avoided.

References
See General References G3, G9, G12, G14, G25 and G32

1. Bruno M *et al*. Preleosibirin, a prefuranic labdane diterpene from *Ballota nigra* subsp. *foetida*. *Phytochemistry* 1986; **25**: 538–9.

2. Savona G *et al*. Structure of ballotinone, a diterpenoid from Ballota nigra. *J Chem Soc Perkin Trans 1* 1976; 1607–9.

3. Savona G *et al*. The structure of ballotenol, a new diterpenoid from Ballota nigra. *J Chem Soc Perkin Trans 1* 1977; 497–9.

HOREHOUND, WHITE

Species (Family)
Marrubium vulgare L. (Labiatae)

Synonym(s)
Common Hoarhound, Hoarhound, Horehound, Marrubium

Part(s) Used
Flower, Leaf

Pharmacopoeial Monographs
BHP 1983
BHP 1990
BPC 1934

Legal Category (Licensed Products)
GSL[G14]

Constituents[G1,G2,G19,G31,G32]
Alkaloids (pyrrolidine-type) Betonicine 0.3%, the *cis*-isomer turicine
Flavonoids Apigenin, luteolin, quercetin, and their glycosides[1]
Terpenoids Diterpenes including marrubiin 0.3–1.0%, a lactone, as the main component with lesser amounts of various alcohols (e.g. marrubenol, marrubiol, peregrinol and vulgarol). Marrubiin has also been stated to be an artefact formed from a precursor, premarrubiin, during extraction.[2]
Volatile oils (trace). Bisabolol, camphene, *p*-cymene, limonene, β-pinene, sabinene and others,[2] a sesquiterpene (unspecified)
Other constituents Choline, saponin (unspecified), β-sitosterol (a phytosterol), waxes (C_{26}-C_{34} alkanes)

Food Use
White horehound is listed by the Council of Europe as a natural source of food flavouring (category N2). This category indicates that white horehound can be added to foodstuffs in small quantities, with a possible limitation of an active principle (as yet unspecified) in the final product.[G9]

Herbal Use
White horehound is stated to possess expectorant and antispasmodic properties. Traditionally, it has been used for acute or chronic bronchitis, whooping cough, and specifically for bronchitis with non-productive cough.[G1,G2,G3,G4,G32]

Dose
Dried herb 1–2 g or by infusion three times daily[G2,G3]
Liquid extract (1:1 in 20% alcohol) 2–4 mL three times daily[G2,G3]

Pharmacological Actions
Animal studies Aqueous extracts have been reported to exhibit an antagonistic effect towards hydroxytryptamine *in vivo* in mice, and *in vitro* in guinea-pig ileum and rat uterus tissue.[3] Expectorant and vasodilative properties have been documented for the volatile oil.[4] However, the main active expectorant principle in white horehound is reported to be marrubiin, which is stated to stimulate secretions of the bronchial mucosa.[G30] Marrubiin has also been stated to be cardioactive, possessing anti-arrhythmic properties, although higher doses are reported to cause arrhythmias.[G30] Marrubin acid (obtained from the saponification of marrubiin) has been documented to stimulate bile secretion in rats, whereas marrubiin was found to be inactive.[5] White horehound is stated to possess bitter properties (BI 65 000 compared to gentian BI 10 000–30 000) with marrubiin as the main active component.[G31]

Large doses of white horehound are purgative.[G5,G30] The volatile oil has antischistosomal activity.[6]

Side-effects, Toxicity
The plant juice of white horehound is stated to contain an irritant principle, which can cause contact dermatitis.[G26] No documented toxicity studies were located for the whole plant, although an LD_{50} (rat, by mouth) value for marrubin acid is reported as 370 mg/kg body-weight.[5] The volatile oil is documented to be highly toxic to the flukes *Schistosoma mansoni* and *Schistosoma haematobium*.[6]

Contra-indications, Warnings
None documented. Cardioactive properties and an antagonism of 5-hydroxytryptamine have been documented in animals.
Pregnancy and lactation White horehound is reputed to be an abortifacient and to affect the menstrual cycle.[G12] Uterine stimulant activity in animals has been documented.[G12] In view of this and the lack of safety data, the use of white horehound during pregnancy should be avoided. Excessive use during lactation should be avoided.

Pharmaceutical Comment
The chemistry of white horehound is well documented. Limited pharmacological information is available, although expectorant properties have been reported which support some of the herbal uses. In view of the lack of toxicity data and suggested cardioactive properties, white horehound should not be taken in excessive doses.

References
See General References G1, G2, G3, G4, G5, G9, G12, G14, G19, G24, G26, G30, G31 and G32
1. Kowalewski Z, Matlawska I. Flavonoid compounds in the herb of *Marrubium vulgare* L. *Herba Pol* 1978; **24:** 183–6.
2. Henderson MS, McCrindle R. Premarrubiin. A diterpernoid from *Marrubium vulgare* L. *J Chem Soc* 1969; (C): 2014.
3. Cahen R. Pharmacologic spectrum of *Marrubium vulgare*. *C R Soc Biol* 1970; **164:** 1467–72.
4. Karryev MO *et al*. Some therapeutic properties and phytochemistry of common horehound. *Izv Akad Nauk Turkm SSR Ser Biol Nauk* 1976; **3:** 86–8.
5. Krejčí I, Zadina R. Die Gallentreibende Wirkung von Marrubiin und Marrabinsäure. *Planta Med*; 1959; **7:** 1–7.
6. Saleh MM, Glombitza KW. Volatile oil of *Marrubium vulgare* and its anti-schistosomal activity. *Planta Med* 1989; **55:** 105.

HORSE-CHESTNUT

Species (Family)
Aesculus hippocastanum L. (Hippocastanaceae)

Synonym(s)
Aesculus

Part(s) Used
Seed

Pharmacopoeial Monographs
Martindale 30th edition
Pharmacopoeias—Ger., Port., and Span.

Legal Category (Licensed Products)
GSL (for external use only)[G14]

Constituents[G10,G24,G29,G31,G32]
Coumarins Aesculetin, fraxin (fraxetin glucoside), scopolin (scopoletin glucoside)
Flavonoids Flavonol (kaempferol, quercetin) glycosides including astragalin, isoquercetrin, rutin; leucocyanidin (quercetin derivative)
Saponins A mixture of saponins collectively referred to as 'aescin' (about 13%); α- and β-escin as major glycosides
Tannins Type unspecified but likely to be condensed in view of the epicatechin content (formed during hydrolysis of condensed tannins)
Other constituents Allantoin, amino acids (adenine, adenosine, guanine), choline, citric acid, phytosterol.

Food Use
Horse-chestnut is not used in foods.

Herbal Use
Traditionally, horse-chestnut has been used for the treatment of varicose veins, haemorrhoids, phlebitis, diarrhoea, fever, and enlargement of the prostate gland.[G25]

Dose
Fruit 0.2–1.0 g three times daily[G25]

Pharmacological Actions
Documented studies have concentrated on the actions of the saponins, in particular, aescin.
Animal studies Anti-inflammatory activity in rats has been documented for both a fruit extract and the saponin fraction.[1–4] Anti-inflammatory activity in the rat has been reported to be greater for a total horse-chestnut extract compared to aescin. In addition, an extract excluding aescin also exhibited activity suggesting horse-chestnut contains anti-inflammatory agents other than aescin.[5] No difference in activity was noted when the horse-chestnut extracts were administered prior to and after dextran (inflammatory agent). It has been proposed that aescin affects the initial phase of inflammation by exerting a 'sealing' effect on cap-

illaries and by reducing the number and/or diameter of capillary pores.[3]
In addition, the saponin fraction has been reported to exhibit analgesic and antigranulation activities in rats,[3] to reduce capillary permeability,[6] and to produce an initial hypotension followed by a longer lasting hypertension in anaesthetised animals.[4] Prostaglandin production by venous tissue is thought to be involved in the regulation of vascular reactivity.[7] Prostaglandins of the E series are known to cause relaxation of venous tissues whereas those of the F_α series produce contraction. Increased venous tone induced by aescin *in vitro* was found to be associated with an increased $PGF_{2\alpha}$ synthesis in the venous tissue.
The saponin fraction has been reported to contract the isolated rabbit ileum.[3]
Considerable antiviral activity *in vitro* towards influenza virus (A_2/Japan 305) has been described for aescin.[8]
Metabolism studies of aescin in the rat have concluded that aescin toxicity is reduced by hepatic metabolism.[9]
Flavonoids and tannins are generally recognised as having anti-inflammatory and astringent properties, respectively.
Human studies Results of a controlled double-blind trial over 4 weeks involving 40 patients with chronic venous insufficiency have confirmed the antioedematous effect and beneficial influence on subjective parameters (pain, tiredness, feeling of tension and pruritus in the legs) of a horse-chestnut extract.[10] A randomised placebo-controlled cross-over double-blind trial of 22 patients with chronic venous insufficiency concluded that 1200 mg horse-chestnut extract (standardised to 100 mg aescin) had an antioedematous effect via a decrease in transcapillary filtration.[11]
Glycosaminoglycan hydrolyses are enzymes involved in the breakdown of substances (proteoglycans) that determine capillary rigidity and pore size (thus influencing the passage of macromolecules into the surrounding tissue). Proteoglycans also interact with collagen, stabilising the fibres and regulating their correct biosynthesis.[12] The activity of these enzymes was found to be raised in varicose patients compared to healthy patients. Treatment of 15 varicose patients with a horse-chestnut extract (900 mg daily) for 12 days was found to cause a significant reduction in the activity of these enzymes.[12] The proposed mode of action suggested that horse-chestnut acts at the site of enzyme release, exerting a stabilising effect on the lysosomal membrane.[12]
The cosmetic applications of horse-chestnut have been reviewed[13] and are attributed to properties associated with the saponin constituents.

Side-effects, Toxicity
Two incidences of toxic nephropathy have been reported and were stated as probably secondary to the ingestion of high doses of aescin.[14] In Japan, where horse-chestnut has been used as an anti-inflammatory drug after surgery or trauma, hepatic injury has been described in a male patient who received an intramuscular injection of a proprietary

product containing horse-chestnut.[15] Liver function tests showed a mild abnormality and a diagnosis of giant cell tumour of bone (grade 2) by bone biopsy was made. Other side-effects stated to have been reported for the product include shock, spasm, mild nausea, vomiting, and urticaria.[15]

The effect of aescin, both free and albumin-bound, on renal tubular transport processes has been studied in the isolated, artificially perfused frog kidney.[16] Aescin was found to primarily affect tubular, rather than glomerular, epithelium and that binding to plasma protein (approximately 50%) protects against this nephrotoxicity. Aescin was thought to be neither secreted nor reabsorbed in the tubules and the concentration of unbound aescin filtered through the kidney (13%) was considered to be too low to have toxic effects. The authors commented that the symptoms of acute renal failure in man are caused primarily by interference with glomeruli and in view of this, the nephrotoxic potential of aescin is probably only relevant when the kidneys are already damaged and also if the aescin is displaced from its binding to plasma protein.[16]

A proprietary product containing horse-chestnut (together with phenopyrazone and cardiac glycoside-containing plant extracts) has been associated with the development of a drug-induced auto-immune disease called 'pseudolupus syndrome' in Germany and Switzerland.[17,18] The individual component in the product responsible for the syndrome was not established.

It has been noted that death occurs rapidly in animals given large doses of aescin, due to massive haemolysis. Death is more prolonged in animals given smaller doses of aescin.[4] LD_{50} values for aescin have been estimated in mice, rats and guinea-pigs and range from 134 to 720 mg/kg (by mouth) and from 1.4 to 15.2 mg/kg (intravenous injection).[G25] The total saponin fraction has been reported to be less toxic in mice (intraperitoneal injection) compared to the isolated aescin mixture (LD_{50} 46.5 mg/kg and 9.5 mg/kg, respectively).[3] The haemolytic index of horse-chestnut is documented as 6 000 compared to 9 500 to 12 500 for aescin.[G31]

Contra-indications, Warnings

Horse-chestnut may be irritant to the gastro-intestinal tract due to the saponin constituents. Saponins are generally recognised to possess haemolytic properties but are not usually absorbed from the gastrointestinal tract following oral administration. horse-chestnut may interfere with anticoagulant/coagulant therapy (coumarin constituents). Aescin, the main saponin component in horse-chestnut, binds to plasma protein and may affect the binding of other drugs. horse-chestnut should be avoided by patients with existing renal or hepatic impairment.

Pregnancy and lactation The safety of horse-chestnut during pregnancy and lactation has not been established. In view of the pharmacologically active constituents present in horse-chestnut, use during pregnancy and lactation is best avoided.

Pharmaceutical Comment

Horse-chestnut is traditionally characterised by its saponin components, in particular aescin which represents a mixture of compounds. However, horse-chestnut also contains other pharmacologically active constituents including coumarins and flavonoids. The traditional use of horse-chestnut in peripheral vascular disorders has largely been substantiated by studies in animals and humans, in which anti-inflammatory and capillary stabilising effects have been observed. Many of the documented activities can probably be attributed to the saponin and flavonoid constituents in horse-chestnut.

References

See General References G9, G10, G14, G22, G23, G24, G25, G29, G31 and G32.

1. Farnsworth NR, Cordell GA. A review of some biologically active compounds isolated from plants as reported in the 1974–75 literature. *Lloydia* 1976; **39**: 420–55.

2. Benoit PS *et al*. Biological and phytochemical evaluation of plants. XIV. Antiinflammatory evaluation of 163 species of plants. *Lloydia* 1976; **39**: 160–71.

3. Cebo B *et al*. Pharmacological properties of saponin fractions from Polish crude drugs: Saponaria officinalis, Primula officinalis, and Aesculus hippocastanum. *Herba Pol* 1976; **22**: 154–62.

4. Vogel G *et al*. Untersuchungen zum Mechanismus der therapeutischen und toxischen Wirkung des Rosskastanien-saponins aescin. *Arzneimittelforschung* 1970; **20**: 699–705.

5. Tsutsumi S, Ishizuka S. Anti-inflammatory effects of the extract *Aesculus hippocastanum* and seed. *Shikwa-Gakutto* 1967; **67**: 1324–8.

6. De Pascale V *et al*. Effect of an escin-cyclonamine mixture on capillary permeability. *Boll Chim Farm* 1974; **113**: 600–14.

7. Longiave D *et al*. The mode of action of aescin on isolated veins: Relationship with $PGF_2\alpha$. *Pharmacol Res Comm* 1978; **10**: 145–53.

8. Rao SG, Cochran KW. Antiviral activity of triterpenoid saponins containing acylated β-amyrin aglycones. *J Pharm Sci* 1974; **63**: 471.

9. Rothkopf M. Effects of age, sex and phenobarbital pretreatment on the acute toxicity of the horse chestnut saponin aescin in rats. *Naunyn-Schmiedarchpharm* 1977; **297**(Suppl): R18.

10. Rudofsky G *et al*. Ödemprotektive Wirkung und klinische Wirksamkeit von Rosskastaniensamenextrakt im Doppelblindversuch. *Phlebol Proktol* 1986; **15**: 47–53.

11. Bisler H *et al*. Wirkung von Rosskastaniensamenextrakt auf die transkapilläre Filtration bei chronischer venöser Insuffizienz. *Dtsch Med Wochenschr* 1986; **111**: 1321–9.

12. Kreysel HW *et al*. A possible role of lysosomal enzymes in the pathogenesis of varicosis and the reduction in their serum activity by Venostasin^R. *Vasa* 1983; **12**: 377–82.

13. Proserpio G *et al*. Cosmetic uses of horse-chestnut (*Aesculum hippocastanum*) extracts, of escin and of the cholesterol/escin complex. *Fitoterapia* 1980; **51**: 113–28.

14. Grasso A, Corvaglia E. Two cases of suspected toxic tubulonephrosis due to escine. *Gazz Med Ital* 1976; **135**: 581–4.

15. Takegoshi K *et al*. A case of Venoplant^R-induced hepatic injury. *Gastroenterol Japonica* 1986; **21**: 62–5.

16. Rothkopf M *et al*. Animal experiments on the question of the renal toleration of the horse chestnut saponin aescin. *Arzneimittelforschung* 1977; **27**: 598–605.

17. Grob P *et al*. Drug-induced pseudolupus. *Lancet* 1975; **ii**: 144–8.

18. Russell AS. Drug-induced autoimmune disease. *Clin Immunol Allergy* 1981; **1**: 57–76.

HORSERADISH

Species (Family)

Radicula armoracia (L.) Robinson (Brassicaceae/Cruciferae)

Synonym(s)

Armoracia lopathifolia Gilib., *A. rusticana* (Gaertn.) Mey & Scherb., *Cochlearia armoracia* L., *Nasturtium armoracia* Fries, *Roripa armoracia* Hitch.

Part(s) Used

Root

Pharmacopoeial Monographs

BPC 1934

Legal Category (Licensed Products)

GSL[G14]

Constituents[G18,G24,G25,G28,G31,G32,G35]

Coumarins Aesculetin, scopoletin.[1]

Phenols Caffeic acid derivatives and lesser amounts of hydroxycinnamic acid derivatives. Concentrations of acids are reported to be much lower in the root than in the leaf.[1]

Volatile oils Glucosinolates (mustard oil glycosides) gluconasturtiin and sinigrin (*S*-glucosides), yielding phenylethylisothiocyanate and allylisothiocyanate after hydrolysis. Isothiocyanate content estimated as 12.2–20.4 mg/g freeze dried root.[2,3] Other isothiocyanate types include isopropyl, 3-butenyl, 4-pentenyl, phenyl, 3-methylthiopropyl and benzyl derivatives.[4]

Other constituents Ascorbic acid, asparagin, peroxidase enzymes, resin, starch, sugar

Other plant parts Kaempferol and quercetin have been documented for the leaf.

Food Use

Horseradish is listed by the Council of Europe as a natural source of food flavouring (category N2). This category indicates that horseradish can be added to foodstuffs in small quantities, with a possible limitation of an active principle (as yet unspecified) in the final product.[G9] In the USA, horseradish is listed as GRAS (Generally Regarded As Safe).[G28] Horseradish is commonly used as a food flavouring.

Herbal Use

Horseradish is stated to possess antiseptic, circulatory and digestive stimulant, diuretic, and vulnerary properties.[G20,G25,G32] Traditionally, it has been used for pulmonary and urinary infection, urinary stones, oedematous conditions, and externally for application to inflamed joints or tissues.[G25]

Dose

Root (fresh) 2–4 g before meals[G25]

Pharmacological Actions

Animal studies A marked hypotensive effect in cats has been documented for horseradish peroxidase, following intravenous administration.[5] The effect was completely blocked by aspirin and indomethacin, but was not affected by antihistamines. It was concluded that horseradish peroxidase acts by stimulating the synthesis of arachidonic acid metabolites.

Side-effects, Toxicity

Isothiocyanates are reported to have irritant effects on the skin and also to be allergenic.[G26,G35] Animal poisoning has been documented for horseradish. Symptoms described include inflammation of the stomach or rumen, and excitement followed by collapse.[G13]

Contra-indications, Warnings

It is stated that horseradish may depress thyroid function, and should be avoided by individuals with hypothyroidism or by those receiving thyroxine.[G20,G25] No rationale for this statement is included except that this action is common to all members of the cabbage and mustard family.

Pregnancy and lactation Allylisothiocyanate is extremely toxic and a violent irritant to mucous membranes.[G35] Its use should be avoided during pregnancy and lactation.

Pharmaceutical Comment

The chemistry of horseradish is well established and it is recognised as one of the richest plant sources of peroxidase enzymes.[G24] Little pharmacological information was located, although the isothiocyanates and peroxidases probably account for the reputed circulatory stimulant and wound healing actions, respectively. The oil is one of the most hazardous of all essential oils and it is not recommended for either external or internal use.[G35] Horseradish should not be ingested in amounts exceeding those used in foods.

References

See General References G5, G9, G18, G20, G24, G25, G26, G28, G31, G32 and G35.

1. Stoehr H, Herrman K. Phenolic acids of vegetables. III. Hydroxycinnamic acids and hydroxybenzoic acids of root vegetables. *Z Lebensm-Unters Forsch* 1975: **159**: 219–24.

2. Hansen H. Content of glucosinolates in horseradish (*Armoracia rusticana*). *Tidsskr Planteavl* 1974; **73**: 408–10.

3. Kojima M. Volatile components of Wasabia japonica. II. Voltile components other than isothiocyanates. *Hakko Kogaku Zasshi* 1971; **49**: 650–3.

4. Kojima M *et al.* Studies on the volatile components of *Wasabia japonica, Brassica juncea*, and *Cocholearia armoracia* by gas chromatography-mass spectrometry. *Yakugaku Zasshi* 1973; **93**: 453–9.

5. Sjaastad OV *et al.* Hypotensive effects in cats caused by horseradish peroxidase mediated by metabolites of arachidonic acid. *J Histochem Cytochem* 1984; **32**: 1328–30.

HYDRANGEA

Species (Family)

Hydrangea arborescens L. (Saxifragaceae)

Synonym(s)

Mountain Hydrangea, Seven Barks, Smooth Hydrangea, Wild Hydrangea

Part(s) Used

Rhizome, Root

Pharmacopoeial Monographs

BHP 1983

Legal Category (Licensed Products)

GSL[G14]

Constituents[G10,G18,G19,G24,G32]

Limited information is available on the chemistry of hydrangea. It is stated to contain carbohydrates (e.g. gum, starch, sugars), flavonoids (e.g. kaempferol, quercetin, rutin), resin, saponins, hydrangin, and hydrangenol, a stilbenoid,[1] and to be free from tannins.

Food Use

Hydrangea is not used in foods. In the USA, hydrangea is listed as a 'Herb of Undefined Safety'.[G10]

Herbal Use

Hydrangea is stated to possess diuretic and antilithic properties. Traditionally, it has been used for cystitis, urethritis, urinary calculi, prostatitis, enlarged prostate gland, and specifically for urinary calculi with gravel and cystitis.[G3,G32]

Dose

Dried rhizome/root 2–4 g or by decoction three times daily[G3]

Liquid extract (1:1 in 25% alcohol) 2–4 mL three times daily[G3]

Tincture (1:5 in 45% alcohol) 2–10 mL three times daily[G3]

Pharmacological Actions

Animal studies None documented for hydrangea. Synthesised hydrangenol derivatives have been reported to possess anti-allergic properties, exhibiting a strong inhibitory action towards hyaluronidase activity and histamine release.[2]

Side-effects, Toxicity

Hydrangea has been reported to cause contact dermatitis,[G26] and it is stated that hydrangin may cause gastro-enteritis.[G10] Symptoms of overdose are described as vertigo and a feeling of tightness in the chest.[G10] An extract has been reported to be non-toxic in animals.[3]

Contra-indications, Warnings

None documented.

Pregnancy and lactation The safety of hydrangea has not been established. In view of the lack of phytochemical, pharmacological, and toxicity data, the use of hydrangea during pregnancy and lactation should be avoided.

Pharmaceutical Comment

Limited information is available on the chemistry of hydrangea, although related species have been investigated more thoroughly.[G19] No scientific evidence was located to justify the herbal uses. In view of the lack of toxicity data, excessive use of hydrangea should be avoided.

References

See General References G3, G10, G14, G18, G19, G24, G26 and G32.

1. Harborne JB and Baxter H. Phytochemical Dictionary. London: Taylor and Francis. 1993.

2. Kakegawa H *et al*. Inhibitory effects of hydrangeol derivatives on the activation of hyaluronidase and their anti-allergic activities. *Planta Med* 1988; **54**: 385–9.

3. Der Marderosian A. *J Toxicol Environ Health* 1976; **1**: 939–53.

HYDROCOTYLE

Species (Family)
Centella asiatica (L.) Urban (Umbelliferae)

Synonym(s)
Centella, Gotu Kola, Indian Pennywort, Indian Water Navelwort, *Hydrocotyle asiatica*

Part(s) Used
Herb

Pharmacopoeial Monographs
BHP 1983
Martindale 30th edition
Pharmacopoeias—Chin.

Legal Category (Licensed Products)
GSL (for external use only)[G14]

Constituents[G10,G21,G30,G32]

Amino acids Alanine and serine (major components), aminobutyrate, aspartate, glutamate, histidine, lysine, threonine.[1] The root contains greater quantities than the herb.[1]
Flavonoids Quercetin, kaempferol, and various glycosides[2–4]
Terpenoids Triterpenes, asiaticoside, centelloside, madecassoside, brahmoside and brahminoside (saponin glycosides). Aglycones are referred to as hydrocotylegenin A–E;[5] compounds A–D are reported to be esters of the triterpene alcohol R_1-barrigenol.[5,6] Asiaticentoic acid, centellic acid, centoic acid, and madecassic acid
Volatile oils Various terpenoids including β-caryophyllene, trans-β-farnesene and germacrene D (sesquiterpenes) as major components, α-pinene and β-pinene. The major terpenoid is stated to be unidentified.
Other constituents Hydrocotylin (an alkaloid), vallerine (a bitter principle), fatty acids (e.g. linoleic acid, linolenic acid, lignocene, oleic acid, palmitic acid, stearic acid), phytosterols (e.g. campesterol, sitosterol, stigmasterol),[7] resin, tannin

The underground plant parts of hydrocotyle have been reported to contain small quantities of at least 14 different polyacetylenes.[8–10]

Food Use
Hydrocotyle is not used in foods.

Herbal Use
Hydrocotyle is stated to possess mild diuretic, antirheumatic, dermatological, peripheral vasodilator, and vulnerary properties. Traditionally it has been used for rheumatic conditions, cutaneous affections, and by topical application, for indolent wounds, leprous ulcers, and cicatrisation after surgery.[G3,G32]

Dose
Dried leaf 0.6 g or by infusion three times daily[G3]

Pharmacological Actions
Animal studies The triterpenoids are regarded as the active principles in hydrocotyle.[7] Asiaticoside is reported to possess wound healing ability, by having a stimulating effect on the epidermis and promoting keratinisation.[11] Asiaticoside is thought to act by an inhibitory action on the synthesis of collagen and mucopolysaccharides in connective tissue.[11]
Both asiaticoside and madecassoside are documented to be anti-inflammatory, and the total saponin fraction is reported to be active in the carrageenan rat paw oedema test.[12]
In-vivo studies in rats have shown that asiaticoside exhibits a protective action against stress-induced gastric ulcers, following subcutaneous administration,[13] and accelerates the healing of chemical-induced duodenal ulcers, after oral administration.[14] It was thought that asiaticoside acted by increasing the ability of the rats to cope with a stressful situation, rather than via a local effect on the mucosa.[13]
In-vivo studies in mice and rats using brahmoside and brahminoside, by intraperitoneal injection, have shown a CNS-depressant effect.[15] The compounds were found to decrease motor activity, increase hexobarbitone sleeping time, slightly decrease body temperature, and were thought to act via a cholinergic mechanism.[15] A hypertensive effect in rats was also observed, but only following large doses.[15]
In-vitro studies with brahmoside and brahminoside indicated a relaxant effect on the rabbit duodenum and rat uterus, and an initial increase, followed by a decrease, in the amplitude and rate of contraction of the isolated rabbit heart.[15] Higher doses were found to cause cardiac arrest, although subsequent intravenous administration in dogs caused no marked change in an ECG.[15]
In-vitro antifertility activity against human and rat sperm has been described for the total saponin fraction.[16] Asiaticoside and brahminoside are thought to be the active components, although no spermicidal or spermostatic action could be demonstrated for the pure saponins.[16] A crude hydrocotyle extract has been reported to significantly reduce the fertility of female mice when administered orally.[10] No mechanism of action was investigated.
Teratogenicity studies in the rabbit have reported negative findings for a hydrocotyle extract containing asiatic acid, madecassic acid, madasiatic acid, and asiaticoside.[17]
Fresh plant juice is reported to be devoid of antibacterial activity,[18] although asiaticoside has been reported to be active versus *Mycobacterium tuberculosis*, *Bacillus leprae*, and *Entamoeba histolytica*, and oxyasiaticoside was documented to be active against tubercle bacillus.[16,18] The fresh plant juice is also stated not to exhibit antitumour or antiviral activities, but to possess a moderate cytotoxic action in human ascites tumour cells.[18]

Human studies Several studies describing the use of hydrocotyle to treat wounds and various skin disorders have been documented. A cream containing a hydrocotyle extract was found to be successful in the treatment of psoriasis in seven patients to whom it was applied.[19] An aerosol preparation, containing a hydrocotyle extract, was reported to improve the healing in 19 of 25 wounds that had proved refractory to other forms of treatment.[11] A hydrocotyle extract containing asiaticoside (40%), asiatic acid (29–30%), madecassic acid (29–30%), and madasiatic acid (1%) was stated to be successful as both a preventive and curative treatment, when given to 227 patients with keloids or hypertrophic scars.[17] The effective dose in adults was reported to be between 60 and 90 mg. It was proposed that the triterpene constituents in the hydrocotyle extract act in a similar manner to cortisone, with respect to wound healing, and interfere with the metabolism of abnormal collagen.[17]

The triterpene constituents are reported to be metabolised primarily in the faeces in a period of 24 to 76 hours, with a small percentage metabolised via the kidneys.[17] An extract containing asiatic acid, madecassic acid, madasiatic acid and asiaticoside reached peak plasma concentrations in 2 to 4 hours, irrespective of whether it is administered in tablet, oily injection, or ointment formulations.[17]

Hydrocotyle has been used in the treatment of patients with chronic lesions such as cutaneous ulcers, surgical wounds, fistulas, and gynaecological wounds.[G21,G22] Hydrocotyle has also been reported to improve the blood circulation in the lower limbs. Stimulation of collagen synthesis in the vein wall resulted in an increase in vein tonicity and a reduction in the capacity of the vein to distend.[10]

The juice of the leaves or the whole plant is documented to be effective for relieving the itching associated with prickly heat.[G26]

Asiaticoside has also been documented to improve the general ability and behavioural pattern of 30 mentally retarded children, when given over a period of 12 weeks. It also increased the mean concentrations of blood sugar, serum cholesterol, and total protein, and lowered blood urea and serum acid phosphatase concentrations, in 43 adults.[16] Vital capacity was also increased.

Side-effects, Toxicity

A burning sensation was reported by 4 of 20 patients, during the period of application of an aerosol preparation containing hydrocotyle.[11] However, it is not clear whether other components in the formulation contributed to this reaction. Ingestion of hydrocotyle is stated to have produced pruritus over the whole body.[G26]

Contra-indications, Warnings

It is stated that hydrocotyle may produce photosensitisation.[G3] Excessive doses may interfere with existing hypoglycaemic therapy and increase serum-cholesterol concentrations; hyperglycaemic and hypercholesterolaemic activities have been reported for asiaticoside in humans. Brahmoside and brahminoside have been reported to exert a CNS-depressant action in animal studies.[15]

Pregnancy and lactation Hydrocotyle is reputed to be an abortifacient and to affect the menstrual cycle.[G12] Relaxation of the isolated rat uterus has been documented for brahmoside and brahminoside.[15] Triterpene constituents have been reported to lack any teratological effects in rabbits.[17] In view of the lack of toxicity data, the use of hydrocotyle during pregnancy should be avoided. Excessive use should be avoided during lactation.

Pharmaceutical Comment

The chemistry of hydrocotyle is well studied and its pharmacological activity seems to be associated with the triterpenoid constituents. Documented clinical and animal data support the herbal use of hydrocotyle as a dermatological agent, and warrants further research into the potential role of hydrocotyle in wound management. In view of the lack of toxicity data, excessive ingestion of hydrocotyle should be avoided.

References

See General References G3, G10, G12, G14, G21, G22, G23, G26, G30 and G32.

1. George VK, Gnanarethinam JL. Free amino acids in *Centella asiatica*. *Curr Sci* 1975; **44:** 790.

2. Rzadkowska-Bodalska H. Flavonoid compounds in herb pennywort (*Hydrocotyle vulgaris*). *Herba Pol* 1974; **20:** 243–6.

3. Voigt G *et al*. Zur Struktur der Flavonoide aus *Hydrocotyle vulgaris* L. *Pharmazie* 1981; **36:** 377–9.

4. Hiller K *et al*. Isolierung von Quercetin-3-*O*-(6-*O*-α-L-arabinopyranosyl)-β-D-galaktopyranosid, einem neuen Flavonoid aus *Hydrocotyle vulgaris* L. *Pharmazie* 1979; **34:** 192–3.

5. Hiller K *et al*. Saponins of *Hydrocotyle vulgaris*. *Pharmazie* 1971; **26:** 780.

6. Hiller K *et al*. Zur Struktur des Hauptsaponins aus *Hydrocotyle vulgaris* L. *Pharmazie* 1981; **36:** 844–6.

7. Asakawa Y *et al*. Mono- and sesquiterpenoids from *Hydrocotyle* and *Centella* species. *Phytochemistry* 1982; **21:** 2590–2.

8. Bohlmann F, Zdero C. Polyacetylenic compounds. 230. A new polyyne from Centella species. *Chem Ber* 1975; **108:** 511–14.

9. Schulte KE *et al*. Constituents of medical plants. XXVII. Polyacetylenes from *Hydrocotyle asiatica*. *Arch Pharm (Weinheim)* 1973; **306:** 197–209.

10. Gotu Kola. *Lawrence Review of Natural Products*, 1988.

11. Morisset T *et al*. Evaluation of the healing activity of hydrocotyle tincture in the treatment of wounds. *Phytotherapy Res* 1987; **1:** 117–21.

12. Jacker H-J *et al*. Zum antiexsudativen Verhalten einiger Triterpensaponine. *Pharmazie* 1982; **37:** 380–2.

13. Ravokatra A, Ratsimamanga AR. Action of a pentacyclic triterpenoid, asiaticoside, obtained from *Hydrocotyle madagascariensis* or *Centella asiatica* against gastric ulcers of the Wistar rat exposed to cold (2°). *C R Acad Sci (Paris)* 1974; **278:** 1743–6.

14.   Ravokatra A *et al.* Action of asiaticoside extracted from hydrocyte on duodenal ulcers induced with mercaptoethylamine in male wistar rats. *C R Acad Sci (Paris)* 1974; **278:** 2317–21.

15.   Ramaswamy AS *et al.* Pharmacological studies on *Centella asiatica* Linn. (*Brahma manduki*) (N.O. Umbelliferae). *J Res Indian Med* 1970; **4:** 160–75.

16.   Oliver-Bever B. Medicinal plants in tropical West Africa. Cambridge: Cambridge University Press, 1986.

17.   Bossé J-P *et al.* Clinical study of a new antikeloid agent. *Ann Plast Surg* 1979; **3:** 13–21.

18.   Lin Y-C *et al.* Search for biologically active substances in Taiwan medicinal plants. 1. Screening for anti-tumor and anti-microbial substances. *Chinese J Microbiol* 1972; **5:** 76–81.

19.   Natarajan S, Paily PP. Effect of topical *Hydrocotyle asiatica* in psoriasis. *Indian J Dermatol* 1973; **18:** 82–5.

ISPAGHULA

Species (Family)
Plantago ovata Forsk. (Plantaginaceae)

Synonyms
Blond Psyllium, Indian Plantago, Ispagol, Pale Psyllium, Spogel

Part(s) Used
Seed

Pharmacopoeial Monographs
BHP 1983
BHP 1990
BPC 1973 (Ispaghula husk)
Martindale 30th edition
Pharmacopoeias—U.S. under the title Plantago Seed

Legal Category (Licensed Products)
GSL[G14]

Constituents[G1,G2,G19,G29,G32]
Alkaloids (monoterpene-type). (+)-boschniakine (indicaine), (+)-boschniakinic acid (plantagonine), indicainine
Mucilages (10–30%). Mixture of polysaccharides with *d*-xylose as the major component, others include *l*-arabinose and aldobiouronic acid. Present mainly in the seed husk
Other constituents Aucubin (iridoid glucoside), sugars (fructose, glucose, sucrose), planteose (trisaccharide), sterols (campesterol, β-sitosterol, stigmasterol), triterpenes (α- and β-amyrin), fatty acids (e.g. linoleic, oleic, palmitic, stearic), tannins

Food Use
In food manufacture, ispaghula may be used as a thickener or stabiliser.[G19]

Herbal Use
Ispaghula is stated to possess demulcent and laxative properties. Traditionally, ispaghula has been used in the treatment of chronic constipation, dysentery, diarrhoea, and cystitis. Topically, a poultice has been used for furunculosis.[G1,G2,G3,G4,G32]

Dose
Seeds 5–10 g (3 g in children) three times daily.[G2,G3] Seeds should be soaked in warm water for several hours before taking.
Liquid extract (1:1 in 25% alcohol) 2–4 mL three times daily[G2,G3]
Husk 3–5 g.[G23] Seeds and husk should be soaked in warm water for several hours before administration.

Pharmacological Actions
The principal pharmacological actions of ispaghula can be attributed to the mucilage component.
Animal studies An alcoholic extract lowered the blood pressure of anaesthetised cats and dogs, inhibited isolated rabbit and frog hearts, and stimulated rabbit, rat and guinea pig ileum.[G19] The extract exhibited cholinergic activity.[G19] A mild laxative action has also been reported in mice administered iridoid glycosides, including aucubin.[1]

Ispaghula husk depressed the growth of chickens by 15% when added to their diet at 2%.[G19]

Ispaghula seed powder is stated to have strongly counteracted the deleterious effects of adding sodium cyclamate (2%), FD & C Red No. 2 (2%), and polyoxyethylene sorbitan monostearate (4%) to the diet of rats.[G19]

Human studies Ispaghula is used as a bulk laxative. The swelling properties of the mucilage enable it to absorb water in the gastro-intestinal tract, thereby increasing the volume of the faeces and promoting peristalsis. Bulk laxatives are often used for the treatment of chronic constipation and when excessive straining must be avoided following anorectal surgery or in the management of haemorrhoids. Ispaghula is also used in the management of diarrhoea and for adjusting faecal consistency in patients with colostomies and in patients with diverticular disease or irritable bowel syndrome. The effect of ispaghula is usually apparent after 24 hours.[23]

In China, the seeds of related *Plantago* species have been used to treat hypertension with about 50% success in clinical trials.[G19]

Side-effects, Toxicity
In common with all bulk laxatives, ispaghula may temporarily increase flatulence and abdominal distension, and may cause intestinal obstruction. If swallowed dry, ispaghula may cause oesophageal obstruction.

Contra-indications, Warnings
In common with all bulk laxatives, ispaghula should not be given to patients with intestinal obstruction or conditions that may lead to intestinal obstruction, such as spastic bowel conditions. Ispaghula should always be taken with plenty of fluid to avoid oesophageal obstruction or faecal impaction. Bulk laxatives lower the transit time through the gastro-intestinal tract and therefore may affect the absorption of other drugs.[G22]

Pregnancy and lactation Ispaghula may be used during pregnancy and lactation.

Pharmaceutical Comment
The characteristic component of ispaghula is the mucilage which provides ispaghula with its bulk laxative action. Many of the herbal uses are therefore supported although no published information was located to justify the use of ispaghula in cystitis or infective skin conditions. Adverse effects and precautions generally associated with bulk laxatives apply to ispaghula.

References
See General References G1, G2, G3, G4, G7, G14, G19, G22, G23, G29 and G32

1. Inouye H *et al*. Purgative activities of iridoid glycosides. *Planta Med* 1974; **25**: 285–8.

JAMAICA DOGWOOD

Species (Family)

Piscidia erythrina L. (Leguminosae)

Synonym(s)

Ichthymethia piscipula (L.) A.S. Hitchc. ex. Sarg., *Piscidia communis* Harms, *Piscidia piscipula* (L.) Sarg., Fish Poison Bark, West Indian Dogwood

Part(s) Used

Root Bark

Pharmacopoeial Monographs

BHP 1983
BHP 1990
BPC 1934

Legal Category (Licensed Products)

GSL[G14]

Constituents[G2,G10,G18,G19,G32]

Acids Piscidic acid (*p*-hydroxybenzyltartaric) and its mono and diethyl esters,[1] fukiic acid and the 3'-*O*-methyl derivative; malic acid, succinic acid, and tartaric acid

Isoflavonoids Ichthynone, jamaicin, piscerythrone, piscidone and others. Milletone, isomillettone, dehydromillettone, rotenone and sumatrol (rotenoids), and lisetin (coumaronochrome)[2–5]

Glycosides Piscidin, reported to be a mixture of two compounds, saponin glycoside (unidentified)[6]

Other constituents Alkaloid (unidentified, reported to be from the stem), resin, voltile oil 0.01%, β-sitosterol, tannin (unspecified)[6]

Food Use

Jamaica dogwood is stated by the Council of Europe to to be toxicologically unacceptable for use as a natural food flavouring.[G9]

Herbal Use

Jamaica dogwood is stated to possess sedative and anodyne properties. Traditionally, it has been used for neuralgia, migraine, insomnia, dysmenorrhoea, and specifically for insomnia due to neuralgia or nervous tension.[G2,G3,G4,G32]

Dose

Dried root bark 1–2 g or by decoction three times daily[G2,G3]

Liquid extract (1:1 in 30% alcohol) 1–2 mL three times daily[G2,G3]

Liquid Extract of Piscidia (BPC 1934) 2–8 mL

Pharmacological Actions

Animal studies Results of early studies reported Jamaica dogwood to possess weak cannabinoid and sedative activities in the mouse, guinea-pig, and cat.[6–8] In addition, *in-vitro* antispasmodic activity on rabbit intestine, and guinea-pig and rat uterine muscle[6,9,10] were noted and in *in-vivo* uteroactivity in the cat and monkey were documented.[6,7,10,11] In some instances, *in-vitro* antispasmodic activity was found to be comparable to, or greater than, that observed for papaverine.

More recent work has supported these findings and reported that the antispasmodic activity of Jamaica dogwood on uterine smooth muscle is attributable to two isoflavone constituents, one being equipotent to papaverine.[11]

Jamaica dogwood extracts have also been documented to exhibit antitussive, antipyretic, and anti-inflammatory activities in various experimental animals.[7]

Rotenone is an insecticide that has been used in agriculture for the control of lice, fleas, and as a larvicide.[G22] Jamaica dogwood has been used extensively throughout Central and South America as a fish poison;[6] the wood contains two piscicidal principles, rotenone and ichthynone. Rotenone is relatively harmless to warm-blooded animals.[12]

Rotenone has reported exhibited anticancer activity towards lymphocytic leukaemia and human epidermoid carcinoma of the nasopharynx.[G10] Rotenone is also documented to be carcinogenic.[G10]

Side-effects, Toxicity

Symptoms of overdose are stated to include numbness, tremors, salivation, and sweating.[G10] Jamaica dogwood has been found to be toxic when administered parenterally to rats and rabbits but non-toxic when given orally, with doses exceeding 90 g dried extract/kg tolerated.[6] An LD_{50} (mice, intravenous injection) of an unidentified saponin constituent has been reported as 75 μg/kg body-weight.[9] Oral doses of up to 1.5 mg/kg were stated to have no effect.[6]

Jamaica dogwood is stated to be irritant and toxic to humans.[G26]

Contra-indications, Warnings

It is recommended that Jamaica dogwood should be used with great care, and only by trained practitioners.[G25] Jamaica dogwood may potentiate sedative effects of existing therapy.

Pregnancy and lactation Jamaica dogwood has been reported to exhibit a potent depressant action on the uterus both in *in vitro* and *in vivo*. In view of this and the general warnings regarding the use of Jamaica dogwood, it should not be used during pregnancy and lactation.

Pharmaceutical Comment

Jamaica dogwood is characterised by various isoflavone constituents, to which the antispasmodic properties described for the wood have been attributed. In addition, sedative and narcotic activities have been documented that justify the reputed herbal uses. Although jamaica dogwood is reported to be of low toxicity in various animal species, it is also documented as toxic to humans [G26] and is recommended to be used with great care.[G25] In view of this, excessive use of Jamaica dogwood should be avoided.

References

See General References G2, G3, G4, G9, G10, G14, G18, G19, G22, G25, G26 and G32.

1. Bridge W *et al*. Constituents of "Cortex Piscidiae Erythrinae". Part I. The structure of piscidic acid. *J Chem Soc* 1948; 257.

2. Falshaw CP *et al*. The Extractives of Piscidia Erythrina L. III. The constitutions of lisetin, piscidone and piscerythrone. *Tetrahedron* 1966; Suppl 7: 333-48.

3. Redaelli C, Santaniello E. Major isoflavonoids of the Jamaican dogwood *Piscidia erythrina*. *Phytochemistry* 1984; **23**: 2976–7.

4. Delle Monache F *et al*. Two isoflavones from *Piscidia erythrina*. *Phytochemistry* 1984; **23**: 2945–7.

5. Harborne JB, Mabry TJ, eds. The Flavonoids. New York: Chapman & Hall, 1982; 606.

6. Costello CH, Butler CL. An investigation of *Piscidia erythrina* (Jamaica Dogwood). *J Am Pharm Assoc* 1948; **37**: 89–96.

7. Aurousseau M *et al*. Certain pharmacodynamic properties of *Piscidia erythrina*. *Ann Pharm Fr* 1965; **23**: 251–7.

8. Della-Loggia R *et al*. Evaluation of the activity on the mouse CNS of several plant extracts and a combination of them. *Riv-Neurol* 1981; **51**: 297–310.

9. Pilcher JD *et al*. The action of the so-called female remedies on the excised uterus of the guinea-pig. *Arch Int Med* 1916; **18**: 557–83.

10. Pilcher JD, Mauer RT. The action of female remedies on the intact uteri of animals. *Surg Gynecol Obstet* 1918; 97–9.

11. Della Loggia R *et al*. Isoflavones as spasmolytic principles of *Piscidia erythrina*. *Prog Clin Biol Res* 1988; **280**: 365–8.

12. Claus E *et al* editors. Pesticides. In: Pharmacognosy. Philadelphia: Lea & Febiger, 1970; 486–7.

JUNIPER

Species (Family)
Juniperus communis L. (Pinaceae)

Synonym(s)
Baccae Juniperi, Genièvre, Wacholderbeeren, Zimbro

Part(s) Used
Fruit (berry)

Pharmacopoeial Monographs
BHP 1983
BPC 1934
Martindale 30th edition
National pharmacopoeias—Aust., Belg., Cz., Ger., Hung., Port., Rom., Rus., Swiss, and Yug.

Legal Category (Licensed Products)
GSL[G14]

Constituents[G1,G10,G19,G27,G31,G32,G35]
Acids Diterpene acids, ascorbic acid, glucuronic acid
Flavonoids Amentoflavone,[1] quercetin, isoquercitrin, apigenin and various glycosides
Tannins Proanthocyanidins (condensed), gallocatechin, epigallocatechin[2]
Volatile oils (0.2–3.42%). Primarily monoterpenes (about 58%) including α-pinene, myrcene and sabinene (major), and camphene, camphor, 1,4-cineole, *p*-cymene, α- and γ-cadinene, limonene, β-pinene, γ-terpinene, terpinen-4-ol, terpinyl acetate, α-thujene, borneol; sesquiterpenes including caryophyllene, epoxydihydrocaryophyllene, and β-elemem-7α-ol[3,4]
Other constituents Geijerone (C_{12} terpenoid), junionone (monocyclic cyclobutane monoterpenoid,[5] desoxypodophyllotoxin (lignan),[6] resins, sugars

Food Use
Juniper berries are widely used as a flavouring component in gin. Juniper is listed by the Council of Europe as a natural source of food flavouring (fruit N2, leaf and wood N3). Category N2 indicates that the berries can be added to foodstuffs in small quantities, with a possible limitation of an active principle (as yet unspecified) in the final product. Category N3 indicates that there is insufficient information available for an adequate assessment of potential toxicity to be made.[G9]

Herbal Use
Juniper is stated to possess diuretic, antiseptic, carminative, stomachic, and antirheumatic properties. Traditionally, it has been used for cystitis, flatulence, colic, and applied topically for rheumatic pains in joints or muscles.[G1,G3,G32]

Dose
Dried ripe fruits 100 mL as an infusion (1:20 in boiling water) three times daily[G3]
Fruit 1–2 g or equivalent three times daily
Liquid extract (1:1 in 25% alcohol) 2–4 mL three times daily[G3]
Tincture (1:5 in 45% alcohol) 1–2 mL three times daily[G3]
Oil (1:5 in 45% alcohol) 0.03–0.2 mL three times daily

Pharmacological Actions
Pharmacological actions that have been documented for juniper are primarily associated with the volatile oil components.
Animal studies The volatile oil is documented to possess diuretic, gastro-intestinal antiseptic, and irritant properties.[G19]
The diuretic activity of juniper has been attributed to the volatile oil component, terpinen-4-ol, which is reported to increase the glomerular filtration rate.[G30] Terpenin-4-ol is also stated to be irritant to the kidneys although in a later review by the same author there is no such statement and the oil is stated to represent no hazards.[G35]
An antifertility effect has been described for a juniper extract, administered to rats (300/500 mg, by mouth) on days 1 to 7 of pregnancy.[8]. An abortifacient effect was also noted at both dose levels when the extract was administered on days 14 to 16.[8] No evidence of teratogenicity was reported. Anti-implantation activity has been reported as 60 to 70% [9] and as dose dependent[8]. Juniper is reported to have both a significant[10] and no[9] antifertility effect. A uterine stimulant activity has been documented for the volatile oil.[G12]
A potent and non-toxic inhibition of the cytopathogenic effects of *Herpes simplex* virus type 1 in primary human amnion cell culture has been described for a juniper extract.[6,11] The active component isolated from the active fraction was identified as a lignan, desoxypodophyllotoxin.[6] Antiviral activities documented for the volatile oil have also been partly attributed to the flavonoid amentoflavone.[1]
Anti-inflammatory activity of 60% compared to 45% for the indomethacin control has been reported for juniper berry extract.[12] Both test and control were administered orally to rats (100 mg/kg and 5 mg/kg respectively) one hour before eliciting foot oedema.
A transient hypertensive effect followed by a more prolonged hypotensive effect has been reported for a juniper extract in rats (25 mg/kg, intravenous injection).[13]
A fungicidal effect against *Penicillium notatum* has been documented.[14]
An astringent activity is generally associated with tannins, which have been documented as components of juniper. The aqueous decoction of the berries has a hypoglycaemic effect in rats.[15].

Side-effects, Toxicity

The volatile oil is reported to be generally non-sensitising and non-phototoxic, although slightly irritant when applied externally to human and animal skin.[G19,G35] Excessive doses of terpinen-4-ol, the diuretic principle in the volatile oil, may cause kidney irritation.[G10]

Dermatitic reactions have been recognised with juniper and positive patch test reactions have been documented.[16,G26] The latter are attributed to the irritant nature of the juniper extract.[16]

Symptoms of poisoning following external application of the essential oil are described as burning, erythema, inflammation with blisters, and oedema.[G10] Internally, symptoms from overdose are documented as pain in or near the kidneys, strong diuresis, albuminuria, haematuria, purplish urine, tachycardia, hypertension, and rarely convulsions, metrorrhagia, and abortion.[G10]

The acute toxicity of juniper has been investigated in rats who were administered extracts for seven days.[12] An oral dose of 2.5 g/kg was tolerated with no mortalities or side-effects noted. A dose of 3 g/kg induced hypothermia and mild diarrhoea in 10 to 30% of animals.[12] An LD_{50} value (mice, intraperitoneal injection) has been stated as 3 g/kg.[4]

Contra-indications, Warnings

Juniper is contra-indicated in individuals with existing renal disease.[G3,G20,G25] The internal use of the oil should be restricted to professionals.[G20] External application of the oil may cause an irritant reaction. However, this has been refuted and the oil is stated to have no hazards and is not contra-indicated.[G35] Juniper has been confused with savin (*Juniperus sabina*) in the literature and this may be the reason for believing that the oil is toxic.[G35] Juniper may potentiate existing hypoglycaemic and diuretic therapies; prolonged use may result in hypokalaemia.

Pregnancy and lactation Juniper is contra-indicated in pregnancy.[G3,G10,G25] Juniper is reputed to be an abortifacient and to affect the menstrual cycle.[G12]

A juniper fruit extract has exhibited abortifacient, antifertility, and anti-implantation activities (*see* Animal studies).

Pharmaceutical Comment

Many of the traditional uses documented for juniper can be supported by documented pharmacological actions or known constituents. There is evidence that the berries are abortifacient and since this is believed not to be due to the oil there must be other toxic constituents present. It is recommended that use should not exceed levels specified in food legislation.

References

See General References G1, G3, G5, G9, G10, G12, G14, G19, G20, G22, G23, G25, G26, G27, G30, G31, G32 and G35.

1. Chandler RF. An inconspicuous but insidious drug. *Rev Pharm Can* 1986; 563–6.

2. Friedrich H, Engelshowe R. Tannin producing monomeric substances in *Juniperus communis*. *Planta Med* 1978; **33**: 251–7.

3. Wagner H, Wolff P, editors. New natural products and plant drugs with pharmacological, biological or therapeutical activity. Berlin: Springer-Verlag, 1977.

4. Fenaroli's handbook of flavor ingredients, 2nd edn. Boca Raton: CRC Press, 1975.

5. Thomas AF, Ozainne M. "Junionone" [1-(2,2-Dimethylcyclobutyl)but-1-en-3-one], the first vegetable monocyclic cyclobutane monoterpenoid. *J C S Chem Comm* 1973; 746.

6. Markkanen, T *et al*. Antiherpetic agent from juniper tree (*Juniperus communis*), its purification, identification, and testing in primary human amnion cell cultures. *Drugs Exp Clin Res* 1981; **7**: 691–7.

8. Agrawal OP *et al*. Antifertility effects of fruits of *Juniperus communis*. *Planta Med* 1980; **40** (Suppl): 98–101.

9. Prakash AO *et al*. Anti-implantation activity of some indigenous plants in rats. *Acta Eur Fertil* 1985; **16**: 441–8.

10. Prakash AO. Biological evaluation of some medicinal plant extracts for contraceptive efficacy. *Contracept Deliv Syst* 1984; **5**: 9.

11. Marrkanen T. Antiherpetic agent(s) from juniper tree (*Juniperus communis*). preliminary communication. *Drugs Exp Clin Res* 1981; **7**: 69–73.

12. Mascolo N *et al*. Biological screening of Italian medicinal plants for anti-inflammatory activity. *Phytotherapy Res* 1987; **1**: 28–31.

13. Lasheras B *et al*. Étude pharmacologique préliminaire de *Prunus spinosa* L. *Amelanchier ovalis* Medikus, *Juniperus communis* L. et *Urtica dioica* L. *Plant Méd Phytothér* 1986; **20**: 219–26.

14. Hejtmánková N *et al*. The antifungal effects of some Cupressaceae. *Acta Univ Palacki Olomuc Fac Med* 1973; **60**: 15–20.

15. Sanchez de Medina, F *et al*. Hypoglycaemic activity of Juniper berries. *Planta Med* 1994; **60**: 197–200.

16. Mathias CGT *et al*. Plant dermatitis — patch test results (1975–78). Note on *Juniperus* extract. *Contact Dermatitis* 1979; **5**: 336–7.

LADY'S SLIPPER

Species (Family)

Cypripedium pubescens Willd. and other related species (Orchidaceae)

Synonym(s)

American Valerian, Cypripedium, Nerve Root, *Cypripedium calceolus* var. *pubescens* R Br.

Related species also referred to as Lady's Slipper include *Calypso bulbosa* (L.) Oakes (*Cypripedium bulbosum* L.) and *Cypripedium parviflorum* Salish

Part(s) Used

Rhizome, Root

Pharmacopoeial Monographs

BHP 1983
BPC 1923

Legal Category (Licensed Products)

GSL (Cypripedium)[G14]

Constituents[G10,G24,G32]

Little chemical information has been documented. Lady's slipper is stated to contain glycosides, resin, tannic and gallic acids (usually associated with hydrolysable tannins), tannins, and a volatile oil.

Several quinones have been reported including cypripedin, stated to belong to a group of rare non-terpenoid phenanthraquinones and not previously isolated from natural sources.[1]

Food Use

Lady's slipper is not used in foods.

Herbal Use

Lady's slipper is stated to possess sedative, mild hypnotic, antispasmodic, and thymoleptic properties. Traditionally, it has been used for insomnia, hysteria, emotional tension, anxiety states, and specifically for anxiety states with insomnia.[G3,G32]

Dose

Dried rhizome/root 2–4 g or by infusion three times daily[G3]

Liquid extract (1:1 in 45% alcohol) 2–4 mL three times daily[G3]

Pharmacological Actions

None documented.

Side-effects, Toxicity

It has been stated that the roots may cause psychedelic reactions and large doses may result in giddiness, restlessness, headache, mental excitement, and visual hallucinations.[G10] Lady's slipper is stated to be allergenic and contact dermatitis has been documented.[G26] The sensitising property of Lady's slipper has been attributed to the quinone constituents.[1]

Contra-indications, Warnings

Lady's slipper may cause an allergic reaction in sensitive individuals.

Pregnancy and lactation The safety of lady's slipper has not been established. In view of the lack of phytochemical, pharmacological, and toxicological information the use of lady's slipper during pregnancy and lactation should be avoided.

Pharmaceutical Comment

Virtually no phytochemical or pharmacological data are available for lady's slipper to justify its use as a herbal remedy. In view of the lack of toxicity data, excessive use should be avoided.

References

See General References G3, G10, G14, G24, G26, and G32.

1. Schmalle H, Hausen BM. A new sensitizing quinone from lady slipper (*Cypripedium calceolus*). *Naturwissenschaften* 1979; **66**: 527–8.

LEMON VERBENA

Species (Family)

Aloysia triphylla (L'Her.) Britton (Verbenaceae)

Synonym(s)

Aloysia citriodora (Cav.) Ort., *Lippia citriodora* (Ort.) HBK, *Verbena citriodora* Cav., *Verbena triphylla* L'Her.

Part(s) Used

Flowering Top, Leaf

Pharmacopoeial Monographs

None

Legal Category (Licensed Products)

Lemon verbena is not included on the GSL[G14]

Constituents[G10,G15,G28,G32]

Flavonoids Flavones including apigenin, chrysoeriol, cirsimaritin, diosmetin, eupafolin, eupatorin, hispidulin, luteolin and derivatives, pectolinarigenin, and salvigenin.[1]

Volatile oils Terpene components include borneol, cineol, citral, citronellal, cymol, eugenol, geraniol, limonene, linalool, β-pinene, nerol, and terpineol (monoterpenes), and α-caryophyllene, β-caryophyllene, myrcenene, pyrollic acid, and isovalerianic acid (sesquiterpenes).[2]

Food Use

In the USA, lemon verbena is listed as GRAS (Generally Regarded As Safe) for human consumption in alcoholic beverages. Lemon verbena is also used in herbal teas.[G28]

Herbal Use

Lemon verbena is reputed to possess antispasmodic, antipyretic, sedative, and stomachic properties. Traditionally, it has been used for the treatment of asthma, cold, fever, flatulence, colic, diarrhoea, and indigestion.[G16,G28,G32]

Dose

Decoction 45 mL taken several times daily.[G15]

Pharmacological Actions

None documented.

Side-effects, Toxicity

None documented for lemon verbena. Terpene-rich volatile oils are generally regarded as irritant and may cause kidney irritation during excretion.

Contra-indications, Warnings

Individuals with existing renal disease should avoid excessive doses of lemon verbena in view of the possible irritant nature of the volatile oil.

Pregnancy and lactation In view of the lack of pharmacological and toxicity data, and the potential irritant nature of the volatile oil, excessive doses of lemon verbena are best avoided during pregnancy and lactation.

Pharmaceutical Comment

Limited information is available on lemon verbena. The traditional uses documented for lemon verbena are probably attributable to the volatile oil, for which many components have been identified, and to the flavone constituents. In the UK, lemon verbena is mainly used as an ingredient of herbal teas.

References

See General References G10, G15, G16, G28, and G32.

1. Skaltsa H, Shammas G. Flavonoids from *Lippia citriodora*. *Planta Med* 1988; **54**: 465.

2. Montes M *et al*. Sur la composition de l'essence d'*Aloysia triphylla* (Cedron). *Planta Med* 1973; **23**: 119–24.

LIFEROOT

Species (Family)
Senecio aureus L. (Asteraceae/Compositae)

Synonym(s)
Golden Senecio, Golden Ragwort, Squaw Weed

Part(s) Used
Herb

Pharmacopoeial Monographs
BHP 1983
Martindale 30th edition (Senecio)

Legal Category (Licensed Products)
Liferoot is not included on the GSL[G14]

Constituents [G32,G33]
Limited information is documented regarding the constituents of liferoot, although it is well recognised that *Senecio* species contain pyrrolizidine alkaloids.
Pyrrolizidine alkaloids Floridanine, florosenine, otosenine, senecionine.[1,2]
The volatile oil composition of various *Senecio* species (but not *S. aureus*) has been investigated.[3]

Food Use
Liferoot is not used as a food, although many *Senecio* species are used as a form of spinach in South Africa.

Herbal Use
Liferoot is stated to possess uterine tonic, diuretic, and mild expectorant properties. Traditionally, it has been used in the treatment of functional amenorrhoea, menopausal neurosis, and leucorrhoea (as a douche).[G3,G32]

Dose
Herb 14 g or by infusion three times daily[G3]
Liquid extract 14 mL (1:1 in 25% alcohol) three times daily[G3]

Pharmacological Actions
No documented studies were located.

Side-effects, Toxicity
Liferoot contains pyrrolizidine alkaloids. The toxicity, primarily hepatic, of this class of compounds is well recognised in both animals and humans[G33] (*see* Comfrey).

Contra-indications, Warnings
In view of the hepatotoxic pyrrolizidine alkaloid constituents, liferoot should not be ingested.[G33]
Pregnancy and lactation In view of the toxic constituents, liferoot is contraindicated during pregnancy and lactation.[G25] Furthermore, liferoot is traditionally reputed to be an abortifacient, emmenagogue, and uterine tonic.[G3,G10] In animals, placental transfer and secretion into breast milk[4] has been documented for unsaturated pyrrolizidine alkaloids.

Pharmaceutical Comment
Little information is documented for liferoot. No pharmacological studies were found to substantiate the traditional uses. The *Senecio* genus is characterised by unsaturated pyrrolizidine alkaloid constituents and the hepatotoxicity of this class of compounds is well recognised (*see* Comfrey). In view of this, liferoot is not suitable for use as a herbal remedy.

References
See General References G3, G10, G22, G23, G25, and G32.

1. Pyrrolizidine alkaloids. Environmental Health Criteria 80. Geneva: WHO, 1988.

2. Roder E *et al*. Pyrrolizidinalkaloide aus *Senecio aureus*. *Planta Med* 1983; **49**: 57–59.

3. Dooren B *et al*. Composition of essential oils of some *Senecio* species. *Planta Med* 1981; **42**: 385–9.

4. Mattocks AR. Chemistry and toxicology of pyrrolizidine alkaloids. London: Academic Press, 1986, 1–393.

LIME FLOWER

Species (Family)
(i) *Tilia cordata* Mill. (Tiliaceae)
(ii) *Tilia platyphyllos* Scop.
(iii) *Tilia × europaea* — hybrid of (i) and (ii)

Synonym(s)
Lime Tree, Linden Tree

Part(s) Used
Flowerheads

Pharmacopoeial Monographs
BHP 1983
BHP 1990
BPC 1949
Martindale 30th edition (Tilia)
Pharmacopoeias—Aust., Cz., Egypt., Fr., Ger., Hung., Rom., Rus., Swiss, and Yug.

Legal Category (Licensed Products)
GSL[(G14)]

Constituents[(G1,G2,G10,G25,G31,G32)].
Acids Caffeic acid, chlorogenic acid, *p*-coumaric acid
Amino acids Alanine, cysteine, cystine, isoleucine, leucine, phenylalanine, serine
Carbohydrates Mucilage polysaccharides (3%). Five fractions identified yielding arabinose, galactose, rhamnose, with lesser amounts of glucose, mannose, and xylose; galacturonic and glucuronic acids;[(1)] gum
Flavonoids Kaempferol, quercetin, myricetin, and their glycosides
Volatile oil Many components including alkanes, phenolic alcohols and esters, and terpenes including citral, citronellal, citronellol, eugenol, limonene, nerol, α-pinene, and terpineol (monoterpenes), and farnesol (sesquiterpene).
Other constituents Saponin (unspecified), tannin (condensed), tocopherol (phytosterol)

Food Use
Lime flower is listed by the Council of Europe as a natural source of food flavouring (category N2). This category indicates that lime flower can be added to foodstuffs in small quantities, with a possible limitation of an active principle (as yet unspecified) in the final product.[(G9)]

Herbal Use
Lime flower is stated to possess sedative, antispasmodic, diaphoretic, diuretic, and mild astringent properties. Traditionally it has been used for migraine, hysteria, arteriosclerotic hypertension, feverish colds, and specifically for raised arterial pressure associated with arteriosclerosis and nervous tension.[(G1,G2,G3,G4,G32)]

Dose
Flowerhead 2–4 g by infusion
Liquid extract (1:1 in 25% alcohol) 2–4 mL
Tincture (1:5 in 45% alcohol) 1–2 mL

Pharmacological Actions
Animal studies In vitro, lime flower has been reported to exhibit antispasmodic activity followed by a spasmogenic effect on rat duodenum.[(2)] The actions were inhibited by atropine and papaverine, and reinforced by acetylcholine. The diaphoretic and antispasmodic properties claimed for lime flower have been attributed to *p*-coumaric acid and the flavonoids.[(G17,G30)] In addition, a number of actions have been associated with volatile oils including diuretic, sedative, and antispasmodic effects, which may also account for some of the reputed uses of lime flower.[(3,4,5)] Volatile oils are not thought to possess any true diuretic activity, but to act as a result of certain terpenoid components having an irritant action on the kidneys during renal excretion.
Lime flower has been documented to possess a restricted range of antifungal activity.[(6)]

Side-effects, Toxicity
Excessive use of lime flower tea may result in cardiac toxicity.[(G30)] However, the rationale for this statement is not included by the author.

Contra-indications, Warnings
It is advised that lime flower should be avoided by individuals with an existing cardiac disorder.[(G10,G17,G30)]
Pregnancy and lactation The safety of lime flower has not been established. In view of the lack of toxicological data, excessive use of lime flower during pregnancy and lactation should be avoided.

Pharmaceutical Comment
The chemistry of lime flower is well documented. Little scientific information was located to justify the reputed herbal uses of lime flower, although some correlation can be made with the known pharmacological activities of the reported constituents. The lack of toxicological data, together with a warning concerning cardiac toxicity, indicates that excessive use of lime flower should be avoided.

References
See General References G1, G2, G3, G4, G6, G9, G10, G14, G17, G22, G23, G25, G30, G31 and G32.

1. Kram G, Franz G. Structural investigations on the water soluble polysaccharides of lime tree flowers (*Tilia cordata* L.) *Pharmazie* 1985; **40**: 501.

2. Lanza JP, Steinmetz M. Actions comparees des exraits aqueux de graines de *Tilia platyphylla* et de *Tilia vulgaris* sur l'intestin isolé de rat. *Fitoterapia* 1986; **57**: 185.

3. Taddei I *et al*. Spasmolytic activity of peppermint, sage and rosemary essences and their major constituents. *Fitoterapia* 1988; **59:** 463–8.

4.   Svendsen AB, Scheffer JJC. *Essential oils and aromatic plants*. Proceedings of the 15th international symposium on essential oils. Dordrecht: Martinus Nijhoff, 1984; 225–6.

5.   Sticher O. Plant mono-, di- and sesquiterpenoids with pharmacological and therapeutical activity. In: New natural products with pharmacological, biological or therapeutical activity. H Wagner and P Wolff eds. Berlin: Springer-Verlag, Berlin 1977, 137–176.

6.   Guerin J-C, Reveillere H-P. Antifungal activity of plant extracts used in therapy. I Study of 41 plant extracts against 9 fungi species. *Ann Pharm Fr* 1984; **B:** 553–9

LIQUORICE

Species (Family)
Glycyrrhiza glabra L. (Leguminosae)

Synonym(s)
Licorice

Part(s) Used
Root, Stolon

Pharmacopoeial Monographs
BHP 1983
BPC 1973
Martindale 30th edition
Pharmacopoeias—Aust., Br., Braz., Chin., Cz., Egypt., Eur., Fr., Ger., Gr., Hung., Ind., It., Jpn, Neth., Nord., Rom., Rus., Swiss, and Yug. Many allow peeled or unpeeled liquorice. Br. also describes Powdered Liquorice.

Legal Category (Licensed Products)
GSL[G14]

Constituents[G1,G2,G19,G24,G32]
Coumarins Glycyrin, heniarin, liqcoumarin, umbelliferone, GU-7 (3-arylcoumarin derivative)[1]
Flavonoids Flavonols and isoflavones including formononetin, glabrin, glabrol, glabrone, glyzarin, glycyrol, glabridin and derivatives, kumatakenin, licoflavonol, licoisoflavones A and B, licoisoflavanone, licoricone, liquiritin and derivatives, phaseollinisoflavan;[2] chalcones including isoliquiritigenin, licuraside, echinatin, licochalcones A and B, neolicuroside[3]
Terpenoids Glycyrrhizin glycoside (1–24%) also known as glycyrrhizic or glycyrrhizinic acid yielding glycyrrhetinic (or glycyrrhetic) acid and glucuronic acid following hydrolysis;[4] glycyrrhetol, glabrolide, licoric acid, liquiritic acid, β-amyrin
Volatile oils (0.047%).[5] More than 80 components identified including anethole, benzaldehyde, butyrolactone, cumic alcohol, eugenol, fenchone, furfuryl alcohol, hexanol, indole, linalool, γ-nonalactone, oestragole, propionic acid, α-terpineol, and thujone[5]
Other constituents Amino acids, amines, gums, lignin, starch, sterols (β-sitosterol, stigmasterol), sugars, wax
Other plant parts Components documented for the leaves of *G. glabra* L. include flavonoids (kaempferol and derivatives, isoquercetin, quercetin and derivatives, phytoalexins), coumarins (bergapten, xanthotoxin), phytoestrogen, β-sitosterol, saponaretin[6]

Food Use
Liquorice is widely used in foods as a flavouring agent. Liquorice root is listed by the Council of Europe as a natural source of food flavouring (category N2). This category indicates that liquorice can be added to foodstuffs in small quantities, with a possible limitation of an active principle (as yet unspecified) in the final product.[G9] In the USA, liquorice is listed as GRAS (Generally Regarded As Safe).[G19]

Herbal Use
Liquorice is stated to possess expectorant, demulcent, antispasmodic, anti-inflammatory, and laxative properties. Traditionally, it is aloso reported to affect the adrenal glands. It has been used for bronchial catarrh, bronchitis, chronic gastritis, peptic ulcer, colic, and primary adrenocortical insufficiency.[G1,G2,G3,G4,G5,G32]

Dose
Powdered root 1–4 g or by decoction three times daily[G2,G3]
Liquorice Extract (BPC 1973) 0.6–2.0 g

Pharmacological Actions
The pharmacological actions of liquorice have been reviewed.[7,8]
Animal studies Much has been documented regarding the steroid-type actions of liquorice (*see* Side-effects, Toxicity). Both glycyrrhizin and glycyrrhetinic acid (GA) have been reported to bind to glucocorticoid and mineralocorticoid receptors with moderate affinity, and to oestrogen receptors, sex-hormone-binding globulin and corticosteroid-binding globulin with very weak affinity.[9–11] It has been suggested that glycyrrhizin and glycyrrhetinic acid may influence endogenous steroid activity via a receptor mechanism, with displacement of corticosteroids or other endogenous steroids.[9].
The anti-oestrogenic action documented for glycyrrhizin at relatively high concentrations has been associated with a blocking effect that would be caused by glycyrrhizin binding at oestrogen receptors.[9] However, oestrogenic activity has also been documented for liquorice and attributed to the isoflavone constituents.[8] Liquorice exhibits an alternative action on oestrogen metabolism, causing inhibition if oestrogen concentrations are high and potentiation when concentrations are low.[8]
The relatively low affinity of glycyrrhizin and glycyrrhetinic acid for binding to mineralocorticoid receptors together with the fact that liquorice does not exert its mineralocortoid activity in adrenalectomised animals, indicates that a direct action at mineralocortoid receptors is not the predominant mode of action.[12] It has been suggested that glycyrrhizin and glycyrrhetinic acid may exert their mineraolcortoid effect via an inhibition of 11β-hydroxysteroid dehydrogenase (11β-OHSD).[12] 11β-OHSD is a microsomal enzyme complex found predominantly in the liver and kidneys which catalyses the conversion of cortisol (potent mineralcortoid activity) to the inactive cortisone. Deficiency of 11β-OHSD results in increased concentrations of urinary

free cortisol and cortisol metabolites. Glycyrrhetinic acid has been shown to inhibit renal 11β-OHSD in rats.[12] It has also been proposed that glycyrrhizin and glycyrrhetinic acid may displace cortisol from binding to transcortin.[13]

Antiplatelet activity *in vitro* has been documented for a 3-arylcoumarin derivative, GU-7, isolated from liquorice.[1] GU-7 was thought to inhibit platelet aggregation by increasing intraplatelet cyclic AMP concentration.

Isoliquiritigenin has been reported to inhibit aldose reductase, the first enzyme in the polyol pathway which reduces glucose to sorbitol.[14] Isoliquiritigenin was subsequently found to inhibit sorbitol accumulation in human red blood cells *in vitro*, and in red blood cells, the sciatic nerve and the lens of diabetic rats administered isoliquirigenin intragastrically.[14,15] Many diabetic complications, such as cataracts, peripheral neuropathy, retinopathy, and nephropathy have been associated with the polyol pathway and have shown improvement with inhibitors of aldose reductase.[14, 15]

Significant anti-inflammatory action is exhibited by glycyrrhetinic acid against UV erythema.[16] 18α-Glycyrrhetinic acid has exhibited stronger anti-inflammatory action compared to its stereoisomer 18β-glycyrrhetinic acid.[17] Chalcones isolated from *G. inflata* Bat. have been reported to inhibit leukotriene production and increase cyclic AMP concentrations in human polymorphonuclear neutrophils *in vitro*.[18] Glycyrrhetinic acid derivatives, but not glycyrrhetinic acid, have exhibited inhibitory effects on writhing and vascular permeability tests and on type IV allergy in mice.[19] The dihemiphthalate derivatives were especially active with respect to the two former activities and have previously been found to inhibit lipoxygenase and cyclooxygenase activities, and to prevent formation of gastric ulcer.[19]

Glycyrrhetinic acid is known to inhibit Epstein-Barr virus activation by tumour promotors.[20]

Antimicrobial activity versus *Staphylococcus aureus*, *Mycobacterium smegmatis*, and *Candida albicans* has been documented for liquorice and attributed to isoflavonoid constituents (glabridin, glabrol and their derivatives).[2] Antiviral activty has been described for glycyrrhetinic acid, which interacts with virus structures producing different effects according to the viral stage affected.[21] Activity was observed against vaccinia, herpes simplex 1, Newcastle disease and vesicular stomatitis viruses, with no activity demonstrated towards poliovirus 1.[21]

In-vitro hepatoprotective activity against CCl_4-induced toxicity has been reported to be greater for glycyrrhetinic acid compared to glycyrrhizin.[22] Glycyrrhetinic acid is thought to act by inhibition of the cytochrome P-450 system required for the metabolism of CCl_4 to the highly reactive radical CCl_3.[22] *Glycyrrhiza uralensis* Fisch is used to treat hepatitis B in China, with a success rate reported to be greater than 70%.[23] Other activities documented for *G. uralensis* are anti-inflammatory and anti-allergic, treatment of jaundice, inhibition of fibrosis of the liver, corticosteroid-like immunosuppressing effect and a detoxifying effect.[23]

Screening of several plant extracts for antifertility activity reported liquorice to be ineffective following oral administration to rats in days 1–7 of pregnancy.[24]

Human studies Carbenoxolone, an ester derivative of glycyrrhetinic acid, has been used in the treatment of gastric and oesophageal ulcers. It is thought to exhibit a mucosal-protecting effect by beneficially interfering with gastric prostanoid synthesis, and increasing mucous production and mucosal blood flow.[25]

Liquorice is thought to exert its mineralocorticoid effect by inhibition of the enzyme 11β-OHSD, which catalyses the conversion of cortisol to the inactive cortisone (see Animal Studies). Administration of liquorice to healthy volunteers has resulted in a disturbance of cortisol metabolism and a significant rise in urinary free cortisol, despite there being no change in plasma concentrations. These changes are consistent with this hypothesis, being indicative of 11β-OHSD deficiency.[12] Liquorice has also been found to suppress both plasma renin activity and aldosterone secretion.[26–28]

The pharmacokinetic profile of glycyrrhizin in rats has been found to be similar to that observed in humans.[29] Glycyrrhizin is primarily (80%) excreted into the bile from the liver against a concentration gradient.[29] This process is saturable and can therefore affect the excretion rate of glycyrrhizin. In addition, enterohepatic recycling occurs with reabsorption of bile-excreted glycyrrhizin from the intestinal tract.[29] Subjects consuming 100–200 g liquorice/day have been reported to achieve plasma-glycyrrhetinic acid concentrations of 80–480 ng/mL.[12]

Side-effects, Toxicity

Apart from confectionery, liquorice can also be ingested from infusions and by chewing tobaccos. Excessive or prolonged liquorice ingestion has resulted in symptoms typical of primary hyperaldosteronism, namely hypertension, sodium, chloride and water retention, hypokalaemia and weight gain, but also in low levels of plasma renin activity, aldosterone and antidiuretic hormone.[13,26,30]

Raised concentrations of atrial natriuretic peptide (ANP), which is secreted in response to atrial stretch and has vasodilating, natriuretic and diuretic properties, has also been observed in healthy subjects following the ingestion of liquorice.[13] Individuals consuming between 10–45g liquorice/day have exhibited raised blood pressure, together with a block of the aldosterone/renin axis and electrocardiogram changes, which resolved one month after withdrawal of the liquorice.[31] Individuals consuming vastly differing amounts of liquorice have exhibited similar side-effect symptoms, indicating that the mineralocorticoid effect of liquorice is not dose dependent and is a saturable process.[31]

Hypokalaemic myopathy has also been associated with liquorice ingestion.[32–36] Severe hypokalaemia with rhabdomyolysis has been documented in a male patient following the ingestion of an alcohol-free beverage containing only small amounts of glycyrrhetinic acid (0.35g/day).[32] The patient had known liver cirrhosis due to alcohol consumption and it was suggested that cirrhotic patients may be more susceptible to the mineralocorticoid side-effects of liquorice.[32] In one case[34], the myoglobinaemia led to glomerulopathy and tubulopathy but with no clinical evidence of acute renal failure (ARF). The latter was attributed to the volume expansion also caused by the liquorice ingestion.

Rhabdomyolysis without myoglobinuria has been described.[37] In addition, severe congestive heart failure and pulmonary oedema have been reported in a previously healthy man who had ingested 700g liquorice over 8 days.[30] Liquorice extract given orally has been reported to have a similar but longer lasting action to intravenous deoxycortone and it has been noted that sodium, chloride and water retention do not have to be accompanied by clinical oedema.[38] Amenorrhoea has been associated with liquorice ingestion (anti-oestrogenic action), with the menstrual cycle re-appearing following the withdrawal of liquorice.[31]

It has been noted that symptoms of hyperaldosteronism often resolve quickly, within a few days to two weeks, following the withdrawal of liquorice, even in individuals who have ingested the substance for many years.[28]

A case has been described where a patient presented with symptoms related to hyperglycaemia and myopathy secondary to liquorice-induced hypokalaemia. An inverse relationship was observed between the concentrations of fasting serum glucose and serum potassium.[39] Interestingly, animal studies have indicated that liquorice may reduce diabetic complications associated with intracellular accumulation of sorbitol.[19]

Contra-indications, Warnings

Numerous instances have been documented where liquorice ingestion has resulted in symptoms of primary hyperaldosteronism, such as water and sodium retention and hypokalaemia. Liquorice should therefore be avoided completely by individuals with an existing cardiovascular-related disorder, and ingested in moderation by other individuals. Hypokalaemia is known to aggravate glucose intolerance and liquorice ingestion may therefore interfere with existing hypoglycaemic therapy. Liquorice may interfere with existing hormonal therapy (oestrogens and antioestrogenic activities documented *in vivo*).

Pregnancy and lactation In view of the oestrogenic and steroid effects associated with liquorice, which may exacerbate pregnancy-related hypertension, excessive ingestion during pregnancy and lactation should be avoided. In addition, liquorice has exhibited a uterine stimulant activity in animal studies, and is traditionally reputed to be an abortifacient and to affect the menstrual cycle (emmenagogue).[G12]

Pharmaceutical Comment

The phytochemistry is well documented for liquorice and it is particularly characterised by triterpenoid components. Many of the traditional uses of liquorice are supported by documented pharmacological data although limited evidence of antispasmodic activity was found. Carbenoxolone, an ester derivative of a triterpenoid constituent in liquorice, is well known for its use in ulcer therapy. Much has been written concerning the steroid-type adverse effects associated with liquorice ingestion. Liquorice ingestion should

therefore be avoided by individuals with an existing cardiovascular disorder and moderate consumption should be observed by other individuals.

References

See General References G1, G2, G3, G4, G7, G9, G11, G12, G14, G19, G22, G23, G24 and G32.

1. Tawata M *et al*. Anti-platelet action of GU-7, a 3-arylcoumarin derivative, purified from *Glycyrrhizae radix*. *Planta Med* 1990; **56:** 259–63.

2. Mitscher LA *et al*. Antimicrobial agents from higher plants. Antimicrobial isoflavanoids and related substances from *Glycyrrhiza glabra* L. var. *typica*. *J Nat Prod* 1980; **43:** 259–69.

3. Miething H, Speicher-Brinker A. Neolicuroside — A new chalcone glycoside from the roots of *Glycyrrhiza glabra*. *Arch Pharm (Weinheim)* 1989; **322:** 141–3.

4. Takino Y *et al*. Quantitative determination of glycyrrhizic acid in liquorice roots and extracts by TLC-densitometry. *Planta Med* 1979; **36:** 74–8.

5. Kameoka H, Nakai K. Components of essential oil from the root of *Glycyrrhiza glabra*. *Nippon Nogeikagaku Kaishi [J Ag Chem Soc Japan]* 1987; **61:** 1119–21.

6. Jimenez J *et al*. Flavonoids of *Helianthemum cinereum*. *Fitoterapia* 1989; **60:** 189.

7. Chandler RF. Licorice, more than just a flavour. *Can Pharm J* 1985; **118:** 421–4.

8. Pizzorno JE, Murray AT. Glycyrrhiza glabra. A textbook of natural medicine. Seattle, WA: John Bastyr College Publications, 1985 (looseleaf).

9. Tamaya MD *et al*. Possible mechanism of steroid action of the plant herb extracts glycyrrhizin, glycyrrhetinic acid, and paeoniflorin: Inhibition by plant herb extracts of steroid protein binding in the rabbit. *Am J Obstet Gynecol* 1986; **155:** 1134–9.

10. Armanini D *et al*. Binding of agonists and antagonists to mineralocorticoid receptors in human peripheral mononuclear leucocytes. *J Hypertens* 1985; **3**(Suppl 3): S157–9.

11. Armanini D *et al*. Affinity of liquorice derivatives for mineralocorticoid and glucocorticoid receptors. *Clin Endocrinol* 1983; **19:** 609–12.

12. Stewart PM *et al*. Mineralocorticoid activity of liquorice: 11-Beta-hydroxysteroid dehydrogenase deficiency comes of age. *Lancet* 1987; **ii:** 821–4.

13. Forslund T *et al*. Effects of licorice on plasma atrial natriuretic peptide in healthy volunteers. *J Intern Med* 1989; **225:** 95–9.

14. Aida K *et al*. Isoliquiritigenin: A new aldose reductase inhibitor from *Glycyrrhizae radix*. *Planta Med* 1990; **56:** 254–8.

15. Yun-ping Z, Jia-qing Z. Oral baicalin and liquid extract of licorice reduce sorbitol levels in red blood cell of diabetic rats. *Chin Med J* 1989; **102:** 203–6.

16. Fujita H *et al*. Antiinflammatory effect of glycyrrhizinic acid. Effects of glycyrrhizinic acid against carrageenin-induced edema, UV-erythema and skin reaction sensitised with DCNB. *Pharmacometrics* 1980; **19:** 481–4.

17.   Amagaya S *et al*. Separation and quantitative analysis of 18α-glycyrrhetinic acid and 18β-glycyrrhetinic acid in *Glycyrrhizae radix* by gas-liquid chromatography. *J Chromatogr* 1985; **320:** 430–4.

18.   Kimura Y *et al*. Effects of chalcones isolated from licorice roots on leukotriene biosynthesis in human polymorphonuclear neutrophils. *Phytotherapy Res* 1988; **2:** 140–5.

19.   Inque H *et al*. Pharmacological activities of glycerrhetinic acid derivatives: Analgesic and anti-type IV allergic effects. *Chem Pharm Bull* 1987; **35:** 3888–93.

20.   Tokuda H *et al*. Inhibitory effects of ursolic and oleandolic acid on skin tumor promotion by 12-*O*-tetradecanoylphorbol-13-acetate. *Cancer Lett* 1986; **33:** 279–85.

21.   Pompei R *et al*. Antiviral activity of glycyrrhizic acid. *Experientia* 1980; **36:** 304.

22.   Kiso Y *et al*. Mechanism of antihepatotoxic activity of glycyrrhizin, I: Effect on free radical generation and lipid peroxidation. *Planta Med* 1984; **:50**: 298–302.

23.   Chang HM *et al*. Advances in Chinese Medicinal Materials Research. Singapore: World Scientific, 1985.

24.   Sharma BB *et al*. Antifertility screening of plants. Part I. Effect of ten indigenous plants on early pregnancy in albino rats. *Int J Crude Drug Res* 1983; **21:** 183–7.

25.   Guslandi M. Ulcer-healing drugs and endogenous prostaglandins. *Int J Clin Pharmacol Ther Toxicol* 1985; **23:** 398–402.

26. Conn J *et al*. Licorice-induced pseudoaldosteronism. Hypertension, hypokalaemia, aldosteronopenia and suppressed plasma renin activity. *JAMA* 1968; **205:** 492–6.

27.   Epstein MT *et al*. Effect of eating liquorice on the renin-angiotensin aldosterone axis in normal subjects. *Br Med J* 1977; **1:** 488–90.

28.   Mantero F. Exogenous mineralocorticoid-like disorders. *Clin Endocrinol Metab* 1981; **10:** 465–78.

29. Ichikawa T *et al*. Biliary excretion and enterohepatic cycling of glycyrrhizin in rats. *J Pharm Sci* 1986; **75:** 672–5.

30.   Chamberlain TJ. Licorice poisoning, pseudoaldosteronism, heart failure. *JAMA* 1970; **213:** 1343.

31.   Corrocher R *et al*. Pseudoprimary hyperaldosteronism due to liquorice intoxication. *Eur Rev Med Pharmacol Sci* 1983; **5:** 467–70.

32.   Piette, A M *et al*. Hypokaliémie majeure avec rhabdomyolase secondaire à l'ingestion de pastis non alcoolisé. *Ann Med Interne (Paris)* 1984; **135:** 296–8.

33.   Cibelli G *et al*. Hypokalemic myopathy associated with liquorice ingestion. *Ital J Neurol Sci* 1984; **5:** 463–6.

34.   Heidermann HT, Kreuzfelder E. Hypokalemic rhabdomyolysis with myoglobinuria due to licorice ingestion and diuretic treatment. *Klin Wochenschr* 1983; **61:** 303–5.

35.   Ruggeri CS *et al*. L. Carnetina cloruro e KCl nel trattamento di un caso di rabdomiolisi atraumatica senza mioglobinuria da ingestione di liquerizia. *Minn Med* 1985; **76:** 725–8.

36.   Bannister B *et al*. Cardiac arrest due to liquorice induced hypokalaemia. *Br Med J* 1977; **2:** 738–9.

37.   Maresca MC *et al*. Low blood potassium and rhabdomyolosis. Description of three cases with different aetiologies. *Minerva Med* 1988; **79:** 79–81.

38.   Molhuysen JA. A liquorice extract with deoxycortone–like action. *Lancet* 1950; **ii:** 381–6.

39.   Jamil A *et al*. Hyperglycaemia related to licorice-induced hypokalaemia. *J Kwt Med Assoc* 1986; **20:** 69–71.

LOBELIA

Species (Family)
Lobelia inflata L. (Campanulaceae)

Synonym(s)
Indian Tobacco

Part(s) Used
Herb

Pharmacopoeial Monographs
BHP 1983
BHP 1990
BPC 1973
BP 1988
Martindale 30th edition
Pharmacopoeias—Aust., Braz., Egypt., and Fr. Chin. specifies *Lobelia chinensis*.

Legal Category (Licensed Products)
GSL[G14]

Constituents[G2,G10,G19,G32]
Alkaloids (piperidine-type) (0.48%). Lobeline (major); others include lobelanine, lobelanidine, norlobelanine, lelobanidine, norlelobanidine, norlobelanidine, lobinine
Other constituents Bitter glycoside (lobelacrin), chelidonic acid, fats, gum, resin, volatile oil

Food Use
Lobelia is not generally used as a food.

Herbal Use
Lobelia is stated to possess respiratory stimulant, antasthmatic, antispasmodic, expectorant, and emetic properties. Traditionally, it has been used for bronchitic asthma, chronic bronchitis, and specifically for spasmodic asthma with secondary bronchitis. It has also been used topically for myositis and rheumatic nodules.[G2,G3,G4,G32]

Dose
Dried herb 0.2–0.6 g or by infusion or decoction three times daily[G2,G3]
Liquid extract (1:1 in 50% alcohol) 0.2–0.6 mL three times daily[G2,G3]

Simple Tincture of Lobelia (BPC 1949) 0.6–2.0 mL

Tincture Lobelia Acid (1:10 in dilute acetic acid) 1–4 mL three times daily[G2,G3]

Pharmacological Actions
The pharmacological activity of lobelia can be attributed to the alkaloid constituents, principally lobeline. Lobeline has peripheral and central effects similar to those of nicotine, but is less potent. Hence, lobeline initially causes CNS stimulation followed by respiratory depression. Lobeline is also reported to possess expectorant properties.

Side-effects, Toxicity
Side-effects of lobeline and lobelia are similar to those of nicotine and include nausea and vomiting, diarrhoea, coughing, tremors, and dizziness. Symptoms of overdosage are reported to include profuse diaphoresis, tachycardia, convulsions, hypothermia, hypotension, and coma, and may be fatal.[G22]

Contra-indications, Warnings
The pharmacological actions of lobeline are similar to those of nicotine.
Pregnancy and lactation Lobelia should not be used during pregnancy or lactation.

Pharmaceutical Comment
The principal constituent of lobelia is lobeline, an alkaloid with similar pharmacological properties to nicotine. Lobelia has previously been used in herbal preparations for the treatment of asthma and bronchitis, and in anti-smoking preparations aimed to lessen nicotine withdrawal symptoms. However, in view of its potent alkaloid constituents, excessive use of lobelia is not recommended.

References
See General References G2, G3, G4, G7, G10, G14, G19, G22, G23, G24 and G32.

MARSHMALLOW

Species (Family)
Althaea officinalis L. (Malvaceae)

Synonym(s)
Althaea

Part(s) Used
Leaf, Root

Pharmacopoeial Monographs
BHP 1983 (Leaf, Root)
BHP 1990 (Root)
BPC 1934
Martindale 30th edition
Pharmacopoeias—Aust., Cz., Fr., Ger., Hung., Rom., Rus., Swiss, and Yug. describe the root.
Althaea Leaf is included in Aust., Cz., Fr., Hung., Rom., and Yug.
Althaea Flower is in Fr.

Legal Category (Licensed Products)
GSL[G14]

Constituents[G1,G2,G19,G24,G30,G32]
Mucilages (about 25–35%). Galacturonic acid, glucuronic acid and rhamnose as major components;[1] others include arabinose, galactose, glucose, mannose, and xylose
Other constituents Asparagine 2%, calcium oxalate, pectin, starch, tannin, phenolic acids (caffeic, ferulic, syringic)

Food Use
Marshmallow is listed by the Council of Europe as a natural source of food flavouring (category N2). This category indicates that marshmallow can be added to foodstuffs in small quantities, with a possible limitation of an active principle (as yet unspecified) in the final product.[G9] In the USA, marshmallow is approved for use in foods.[G19]

Herbal Use
Marshmallow is stated to possess demulcent, expectorant, emollient, diuretic, antilithic, and vulnerary properties. Traditionally, it has been used internally for the treatment of respiratory catarrh and cough, peptic ulceration, inflammation of the mouth and pharynx, enteritis, cystitis, urethritis and urinary calculus, and topically for abscesses, boils, and varicose and thrombotic ulcers.[G1,G2,G3,G4,G32]

Dose
Dried leaf 2–5 g or by infusion three times daily[G2,G3]
Leaf, Liquid extract 2–5 mL (1:1 in 25% alcohol) three times daily[G2,G3]
Ointment 5% Powdered Althaea Leaf in usual ointment base three times daily[G2,G3]

Dried root 2–5 g or by cold extraction three times daily[G2,G3]
Root, Liquid extract 2–5 mL (1:1 in 25% alcohol) three times daily[G2,G3]
Syrup of Althaea (BPC 1949) 2–10 mL three times daily[G2,G3]

Pharmacological Actions
Animal studies Antimicrobial activity towards *Pseudomonas aeruginosa*, *Proteus vulgaris*, and *Staphylococcus aureus* has been documented for marshmallow.[2] The mucilage has demonstrated considerable hypoglycaemic activity in non-diabetic mice.[3] A lack of anti-inflammatory activity has been observed for marshmallow in the carrageenan rat paw oedema test.[4]

Side-effects, Toxicity
None documented.

Contra-indications, Warnings
Marshmallow may interfere with existing hypoglycaemic therapy.
Pregnancy and lactation There are no known problems with the use of marshmallow during pregnancy or lactation.

Pharmaceutical Comment
The major constituent of marshmallow is mucilage, which therefore supports the reputed demulcent action. However, little documented information is available to justify the additional herbal uses. Although no toxicity data were located, the chemistry of marshmallow and its use in foods indicate that there should not be any reason for concern regarding safety.

References
See General References G1, G2, G3, G4, G5, G9, G14, G22, G23, G24, G30 and G32.

1. Blaschek W, Franz G. A convenient method for the quantitative determination of mucilage polysaccharides in *Althaeae radix*. *Planta Med* 1986; **52** (Suppl): 537.

2. Recio MC *et al.* Antimicrobial activity of selected plants employed in the Spanish Mediterranean area Part II. *Phytotherapy Res* 1989; **3**: 77–80.

3. Tomodo M *et al.* Hypoglycaemic activity of twenty plant mucilages and three modified products. *Planta Med* 1987; **53**: 8–12.

4. Mascolo N *et al.* Biological screening of Italian medicinal plants for anti-inflammatory activity. *Phytotherapy Res* 1987; **1**: 28–31.

MATÉ

Species (Family)
Ilex paraguariensis St. Hil. (Aquifoliaceae)

Synonym(s)
Ilex, Jesuit's Brazil Tea, Paraguay Tea, St. Bartholomew's Tea, Yerba Maté

Part(s) Used
Leaf

Pharmacopoeial Monographs
BHP 1983
BPC 1934
Martindale 30th edition

Legal Category (Licensed Products)
GSL[G14]

Constituents[G1,G10,G22,G24,G32]
Alkaloids(xanthine-type) Caffeine 0.2–2.0%, theobromine 0.1–0.2%, theophylline 0.05%
Flavonoids Kaempferol, quercetin, and their glycosides including rutin[1]
Tannins 4–16%
Terpenoids Ursolic acid (major), β-amyrin, ilexoside A, ilexoside B methyl ester[2]
Other constituents Choline and trigonellin (amines), amino acids,[1] riboflavine (vitamin B_2), pyridoxine (vitamin B_6), niacin, pantothenic acid, vitamin C, resins
Other Ilex species Triterpenoid saponins termed ilexsaponins B_1, B_2, and B_3 have been isolated from *Ilex pubescens* Hook. et Arn.[3]
A cyanogenetic glucoside has been isolated from *Ilex aquifolium*.[4]

Food Use
Maté is listed by the Council of Europe as a natural source of food flavouring (category N2). This category indicates that maté can be added to foodstuffs in small quantities, with a possible limitation of an active principle (as yet unspecified) in the final product.[G9] Maté is commonly consumed as a beverage. It is stated to be less astringent than tea.[G22]

Herbal Use
Maté is stated to possess CNS stimulant, thymoleptic, diuretic, antirheumatic, and mild analgesic properties. Traditionally, it has been used for psychogenic headache and fatigue, nervous depression, rheumatic pains, and specifically for headache associated with fatigue.[G1,G3,G4,G32]

Dose
Dried leaf 2–4 g or by infusion three times daily[G2,G3]

Liquid extract (1:1 in 25% alcohol) 2–4 mL three times daily[G2,G3]

Pharmacological Actions
Animal studies In-vivo hypotensive activity in rats has been reported for an aqueous extract of *Ilex pubescens* (commonly referred to as maodongqing or MDQ) It was concluded that intravenous administration of MDQ releases histamine.[5]
Human studies The xanthine constituents, in particular caffeine, are the active principles in maté. The pharmacological actions of caffeine are well documented and include stimulation of the CNS, respiration, and skeletal muscle, in addition to cardiac stimulation, coronary dilation, smooth muscle relaxation, and diuresis.[G19] Reduction of appetite has been documented for maté.[1]
In China, MDQ is used parenterally for the treatment of cardiovascular diseases (hypotensive action).[1]

Side-effects, Toxicity
Side-effects generally associated with xanthine-containing beverages include sleeplessness, anxiety, tremor, palpitations, and withdrawal headache.
Veno-occlusive disease of the liver in a young woman has been attributed to the consumption of large quantities of maté over a number of years.[G22] The association between consumption of maté infusions and oesophageal cancer has been investigated in Uruguay, where oesophageal cancer constitutes a major public health problem.[6,7] Heavy consumption was reported to elevate the relative risk of oesophageal cancer by 6.5 and 34.6 in men and women, respectively.
The fatal dose of caffeine in man is stated to be 10 g.[G19]

Contra-indications, Warnings
Warnings generally associated with caffeine are applicable, such as restricted intake by individuals with hypertension or a cardiac disorder.
Pregnancy and lactation It is generally recommended that caffeine consumption should be restricted during pregnancy, although conflicting results have been documented concerning the association between birth defects and caffeine consumption. In view of this, excessive consumption of maté during pregnancy should be avoided. Caffeine is excreted in breast milk, but at concentrations too low to represent a hazard to breast-fed infants.[G22] As with all xanthine-containing beverages, excessive consumption of maté by breast-feeding mothers should be avoided.

Pharmaceutical Comment
Maté is characterised by the xanthine constituents, which also represent the active principles. The herbal uses of maté can be attributed to the pharmacological actions of caffeine, which are well documented. Side-effects and warnings

associated with other xanthine-containing beverages, such as tea and coffee, are applicable to maté.

References

See General References G1, G3, G4, G5, G9, G10, G14, G19, G22, G23, G24 and G32.

1.   Ohem N, Holzl J. Some new investigations on *Ilex para-guariensis* — Flavonoids and triterpenes. *Planta Med* 1988; **54:** 576.

2.   Inada A. Two new triterpenoid glycosides from the leaves of *Ilex chinensis. Chem Pharm Bull* 1987; **37:** 884–5.

3.   Hidaka K *et al.* New triterpene saponins from *Ilex pubescens. Chem Pharm Bull* 1987; **35:** 524–9.

4.   Willems M. Quantitification and distribution of a novel cyanogenic glycoside in *Ilex aquifolium. Planta Med* 1989; **55**: 114.

5.   Yang ML, Pang PKT. The vascular effects of *Ilex pubescens. Planta Med* 1986; **52:** 262–5.

6.   Morton JF. The potential carcinogenicity of herbal tea. *Envir Carcino Rev. J Envir Sci Hlth* 1986; **C4:** 203–223.

7.   Vassallo A *et al.* Esophageal cancer in Uruguay : a case control study. *J National Cancer Institute* 1985; **75:** 1005-9.

MEADOWSWEET

Species (Family)
Filipendula ulmaria (L.) Maxim. (Rosaceae)

Synonym(s)
Dropwort, Filipendula, Queen of the Meadow, *Spiraea ulmaria* L.

Part(s) Used
Herb

Pharmacopoeial Monographs
BHP 1983
BHP 1990

Legal Category (Licensed Products)
GSL[G14]

Constituents[G1,G2,G10,G20,G31,G32]

Flavonoids Flavonols, flavones, flavanones, and chalcone derivatives (e.g. hyperoside[1] and spireoside[2], kaempferol glucoside,[3] avicularin[4]

Salicylates Main components of the volatile oil including salicylaldehyde (major, up to 70%), gaultherin, isosalicin, methyl salicylate, monotropitin, salicin, salicylic acid, spirein[5–8]

Tannins 1% (alcoholic extract), 12.5% (aqueous extract).[5] Hydrolysable type;[9] leaf extracts have also yielded catechols,[1] compounds normally associated with condensed tannins.

Volatile oils Many phenolic components including salicylates (*see above*), benzyl alcohol, benzaldehyde, ethyl benzoate, heliotropin, phenylacetate, vanillin.[4,5]

Other constituents Coumarin (trace),[1] mucilage, carbohydrates, ascorbic acid (vitamin C)

Food Use
Meadowsweet is listed by the Council of Europe as a natural source of food flavouring (category N2). This category indicates that meadowsweet can be added to foodstuffs in small quantities, with a possible limitation of an active principle (as yet unspecified) in the final product.[G9] In the USA, meadowsweet is listed by the FDA as a Herb of Undefined Safety.[G10]

Herbal Use
Meadowsweet is stated to possess stomachic, mild urinary antiseptic, antirheumatic, astringent, and antacid properties. Traditionally, it has been used for atonic dyspepsia with heartburn and hyperacidity, acute catarrhal cystitis, rheumatic muscle and joint pains, diarrhoea in children, and specifically for the prophylaxis and treatment of peptic ulcer.[G1,G2,G3,G4,G32]

Dose
Dried herb 4–6 g or by infusion three times daily[G2,G3]
Liquid extract (1:1 in 25% alcohol) 1.5–6.0 mL three times daily[G2,G3]
Tincture (1:5 in 45% alcohol) 2–4 mL three times daily[G2,G3]

Pharmacological Actions
Animal studies Lowering of motor activity and rectal temperature, myorelaxation, and potentiation of narcotic action have been documented for meadowsweet.[5] In addition, flower extracts have been reported to prolong life expectancy of mice, lower vascular permeability, and prevent the development of stomach ulcers in rats and mice.[5,10,11] However, meadowsweet has also been reported to potentiate the ulcerogenic properties of histamine in the guinea-pig.[10] The anti-ulcer action documented for meadowsweet is associated with the aqueous extract and greatest activity has been observed with the flowers.[9,11] Meadowsweet has been reported to increase bronchial tone in the cat[9] and to potentiate the bronchospastic properties of histamine in the guinea-pig.[9] *In-vitro*, meadowsweet has been reported to increase intestinal tone in the guinea-pig and uterine tone in the rabbit.[9]

Bacteriostatic activity against *Staphylococcus aureus*, *Staphylococcus epidermidis*, *Escherichia coli*, *Proteus vulgaris*, and *Pseudomonas aeruginosa* has been documented for flower extracts.[12]

Tannins are generally considered to possess astringent properties and have been reported as constituents of meadowsweet. Meadowsweet is stated to promote uric acid excretion.[G20]

Side-effects, Toxicity
None documented.

Contra-indications, Warnings
Salicylate constituents have been documented and therefore the usual precautions recommended for salicylates are relevant for meadowsweet (*see* Willow). Meadowsweet is stated to be used for the treatment of diarrhoea in children but in view of the salicylate constituents, this is not advisable.

Bronchospastic activity has been documented and meadowsweet should therefore be used with caution by asthmatics.

Aqueous extracts have been reported to contain high tannin concentrations and excessive consumption should therefore be avoided.

Pregnancy and lactation In-vitro uteroactivity has been documented for meadowsweet. In view of the salicylate constituents and the lack of toxicity data, the use of meadowsweet during pregnancy and lactation should be avoided.

Pharmaceutical Comment

The chemistry of meadowsweet is characterised by a number of phenolic constituents including flavonoids, salicylates, and tannins. Documented scientific evidence justifies some of the antiseptic, antirheumatic, and astringent actions, although no human data were available. No documented toxicity data were located for meadowsweet and in view of this, excessive use should be avoided.

References

See General References G1, G2, G3, G4, G9, G10, G14, G20, G31 and G32.

1.   Genic AY and Ladnaya LY. Phytochemical study of Filipendula ulmaria Maxim. and Filipendula hexapetala Gilib. of flora of the Lvov region. *Farm Zh (Kiev)* 1980; **1:** 50–2.

2.   Novikova NN. Use of Filipendula ulmaria in medicine. *Tr Perm Farm Inst* 1969; 267–70.

3.   Scheer T and Wichtl M. Zum Vorkommen von Kämpferol-4'-*O*-β-D-glucopyranoside in *Filipendula ulmaria* und *Allium cepa*. *Planta Med* 1987 **53:** 573–4.

4.   Syuzeva ZF and Novikova NN. Flavonoid composition of Filipendula ulmaria queen-of-the-meadow. *Nauch Tr Perm Farm Inst* 1973; **5:** 2–26.

5.   Barnaulov OD *et al.* Chemical composition and primary evaluation of the properties of preparations from Filipendula ulmaria (L.) Maxim flowers. *Rastit Resur* 1977; **13:** 661–9.

6.   Saifullina NA and Kozhina IS. Composition of essential oils from flowers of Filipendula ulmaria, F. denudata, and F. stepposa. *Rastit Resur* 1975; **11:** 542–4.

7.   Thieme H. Isolierung eines neuen phenolischen glykosids aus den blüten von *Filipendula ulmaria* (L.) Maxim. *Pharmazie* 1966; **21:** 123.

8.   Valle MG *et al.* Das ätherische öl aus *Filipendula ulmaria*. *Planta Med* 1988; **54:** 181–2.

9.   Barnaulov OD *et al.* Preliminary evaluation of the spasmolytic properties of some natural compounds and galenic preparations. *Rastit Resur* 1978; **14:** 573–9.

10.   Barnaulov OD, Denisenko PP. Antiulcerogenic action of the decoction from flowers of *Filipendula ulmaria* (L.). *Pharmakol-Toxicol* (Moscow) 1980; **43:** 700–5.

11.   Yanutsh AY *et al.* A study of the antiulcerative action of the extracts from the supernatant part and roots of *Filipendula ulmaria*. *Farm Zh* (Kiev) 1982; **37:** 53–6.

12.   Catanicin-Hintz I *et al.*   Action of some plant extracts on the bacteria involved in urinary infections. *Clujul-Med* 1983; **56:** 381–4.

MISTLETOE

Species (Family)
Viscum album L. (Loranthaceae)

Synonym(s)
Viscum

Part(s) Used
Leaf, Fruit (Berry), Twig

Pharmacopoeial Monographs
BHP 1983
BPC 1934
Martindale 30th edition

Legal Category (Licensed Products)
Mistletoe is not included on the GSL[G14]

Constituents[G1,G10,G32]

Acids Fatty acids (C_{12}-C_{22}), 80% oleic and palmitic;[1] phenolic acids (e.g. anisic, caffeic, *p*-coumaric, ferulic, gentisic, myristic, *p*-hydroxybenzoic, *p*-hydroxyphenylacetic, protocatechuic, shikimic, sinapic, quinic, vanillic);[1,2]
Alkaloids[3] It has been suggested that alkaloids can be passed on from hosts to parasitic plants like mistletoe (e.g. nicotine alkaloids have been isolated from mistletoe growing on Solanaceae shrubs).[4]
Amines Acetylcholine, choline, β-phenylethylamine, histamine, propionylcholine, tyramine.[5]
Flavonoids Flavonol (e.g. quercetin) derivatives,[3] chalcone derivatives,[6] flavonone derivatives[6]
Lectins Mixture of high-molecular-weight polypeptides. Quoted molecular weights include 160 000,[7] 115 000 (4 chains),[7,8] 60 000 (2 chains).[9] Three lectins have been isolated which possess either 2 chains (LII, LIII) or 4 chains (LI).[10]
Terpenoids β-Amyrin, betulinic acid, lupeol and ester combinations, oleanolic acid, resin acids, ursolic acid, β-sitosterol, dihydro-β-sitosterol, stigmasterol, sterol A, phytosterol glucoside[6,11]
Viscotoxins Mixture of low-molecular-weight polypeptides including the pure proteins viscotoxins A_2, A_3, and B[12–14]
Other constituents Mucilage, polyols (e.g. mannitol, dulcitol, xylitol, inositol, pinitol, quebrachitol, quercitol),[15] sugars (e.g. fructose, glucose, raffinose, sucrose),[13] starch, syringin (a phenolic glucoside),[6] tannin

Food Use
Mistletoe is not generally used as a food. The branches and berries of mistletoe are listed by the Council of Europe as natural sources of food flavouring (category N3).[G9] This category indicates that mistletoe may be added to foodstuffs in the traditionally accepted manner, although there is insufficient information available for an adequate assessment of potential toxicity.

Herbal Use
Mistletoe is stated to possess hypotensive, cardiac depressant, and sedative properties. Traditionally, it has been used for high blood pressure, arteriosclerosis, nervous tachycardia, hypertensive headache, chorea, and hysteria.[G1,G3,G32]

Dose
Dried Leaves 2–6 g or by infusion three times daily[G3]
Liquid Extract (1:1 in 25% alcohol) 1–3 mL three times daily[G3]
Tincture (1:5 in 45% alcohol) 0.5 mL three times daily[G3]
Infusion (1:20 in cold water) (40–120 mL) daily[G3]
Soft extract (1:8 infusion or tincture) 0.3–0.6 mL three times daily [G3]

Pharmacological Actions
Documented pharmacological studies for mistletoe have concentrated on the cytotoxic and immunostimulant properties of the plant. The pharmacological actions of mistletoe have been reviewed extensively.[4,5,12,15–17]
Animal studies Much has been documented concerning the possible role of mistletoe in the treatment of cancer, in particular, a proprietary product Iscador™, which is produced from naturally fermented mistletoe plant juice. The immunostimulant and cytotoxic effects exhibited by mistletoe are thought to play an important role in the cancerostatic action.[18]
Cytotoxic activity has been exhibited both *in vitro* and *in vivo* by the crude plant juice, Iscador™, glycoprotein fractions (lectins, viscotoxins), and alkaloid fractions.[3,18,19] Significant antitumour activity has been observed *in vivo* for mistletoe extracts against murine tumours, Lewis lung carcinoma, colon adenocarcinoma 38, and C3H mammary adenocarcinoma 16/C.[4] Researchers in Korea have isolated cytotoxic alkaloids from twigs and leaves of Korean mistletoe (*V. album, coloratum*) with activity reported against L1210 (*in vitro*) and P388 (*in vivo*) test systems.[3] The authors commented that preliminary studies indicated the presence of some of these cytotoxic alkaloids in the European mistletoe (*V. album*). The anticancer activities of various mistletoe extracts and the contribution of the alkaloidal components towards this activity has been reviewed.[4] Alkaloidal components in mistletoe are thought to form glycoconjugates with lectins and viscotoxins, and help maintain the specific structures of these molecules necessary for therapeutic activity.[4]

The mode of action for cytotoxic activity of mistletoe has been linked to the ability of the basic amino acids present in mistletoe to maintain cell differentiation.[18] Sensitivity to mistletoe extracts has been documented for acute lymphoblastic leukaemia cells resistant to methotrexate and cytarabine.[20]

The optimum dose of Iscador™ for tumour inhibition in mice weighing approximately 30 g, has been estimated at 0.11 mg and 0.153 mg.[18] The degree of inhibition compared to controls was stated as 20 to 50%.[18]

In-vivo **immunostimulant activity** in mice (humoral and cellular), demonstrated by an enhancement of delayed hypersensitivity and antibody formation to sheep red blood cells, has been documented for the crude plant juice, Iscador™ and for a polysaccharide fraction isolated from the berries.[21] Activity was attributed to stimulation of the monophagocytic system and to induction of inflammation. The results indicated that the immunostimulant property of mistletoe is not solely attributable to the polysaccharides found in the berries (plant juice also active) or to the Lactbacilli content of the fermented plant juice (crude extract also active). Non-specific immunological effects with mistletoe extracts are reported to be dependent on the frequency and quantity of the applied extract.[22]

Agglutinating activity that is preferential towards tumour cells over erythrocytes has been exhibited by Iscador™ and by a lectin fraction. [23–25] The lectins have been shown to bind to a number of cells including erythrocytes (non-specific to blood type),[7,10] lymphocytes, leucocytes, macrophages, glycoproteins, and plasma proteins.[9,10] Binding has been found to be stereospecific towards units containing a D-galactose molecule,[8,9,25] although D-galactose units with unmodified hydroxyl groups at C_2, C_3, and C_4 inhibit erythrocyte agglutination.[26] Tyrosine residues are also thought to be involved in the agglutination process.[8] Plasma proteins compete for the lectin receptor site and, therefore, decrease the agglutination of erythrocytes and tumour cells.[27] Unlike many other sugars, lactose units have also been found to inhibit erythrocyte agglutination.[26]

Mistletoe lectins have been reported to prevent viscotoxin- and allergen-stimulated histamine release from human leucocytes.[28]

The **hypotensive** effect documented for mistletoe has been attributed to various biologically active constituents such as acetylcholine, histamine, GABA, tyramine, and flavones.[G11] The exact nature of the hypotensive effect of mistletoe seems unclear: it has been reported that activity is mainly due to an inhibitory action on the excitability of the vasomotor centre in the medulla oblongata.[29] However, it has also been stated that the hypotensive action of mistletoe is mainly of a reflex character, exerting a normalising effect on both hypertensive and hypotensive states.[29] The effect of different mistletoe plant parts and host-plant on the hypotensive activity has been studied with highest activity reported for mistletoe leaves parasitising on willow.[29]

Human studies Iscador™ has been administered to patients with cancer of the breast, cervix, colon, rectum, and stomach.[18] Treated groups were reported to show a slight improvement over controls, the best results being obtained with cancer of the colon. It has been suggested that the relatively weak antitumour effects of Iscador may provide a useful adjunct to conventional surgery and radiotherapy.[18]

Intrapleural instillation of Iscador™ has been used to dry out malignant pleural exudations[30,31] and it has been reported to increase life span in a fatal case of small-cell lung cancer.[41]

Cells responsible for natural killer (NK) **cytolytic activity** have been shown to be large granular lymphocytes (LGL).[32] The cytolytic activity of NK cells is regulated by a number of factors including polymorphonuclear leucocytes (PMN). A significant increase in NK cell cytotoxicity and antibody dependent cell-mediated cytotoxicity, with augmented concentrations of LGL, has been noted in peripheral blood samples taken from breast cancer patients given a single infusion of Iscador™.[33] A decrease in NK and LGL values has been shown to be paralleled by an increase in PMN concentrations in peripheral blood post-Iscador™ infusion.[32] Interferons, interleukin-2, and some other lymphokines have previously been described as modifiers of the spontaneous cytotoxicity of NK cells and of monocytes.[34] The effect of Iscador™ on immunological parameters is stated to follow a kinetic pattern similar to that seen after treatment with α-interferon.[33] Stimulation of cell-mediated immunity has been observed in female patients with arthrosis administered weekly injections (ic) of mistletoe extract.[22] A depressive action was observed in patients receiving daily administration of higher doses.[22]

Extracts of mistletoe have been shown to strongly increase the cytolytic activity of NK cells using human peripheral blood mononuclear cells and a human cell line (K562 leukaemia).[34] The active component in the mistletoe extract is stated not to be a protein, thus excluding lectins and viscotoxins, and is thought to be a complex polysaccharide.[34] Mistletoe extract is not itself cytolytic but must be present during the NK cell-mediated tumour cell lysis to elicit enhancement.[34] Galacturonic acid inhibits this enhancement of NK cell cytotoxicity by acting at the effector cell specific site.[34] Two mechanisms have been proposed for the enhancement of NK cell cytotoxicity by mistletoe; one involves a bridging mechanism between the effector (NK) and target (tumour) cells, and another involves an immediate trigger of receptor expression on effector cells for target cell recognition.[34]

Side-effects, Toxicity

Hepatitis has been documented in a woman who had ingested a herbal preparation containing kelp, motherwort, skullcap, and mistletoe.[35] Mistletoe was assumed to be the causal factor since it was the only known toxic ingredient in the remedy.[35] However, no other instances of hepatotoxicity have been documented for mistletoe and, more recently, hepatitis has been documented with scullcap (*see* Scullcap monograph).

Symptoms of toxicity documented following the ingestion of mistletoe include hypotension, coma, seizures, myosis, mydriasis, and death.[36] Hypertension leading to cardiovascular collapse has been reported for American mistletoe (*Phoradendron* species).[36] It has been stated that no serious side-effects have been reported for Iscador™ following its administration to at least 1000 patients, although mild pyrexia and mild leucocytosis have been documented.[18] In contrast to the immunosuppression normally associated with cytotoxic therapy, Iscador™ has exhibited immunostimulant actions.

Toxic actions in animals have been documented for mistletoe lectins and viscotoxins.

Intravenous administration of viscotoxin to cats (35 µg/kg) resulted in a negative inotropic effect on cardiac muscle, reflex bradycardia, and hypotension.[37] Viscotoxins A_3 and B have also caused muscle contracture and progressive depolarisation in isolated smooth, skeletal and cardiac muscle preparations.[38] The mode of action was thought to involve the displacement of calcium from cell membrane bound sites. The viscotoxins precipitate histamine release from human leucocytes in an irritant manner without destroying the cells.[28] Viscotoxin is toxic on parenteral administration and an LD_{50} value (mice, intraperitoneal injection) has been estimated as 0.7 mg/kg.[39]

Mistletoe lectins inhibit protein synthesis in both cells and cell-free systems.[40] In common with other known toxic lectins (e.g. ricin), mistletoe lectins bind to plasma proteins, are specific towards D-galactose, possess some cytotoxic activity and have caused macroscopic lesions in rats (e.g. ascites, congested intestine, pancreatic haemorrhages).[21] An LD_{50} (mice) value for mistletoe lectin fraction is reported as 80 µg/kg compared with 3 µg/kg for ricin.[40]

Documented LD_{50} values (mice, intraperitoneal injection) are greater than 2.25 mg for the polysaccharide fraction from the berries, 32 mg for the crude plant juice, and 276 mg for Iscador™.[21]

Contra-indications, Warnings

Mistletoe berries are highly poisonous and it is advised that the herb should only be prescribed by a registered herbal practitioner.[G20] Mistletoe may interfere with existing cardiac, immunosuppressant, hypo/hypertensive, antidepressant, and anticoagulant/coagulant therapies.

Pregnancy and lactation The use of mistletoe is contra-indicated in view of the toxic constituents. Tyramine and a cardioactive principle isolated from mistletoe have both exhibited uterine stimulant activity in animal studies.

Pharmaceutical Comment

The constituents of mistletoe have been well investigated and to some extent are thought to be dependent on the host-plant on which mistletoe is a parasite. Mistletoe is reputed to be a cardiac depressant. Cardioactive constituents are not generally recognised as constituents of mistletoe, although this may depend on the nature of the host plant.

Documented literature for mistletoe has centred primarily on the pharmacological and toxic actions of the lectin and viscotoxin constituents. Much interest has been generated by the immunostimulant and cytotoxic actions documented for mistletoe and its potential role in treating conditions involving the immune system. Mistletoe seems to have the unusual combination of being both cytotoxic and immunostimulating. Further research is required to establish the true usefulness of mistletoe in these therapeutic areas.

The toxic nature of the mistletoe constituents (e.g. alkaloids, lectins, viscotoxins) indicates that it is unsuitable for self-medication. Mistletoe berries may only be supplied from pharmacies.[42]

References

See General References G1, G3, G5, G9, G10, G20, G22, G23 and G32.

1.   Krzaczek, T. Pharmacobotanical studies of the subspecies *Viscum album* L. IV. *Ann Univ Mariae Curie-Sklodowska, Sect D* 1977; **32:** 281–91.

2.   Becker H, Exner J. Comparative studies of flavonoids and phenylcarboxylic acids of mistletoes from different host trees. *Z Pflanzenphysiol* 1980; **97:** 417–28.

3.   Khwaja TA *et al.* Isolation of biologically active alkaloids from Korean mistletoe *Viscum album, coloratum*. *Experientia* 1980; **36:** 599–600.

4.   Khwaja TA *et al.* Recent studies on the anticancer activities of mistletoe (*Viscum album*) and its alkaloids. *Oncology* 1986; **43**(Suppl 1): 42–50.

5.   Graziano MN *et al.* Isolation of tyramine from five Argentine species of Loranthaceae. *Lloydia* 1967; **30:** 242–4.

6.   Fukunaga T *et al.* Studies on the constituents of the European mistletoe, *Viscum album* L. *Chem Pharm Bull* 1987; **35:** 3292–7.

7.   Ziska P *et al.* The lectin from *Viscum album* L. purification by biospecific affinity chromatography. *Experientia* 1978; **34:** 123–4.

8.   Ziska P *et al.* Chemical modification studies on the D-galactopyranosyl binding lectin from the mistletoe *Viscum album* L. *Acta Biol Med Ger* 1979; **38:** 1361–3.

9.   Luther P *et al.* The lectin from *Viscum album* L. — isolation, characterization, properties and structure. *Int J Biochem* 1980; **11:** 429–35.

10.   Franz H *et al.* Isolation and properties of three lectins from mistletoe (*Viscum album* L.). *Biochem J* 1981; **195:** 481–4.

11.   Krzaczek, T. Pharmacobotanical studies of the subspecies *Viscum album* L. III. Terpenes and sterols. *Ann Univ Mariae Curie-Sklodowska, Sect D* 1977; **32:** 125–34.

12.   Samuelsson G. Misteltoe toxins. *Syst Zool* 1973; **22:** 566–9.

13.   Olson T. The disulphide bonds of viscotoxin A2 from the European mistletoe (*Viscum album* L. Loranthaceae). *Acta Pharm Suec* 1974; **11:** 381–6.

14.   Samuelsson G, Jayawardene AL. Isolation and characterization of viscotoxin 1-Ps from *Viscum album* L. ssp. *austriacum* (Wiesb.) Vollmann, growing on *Pinus silvestris*. *Acta Pharm Suec* 1974; **11:** 175–84.

15.   Krzaczek T. Pharmacobotanical studies of the sub-species *Viscum album* L. II. Saccharides. *Ann Univ Mariae Curie-Sklodowska Sect D* 1976; **31:** 281–90.

16.   Locock RA. Mistletoe. *Can Pharm J* 1986; **119:** 125–127.

17.   Anderson LA, Phillipson JD. Mistletoe — the magic herb. *Pharm J* 1982; **229:** 437–9.

18.   Evans MR, Preece AW. *Viscum album* — A possible treatment for cancer? *Bristol MedicoChir J* 1973; **88:** 17–20.

19.   Konopa J *et al.* Isolation of viscotoxins. Cytotoxic basic polypeptides from *Viscum album* L. *Hoppe-Seyler's Z Physiol Chem* 1980; **361**: 1525–33.

20.   Hülsen H, Mechelke F. *In vitro* effectiveness of a mistletoe preparation on cytostatic-drug-resistant human leukemia cells. *Naturwissenschaften* 1987; **74**: 144–145.

21.   Bloksma N *et al.* Stimulation of humoral and cellular immunity by *Viscum* preparations. *Planta Med* 1982; **46**: 221–7.

22.   Coeugniet EG, Elek E. Immunomodulation with *Viscum album* and *Echinacea purpurea* extracts. *Onkologie* 1987; **10**(Suppl 3): 27–33.

23.   Luther P, Mehnert WH. Zum serologischen Verhalten einiger handelsüblicher Präparate aus *Viscum album* L., insbesondere des Iscador, in bezug aug menschliche Blutzellen und Aszites-Tumorzellen von Mäusen. *Acta Biol Med Ger* 1974; **33**: 351–7.

24.   Luther P *et al.* Isolation and characterization of mistletoe extracts. II. Action of agglutinating and cytotoxic fractions on mouse ascites tumor cells. *Acta Biol Med Germ* 1977; **36**: 119–25.

25.   Luther P *et al.* Reaktionen einiger antikörperähnlicher Substanzen aus Insekten (Protektine) und Pflanzen (Lektine) mit Aszites-Tumorzellen. *Acta Biol Med Ger* 1973; **31**: K11–18.

26.   Ziska P and Franz H. Studies on the interaction of the mistletoe lectin I with carbohydrates. *Experientia* 1981; **37**: 219.

27.   Franz H *et al.* Isolation and characterization of mistletoe extracts. I. Affinity chromatography of mistletoe crude extract on insolubilized plasma proteins. *Acta Biol Med Ger* 1976; **36**: 113–17.

28.   Luther P *et al.* Allergy and lectins: Interaction between IgE-mediated histamine release and glycoproteins from *Viscum album* L. (mistletoe). *Acta Biol Med Ger* 1978; **37**: 1623–8.

29.   Petkov V. Plants with hypotensive, antiatheromatous and coronarodilatating action. *Am J Chin Med* 1979; **7**(3); 197–236.

30.   Salzer G. The local treatment of malignant pleural exudations with Iscador (a drug obtained from mistletoe). Preliminary report. *Osterr Z Onkol* 1977; **4**: 13–14.

31.   Salzer G. Pleura carcinosis. Cytomorphological findings with the mistletoe preparation Iscador and other pharmaceuticals. *Oncology* 1986; **43**(Suppl 1): 66–70.

32.   Hajto T, Hostanska K. An investigation of the ability of *Viscum album*-activated granulocytes to regulate natural killer cells *in vivo*. *Clin Trials J* 1986; **23**: 345–57.

33.   Hajto T. Immunomodulatory effects of Iscador: a *Viscum album* preparation. *Oncology* 1986; **43**(Suppl 1): 51–65.

34.   Mueller EA *et al.* Biochemical characterization of a component in extracts of *Viscum album* enhancing human NK cytotoxicity. *Immunopharmacology* 1989; **17**: 11–18.

35.   Harvey J, Colin-Jones DG. Mistletoe hepatitis. *Br Med J* 1981; **282**: 186–7.

36.   Hall AH *et al.* Assessing mistletoe toxicity. *Ann Emerg Med* 1986; **15**: 1320–3.

37.   Rosell S, Samuelsson G. Effect of mistletoe viscotoxin and phoratoxin on blood circulation. *Toxicon* 1966; **4**: 107–110.

38.   Andersson K-E, Jóhannsson M. Effects of viscotoxin on rabbit heart and aorta, and on frog skeletal muscle. *Eur J Pharmacol* 1973; **23**: 223–31.

39.   Samuelsson G. Screening of plants of the family Loranthaceae for toxic proteins. *Acta Pharm Suec* 1966; **3**: 353–62.

40.   Stirpe F *et al.* Inhibition of protein synthesis by a toxic lectin from *Viscum album* L. (mistletoe). *Biochem J* 1980; **190**: 843–5.

41.   Bradley GW, Clover A. Apparent response of small cell lung cancer to an extract of mistletoe and homoeopathic treatment. *Thorax* 1989; **44**: 1047–8

42.   The Medicines (Retail Sale or Supply of Herbal Medicines) Order 1977, SI 1977: 2130.

MOTHERWORT

Species (Family)
Leonurus cardiaca L. and various other *Leonurus* species (Labiatae)

Synonym(s)
Leonurus

Part(s) Used
Herb

Pharmacopoeial Monographs
BHP 1983
BHP 1990
Martindale 25th edition

Legal Category (Licensed Products)
GSL[G14]

Constituents[G2,G10,G18,G25,G32]
Alkaloids (0.35%). Stachydrine (a pyrrolidine-type alkaloid), betonicine and turicin (stereoisomers of 4-hydroxystachydrine), leonurine 0.0068% (a guanidine derivative),[1] leonuridin, leonurinine. The presence of leonurine in *L. cardiaca* has been disputed, although it has been documented for other *Leonurus* species.
Flavonoids Glycosides of apigenin, kaempferol, and quercetin (e.g. hyperoside, kaempferol-3-D-glucoside, genkwanin, quinqueloside, quercitrin, rutin)[2,3]
Iridoids Ajugol, ajugoside, galiridoside, leonurid and 3 or 4 more unidentified glycosides[4]
Tannins (2–8%). Type not specified. Pseudotannins (e.g. pyrogallol, catechins)
Terpenoids Volatile oil 0.05%, resin, wax, ursolic acid, leocardin (a labdane diterpene)[5] as an epimeric mixture, and a diterpene lactone similar to marrubiin[2]
Other constituents Citric acid, malic acid, oleic acid, bitter principles,[6,7] carbohydrates 2.89%, choline, a phenolic glycoside (caffeic acid 4-rutinoside).[8] Cardiac glycosides (bufadienolide/bufanolide type) have been documented although their presence in motherwort has not been confirmed.
A *Cad*-specific lectin has been isolated from the seeds.[9]

Food Use
Motherwort is not used in foods. In the USA, motherwort is listed by the FDA as a 'Herb of Undefined Safety'.[G10]

Herbal Use
Motherwort is stated to possess sedative and antispasmodic properties. Traditionally, it has been used for cardiac debility, simple tachycardia, effort syndrome, amenorrhoea, and specifically for cardiac symptoms associated with neurosis.[G2,G3,G4,G32]

Dose
Dried herb 2–4 g or by infusion three times daily[G2,G3]
Liquid extract (1:1 in 25% alcohol) 2–4 mL three times daily[G2,G3]
Tincture (1:5 in 45% alcohol) 2–6 mL three times daily[G2,G3]

Pharmacological Actions
Animal studies The uterotonic principle in motherwort is unclear, although leonurine is reported to be the uteroactive constituent in various *Leonurus* species. In addition, oxytocic activity documented for *L. cardiaca* has been attributed to another alkaloid constituent, stachydrine.[G12] Uterotonic activity has been reported for leonurine in various *in-vitro* preparations including human myometrial strips and isolated rat uterus.[10,11]
In-vitro cardioactivity has been documented for motherwort.[12] An alcoholic extract was found to have a direct inhibitory effect on myocardial cells: antagonistic action towards calcium chloride (provided that the extract was administered before calcium chloride), and towards both α- and β-adrenoceptor stimulation was observed. No significant effect on the cardiac activity of the isolated guinea-pig heart was noted for caffeic acid 4-rutinoside.[8]
A related species, *Leonurus heterophyllus*, has been stated to prevent platelet aggregation, although no such documented action was located for motherwort.[13]
Ursolic acid has been reported to possess antiviral, tumour-inhibitory, and cytotoxic activities.[14,15] Ursolic acid was found to inhibit the Epstein-Barr virus *in vitro* and to inhibit tumour production by TPA in mouse skin, with activity comparable to that of retinoic acid, a known tumour-promoter inhibitor.[15] *In-vitro* cytotoxicity was documented in lymphocytic leukaemia (P-388, L-1210), human lung carcinoma (A-549), KB cells, human colon (HCT-8), and mammary tumour (MCF-7).[14]

Side-effects, Toxicity
It has been stated that the leaves of motherwort may cause contact dermatitis and that the lemon-scented oil may result in photosensitisation.[G26] No documented toxicity studies were located. Cytotoxic activities have been reported for ursolic acid (*see* Animal studies).

Contra-indications, Warnings
Excessive use may interfere with existing therapy for a cardiac disorder (cardiac glycoside constituents, *in-vitro* activity). Sensitive individuals may experience an allergic reaction.
Pregnancy and lactation Motherwort is reputed to affect the menstrual cycle.[G10] In view of the lack of toxicity data and the documented *in-vitro* uterotonic activity,[G12] the use of motherwort during pregnancy and lactation should be avoided.

Pharmaceutical Comment

The common name motherwort may be applied to one of many *Leonurus* species. *L. cardiaca* is the typical European species utilised, whereas *Leonurus artemisia* is commonly used in traditional Chinese medicine. Other species referred to as motherwort include *Leonurus sibirious* and *L. heterophyllus*. The chemistry of *L. cardiaca* is well studied although the presence of the uterotonic principle leonurine has been disputed. Cardioactive properties in animals have been reported for motherwort (*L. cardiaca*), which thus support some of the stated herbal uses. However, any symptoms of cardiac disorder are not suitable for self-diagnosis and treatment with a herbal remedy. In view of the lack of toxicity data and possible cardioactivity, excessive use of motherwort should be avoided.

References

See General References G2, G3, G4, G10, G12, G14, G18, G25, G26 and G32.

1   Gulubov AZ. Structure of alkaloids from *Leonurus cardiaca*. *Nauch Tr Vissh Predagog Inst Plovdiv Mat Fiz Khim Biol* 1970; **8:** 129–32.

2.   Scott JH *et al*. Components of *Leonurus cardiaca*. *Sci Pharm* 1973; **41:** 149–55.

3.   Kartnig T *et al*. Flavonoid-*O*-glycosides from the herbs of *Leonurus cardiaca*. *J Nat Prod* 1985; **48:** 494–507.

4.   Buzogany K, Cucu V. Comparative study between the species of *Leonurus quinquelobatus*. Part II Iridoids. *Clujul Med* 1983; **56:** 385–8.

5.   Malakov P *et al*. The structure of leocardin, two epimers of a diterpenoid from *Leonurus cardiaca*. *Phytochemistry* 1985; **24:** 2341–3.

6.   Brieskorn CH, Hofmann R. Labiatenbitterstoffe: Ein clerodan-derivat aus *Leonurus cardiaca* L. *Tetrahedron Lett* 1979; **27:** 2511–12.

7.   Brieskorn CH, Broschek W. Bitter principles and furanoid compounds of *L. cardiaca*. *Pharm Acta Helv* 1972; **47:** 123–32.

8.   Tschesche R *et al*. Caffeic acid 4-rutinoside from *Leonurus cardiaca*. *Phytochemistry* 1980; **19:** 2783.

9.   Bird GWG, Wingham J. Anti-Cad lectin from the seeds of *Leonurus cardiaca*. *Clin Lab Haematol* 1979; **1:** 57–9.

10.   Yeung HW *et al*. The structure and biological effect of leonurine — A uterotonic principle from the Chineses drug, I-mu Ts'ao. *Planta Med* 1977; **31:** 51–6.

11.   Kong YC *et al*. Isolation of the uterotonic principle from *Leonorus artemisia*, the Chinese motherwort. *Am J Chin Med* 1976; **4:** 373–82.

12.   Yanxing X. The inhibitory effect of motherwort extract on pulsating myocardial cells in vitro. *J Trad Chin Med* 1983; **3:** 185–8.

13.   Chang CF, Li CZ. Experimental studies on the mechanism of anti-platelet aggregation action of motherwort. *Chung-Hoi-I-Chich-Ho-TSQ Chin* 1986; **6:** 39–40.

14.   Kuo-Hsiung L *et al*. The cytotoxic principles of *Prunella vulgaris*, *Psychotria serpens*, and *Hyptis capitata*: Ursolic acid and related derivatives. *Planta Med* 1988; **54:** 308.

15.   Tokuda H *et al*. Inhibitory effects of ursolic and oleanolic acid on skin tumor promotion by 12-*O*-tetradecanoylphorbol-13-acetate. *Cancer Lett* 1986; **33:** 279–85.

MYRRH

Species (Family)

(i) *Commiphora molmol* Engl. (Burseraceae)
(ii) *Commiphora abyssinica* (Berg) Engl.
(iii) Other *Commiphora* species

Synonym(s)

(i) Balsamodendron Myrrha; Commiphora, *Commiphora myrrha* (Nees) Engl., African and Somali myrrh
(ii) Arabian and Yemen myrrh

Part(s) Used

Oleo-gum-resin

Pharmacopoeial Monographs

BHP 1983
BHP 1990
BPC 1973
Martindale 30th edition
Pharmacopoeias—Aust., Cz., Ger., and Swiss.

Legal Category (Licensed Products)

GSL[G14]

Constituents[G1,G2,G19,G24,G32]

Carbohydrates Up to 60% gum yielding arabinose, galactose, xylose, and 4-*O*-methylglucuronic acid following hydrolysis
Resins Up to 40% (average 20%) consisting of α-, β-, and γ-commiphoric acids, commiphorinic acid, α- and β-heerabomyrrhols, heeraboresene, commiferin
Steroids Campesterol, cholesterol, β-sitosterol
Terpenoids α-Amyrin. Nine sesquiterpenoid hydrocarbons, a sesquiterpene alcohol (elemol), and five furanosesquiterpenoids have been isolated from *C. abyssinica*.[1]
Volatile oils (1.5–17%). Dipentene, cadinene, heerabolene, limonene, pinene, eugenol, *m*-cresol, cinnamaldehyde, cuminaldehyde, cumic alcohol, and others.

Food Use

Myrrh is listed by the Council of Europe as a natural source of food flavouring (category N2). This category indicates that myrrh can be added to foodstuffs in small quantities, with a possible limitation of an active principle (as yet unspecified) in the final product.[G9]

Herbal Use

Myrrh is stated to possess antimicrobial, astringent, carminative, expectorant, anticatarrhal, antiseptic, and vulnerary properties. Traditionally, it has been used for aphthous ulcers, pharyngitis, respiratory catarrh, common cold, furunculosis, wounds and abrasions, and specifically for mouth ulcers, gingivitis, and pharyngitis.[G1,G2,G3,G4,G32]

Dose

Myrrh Tincture (BPC 1973) 2.5–5.0 mL

Tincture Myrrh Co. (Thompsons) (1 part Capsicum Tincture BPC 1973 to 4 parts Myrrh Tincture BPC 1973) 1.0–2.5 mL

Pharmacological Actions

Animal studies Anti-inflammatory (carrageenan-induced inflammation and cotton pellet granuloma)[2] and antipyretic activities in mice[2,3] have been documented for *C. molmol*. Hypoglycaemic activity in both normal and diabetic rats has been reported for a myrrh extract.[4,5] Together with an aloe gum extract, myrrh was found to be an active component of a multi-plant extract that exhibited antidiabetic activity. The mode of action was thought to involve a decrease in gluconeogenesis and an increase in peripheral utilisation of glucose in diabetic rats.

Myrrh is stated to have astringent properties on mucous membranes[G22] and to have antimicrobial activities *in vitro*.[G19]

Anti-inflammatory and hypocholesterolaemic activities have been reported for an Indian plant, *Commiphora mukul*, commonly known as guggulipid. Anti-inflammatory activity was described for a crystalline steroidal fraction of guggulipid in both acute (carrageenan-induced rat paw oedema test) and chronic (adjuvant arthritis) models of inflammation.[6] A ketosteroid has been identified as the active hypocholesterolaemic principle in guggulipid.[7] In some animal species, thyroid suppression is required as well as cholesterol administration in order to achieve experimental hypercholesterolaemia. Results of studies in chicks administered a thyroid suppressant and cholesterol indicated that guggulipid prevents endogenous hypercholesterolaemia via stimulation of the thyroid gland.[7] When fed to rabbits, guggulipid has been found to reverse the decrease in catecholamine concentrations and dopamine-β-decarboxylase activity that are associated with hyperlipidaemia.[8]

Human studies No documented studies were located for myrrh. Guggulipid has been reported to lower the concentration of total serum lipids, serum cholesterol, serum triglycerides, serum phospholipids, and β-lipoproteins in 20 patients.[9] This effect was comparable to two other known lipid-lowering drugs also used in the study.

Side-effects, Toxicity

No reported side-effects were located for *C. molmol* or *C. abyssinica*. Hiccup,[9] diarrhoea,[7] restlessness, and apprehension,[9] were documented as side-effects for guggulipid when administered to 20 patients.[9] Myrrh has been reported to be non-irritating, non-sensitising, and non-phototoxic to human and animal skins.[G19]

Contra-indications, Warnings

Myrrh may interfere with existing antidiabetic therapy, as hypoglycaemic properties have been documented. Thyroid stimulation and lipid lowering properties have been documented for the related species, *Commiphora mukul*.

Pregnancy and lactation Myrrh is reputed to affect the menstrual cycle[G19] and the safety of myrrh taken during pregnancy has not been established. Excessive use of myrrh during pregnancy should be avoided.

Pharmaceutical Comment

The volatile oil, gum, and resin components of myrrh are well documented. The anti-inflammatory and antipyretic activities documented in animals support some of the traditional uses. Phenol components of the volatile oil may account for the antimicrobial properties of myrrh, although no documented studies were located. Lipid-lowering properties via a stimulant action on the thyroid gland have been documented for *C. mukul* in both animals and humans. In view of the lack of toxicity data, excessive use of myrrh should be avoided.

References

See General References G1, G2, G3, G4, G7, G9, G14, G19, G22, G23, G24 and G32.

1.   Brieskorn CH and Noble P. Constituents of the essential oil of myrrh. II: Sesquiterpenes and furanosesquiterpenes. *Planta Med* 1982; **44:** 87–90.

2.   Tariq M *et al*. Anti-inflammatory activity of *Commiphora molmol*. *Agents Actions* 1986; **17:** 381–2.

3.   Mohsin A *et al*. Analgesic, antipyretic activity and phytochemical screening of some plants used in traditional Arab system of medicine. *Fitoterapia* 1989; **60:** 174–7.

4.   Al-Awadi FM, Gumaa KA. Studies on the activity of individual plants of an antidiabetic plant mixture. *Acta Diabetol Lat* 1987; **24:** 37–41.

5.   Al-Awadi FM *et al*. On the mechanism of the hypoglycaemic effect of a plant extract. *Diabetologia* 1985; **28:** 432–4.

6.   Arora RB *et al*. Anti-inflammatory studies on a crystalline steroid isolated from *Commiphora mukul*. *Indian J Med Res* 1972; **60:** 929–31.

7.   Tripathi SN *et al*. Effect of a keto-steroid of *Commifora mukul* L. on hypercholesterolemia and hyperlipidemia induced by neomercazole and cholesterol mixture in chicks. *Indian J Exp Biol* 1975; **13:** 15–18.

8.   Srivastava M *et al*. Effect of hypocholesterolemic agents of plant origin on catecholamine biosynthesis in normal and cholesterol fed rabbits. *J Biosci* 1984; **6:** 277–82.

9.   Malhotra SC, Ahuja MMS. Comparative hypolipidaemic effectiveness of gum guggulu (*Commiphora mukul*) fraction 'A', ethyl-*p*-chlorophenoxyisobutyrate and Ciba-13437-Su. *Indian J Med Res* 1971; **59:** 1621-32.

NETTLE

Species (Family)
Urtica dioica L. (Urticaceae)

Synonym(s)
Stinging Nettle, Urtica

Part(s) Used
Herb

Pharmacopoeial Monographs
BHP 1983
BHP 1990
Martindale 28th edition

Legal Category (Licensed Products)
GSL[G14]

Constituents[G2,G10,G32]
Acids Carbonic acid, formic acid, silicic acid, citric acid, fumaric acid, glyceric acid, malic acid, oxalic acid, phosphoric acid, quinic acid, succinic acid, threonic acid, and threono-1,4-lactone[1]
Amines Acetylcholine, betaine, choline, lecithin, histamine, serotonin,[2] a glycoprotein[3]
Flavonoids Flavonol glycosides (e.g. isorhamnetin, kaempferol, quercetin)[4]
Other constituents Choline acetyltransferase,[5] scopoletin,[4] β-sitosterol, tannin
Other plant parts The rhizome contains lectin (UDA) composed of six isolectins,[6,7] coumarin (scopoletin), triterpenes, β-sitosterol, its glucoside, and six stearyl derivatives),[8,9] two phenylpropane derivatives, and six lignans.[10]

Food Use
Nettle is listed by the Council of Europe as a natural source of food flavouring (category N3). This category indicates that insufficient information is available on nettle for an adequate assessment of potential toxicity.[G9] Nettle is used in soups and herbal teas. In the USA, nettle is listed by the FDA as a Herb of Undefined Safety.[G10]

Herbal Use
Nettle is stated to possess antihaemorrhagic and hypoglycaemic properties. Traditionally, it has been used for uterine haemorrhage, cutaneous eruption, infantile and psychogenic eczema, epistaxis, melaena, and specifically for nervous eczema.[G2,G3,G4,G32]

Dose
Dried herb 2–4 g or by infusion three times daily[G2,G3]
Liquid extract (1:1 in 25% alcohol) 3–4 mL three times daily[G2,G3]
Tincture (1:5 in 45% alcohol) 2–6 mL three times daily[G2,G3]

Pharmacological Actions
Animal studies CNS-depressant activity has been documented for nettle. It has been shown to produce a reduction in spontaneous activity in rats and mice,[11,12] inhibition of drug-induced convulsions, and a lowering of body temperature in rats.[11] Nettle has been reported to have no effect on the blood pressure of mice,[12] whereas in cats, it has produced a marked hypotensive effect and bradycardia.[13] Atropine was reported to have no effect on these latter actions and a mode of action via α-adrenoceptors was suggested.[13]

Nettle is stated to contain both hypoglycaemic and hyperglycaemic principles.[14] The hypoglycaemic component has been termed 'urticin' and nettle has been reported to lower the blood-sugar concentration in hyperglycaemic rabbits.[14] Uteroactivity has been documented for nettle in pregnant and non-pregnant mice; betaine and serotonin were stated to be the active constituents.[15] A nettle extract was reported to be devoid of antifertility activity following oral administration to mice (250 mg/kg).[16] Analgesic activity in mice has been documented.[12]

The isolectins isolated from the rhizome are reported to cause nonspecific agglutination of erythrocytes and to induce the synthesis of interferon by human lymphocytes.[6,7] UDA and the individual isolectins are documented to have the same carbohydrate-binding properties.[6,7]

Human studies Clinical studies have confirmed haemostatic properties documented for nettle,[G10] although no further details were stated.

Side-effects, Toxicity
Consumption of nettle tea has caused gastric irritation, a burning sensation of the skin, oedema, and oliguria.[G10] The leaves are extremely irritant in view of their acetylcholine- and histamine-containing glandular hairs. An LD_{50} (mice, intraperitoneal injection) value of 3.625 g/kg body-weight has been documented for nettle.[12]

Contra-indications, Warnings
In view of the documented pharmacological actions for nettle, excessive use may interact with concurrent therapy for diabetes, high or low blood pressure, and may potentiate drugs with CNS depressant actions. Gastro-intestinal irritation has been documented.

Pregnancy and lactation Nettle is reputed to be an abortifacient and to affect the menstrual cycle.[G12] Uteroactivity has been documented in animal studies. In view of this, the use of nettle during pregnancy should be avoided. Excessive use is best avoided during lactation.

Pharmaceutical Comment

The chemistry of nettle is well documented. Limited pharmacological data are available to support the traditional herbal uses although hypoglycaemic activity *in vivo* has been reported. Irritant properties have been documented for nettle and excessive use should be avoided.

References

See General References G2, G3, G4, G9, G10, G12, G14, G21, and G32.

1.   Bakke ILF *et al* Water-soluble acids from Urtica dioica L. *Medd Nor Farm Selsk* 1978; **40:** 181–8.

2.   Adamski R and Bieganska J. Studies on substances present in *Urtica dioica* L. leaves II. Analysis for protein amino acids and nitrogen containing non-protein amino acids. *Herba Polonica* 1984; **30:** 17–26.

3.   Andersen S and Wold JK. Water-soluble glycoprotein from *Urtica dioica* leaves. *Phytochem* 1978; **17:** 1875–7.

4.   Chaurasia N and Wichtl M. Flavonolglykoside aus *Urtica dioica*. *Planta Med* 1987; **53:** 432–4.

5.   Barlow RB and Dixon ROD. Choline aceytltransferase in the nettle *Urtica dioica* L. *Biochem J* 1973; **132:** 15–18.

6.   Shibuya N *et al*. Carbohydrates binding properties of the stinging nettle (*Urtica dioica*) rhizome lectin. *Archiv Biochem Biophys* 1986; **249:** 215–224.

7.   Damme EJM *et al*. The *Urtica dioica* agglutinin is a complex mixture of isolectins. *Plant Physiol* 1988; **86:** 598–601.

8.   Chaurasia N and Wichtl M. Scopoletin, 3-β-sitosterin und 3- β-D-glucosid aus Brennesselwurzel (Urticae radix). *Dtsch Apothek Zeitung* 1986; **126:** 81–3.

9.   Chaurasia N and Wichtl M. Sterols and steryl glycosides from *Urtica dioica*. *J Nat Prod* 1987; **50:** 881–5.

10.   Chaurasia N and Wichtl M. Phenylpropane und lignane aus der wurzel von Urtica dioica L. *Dtsch Apothek Zeitung* 1986; **126:** 1559–63.

11.   Broncano J *et al*. Estudio de diferentes preparados de *Urtica dioica* L sobre SNC. *An R Acad Farm* 1987; **53:** 284–91.

12.   Lasheras B *et al*. Étude pharmacologique préliminaire de *Prunus spinosa* L. *Amelanchier ovalis* medikus *Juniperus communis* L. et *urtica dioica* L. *Plant méd phytothér* 1986; **20:** 219–26.

13.   Broncano FJ *et al*. Étude de l'effet sur le centre cardiovasculaire de quelques préparations de l'*Urtica dioica* L. *Planta Med* 1983; **17:** 222–9.

14.   Oliver-Bever B, Zahland GR. Plants with oral hypoglycaemic activity. *Quart J Crude Drug Res* 1979; **17:** 139–96.

15.   Broncano FJ *et al*. Estudio de efecto sobre musculatura lisa uterina de distintos preparados de las hojas de *Urtica dioica* L. *An R Acad Farm* 1987; **53:** 69–76.

16.   Sharma BB *et al*. Antifertility screening of plants. Part I. Effect of ten indigenous plants on early pregnancy in albino rats. *Int J Crude Drug Res* 1983; **21:** 183–7.

PARSLEY

Species (Family)
Petroselinum crispum (Mill.) Nyman (Apiaceae/Umbelliferae)

Synonym(s)
Apium petroselinum L., *Carum petroselinum* (L.) Benth, *Petroselinum sativum* Hoffin.

Part(s) Used
Leaf, Root, Seed

Pharmacopoeial Monographs
BHP 1983
BHP 1990
Martindale 28th edition

Legal Category (Licensed Products)
GSL[G14]

Constituents[G1,G2,G10,G19,G24,G32,G35]
Flavonoids Glycosides of apigenin, luteolin (e.g. apiin, luteolin-7-apiosyl-glucoside, apigenin-7-glucoside (leaf only), luteolin-7-diglucoside (leaf only))
Furanocoumarins Bergapten and oxypeucedanin as major constituents (up to 0.02% and 0.01% respectively); also 8-methoxypsoralen, imperatorin, isoimperatorin, isopimpinellin, psoralen, xanthotoxin (up to 0.003%)[1]
Volatile oils (2–7% in seed, 0.05% in leaf). The seed contains apiole, myristicin, tetramethoxyallylbenzene, various terpene aldehydes, ketones, and alcohols. The leaf contains myristicin (up to 85%), apiole, 1,3,8-*p*-menthatriene, 1-methyl-4-isopropenylbenzene, methyl disulphide, monoterpenes (e.g. α-and β-pinene, β-myrcene, β-ocimene, β-phellandrene, *p*-terpinene, α-terpineol), sesquiterpenes (e.g. α-copaene, carotol, caryophyllene).
Other constituents Fixed oil, oleo-resin, proteins, carbohydrates, and vitamins (especially vitamins A and C).
A detailed vitamin and mineral analysis is given in reference.[G10]

Food Use
Parsley is listed by the Council of Europe as natural source of food flavouring (category N2). This category indicates that parsley can be added to foodstuffs in small quantities, with a possible limitation of an active principle (as yet unspecified) in the final product.[G9] Parsley is commonly used in foods.

Herbal Use
Parsley is stated to possess carminative, antispasmodic, diuretic, emmenagogue, expectorant, antirheumatic, and antimicrobial properties. Traditionally, it has been used for flatulent dyspepsia, colic, cystitis, dysuria, bronchitic cough in the elderly, dysmenorrhoea, functional amenorrhoea, myalgia, and specifically for flatulent dyspepsia with intestinal colic.[G1,G2,G3,G4,G32]

Dose
Leaf/Root 2–4 g or by infusion
Seed 1–2 g
Dried root 2–4 g or by infusion three times daily[G2,G3]
Liquid extract (1:1 in 25% alcohol) 2–4 mL three times daily[G2,G3]

Pharmacological Actions
Animal studies Parsley extract (0.25–1.0 mL/kg, by intravenous injection) has been reported to lower the blood pressure of cats by more than 40%,[2] and to decrease both respiratory movements and blood pressure in anaesthetised dogs.[3] Parsley exhibits a tonic effect on both intestinal and uterine muscle.[3] This uterine effect has been attributed to the apiole content,[G12] but has also been observed with apiole-free aqueous extracts.[3] An aqueous extract of parsley has been documented to contain an antithiamine substance which was unaffected by cooking or contact with gastric juice.[3] Myristicin and apiole are both effective insecticides.[4]
Parsley seed oil has been reported to stimulate hepatic regeneration.[5]
Human studies Myristicin is the hallucinogenic principle present in nutmeg seed. It has been hypothesised that myristicin is converted in the body to amphetamine, to which it is structurally related.[4] Myristicin has a structural similarity with sympathetic amines and it is thought that it may compete for monoamine oxidase enzymes, thereby exhibiting a monoamine oxidase inhibitor (MAOI)-like action.[6] Parsley oil has been included in the diet of pregnant women and is reported to increase diuresis, and plasma-protein and plasma-calcium concentrations.[4]
The diuretic effect associated with the consumption of parsley is probably attributable to the pharmacological activities of myristicin (sympathetic action) and apiole (irritant effect).

Side-effects, Toxicity[G35]
Chronic and excessive consumption of fresh parsley (170 g daily for 30 years) has been associated with generalised itching and pigmentation of the lower legs in a 70-year-old woman.[6] The symptoms were attributed to excessive ingestion of parsley in the presence of chronic liver disease. The aetiology of the chronic hepatitis was unknown, but considered possibly related to the chronic exposure to the psoralen constituents in parsley.[6] Apiole and myristicin are also documented to be hepatotoxic.
The ingestion of approximately 10 g apiole has been reported to cause acute haemolytic anaemia, thrombocytopenia purpura, nephrosis and hepatic dysfunction. However,

ingestion of 10 g of apiole would require a dose of more than 200 g parsley. The amount of apiole ingested as a result of normal dietary consumption of parsley is not hazardous. Myristicin has been documented to cause giddiness, deafness, hypotension, decrease in pulse rate, and paralysis, followed by fatty degeneration of the liver and kidney.[G10] In addition, myristicin is known to possess hallucinogenic properties. However, when compared to nutmeg, parsley contains a relatively low concentration of myristicin (less than 0.05% in parsley leaf, about 0.4–0.89% in nutmeg); parsley seed is potentially hazardous in view of its higher volatile oil content (about 2–7%) which contains apiole and myristicin.

Parsley contains phototoxic furanocoumarins (see Celery). However, photodermatitis resulting from the oral ingestion of parsley is thought to be unlikely. The ingestion of 50 g parsley provides negligible amounts of bergapten (0.5–0.8 g).[7] The concentration of oxypeucedanin provided was not mentioned. However, a photoactive reaction from topical contact with parsley is possible.

Apiole is an irritant component of the volatile oil and may cause irritation of the kidneys during excretion.

Parsley seed oil has been reported to stimulate hepatic regeneration.[4] Myristicin and apiole are documented to have a similar chemical structure and acute toxicity to safrole, which is known to be carcinogenic and hepatotoxic (see Sassafras).[4] The carcinogenic potential of apiole and myristicin has not been evaluated.[4]

LD_{50} (mice, intravenous injection) values for apiole and myristicin have been documented as 50 mg/kg and 200 mg/kg body-weight, respectively.[4]

Contra-indications, Warnings

Parsley should not be ingested in excessive amounts in view of the documented toxicities of apiole and myristicin. Parsley may cause a photoactive reaction, especially following external contact, may aggravate existing renal disease, and may potentiate existing MAOI therapy.

Pregnancy and lactation Parsley is reputed to affect the menstrual cycle.[G3] Uteroactivity has been documented in humans and animals[G12], and parsley is stated to be contra-indicated during pregnancy.[G25,G35] Myristicin has been reported to cross the placenta and can lead to foetal tachy-cardia.[8] In view of this, parsley should not be taken during pregnancy and lactation in doses that greatly exceed the amounts used in foods.

Pharmaceutical Comment

Parsley is commonly consumed as part of the diet. The pharmacological and toxicological properties of parsley are primarily associated with the volatile oil, particularly the apiole, myristicin, and furanocoumarin constituents. Most of the reported uses of parsley are probably due to the volatile oil; no documented information was located regarding antirheumatic and antimicrobial properties. Parsley should not be consumed in doses that greatly exceed the amounts used in foods, as excessive ingestion may result in apiole and myristicin toxicity.

References

See General References G1, G2, G3, G4, G9, G10, G12, G14, G19, G21, G24, G25, G32 and G35.

1. Chaudhary SK et al. Oxypeucedanin, a major furocoumarin in parsley, *Petroselinum crispum*. *Planta Med* 1986; **52**: 462–4.

2. Petkov V. Plants with hypotensive, antiatheromatous and coronarodilatating action. *Am J Chin Med* 1979; **7**: 197–236.

3. Opdyke DLJ. Parsley seed oil. *Food Cosmetics Toxicol* 1975; **13**(Suppl): 897–8.

4. Buchanan RL. Toxicity of spices containing methylenedioxybenzene derivatives: A review. *J Food Safety* 1978; **1**: 275–93.

5. Gershbein LL. Regeneration of rat liver in the presence of essential oils and their components. *Food Cosmet Toxicol* 1977; **15**: 171–81.

6. Cootes P. Clinical curio: liver disease and parsley. *Br Med J* 1982; **285**: 1719.

7. Zaynoun S et al. The bergapten content of garden parsley and its significance in causing cutaneous photosensitization. *Clin Exp Dermatol* 1985; **10**: 328–31.

8. Lavy G. Nutmeg intoxication in pregnancy. *J Reprod Med* 1987; **32**: 63–4.

PARSLEY PIERT

Species (Family)
Aphanes arvensis L. (Rosaceae)

Synonym(s)
Alchemilla arvensis Scop., Aphanes

Part(s) Used
Herb

Pharmacopoeial Monographs
BHP 1983

Legal Category (Licensed Products)
GSL[G14]

Constituents[G3,G15,G32]
Limited information is available. A related species *Alchemilla vulgaris* (Lady's Mantle) is reported to contain 6–8% tannins (hydrolysable–type);[G19] none have been documented for parsley piert, although it is stated to contain an astringent principle.[G2]

Food Use
Parsley piert is not used in foods.

Herbal Use
Parsley piert is stated to possess diuretic and demulcent properties, and to dissolve urinary deposits. Traditionally, it has been used for kidney and bladder calculi, dysuria, strangury, oedema of renal and hepatic origin, and specifically for renal calculus.[G3,G32]

Dose
Dried herb 2–4 g or by infusion three times daily[G3]
Liquid extract (1:1 in 25% alcohol) 2–4 mL three times daily[G3]
Tincture (1:5 in 45% alcohol) 2–10 mL three times daily[G3]

Pharmacological Actions
None documented.

Side-effects, Toxicity
None documented.

Contra-indications, Warnings
None documented.

Pregnancy and lactation In view of the lack of phytochemical, pharmacological, and toxicity information, the use of parsley piert during pregnancy and lactation should be avoided.

Pharmaceutical Comment
Little chemical information is available on parsley piert. No scientific evidence was found to justify the herbal uses. Parsley piert may exhibit astringent actions. In view of the lack of toxicity data, excessive use of parsley piert should be avoided.

References
See General References G3, G14, G15, G32.

PASSIONFLOWER

Species (Family)
Passiflora incarnata L. (Passifloraceae)

Synonym(s)
Apricot Vine, Grenadille, Maypop, Passiflora, Passion Vine

Part(s) Used
Herb

Pharmacopoeial Monographs
BHP 1983
BHP 1990
Martindale 30th edition
Pharmacopoeias—Egypt., Fr., Ger., and Swiss. Braz. includes the leaves of *Passiflora alata*.

Legal Category (Licensed Products)
GSL[G14]

Constituents[G1,G2,G10,G19,G32]
Alkaloids (indole-type) Harman (major), harmaline, harmalol, harmine, harmol (disputed)
Flavonoids Vitexin, isovitexin and their *C*-glycosides, apigenin, luteolin glycosides (e.g. orientin, homoorientin, lucenin); kaempferol, quercetin, rutin.[1–6]
Other constituents Maltol and ethylmaltol (γ-pyrone derivatives), passicol (a polyacetylene),[7] fatty acids (e.g. linoleic acid, linolenic acid, myristic acid, palmitic acid, oleic acid), formic acid, butyric acid, sitosterol, stigmasterol, sugars, gum
Other plant parts Coumarins scopoletin and umbelliferone are found in the root.
Other Passiflora species Cyanogenetic glycosides passibiflorin, epipassibiflorin, and passitrifasciatin (*Passiflora biflora*, *Passiflora talamancensis*, *Passiflora trifasciata*),[8] linamarin and lotaustralin (*Passiflora lutea*),[9] prunasin (*Passiflora edulis*)[10]

Food Use
Passionflower is listed by the Council of Europe as a natural source of food flavouring (category N3). This category indicates that passionflower can be added to foodstuffs in the traditionally accepted manner, but that there is insufficient information available for an adequate assessment of potential toxicity.[G9]

Herbal Use
Passionflower is stated to possess sedative, hypnotic, antispasmodic, and anodyne properties. Traditionally, it has been used for neuralgia, generalised seizures, hysteria, nervous tachycardia, spasmodic asthma, and specifically for insomnia.[G1,G2,G3,G4,G32] Passionflower is used extensively in homoeopathy.

Dose
Dried herb 0.25–1.0 g or by infusion three times daily[G2,G3]
Liquid extract (1:1 in 25% alcohol) 0.5–1.0 mL three times daily[G2,G3]
Tincture (1:8 in 45% alcohol) 0.5–2.0 mL three times daily[G2,G3]

Pharmacological Actions
Animal studies CNS sedation, potentiation of hexobarbitone sleeping time, anticonvulsant activity (high dose) and a reduction in spontaneous motor activity (low dose) have been documented for maltol and ethylmaltol in mice.[11,12] Subsequent research documenting similar activities in mice was unable to attribute the observed activities to either flavonoid or alkaloid components present in the tested extract.[13] The harman alkaloids are generally known to exhibit central stimulant activity via monoamine oxidase inhibition. It has been suggested that the sedative effects of maltol and ethylmaltol mask the stimulant actions of these alkaloids.[11] The CNS depressant effect exhibited by *P. edulis* has been attributed to alkaloid and flavonoid compounds[14] and to a protein-like substance.[15]
Passicol exhibits antimicrobial activity towards a wide variety of moulds, yeasts, and bacteria.[7] Group A haemolytic streptococci are stated to be more susceptible than *Staphylococcus aureus*, with *Candida albicans* of intermediate susceptibility.[7]

Side-effects, Toxicity
No reported side effects to passionflower were located. The acute toxicity of a fluid extract in mice (intraperitoneal injection) is stated as greater than 900 mg/kg.[13]
Cyanogenetic glycosides have been documented for related *Passiflora* species.

Contra-indications, Warnings
Excessive doses of passionflower may cause sedation and may potentiate MAOI therapy.
Pregnancy and lactation Both harman and harmaline have exhibited uterine stimulant activity in animal studies.[G12] No other data regarding the use of passionflower during pregnancy or lactation were located. In view of this, excessive use of passionflower during pregnancy and lactation should be avoided.

Pharmaceutical Comment
Passionflower is characterised by the harman alkaloid and *C*-glycoside flavonoid constituents. Despite traditional use as a sedative and anticonvulsant, few pharmacological studies have been undertaken. However, CNS sedative properties have been documented thus supporting the traditional uses, although the active constituents have not been clearly identified. In view of the lack of toxicity data, excessive use should be avoided.

References

See General Reference G1, G2, G3, G4, G9, G10, G12, G14, G19, G22, G24 and G32.

1. Quercia V *et al.* Identification and determination of vitexin and isovitexin in *Passiflora incarnata* extracts. *J Chromatogr* 1978; **161**: 396–402.

2. Pietta P *et al.* Isocratic liquid chromatographic method for the simultaneous determination of *Passiflora incarnata* L. and *Crataegus monogyna* flavonoids in drugs. *J Chromatogr* 1986; **357**: 233–8.

3. Geiger H *et al.* The *C*-Glycosylfavone pattern of *Passiflora incarnata* L. *Z Naturforsch* 1986; (Sept/Oct): 949–50.

4. Proliac A, Raynaud J. The presence of *C*-β-D-6-glucopyranosyl-*C*-α-L-arabinopyranosyl-8-apigenin in leafy stems of *Passiflora incarnata* L. *Pharmazie* 1986; **41**: 673–4.

5. Congora C *et al.* Isolation and identification of two mono-*C*-glucosyl-luteolins and of the di-*C*-substituted 6,8-diglucosyl-luteolin from the leavy stalks of *Passiflora incarnata* L. *Helv Chim Acta* 1986; **69**: 251–3.

6. Proliac A, Raynaud J. *O*-glucosyl-2"-*C*-glucosyl-6 apigénine de *Passiflora incarnata* L. (Passifloraceae). *Pharm Acta Helv* 1988; **63**: 174–5.

7. Nicholls JM *et al.* Passicol, an antibacterial and antifungal agent produced by *Passiflora* plant species: qualitative and quantitative range of activity. *Antimicrob Agents Chemother* 1973; **3**: 110–17.

8. Spencer KC, Seigler DS. Passibiflorin, epipassibiflorin and passitrifasciatin: Cyclopentenoid cyanogenic glycosides from *Passiflora*. *Phytochemistry* 1985; **24**: 981–6.

9. Spencer KC, Siegler DS. Co-occurrence of valine/isoleucine derived cyclopentenoid cyanogens in a *Passiflora* species. *Biochem Syst Ecol* 1985; **13**: 303–4.

10. Spencer KC, Seigler DS. Cyanogenesis of *Passiflora edulis*. *J Agric Food Chem* 1983; **31**: 794–6.

11. Aoyagi N *et al.* Studies on *Passiflora incarnata* dry extract. I. Isolation of maltol and pharmacological action of maltol and ethyl maltol. *Chem Pharm Bull* 1974; **22**: 1008–13.

12. Kimura R *et al.* Central depressant effects of maltol analogs in mice. *Chem Pharm Bull* 1980; **28**: 2570–2579.

13. Speroni E, Minghetti A. Neuropharmacological activity of extracts from *Passiflora incarnata*. *Planta Med* 1988; **54**: 488–91.

14. Lutomski J *et al.* Pharmacochemical investigation of the raw materials from *Passiflora* genus. *Planta Med* 1975; **27**: 112–21.

15. Dovale NB *et al.* Psychopharmacological effects of preparations of *P.edulis* Passionflower. *Cienc Cult* 1983; **35**: 11–24.

PENNYROYAL

Species (Family)
(i) *Mentha pulegium* L. (Labiatae)
(ii) *Hedeoma pulegoides* (L.) Pers.

Synonym(s)
Pulegium,
(i) European Pennyroyal,
(ii) American Pennyroyal

Part(s) Used
Herb

Pharmacopoeial Monographs
BHP 1983
Martindale 30th edition (Pulegium Oil)

Legal Category (Licensed Products
Pennyroyal is not included on the GSL[G14]

Constituents[G10,G24,G32,G35]
Volatile oils (1–2%). Pulegone as principal component (60–90%), others include menthone, *iso*-menthone, 3-octanol, piperitenone, *trans-iso*-pulegone.

Food Use
Pennyroyal is not commonly used in foods. It is listed by the Council of Europe as a natural source of food flavouring (category N3). This category indicates that there is insufficient information is available for an adequate assessment of toxicity (*but see* Toxicity, below).

Herbal Use
Pennyroyal is stated to possess carminative, antispasmodic, diaphoretic, and emmenagogue properties, and has been used topically as a refrigerant, antiseptic, and insect repellent. Traditionally, it has been used for flatulent dyspepsia, intestinal colic, common cold, delayed menstruation, and topically for cutaneous eruptions, formication, and gout.[G3]

Dose
Herb 1–4 g or as infusion three times daily[G3]
Liquid extract (1:1 in 45% alcohol) 1–4 mL three times daily[G3]

Pharmacological Actions
None documented.

Side-effects, Toxicity
The toxicity of pennyroyal oil is well recognised and human fatalities following its ingestion as an abortifacient have been reported.[1–3] Symptoms reported following ingestion of the oil include abdominal pain, nausea, vomiting, diarrhoea, lethargy and agitation, pyrexia, raised blood pressure and pulse rate, and generalised urticarial rash. Generally, doses required for an abortifacient effect are also toxic and fatalities have involved both nephrotoxicity and hepatotoxicity.[2–4] Doses of one ounce and 30 mL[1–3] have proved fatal, whereas individuals have recovered following unsuc-

cessful abortion attempts involving the ingestion of 7.5 mL oil.[3] The mechanism of hepatotoxicity for pennyroyal is not known.[2] A direct hepatoxic action has been suggested for the ketone component, pulegone.[2] Alternatively, metabolic conversion of pulegone to a reactive intermediate, a furan or epoxide, has been proposed.[2]

Acute LD_{50} values for pennyroyal oil are documented as 0.4 g/kg (oral, rats) and 4.2 g/kg (dermal, rabbits).[4] The oil is non- or moderately irritating, non-sensitising, and non-phototoxic.[4] Acute LD_{50} values documented for pulegone, the principal oil component, are not suprisingly similar to those for the oil: 0.47 g/kg (oral, rats), 3.09 g/kg (dermal, rabbits).[5] Steroid (pregnenolone-16α-carbonitrile) treatment has reduced hepatotoxicity observed in female rats fed pulegone whereas triamcinolone has increased it.[5] Toxicity of pulegone is unaffected by partial hepatectomy or ligation of the common bile duct, while partial nephrectomy intensified toxicity.[5]

Contra-indications, Warnings
Pennyroyal oil is irritant and instances of hepatotoxicity and nephrotoxicity have been documented following its ingestion. Both the internal and external use of pennyroyal oil has been contra-indicated.[G35]

Pregnancy and lactation
Pennyroyal is contra-indicated in pregnancy.[G3] Traditionally, it has been employed as an abortifacient, this use probably resulting from the irritant action of the oil on the genito-urinary tract. Fatalities have resulted from the doses of oil required to exert an abortifacient effect.

Pharmaceutical Comment
Interest in penny royal has focussed on the toxicity associated with the volatile oil. No documented reports of the pharmacological actions exhibited by the herb were located. Pennyroyal herb teas have been reported to be used without side-effects,[2] presumably due to lower amounts of oil ingested. In view of its potential toxicity, excessive ingestion of the oil should be avoided. Pennyroyal oil is not suitable for internal or external use.

References
See General References G3, G10, G14, G22, G23, G24, G32, G33 and G35.

1. Vallance WB. Pennyroyal poisoning. A fatal case. *Lancet* 1955; **ii:** 850–1.

2. Sullivan JB *et al.* Pennyroyal oil poisoning and hepatotoxicity. *JAMA* 1979; **242:** 2873.

3. Gunby P. Plant known for centuries still causes problems today. *JAMA* 1979; **241:** 2246–7.

4. Opdyke DLJ. Pennyroyal oil european. *Food Cosmet Toxicol* 1974; **12:** 949–50.

5. Opdyke DLJ. Fragrance raw materials monographs: d-pulegone. 1978; pp. 867-8.

PILEWORT

Species (Family)
Ranunculus ficaria L. (Ranunculaceae)

Synonym(s)
Ficaria, *Ficaria ranunculoides* Moench., Lesser Celandine, Ranunculus

Part(s) Used
Herb

Pharmacopoeial Monographs
BHP 1983
BPC 1934

Legal Category (Licensed Products)
GSL[G14]

Constituents[G18,G20,G32]
Lactones Anemonin (dimer), protoanemonin (precursor to anemonin)
Triterpenoids Glycosides based on the sapogenins hederagenin and oleanolic acid, with arabinose, glucose, and rhamnose, as sugar moieties[1]
Other constituents Tannin, ascorbic acid (vitamin C)

Food Use
Pilewort is not used in foods.

Herbal Use
Pilewort is stated to possess astringent and demulcent properties. Traditionally, it has been used for haemorrhoids, and specifically for internal or prolapsed piles with or without haemorrhage, by topical application as an ointment or a suppository.[G3,G32]

Dose
Dried herb 2–5 g or by infusion three times daily[G3]
Liquid extract (1:1 in 25% alcohol) 2–5 mL three times daily[G3]
Ointment 3% in a suitable basis
Pilewort Ointment (BPC 1934) 30% fresh herb in benzoinated lard

Pharmacological Actions
Animal studies Local antihaemorrhoidal activity has been documented for the saponin constituents.[1] Antibacterial and antifungal properties have been documented for both anemonin and protoanemonin, although anemonin is reported to exhibit much weaker activity.[G13,G24]
The reported presence of tannin constituents[G20] supports the reputed astringent activity of pilewort, although no pharmacological studies were located.

Side-effects, Toxicity
The sap of pilewort is stated to be irritant.[G26] Protoanemonin is stated to be an acrid skin irritant, although it is readily converted into the inactive dimer anemonin.[G13] Protoanemonin is stated to have a marked ability to combine with sulfhydryl (-SH) groups and it is thought that the toxic subdermal properties of protoanemonin may depend on the inactivation of enzymes containing -SH groups.[G13] An LD_{50} value (mice, intraperitoneal injection) for anemonin has been reported as 150 mg/kg body-weight.[G24]

Contra-indications, Warnings
Pilewort is not recommended for internal consumption.[G25] Topical use of pilewort may cause irritant skin reactions.
Pregnancy and lactation The safety of pilewort has not been established. It is not recommended for internal consumption;[G25] in view of this and the potential irritant action, the use of pilewort during pregnancy and lactation is best avoided.

Pharmaceutical Comment
Limited information is available on the chemistry of pilewort. Little scientific information was located to justify the herbal uses, although antihaemorrhoidal activity has been documented for the saponin constituents. In view of the toxic and irritant properties stated for protoanemonin, the excessive use of pilewort is not advisable.

References
See General References G3 ,G5, G13, G14, G18, G20, G24, G25, G28, and G32.

1. Texier O *et al.* A triterpenoid saponin from *Ficaria ranunculoides* tubers. *Phytochemistry* 1984; **23:** 2903–5.

PLANTAIN

Species (Family)
Plantago major L. (Plantaginaceae)

Synonym(s)
Common Plantain, General Plantain, Greater Plantain

Part(s) Used
Leaf

Pharmacopoeial Monographs
BHP 1983
Martindale 30th edition (Plantain Seed)
Pharmacopoeias—Jpn describes the seed

Legal Category (Licensed Products)
Plantain is not included on the GSL[G14]

Constituents[G1,G10,G18,G26,G31,G32]
Acids Benzoic acid, caffeic acid, chlorogenic acid, cinnamic acid, *p*-coumaric acid, ferulic acid, fumaric acid, gentisic acid, *p*-hydroxybenzoic acid, neochlorogenic acid, salicylic acid, syringic acid, ursolic acid, vanillic acid;[1,2] oleanolic acid, ascorbic acid
Alkaloids Trace (unspecified),[3,4] boschniakine and the methyl ester of boschniakinic acid[5]
Amino acids DL-α-alanine, asparagine, L-histidine, DL-lysine, DL-leucine, serine, tryptophan[6]
Carbohydrates L-Fructose, D-glucose, planteose, saccharose, stachyose, *d*-xylose, sorbitol, tyrosol, mucilage, gum[7]
Flavonoids Apigenin, baicalein, scutellarein, baicalin, homoplantaginin, nepitrin, luteolin, hispidulin, plantagoside[8–10]
Iridoids Aucubin, aucubin derivatives, plantarenaloside, aucuboside, melitoside[5,11,12]
Tannins (4%). Unspecified
Other constituents Choline, allantoin, invertin and emulsin (enzymes), fat 10–20%, resin, saponins, steroids,[13] thioglucoside

Food Use
Plantain leaf is not used in foods. A related species, *Plantago lanceolata* L., is listed by the Council of Europe as a natural source of food flavouring (category N2). This category indicates that *P. lanceolata* can be added to foodstuffs in small quantities, with a possible limitation of an active constituent (as yet unspecified) in the final product.[G9] In the USA, plantain is listed by the FDA as a 'Herb of Undefined Safety'.[G10]

Herbal Use
Plantain is stated to possess diuretic and antihaemorrhagic properties. Traditionally, it has been used for cystitis with haematuria, and specifically for haemorrhoids with bleeding and irritation.[G1,G3,G20,G32]

Dose
Dried leaf 2–4 g or by infusion three times daily[G3]
Liquid extract (1:1 in 25% alcohol) 2–4 mL three times daily[G3]
Tincture (1:5 in 45% alcohol) 2–4 mL three times daily[G3]

Pharmacological Actions
Animal studies An aqueous extract has been reported to possess bronchodilatory activity in guinea-pigs. It was more effective against acetylcholine-induced contraction, than towards constriction induced by histamine or serotonin.[14] The bronchodilatory activity of plantain in guinea-pigs has been reported to be less active and of shorter duration compared to salbutamol or atropine.[15]

Hypotensive activity in normotensive, anaesthetised dogs has been documented; 125 mg/kg extract was found to decrease arterial blood pressure by 20–40 mmHg.[16]

An aqueous extract, reported to contain flavonoids, saponins, steroids and alkaloids, was shown to possess anti-inflammatory activity in the rat using various models of inflammation, and a strengthening of capillary vessels has also been documented.[13] However, an extract was found to exhibit minimal (11%) inhibition of carrageenan induced rat paw oedema.[17] Leaf extracts in hexane have shown potent wound-healing activity in rabbits; the effect was primarily attributed to C_{26}-C_{30} alcohols present in the extract.[18] Both the anti-inflammatory and wound healing activities of plantain have been attributed to the high content of chlorogenic and neochlorogenic acids.[2]

Aucubin and a haemolytic saponin fraction have exhibited antibiotic activity towards *Micrococcus flavus* and *Staphylococcus aureus* (aucubin only).[19] Antibacterial activity towards *Bacillus subtilis* has been documented for the fresh plant juice, which was also found to lack activity towards Gram-positive organisms and fungi.[20] A negative response to cytotoxic, antitumour, and antiviral activity was also reported for the plant juice.[20]

A mild laxative action has been reported in mice administered iridoid glycosides, including aucubin.[21] Plantain seed is sometimes used as a substitute for ispaghula (a bulk laxative).[G22]

Plantain has been documented to lower concentrations of total plasma lipids, cholesterol, β-lipoproteins, and triglycerides in rabbits with experimental atherosclerosis.[22] Plantain has been reported to be useful in lowering plasma-cholesterol concentrations.[23]

A tonus-raising effect on isolated guinea-pig and rabbit uterus tissue has been documented for an aqueous extract at a dose of 1–2 mg/cm³.[24]

Aucubin has been stated to be the active principle responsible for a hepatoprotective effect documented for plantain.[25]

Human studies Plantain has been reported to be effective in the treatment of chronic bronchitis of a spastic or non-spastic nature.[14,26,27] A pronounced improvement in both subjective and objective symptoms of the common cold following treatment with plantain has also been reported.[28] Plantain, in combination with agrimony, German chamomile, peppermint, and St. John's wort, has been documented to provide pain relief in patients with chronic gastroduodenitis.[29] Following treatment, previously diagnosed erosions and haemorrhagic mucous changes were stated to have disappeared.

Side-effects, Toxicity

Allergic contact dermatitis to plantain has been reported.[G26] The green parts of the plant are thought to yield a mustard oil-type of thioglucoside, which releases an irritant principle (isothiocyanate) upon enzymatic hydrolysis.[G26] The seed may also cause sensitisation and dermatitis. Plantain is reported to be of low toxicity with LD_{50} values in the rat documented as 1 g/kg (intraperitoneal injection) and greater than 4 g/kg (by mouth).[15]

Contra-indications, Warnings

Plantain may cause a contact allergic reaction; it induces the formation of IgE antibodies, which may cross-react to psyllium.[30] Excessive doses may exert a laxative effect and a hypotensive effect.
Pregnancy and lactation In-vitro uterotonic activity has been documented for plantain. In view of this, excessive use of plantain, which may also exert a laxative effect, should be avoided during pregnancy.

Pharmaceutical Comment

The constituents of plantain are well documented and the reputed antihaemorrhagic properties are probably attributable to the tannin constituents. In addition, bronchospastic activity has been documented in both animal and human studies, and may warrant further research. The toxicity of plantain is reported to be low but excessive ingestion should be avoided. The bulk laxative ispaghula consists of the dried seeds of related species *Plantago psyllium, P. ovata,* and *P. indica.*[G22]

References

See General References G1, G3, G9, G10, G14, G18, G20, G22, G23, G26, G31, and G32.

1. Andrzejewska-Golec E, Swiatek K. Chemotaxonomic studies on the genus *Plantago* II. Analysis of phenolic acid fraction. *Herba Pol* 1986; **32:** 19–31.

2. Maksyutina NP. Hydroxycinnamic acids of *Plantago major* and *Pl. lanceolata. Khim Prirodn Soedin* 1971; **7:** 795.

3. Smolenski SJ *et al.* Alkaloid screening.IV. *Lloydia* 1974; **37:** 30–61.

4. Pailer M and Haschke-Hofmeister E. Inhaltsstoffe aus Plantago major. *Planta Med* 1969; **17:** 139–45.

5. Popov S *et al.* Cyclopentanoid monoterpenes from *Plantago* species. *Izv Khim* 1981; **14:** 175–80.

6. Maksyutin GV. Amino acids in Plantago (plantain) major leaves and Matricaria recutita inflorescences. *Rastit Resur* 1972; **8:** 110–12.

7. Tomoda M *et al.* Plant mucilages. XXIX. Isolation and characterization of a mucous polysaccharide, plantago-mucilage A, from the seeds of *Plantago major* var. *asiatica. Chem Pharm Bull* 1981; **29:** 2877–84.

8. Lebedev-Kosov VI. Flavonoids of *Plantago major. Khim Prirodn Soedin* 1976; **12:** 730.

9. Lebedev-Kosov VI *et al.* Flavonoids of *Plantago major. Khim Prirodn Soedin* 1977; **13:** 223.

10. Endo T *et al.* The glycosides of *Plantago major* var. *japonica* Nakai. A new flavone glycoside, plantagoside. *Chem Pharm Bull* 1981; **29:** 1000–1004.

11. Oshio H and Inouye H. Two new iridoid glucosides of Plantago asiatica. *Planta Med* 1982; **44:** 204–6.

12. Andrzejewska-Golec E, Swiatek K. Chemotaxonomic studies on the genus *Plantago* I. Analysis of the iridoid fraction. *Herba Pol* 1984; **30:** 9–16.

13. Lambev I *et al.* Study of the anti-inflammatory and capillary restorative activity of a dispersed substance from *Plantago major* L. *Probl Vatr Med* 1981; **9:** 162–9.

14. Koichev A *et al.* Pharmacologic-clinical study of a preparation from *Plantago major. Probl Pneumol Ftiziatr* 1983; **11:** 68–74.

15. Marcov M *et al.* Pharmacologic study of the influence of the disperse substance extracted from Plantago major on bronchial smooth muscles. *Probl Vatr Med* 1980; **8:** 132–9.

16. Kyi KK *et al.* Hypotensive property of *Plantago major* Linn. *J Life Sci* 1971; **4:** 167–71.

17. Mascolo N *et al.* Biological screening of Italian medicinal plants for anti-inflammatory activity. *Phytotherapy Res* 1987: **1:** 28–31.

18. Mironov VA *et al.* Physiologically active alcohols of *Plantago major. Khim-Farm Zh* 1983; **17:** 1321–5.

19. Tarle D. Antibiotic effect of aucubin, saponins and extract of plantain leaf — herba or folium *Plantaginis lanceolata. Farm Glas* 1981; **37:** 351–4.

20. Lin Y-C *et al.* Search for biologically active substances in Taiwan medicinal plants I. Screening for anti-tumor and anti-microbial substances. *Chin J Microbiol* 1972; **5:**76–8.

21. Inouye H *et al.* Purgative activities of iridoid glycosides. *Planta Med* 1974; **25:** 285–8.

22. Maksyutina NP *et al.* Chemical composition and hypocholesterolemic action of some drugs from Plantago major leaves. Part I. Polyphenolic compounds. *Farm Zh (Kiev)* 1978; **(4):** 56–61.

23. Ikram M. Medicinal plants as hypocholesterolemic agents. *JPMA* 1980; **30:** 278–9.

24. Shipochliev T. Extracts from a group of medicinal plants enhancing the uterine tonus. *Vet Med Nauki* 1981; **18** 94–8.

25. Chang I-M and Yun (Choi) HS. Plants with liver-protective activities: pharmacology and toxicology of aucubin. In: Chang HM *et al.* (Eds) *Adv Chin Med Mat Res.* Singapore: World Scientific, 1985; 269.

26.   Koichev A. Complex evaluation of the therapeutic effect of a preparation from Plantago major in chronic bronchitis. *Probl Vatr Med* 1983; **11:** 61–9.

27.   Matev M *et al*. Clinical trial of Plantago major preparation in the treatment of chronic bronchitis. *Vatr Boles* 1982 **21:** 133–7.

28.   Koichev A. Study on the therapeutic effect of different doses from the preparation Plantago major in cold. *Prob Vatr Med* 1982; **10:** 117–24.

29.   Chakarski I *et al*. Clinical study of a herb combination consisting of Agrimonia eupatoria, Hipericum perforatum, Plantago major, Mentha piperita, Matricaria chamomila for the treatment of patients with gastroduodenitis. *Probl Vatr Med* 1982; **10**: 78–84.

30.   Rosenberg S *et al*. Serum IgE antibodies to psyllium in individuals allergic to psyllium and English plantain. *Ann Allergy* 1982; **48:** 294–8.

PLEURISY ROOT

Species (Family)
Asclepias tuberosa L. (Asclepiadaceae)

Synonym(s)
Asclepias

Part(s) Used
Root

Pharmacopoeial Monographs
BHP 1983

Legal Category (Licensed Products)
GSL[G14]

Constituents [G24,G32]
Little chemical information is available for pleurisy root. Cardiac glycosides of the cardenolide type (e.g. afroside, asclepin, calactin, calotropin, gomphoside, syriogenin, syrioside, uscharidin, uscharin, and uzarigenin) have been documented for many *Asclepias* species[1-4] including *A. tuberosa*.[5] Concentrations of cardiac glycosides are reported to vary between *Asclepias* species[1] and individual plant parts,[4] in descending order of latex, stem, leaf, and root.[6]

No other data regarding constituents of the root were located.

Other plant parts Constituents documented for the herb include flavonols (e.g. kaempferol, quercetin) and flavonol glycosides (e.g. rutin and isorhamnetin), amino acids, caffeic acid, chlorogenic acid, choline, carbohydrates (e.g. glucose, fructose, sucrose), β-sitosterol, triterpenes (e.g. α-amyrin and β-amyrin, lupeol, friedelin, viburnitol), volatile oil, resin[G24,7]

Food Use
Pleurisy root is not used in foods.

Herbal Use
Pleurisy root is stated to possess diaphoretic, expectorant, antispasmodic, and carminative properties. It has been used for bronchitis, pneumonitis, influenza, and specifically for pleurisy.[G3,G20,G32]

Dose
Dried root 1–4 g or by infusion three times daily[G3]

Liquid extract (1:1 in 45% alcohol) 1–4 mL three times daily[G3]

Tincture (1:10 in 45% alcohol) 1–5 mL three times daily[G3]

Pharmacological Actions
Animal studies Low doses of extracts of *Asclepias* species including *A. tuberosa* have been documented to cause uterine contractions (*in vivo*) and to exhibit oestrogenic effects.[5,9,10,G12] No effect was observed on blood pressure or respiration (*in vivo*), or on the isolated heart (frog, turtle).[9] Various activities have been reported for related *Asclepias* species. A positive inotropic action (*in vivo* and *in vitro*) has been reported for asclepin (*Asclepias curassavica*), which was found to be more potent, longer-acting, and with a wider safety margin when compared to other cardiac glycosides (including digoxin).[11-13] Asclepin was also reported to exhibit a more powerful activity towards weak cardiac muscle.[13] Plant extracts of *A. curassavica*, *Asclepias engelmanniana* and *Asclepias glaucescens* have exhibited a stimulatory effect on the mammalian CNS, causing an increase in serotonin and noradrenaline concentrations.[14]

Antitumour/cytotoxic activities have been documented for *A. albicans* and were attributed to various cardenolide constituents.[15]

Side-effects, Toxicity
Pleurisy root and other *Asclepias* species have been documented to cause dermatitis; the milky latex is reported to be irritant.[G26] Large doses may cause nausea, vomiting, and diarrhoea.[G3,G20] Various *Asclepias* species, including *A. tuberosa,* are known to be toxic to livestock, with cardenolides implicated as the toxic constituents.[1,5] Toxic effects on the lungs, gastrointestinal tract, kidneys, brain, and spinal cord have been observed in rats and rabbits following intravenous administration of an alcoholic extract.[10]

Toxicity studies involving related *Asclepias* species have also been documented. The cardenolide fraction of *Asclepias eriocarpa* is reported to contain toxic principles. The whole plant, plant extracts, an isolated and purified cardenolide (labriformin), and digoxin were all found to show qualitatively similar signs of toxicity and gross pathology in sheep and guinea-pigs.[16] LD_{50} values (mice, intraperitoneal injection) for cardenolides obtained from *A. curassavica* and *A. eriocarpa* were all estimated at less than 50 mg/kg body-weight. Asclepin (*A. curassavica*) was reported to be safe following a three month toxicity study in rats, using doses of 0.8, 8, and 20 mg/kg (route unspecified).[13] Asclepin has also been documented to have a wider margin of safety than digoxin[11-13] (*see* Animal studies).

Studies in cats have reported asclepin to be less cumulative compared to digoxin.[13]

Contra-indications, Warnings
Pleurisy root may interfere with existing cardiac drug therapy. Excessive doses of pleurisy root may interfere with drug therapies that affect amine concentrations in the brain (e.g. antidepressants) and with hormonal therapy.

Pregnancy and lactation Uterotonic activity (*in vivo*) has been reported for pleurisy root.[5,G12] In view of this and the potential toxicity of pleurisy root, it is best avoided during pregnancy or lactation.

Pharmaceutical Comment

The chemistry of pleurisy root is poorly documented, but phytochemical studies on pleurisy root and related *Asclepias* species have identified many cardiac glycoside constituents. No scientific evidence was found to justify the herbal uses. In view of the potential toxicity of pleurisy root, excessive use is not recommended.

References

See General References G3, G12, G14, G20, G24, G26, and G32.

1.   Seiber JN *et al*. New cardiac glycosides (cardenolides) from *Asclepias* species. *Plant Toxicol. Proceedings of the Aust/USA poisonous plants symposium* 1985; 427–37.

2.   Radford DJ *et al*. Naturally occurring cardiac glycosides. Med J Aust 1986; **144**: P540–4.

3.   Jolad SD *et al*. Cardenolides and a lignan from *Asclepias subulata*. *Phytochemistry* 1986; **25**: 2581–90.

4.   Seiber JN *et al*. Cardenolides in the latex and leaves of seven *Asclepias* species and *Calotropis procera*. *Phytochemistry* 1982; **21**: 2343–8.

5.   Conway GA, Slocumb JC. Plants used as abortifacients and emmenagogues by Spanish New Mexicans. *J Ethnopharmacol* 1979; **1**: 241–61.

6.   Duffey SS, Scudder GGE. Cardiac glycosides in North American Asclepiadaceae, a basis for unpalatability in brightly coloured Hemiptera and Coleoptera. *J Insect Physiol* 1972; **18**: 63–78.

7.   Nelson CJ *et al*. Seasonal and intraplant variation of cardenolide content in the California milkweed *Asclepias eriocarpa* and implications for plant defense. *J Chem Ecol* 1981; **7**: 981–1010.

8.   Pagani F. Plant constituents of *Asclepias tuberosa* (Asclepiadaceae). *Boll Chim Farm* 1975; **114**: 450–6.

9.   Costello CH, Butler CL. The estrogenic and uterine-stimulating activity of *Asclepias tuberosa*. *J Am Pharm Ass Sci Ed* 1949; **39**: 233–7.

10.   Hassan WE, Reed HL. Studies on species of *Asclepias* VI. Toxicology, pathology and pharmacology. *J Am Pharm Ass Sci Ed* 1952; **41**: 298–300.

11.   Patnaik GK, Dhawan BN. Pharmacological investigations on asclepin — a new cardenolide from *Asclepius curassavica*. Part I. Cardiotonic activity and acute toxicity. *Arzneimittelforschung* 1978; **28**: 1095–9.

12.   Patnaik GK, Koehler E. Comparative studies on the inotropic and toxic effects of asclepin, g-strophanthin, digoxin and digitoxin. *Arzneimittelforschung* 1978; **28**: 1368–72.

13.   Dhawan BN, Patnaik GK. Investigation on some new cardioactive glycosides. *Indian Drugs* 1985; **22**: 285–90.

14.   Del Pilar Alvarez Pellitero M. Pharmacological action of medicinal plants in the nervous system. *An Inst Farmacol Espan* 1971; **20**: 299–387.

15.   Koike K *et al*. Potential anticancer agents. V. Cardiac glycosides of *Asclepias albicans* (Asclepiadaceae). *Chem Pharm Bull* 1980; **28**: 401–5.

16.   Benson JM *et al*. Comparative toxicology of cardiac glycosides from the milkweed *Asclepias eriocarpa*. *Toxicol Appl Pharmacol* 1977; **41**: 131–2.

POKEROOT

Species (Family)
Phytolacca americana L. (Phytolaccaceae)

Synonym(s)
Pokeweed, Pocan, Red Plant, *Phytolacca decandra* L.

Part(s) Used
Root

Pharmacopoeial Monographs
BHP 1983
BPC 1934
Martindale 28th edition
Pharmacopoeias—Chin.

Legal Category (Licensed Products)
GSL [G14]

Constituents[G10,G24,G32]

Alkaloids (betalain-type) Betanidine, betanine, isobetanine, isobetanidine, isoprebetanine, phytolaccine, prebetanine

Lectins Pokeweed mitogen (PWM) consisting of five glycoproteins Pa-1 to Pa-5

Saponins Triterpenes — phytolaccosides A-1, D_2, and O,[1–3] aglycones include phytolaccagenin, jaligonic acid, phytolaccagenic acid, aesculentic acid, [2,4–6] acinosolic acid methyl ester;[5] monodesmosidic and bidesmosidic compounds with oleanolic acid and phytolaccagenic acids as aglycone in *P. dodecandra*[7]

Other constituents Isoamericanin A (neo-lignan),[8] (PAP pokeweed antiviral protein)[9], α-spinasterol,[5] histamine, and GABA[10]

Food Use
Pokeroot is not commonly used in foods.   In the USA, the Herb Trade Association has recommended that pokeroot should not be sold as a herbal beverage or food.[11]

Herbal Use
Pokeroot is stated to possess antirheumatic, anticatarrhal, mild anodyne, emetic, purgative, parasiticidal, and fungicidal properties. Traditionally, it has been used for rheumatism, respiratory catarrh, tonsillitis, laryngitis, adenitis, mastitis, mumps, skin infections (e.g. scabies, tinea, sycosis, acne), mammary abscesses, and mastitis.[G3,G32]

Dose
Dried root 0.06–0.3 g or by decoction three times daily[G3]
Liquid extract (1:1 in 45% alcohol) 0.1–0.5 mL three times daily [G3]
Tincture (BPC 1923) 0.2–0.6 mL

Pharmacological Actions

Animal studies Anti-inflammatory activity has been documented for saponin fractions isolated from *P. americana* [2,12] Activity comparable or greater than that of cortisone acetate was observed in the carageenan rat paw oedema test when the extract was administered by intraperitoneal injection. The major aglycone, phytolaccagenin, was reported to exhibit greater activity than glycyrrhetic acid and oleanolic acid, which are both known to be effective in acute inflammation. Oral administration required a six-fold increase in dose for comparable activity.[12] Potency of the saponin extract was reduced to one-eighth of that of cortisone when tested against chronic inflammation (granuloma pouch method).[12] The ED_{50} for saponin and phytolaccagenin fractions against carrageenan-induced oedema in the rat (intraperitoneal injection) has been determined as 15.1 and 26 mg/kg respectively.[12]

Isoamericanin A (a neo-lignan) isolated from the seeds of *P. americana* has been reported to increase prostaglandin I_2 production from the rat aorta by up to about 150 % at a concentration of 10^{-5} and to elicit a moderate inductive effect on the *in-vivo* release of PGI_2.[8]

Hypotensive properties have been described for a pokeroot extract with the activity attributed to histamine and GABA.[10]

A diuretic effect has been described in rats administered pokeroot extract orally at a dose of 500 mg/kg.[13] The effect was reported to be significantly greater than that observed in the saline-treated group of rats, but less than in the frusemide-treated (150 mg/kg) group.

In-vitro contraction of the guinea-pig ileum has been described for pokeroot extracts.[14] Activity was attributed to a single active constituent that proved to be heat resistant.

The properties of pokeweed antiviral protein have been reviewed.[15]

Molluscicidal activity against schistosomiasis-transmitting snails and spermicidal activity have been documented for saponin components obtained from the fruits of the related species, *P. dodecandra*.[7,16,17] An enzyme located in the seeds has been found to be necessary for molluscicidal activity of *P. dodecandra*.[18] Crushing the seeds to release the enzyme is critical for activity. The enzyme is inactivated by heat or alcohol and a cold water extraction of the finely ground fruits was found to provide the greatest molluscicidal activity. The saponin-containing extract of *P. dodecandra* is commonly referred to as 'Endod'.[19] Fruits of *P. americana* also possess molluscicidal properties.[G21]

Abortifacient activity in mice has been exhibited by a related species *P. acinosa* Roxb. with activity strongest in the seed and weakest in the leaf. Activity in the various extracts was destroyed by heat and pepsin suggesting a protein to be the active principle.[20]

Side-effects, Toxicity

Haematological aberrations have been observed in human peripheral blood following oral ingestion of the berries or exposure of broken skin/conjunctival membrane to the berry juice.[21–23] Analysis of peripheral blood revealed plasmacytoid cells, dividing cells, and mature plasmacytes. Eosinophilia was also noted. The mitogenic principles in pokeroot, lectins, are reported to be a mixture of agglutinating and non-agglutinating glycoproteins affecting both T-cell and B-cell lymphocytes.[24]

Pokeroot leaf extracts have been reported to be agglutinating, but lacking in mitogenic activity.[25]

A 43-year old woman suffered the following symptoms 30 minutes after drinking a cup of herbal tea prepared from half a teaspoon of powdered pokeroot: nausea, vomiting, cramping, generalised abdominal pain followed by profound watery diarrhoea, weakness, haematemesis and blood diarrhoea, hypotension, and tachycardia.[26] Chewing the root for the relief of a sore throat and cough has resulted in severe abdominal cramps, protracted vomiting, and profuse watery diarrhoea.[27] Additional symptoms of poisoning that have been documented for pokeroot include difficulty with breathing, spasms, severe convulsions, and death.[28]

The clinical symptoms of pokeroot poisoning have been reviewed.[27]

All parts of the pokeroot plant are considered as potentially toxic, with the root generally recognised as the most toxic part.[27] Toxicity is reported to increase with plant maturity although the young green berries are more toxic compared to the more mature red fruits.[27]

High doses of saponin extracts have produced thymolytic effects in rats.[12]

LD_{50} values for the saponin fraction (intraperitoneal injection) have been determined as 181 mg/kg in mice and 208 mg/kg in rats.[12] In contrast, no deaths were observed in rats administered phytolaccagenin intraperitoneal injection up to a dose of 2 g/kg.[12] Oral doses of saponin up to 1.5 g/kg did not produce any mortalities in treated rats.[12]

The mutagenic potential of *P. americana* and *P. dodecandra* fruit extracts has been tested using *Salmonella typhimurium* strain TM677.[19] No activity was found for any of the extracts tested.

Contra-indications, Warnings

Fresh pokeroot is poisonous and the dried root emetic and cathartic.[G20] The toxic effects documented following the ingestion of pokeroot make it unsuitable for internal ingestion. In addition, external contact with the berry juice should be avoided: systemic symptoms of toxicity have occurred following exposure of broken skin and conjunctival membranes to the juice.

In 1979, the American Herb Trade Association declared that pokeroot should no longer be sold as a herbal beverage or food.[11] It further recommended that all packages containing pokeroot carry an appropriate warning regarding the potential toxicity of pokeroot when taken internally. In the UK, manufacturers of licensed medicinal products are permitted to include pokeroot provided that the dose is restricted and that suitable evidence is given to demonstrate the absence of the toxic protein constituents.

Pregnancy and lactation Pokeroot is reputed to affect the menstrual cycle and is documented to exhibit uterine stimulant activity in animals.[G12]

Pharmaceutical Comment

Apart from its traditional use as a herbal remedy, pokeroot is also known to possess molluscicidal properties. Anti-inflammatory activity documented in animal studies support the traditional use of pokeroot in rheumatism. However, pokeroot is also recognised as a toxic plant. The effects of pokeroot intoxication arise from the ingestion of any or all plant parts, liquid preparations of plant extracts such as herbal teas, or through skin contact with the plant.[27] The main toxic agents are the pokeweed mitogen (lectins) and the glycoside saponins. The toxic properties of these two classes of compounds, mitogenic and irritant respectively, are well recognised. Excessive use of pokeroot cannot be supported in the light of these known toxicities.

References

See General References G3, G5, G10, G12, G14, G20, G21, G24, G32 and G34

1. Woo WS *et al.* Triterpenoid saponins from the roots of *Phytolacca americana*. *Planta Med* 1978; **34:** 87–92.

2. Woo WS *et al.* Constituents of phytolacca species. (I) Antiinflammatory saponins. *Kor J Pharmacog* 1976; **7:** 47–50.

3. Kang SK, Woo WS. Two new saponins from *Phytolacca americana*. *Planta Med* 1987; **53:** 338–4.

4. Kang S, Woo WS. Triterpenes from the berries of *Phytolacca americana*. *J Nat Prod* 1980; **43:** 510–13.

5. Woo WS *et al.* Constituents of *Phytolacca* species (II). Comparative examination on constituents of the roots of *Phytolacca americana, P. esculenta* and *P. insularis. Kor J Pharmacog* 1975; **7:** 51–54.

6. Woo WS and Kang SS. The structure of Phytolaccoside G. *Pharm Soc Korea* 1977; **21:** 159–162.

7. Dorsaz A-C, Hostettmann K. Further saponins from *Phytolacca dodecandra* l'Herit. *Helv Chim Acta* 1986; **69:** 2038–47.

8. Hasegawa T *et al.* Structure of isoamericanin A, a prostaglandin I_2 inducer, isolated from the seeds of *Phytolacca americana* L. *Chem Lett* 1987; **2:** 329–32.

9. Ready MP *et al.* Extracellular localization of pokeweed antiviral protein. *Proc Natl Acad Sci USA* 1986; **83:** 5033–56.

10. Funayama S, Hikino H. Hypotensive principles of *Phytolacca* roots. *J Nat Prod* 1979; **42:** 672–4.

11. Tyler VE *et al.* Poke root. In: Pharmacognosy. 8th edn. Philadelphia: Lea and Febiger, 1981; 493–4.

12. Woo WS, Shin KH. Antiinflammatory action of *Phytolacca* saponin. *J Pharm Soc Korea* 1976; **20:** 149–55.

13. Anokbonggo WW. Diuretic effect of an extract from the roots of *Phytolacca dodecandra* l'Herit in the rat. *Biochem Biol* 1975; **11:** 275–7.

14. Anokbonggo WW. Extraction of pharmacologically active constituents of the roots of *Phytolacca dodecandra*. *Planta Med* 1975; **28**: 69–75.

15. Irvin JD. Pokeweed antiviral protein. *Pharmac Ther* 1983; **21**: 371–87.

16. Adewunmi CO, Marzuis VO. Comparative evaluation of the molluscicidal properties of aridan (*Tetrapleura tetrapleura*) laplapa pupa (*Jatropha gossypyfolia*) endod (*Phytolacca dodecandra*) and bayluscide. *Fitoterapia* 1987; **58**: 325–8.

17. Dorsaz A-C, Hostettmann K. Further saponins from *Phytolacca dodecandra*: their molluscicidal and spermicidal properties. *Planta Med* 1986; **52**: 557–8.

18. Parkhurst RM *et al*. The molluscicidal activity of *Phytolacca dodecandra*. I. Location of the activating esterase. *Biochem Biophys Res Comm* 1989; **158**: 436–9.

19. Pezzuto JM *et al*. Evaluation of the mutagenic potential of endod (*Phytolacca dodecandra*), a molluscicide of potential value for the control of schistosomiasis. *Toxicol Lett* 1984; **22**: 15–20.

20. Yeung HW *et al*. Abortifacient activity in leaves, roots and seeds of *Phytolacca acinosa*. *J Ethnopharmacol* 1987; **21**: 31–5.

21. Barker BE *et al*. Haematological effects of pokeweed. *Lancet* 1967; **i**: 437.

22. Barker BE *et al*. Peripheral blood plasmacytosis following systemic exposure to *Phytolacca americana* (pokeweed). *Pediatrics* 1966; **38**: 490–3.

23. Barker BE *et al*. Mitogenic activity in *Phytolacca americana* (pokeweed). *Lancet* 1965; **i**: 170.

24. McPherson A. Pokeweed and other lymphocyte mitogens. In: Toxic plants. Kinghorn AD, editor. New York: Columbia University Press, 1979; 84–102.

25. Downing HJ *et al*. Plant agglutinins and mitosis. *Nature* 1968; **217**: 655.

26. Lewis WH, Smith PR. Pokeroot herbal tea poisoning. *JAMA* 1979; **242**: 2759–60.

27. Roberge R *et al*. The root of evil — poke weed intoxication. *Ann Emerg Med* 1986; **15**: 470–3.

28. Hardin JW, Arena JM. Human poisoning from native and cultivated plants. 2nd ed. Durham: Duke University Press, 1974: 69–73.

POPLAR

Species (Family)
Populus tremuloides Michx. (Salicaceae)

Synonym(s)
Populus Alba, Quaking Aspen, White Poplar

Part(s) Used
Bark

Pharmacopoeial Monographs
BHP 1983

Legal Category (Licensed Products)
GSL[G14]

Constituents[G2,G17,G18,G32]
Glycosides Salicin (about 2.4%), salicortin, salireposide and various benzoate derivatives including populin (salicin-6-benzoate), tremuloidin (salicin-2-benzoate), tremulacin (salicortin-2-benzoate)

Other constituents Tannins (unspecified), triterpenes including fats, waxes, α-amyrin and β-amyrin, carbohydrates including glucose, fructose and various trisaccharides

Food Use
Poplar is listed by the Council of Europe as a natural source of food flavouring (category N2). This category indicates that poplar can be added to foodstuffs in small quantities, with a possible limitation of an active principle (as yet unspecified) in the final product.[G9]

Herbal Use
Poplar is stated to possess antirheumatic, anti-inflammatory, antiseptic, astringent, anodyne, and cholagogue properties. Traditionally, it has been used for muscular and arthrodial rheumatism, cystitis, diarrhoea, anorexia with stomach or liver disorders, common cold, and specifically for rheumatoid arthritis.[G2,G3,G32]

The buds of *Populus tremula* (European white poplar, aspen) and *Populus nigra* (black poplar) are used, reputedly as expectorant and circulatory stimulant remedies, for upper respiratory-tract infections and rheumatic conditions.[G25]

Dose
Dried bark 1–4 g or by decoction three times daily[G2,G3]

Liquid extract (1:1 in 25% alcohol) 1–4 mL three times daily[G2,G3]

Pharmacological Actions
Animal studies None documented for poplar. *See* Willow for the pharmacological actions associated with salicylates.

Human studies None documented for poplar. The pharmacological actions of salicylates in man are well documented and are applicable to poplar. Salicin is a prodrug that is metabolised to saligenin in the gastro-intestinal tract and to salicylic acid following absorption.

Side-effects, Toxicity
None documented. *See* Willow for side-effects and toxicity associated with salicylates.

Contra-indications, Warnings
See Willow for contra-indications and warnings associated with salicylates.

Pregnancy and lactation The safety of poplar taken during pregnancy has not been established. *See* Willow for contra-indications and warnings regarding the use of salicylates during pregnancy and lactation.

Pharmaceutical Comment
The chemistry of poplar is characterised by the phenolic glycoside components, which support some of the reputed herbal uses. The usual precautions associated with other salicylate-containing drugs are applicable to poplar.

References
See General References G2, G3, G9, G14, G17, G18, G25, G32

PRICKLY ASH, NORTHERN

Species (Family)
Zanthoxylum americanum Miller (Rutaceae)

Synonym(s)
Toothache Bark, Xanthoxylum, Zanthoxylum

Part(s) Used
Bark, Berry

Pharmacopoeial Monographs
BHP 1983
BPC 1934
Martindale 30th edition
Pharmacopoeias—Chin. and Jpn, which include Powdered
Zanthoxylum Fruit.

Legal Category (Licensed Products)
Northern prickly ash is not included on the GSL[G14]

Constituents[G2,G19,G32]
Alkaloids (isoquinoline-type) Lauriflorine and nitidine
(major constituents), candicine, chelerythrine, magnoflorine, tembetarine
Coumarins Xanthyletin, xanthoxyletin, alloxanthoxyletin,
8-(3,3-dimethylallyl)alloxanthoxyletin
Other constituents Resins, tannins, acrid volatile oil
Other plant parts Two furoquinoline alkaloids (γ-fagarine
and skimmianine) have been isolated from the leaves.

Food Use
Prickly ash is listed by the Council of Europe as a natural
source of food flavouring (category N3). This category
indicates that prickly ash can be added to foodstuffs in the
traditionally accepted manner, but that there is insufficient
information available for an adequate assessment of potential toxicity.[G9]

Herbal Use
Prickly ash is stated to possess circulatory stimulant, diaphoretic, antirheumatic, carminative, and sialagogue properties. Traditionally, it has been used for cramps,
intermittent claudication, Raynaud's syndrome, chronic
rheumatic conditions, and specifically for peripheral circulatory insufficiency associated with rheumatic symptoms.
The berries are stated to be therapeutically more active in
circulatory disorders.[G2,G3,G32]

Dose
Dried bark 1–3 g or by decoction three times daily[G2,G3]

Bark, Liquid extract (1:1 in 45% alcohol) 1–3 mL three
times daily[G2,G3]

Bark, Tincture (1:5 in 45% alcohol) 2–5 mL three times
daily[G2,G3] **Dried berry** 0.5–1.5 g[G2,G3]

Berry, Liquid extract (1:1 in 45% alcohol) 0.5–1.5 mL[G2,G3]

Pharmacological Actions
Animal studies None documented for northern prickly ash.
See Southern prickly ash for activities of alkaloid constituents (e.g. chelerythrine and nitidine).

Side-effects, Toxicity
The alkaloid constituents are potentially toxic (*see* Southern
prickly ash).

Contra-indications, Warnings
Excessive ingestion may interfere with anticoagulant therapy in view of the coumarin constituents (*see* Southern
prickly ash).

Pregnancy and lactation The safety of northern prickly ask
has not been established. In view of the pharmacologically
active constituents the use of northern prickly ash during
pregnancy and lactation should be avoided.

Pharmaceutical Comment
Northern prickly ash contains similar alkaloid constituents
to the southern species but varies with respect to other documented components. No pharmacological studies documented specifically for northern prickly ash were located.
However, activities have been reported for individual alkaloid constituents and the monograph for southern prickly
ash should be consulted. There is limited scientific evidence
to support the traditional herbal uses. In view of the pharmacologically active constituents and potential toxicity
associated with the alkaloids, excessive use of northern
prickly ash should be avoided.

References
See General References G2, G3, G5, G9, G14, G19, G22, and G32.

220

PRICKLY ASH, SOUTHERN

Species (Family)
Zanthoxylum clava-herculis L. (Rutaceae)

Synonym(s)
Toothache Bark, Xanthoxylum, Zanthoxylum

Part(s) Used
Bark, Berry

Pharmacopoeial Monographs
BHP 1983
BHP 1990
BPC 1934
Martindale 30th edition
Pharmacopoeias—Chin. and Jpn, which includes Powdered
Zanthoxylum Fruit

Legal Category (Licensed Products)
GSL[G14]

Constituents[G2, G19, G22, G32]
Alkaloids (isoquinoline-type) Chelerythrine and magnoflorine (major constituents), candicine, lauriflorine, nitidine, *N*-acetylanonaine [1], tembetarine
Amides Cinnamamide, herculin, neoherculin
Lignans (−)-Asarinin, (−)-sesamin, γ,γ-dimethylallyl ether of (−)-pluviatilol[1]
Other constituents Resins, tannins, an acrid volatile oil (about 3.3%)

Food Use
Southern prickly ash is listed by the Council of Europe as a natural source of food flavouring (category N3). This category indicates that prickly ash can be added to foodstuffs in the traditionally accepted manner, but that there is insufficient information available for an adequate assessment of potential toxicity.[G9]

Herbal Use
Southern prickly ash is stated to possess circulatory stimulant, diaphoretic, antirheumatic, carminative, and sialogogue properties. Traditionally, it has been used for cramps, intermittent claudication, Raynaud's syndrome, chronic rheumatic conditions, and specifically for peripheral circulatory insufficiency associated with rheumatic symptoms. The berries are stated to be therapeutically more active in circulatory disorders.[G2,G3,G4,G32]

Dose
Dried bark 1–3 g or by decoction three times daily[G2,G3]
Bark, Liquid extract (1:1 in 45% alcohol) 1–3 mL three times daily[G2,G3]

Bark, Tincture (1:5 in 45% alcohol) 2–5 mL three times daily[G2,G3]
Dried berry 0.5–1.5 g[G2,G3]
Berry, Liquid extract (1:1 in 45% alcohol) 0.5–1.5 mL[G2,G3]

Pharmacological Actions
Animal studies Southern prickly ash has been reported to act as a reversible neuromuscular blocking agent. Activity was associated with a neutral fraction of the bark that was thought to act primarily by blockade of endplate receptors.[2]
Various activities have been documented for the benzophenanthridine alkaloids (e.g. chelerythrine, nitidine) present in southern prickly ash. Hypotensive properties in mice have been documented for nitidine chloride, a single dose of 2 mg/kg body-weight lowered the blood pressure by 20% within 90 minutes and persisted for six hours.[3] Nitidine was also found to antagonise the effects of angiotensin induced hypertension.[3] Antileukaemic activity has been documented for nitidine, although preclinical toxicity prevented further investigations.[4,5]
Anti-inflammatory activity in rats has been documented for chelerythrine (10 mg/kg by mouth) comparable to that achieved with indomethacin (5 mg/kg by mouth).[6] Chelerythrine has also been reported to potentiate the analgesic effect of morphine, prolong barbiturate-induced sleep, and cause temporary hypertension followed by hypotension in cats, mice, and rabbits.[7]
Significant antimicrobial activity towards Gram-positive bacteria and *Candida albicans* has been documented for chelerythrine, although conflicting activities have been reported regarding Gram-negative bacteria.[6] Chelerythrine has been shown to interact with Na+K+ ATPase and to inhibit hepatic L-alanine and L-aspartate aminotransferases in the rat, while nitidine has been reported to inhibit *t*-RNA methyltransferase and catechol-*O*-methyltransferase.[5]
The lignan component, asarinin, has been reported to possess antitubercular activity.[G19] Neoherculin is reported to possess insecticidal and sialogogic properties.[1]
Pharmacological activities, including anti-inflammatory, cardiovascular, and antibacterial properties have been documented for various other *Zanthoxylum* (or *Fagara/Xanthoxylum*) species.[5] For example, the root of *Zanthoxylum zanthoxyloides*, a Nigerian species, is commonly used as a chewing stick. These sticks are believed to possess antimicrobial properties and extracts were found to exhibit antimicrobial activity towards more than 20 organisms, including Gram-positive and Gram-negative bacteria, and *Candida* species.[5] Anti-inflammatory activity (carrageenan rat paw oedema test) has been described for fagaramide (piperonyl-4-acrylic isobutylamide), isolated from *Z. zanthoxyloides*.[8] The activity, approximately twenty times less potent than indomethacin, was thought to be partially mediated by inhibition of prostaglandin synthesis.[8]

The essential oil obtained from the Indian species *Zanthoxylum limonella* has been reported to exhibit *in-vitro* anthelmintic activity against earthworms, tapeworms, and hookworms that was stated to be superior to that of piperazine phosphate.[9]

Side-effects, Toxicity

None documented in humans. Ingestion of southern prickly ash by cattle, chicken, and fish has proved lethal. This was attributed to the neuromuscular blocking properties of the bark.[2] Neoherculin is reported to be the major ichthyotoxic principle in an extract of southern prickly ash bark.

The acute and chronic toxicity of chelerythrine in mice is reported to be low.[4] LD_{50} values were stated as 18.5 mg/kg body-weight (intravenous injection) and 95 mg/kg (subcutaneous injection). Oral administration of 10 mg/kg for three days followed by 5 mg/kg for seven days produced no adverse effects.

Contra-indications, Warnings

None documented for southern prickly ash. Chelerythrine has been reported to interact with Na^+K^+ ATPase which may interfere with cardiac glycoside therapy. However the clinical relevance of this with respect to prickly ash is unknown. Hypotensive and sedative activities have been documented in animals. Both chelerythrine and nitidine have been reported to inhibit various hepatic enzymes (*see* Animal studies). The alkaloid constituents in southern prickly ash are potentially toxic.

Pregnancy and lactation The safety of southern prickly ash has not been established. In view of this and the pharmacologically active compounds, the use of southern prickly ash during pregnancy and lactation is best avoided.

Pharmaceutical Comment

The chemistry of southern prickly ash is well documented and particularly characterised by the alkaloid constituents. Limited pharmacological information has been documented for southern prickly ash, although several properties have been described for individual constituents. With the exception of anti-inflammatory and analgesic properties few data have been documented that support the herbal uses. Limited toxicity data are available and some benzophenanthridine alkaloids are associated with cytotoxicity. In view of this, excessive use of prickly ash should be avoided. Northern prickly ash has been used for similar herbal uses but has a different chemical composition compared to the southern species. Refer to northern prickly ash monograph.

References

See General References G2, G3, G4, G5, G9, G14, G19, G22, G23, and G32

1. Rao KV, Davies R. The ichthyotoxic principles of *Zanthoxylum clava-herculis. J Nat Prod* 1986; **49**(2): 340–2.

2. Bowen JM, Cole RJ. Neuromuscular blocking properties of southern prickly ash toxin. *Fed Proc* 1981; **40**: 696.

3. Addae-Mensah I *et al*. Structure and anti-hypertensive properties of nitidine chloride from *Fagara* species. *Planta Med* 1986; **52**:(Suppl) 58.

4. Krane BD *et al*. The benzophenanthridine alkaloids. *J Nat Prod* 1984; **47**: 1–43.

5. Simánek, V. Benzophenanthridine alkaloids. In: Brossi A, editor. The Alkaoids, vol 26. New York: Academic Press, 1985: 185–240.

6. Lenfield J *et al*. Antiinflammatory activity of quaternary benzophenanthridine alkaloids from *Chelidonium majus*. *Planta Med* 1981; **43**: 161–5.

7. Preininger V. In: Manske RHF, editor. The Alkaloids, vol 15. New York: Academic Press, 1975: 242.

8. Oriowo MA. Anti-inflammatory activity of piperonyl-4-acrylic isobutyl amide, an extractive from *Zanthoxylum zanthoxyloides*. *Planta Med* 1982; **44**: 54–6.

9. Kalyani GA *et al*. *In vitro* anthelmintic acitivity of essential oil from the fruits of *Zanthoxylum limonella*. *Fitoterapia* 1989; **60**: 160–2.

PULSATILLA

Species (Family)
(i) *Anemone pulsatilla* L. (Ranunculaceae)
(ii) *Anemone pratensis* L.
(iii) *Anemone patens* L.

Synonym(s)
Pasque Flower, *Pulsatilla nigrans*

Part(s) Used
Herb

Pharmacopoeial Monographs
BHP 1983
BHP 1990
BPC 1934
Martindale 30th edition

Legal Category (Licensed Products)
GSL[G14]

Constituents[G2,G10,G24,G32]
Flavonoids Delphinidin and pelargonidin glycosides
Saponins Hederagenin (as the aglycone)
Volatile oils Ranunculin (a glycoside); enzymatic hydrolysis yields the unstable lactone protoanemonin which readily dimerises to anemonin
Other constituents Carbohydrates (e.g. arabinose, fructose, galactose, glucose, rhamnose), triterpenes (e.g. β-amyrin), β-sitosterol

Food Use
Pulsatilla is not used in foods.

Herbal Use
Pulsatilla is stated to possess sedative, analgesic, antispasmodic, and bactericidal properties. Traditionally, it has been used for dysmenorrhoea, orchitis, ovaralgia, epididymitis, tension headache, hyperactive states, insomnia, boils, skin eruptions associated with bacterial infection, asthma and pulmonary disease, earache, and specifically for painful conditions of the male or female reproductive system.[G2,G3,G4,G32] Pulsatilla is widely used in homoeopathic preparations as well as in herbal medicine.

Dose
Dried herb 0.12–0.3 g by infusion or decoction three times daily[G2,G3]
Liquid extract (1:1 in 25% alcohol) 0.12–0.3 mL three times daily[G2,G3]
Tincture (1:10 in 40% alcohol) 0.3–1.0 mL three times daily[G2,G3]

Pharmacological Actions
Animal studies Uteroactivity (stimulant and depressant) has been documented for pulsatilla.[1,2,G12] *In-vivo* sedative and antipyretic properties in rodents have been documented for anemonin and protoanemonin.[3]

Cytotoxicity (KB tumour system) has been reported for anemonin.[G10]

Side-effects, Toxicity
Fresh pulsatilla is poisonous because of the toxic volatile oil component, protoanemonin. Protoanemonin rapidly degrades to the non-toxic anemonin. Inhalation of vapour from the volatile oil may cause irritation of the nasal mucosa and conjunctiva.[G26] Allergic reactions to pulsatilla have been documented and patch tests have produced vesicular reactions with hyperpigmentation.[G26] Cytotoxicity has been documented for anemonin (*see* Animal studies).

Contra-indications, Warnings
Fresh pulsatilla is poisonous and should not be ingested. External contact with the fresh plant should be avoided. The toxic principle, protoanemonin, rapidly degrades to the non-toxic anemonin during drying of the plant material. Individuals may experience an allergic reaction to pulsatilla, especially those with an existing hypersensitivity.

Pregnancy and lactation Pulsatilla is reputed to affect the menstrual cycle.[G10] Uteroactivity has been documented for pulsatilla (*see* Animal studies). In view of this, the use of pulsatilla during pregnancy should be avoided. Excessive ingestion is best avoided during lactation.

Pharmaceutical Comment
Pulsatilla is widely used in both herbal and homoeopathic preparations, although little documented chemical and pharmacological information is available to assess its true benefit. The fresh plant is known to be irritant; it contains a toxic principle (protoanemonin) and should not be ingested. The dried plant material is not considered to be toxic.

References
See General References G2, G3, G4, G5, G10, G12, G14, G22, G24, G26, and G32.

1. Pilcher JM *et al*. The action of the so-called female remedies on the excised uterus of the guinea-pig. *Arch Intern Med* 1916; **18:** 557–83.

2. Pilcher JM *et al*. The action of "female remedies" on intact uteri of animals. *Surg Gynecol Obstet* 1918; **18:** 97–9.

3. Martin ML *et al*. Pharmacological effects of lactones isolated from *Pulsatilla alpina* subsp. *apiifolia*. *J Ethnopharmacol* 1988; **24:** 185–91.

QUASSIA

Species (Family)
(i) *Picrasma excelsa* (Sw.) Planch. (Simaroubaceae)
(ii) *Quassia amara* L.

Synonym(s)
Bitterwood, Picrasma
(i) Jamaican Quassia, *Picraena excelsa* Lindl.
(ii) Surinam Quassia

Part(s) Used
Stem wood

Pharmacopoeial Monographs
BHP 1983
BHP 1990
BPC 1973
Martindale 30th edition
Pharmacopoeias—Egypt., Fr., and Jpn. All allow Jamaican or Surinam quassia.

Legal Category (Licensed Products)
GSL[G14]

Constituents[G1,G2,G10,G19,G32]
Alkaloids (indole-type) Canthin-6-one, 5-methoxycanthin-6-one, 4-methoxy-5-hydroxycanthin-6-one, *N*-methoxy-1-vinyl-β-carboline[1,2]
Terpenoids Isoquassin (picrasmin) in *P. excelsa*, quassin 0.2%, quassinol, quassimarin,[3] 18-hydroxyquassin, neoquassin, a dihydronorneoquassin[4] and simalikalactone D in *Q. amara*
Coumarins Scopoletin[1]
Other constituents β-Sitosterol, β-sitostenone; thiamine 1.8% (in *P. excelsa*).

Food Use
Quassia is listed by the Council of Europe as a natural source of food flavouring (category N2). This category indicates that quassia can be added to foodstuffs in small quantities, although the concentration of quassin must not exceed 5 mg/kg; a concentration of 50 mg/kg is permitted in alcoholic beverages, and 10 mg/kg in pastilles and lozenges.[G9] In the USA, quassia is regarded by the FDA as GRAS (Generally Regarded As Safe).

Herbal Use
Quassia is stated to possess bitter, orexigenic, sialogogue, gastric stimulant, and anthelmintic properties. Traditionally, it has been used for anorexia, dyspepsia, nematode infestation (by oral or rectal administration), pediculosis (by topical application), and specifically for atonic dyspepsia with loss of appetite.[G1,G2,G3,G4,G32]

Dose
Dried wood 0.3–0.6g or by cold infusion three times daily[G2,G3]
Concentrated Quassia Infusion (BPC 1959) 2–4 mL. **Quassia Infusion** is prepared by diluting one volume of Concentrated Quassia Infusion to eight volumes with water
Tincture of Quassia (BP 1948) 2–4 mL
Enema (infusion with cold water, 1 in 20) 150 mL per rectum on 3 successive mornings together with 16 g magnesium sulphate by mouth.

Pharmacological Actions
The quassinoids are reported to possess bitter properties 50 times greater than quinine.[G10]
Animal studies The β-carboline alkaloids have exhibited positive inotropic activity *in vitro*.[1] Canthin-6-one is reported to possess antibacterial and antifungal activity. Cytotoxic and amoebicidal activities (assessed against guinea-pig keratinocyte and *Entamoeba histolytica* test systems, respectively) have been documented for canthin-6-one and quassin (*P. excelsa*).[5] However, later studies have disputed any amoebicidal action. Quassin is reported to be inactive against P388 leukaemia and 9KB test systems. Significant antitumour activity in mice against the P388 lymphatic leukaemia and *in vitro* against human carcinoma of the nasopharynx (KB) has been documented.[3] Quassimarin and simalikalactone were both isolated from the active extract.
Human studies The successful treatment of 454 patients with head lice has been documented for quassia tincture.[6] Quassia has been used as an enema to expel threadworms.[G21]

Side-effects, Toxicity
No side-effects have been reported in 454 patients who used quassia tincture as a scalp lotion to treat headlice.[6] Large doses of quassia may irritate the stomach and cause vomiting.[G2]

Contra-indications, Warnings
Excessive doses may interfere with existing cardiac and anticoagulant therapies. However, the coumarin concentrations in quassia are not thought to pose a hazard. In addition, large doses of quassia are emetic and therefore excessive consumption is self-limiting.
Pregnancy and lactation In view of the reported cytotoxic and emetic activities, the use of quassia during pregnancy and lactation is best avoided.

Pharmaceutical Comment
The chemistry of quassia is well studied and is characterised by bitter terpenoids (quassinoids) and β-carboline indole alkaloids. Limited data have been documented to justify the traditional herbal uses although the bitter princi-

ples support the use of quassia as an appetite stimulant in anorexia. However, in view of the documented cytotoxic activities and limited toxicological data, quassia in herbal remedies should not be taken in amounts greatly exceeding those used in foods.

References

See General References G1,G2,G3,G4,G7,G9,G10,G14,G19,G21, G22,G23, and G32.

1.   Wagner H *et al*. New constituents of *Picrasma excelsa*, I. *Planta Med* 1979; **36:** 113–18.

2.   Wagner H, Nestler T. *N*-Methoxy-1-vinyl-β-carbolin, ein neues Alkaloid aus *Picrasma excelsa* (Swartz) Planchon. *Tetrahedron Letters* 1978; **31:** 2777–8.

3.   Kupchan SM, Streelman DR. Quassimarin, a new antileukemic quassinoid from *Quassia amara. J Org Chem* 1976; **41:** 3481–2.

4.   Grandolini G *et al*. A new neoquassin derivative from *Quassia amara. Phytochemistry* 1987; **26:** 3085–7.

5.   Harris A, Phillipson JD. Cytotoxic and amoebicidal compounds from *Picrasma excelsa* (Jamaican Quassia). *J Pharm Pharmacol* 1982; **34:** 43P.

6.   Jensen O *et al*. Pediculosis capitis treated with quassia tincture. *Acta Dermat Venereol (Stockholm)* 1978; **58:** 557–9.

QUEEN'S DELIGHT

Species (Family)

Stillingia sylvatica L. (Euphorbiaceae)

Synonym(s)

Queen's Root, Stillingia, *Stillingia treculeana* (Muell. Arg.) Johnst., Yaw Root

Part(s) Used

Root

Pharmacopoeial Monographs

BHP 1983

BPC 1934

Legal Category (Licensed Products)

GSL[G14]

Constituents[G19,G24,G32]

Terpenoids Eight compounds, termed Stillingia factors S_1-S_8 have been isolated and identified as daphnane-type and tigliane-type esters carrying saturated, polyunsaturated or hydroxylated fatty acids.[1]

Other constituents Volatile oil 3–4%, fixed oil, acrid resin (sylvacrol), resinic acid, stillingine (a glycoside), tannin

Other plant parts Hydrocyanic acid (leaf and stem)[1]

Food Use

Queen's delight is not used in foods.

Herbal Use

Queen's delight is stated to possess sialogogue, expectorant, diaphoretic, dermatological, astringent, antispasmodic, and in large doses, cathartic properties. Traditionally, it has been used for bronchitis, laryngitis, laryngismus stridulus, cutaneous eruptions, haemorrhoids, constipation, and specifically for exudative skin eruption with irritation and lymphatic involvement, and laryngismus stridulus.[G3,G32]

Dose

Dried root 1–2 g or by decoction three times daily[G3]

Liquid extract (1:1 in 25% alcohol) 0.5–2.0 mL three times daily[G3]

Tincture (1:5 in 45% alcohol) 1–4 mL three times daily[G3]

Pharmacological Actions

None documented.

Side-effects, Toxicity

Overdose of queen's delight is reported to cause vertigo, burning sensation of the mouth, throat, and gastro-intestinal tract, diarrhoea, nausea and vomiting, dysuria, aches and pains, pruritus and skin eruptions, cough, depression, fatigue, and perspiration.[G10] The diterpene esters are toxic irritant principles known to cause swelling and inflammation of the skin and mucous membranes.[1,G13]

The leaves and stem are documented to be toxic to sheep because of the hydrocyanic acid content.[2]

Contra-indications, Warnings

In view of the irritant nature of the diterpene esters, queen's delight may cause irritation to the mucous membranes. It is stated that queen's delight should be used with care, and never taken in large doses.[G25] It is recommended that the root should not be used after two years of storage.[G25]

Pregnancy and lactation In view of the irritant and potentially toxic constituents, the use of queen's delight during pregnancy and lactation should be avoided.

Pharmaceutical Comment

The Euphorbiaceae plant family is characterised by the diterpene esters. These compounds, known as phorbol, ingenane, or daphnane esters depending on their skeleton type, have been investigated as constituents of genera such as *Euphorbia* and *Croton*, and some of them have been found to be co-carcinogenic and highly irritant to mucous membranes.[G13] No scientific evidence was found to justify the reputed herbal uses. In view of this and the potential toxicity of queen's delight excessive use is not recommended.

References

See General References G3,G5,G10,G13,G14,G19,G24,G25 and G32.

1. Adolf W and Hecker E. New irritant diterpene-esters from roots of *Stillingia sylvatica* L. (Euphorbiaceae). *Tetrahedron Lett* 1980; **21**: 2887–90.

2. Lewis WH and Elvin-Lewis MPF. Medical Botany. New York: Wiley Interscience, 1977.

RASPBERRY

Species (Family)
Rubus idaeus L. (Rosaceae)

Synonym(s)
Rubus

Part(s) Used
Leaf

Pharmacopoeial Monographs
BHP 1983
BPC 1949
Martindale 30th edition

Legal Category (Licensed Products)
GSL[G14]

Constituents[G1,G29,G31,G32]
Limited phytochemical information is available for raspberry. Documented constituents include acids, polypeptides, tannins, and flavonoids (e.g. rutin).[1]

Food Use
Both the leaf and fruit are listed by the Council of Europe as natural sources of food flavouring (categories N2 and N1 respectively). Category N2 allows the addition of the leaf to foodstuffs in small quantities, with a possible limitation of an active principle (as yet unspecified) in the final product. Category N1 indicates that no restrictions apply to the fruit.[G9] Raspberry fruit is commonly used in foods.

Herbal Use
Raspberry is stated to possess astringent and *partus praeparator* properties. Traditionally, it has been used for diarrhoea, pregnancy, stomatitis, tonsillitis (as a mouthwash), conjunctivitis (as an eye lotion), and specifically to facilitate parturition.[G1,G3,G32]

Dose
Dried leaf 4–8 g or by infusion three times daily[G3]
Liquid extract (1:1 in 25% alcohol) 4–8 mL three times daily[G3]

Pharmacological Actions
Animal studies Uteroactivity has been documented for a leaf infusion in both pregnant and non-pregnant rat and human uteri.[2] The extract was reported to have little or no effect on the uterine strips from non-pregnant rats, but inhibited contractions of those from pregnant rats. Similarly, the extract had no effect on strips from non-pregnant human uteri, but initiated contractions in strips from human uteri at 10 to 16 weeks of pregnancy. The intrinsic rhythm of the uteri in which a pharmacological effect was observed (pregnant rat and human uteri) was reported to become more regular, with contractions, in most cases, less frequent.[2] Aqueous extracts of raspberry leaves have been reported to contain a number of active constituents, including a smooth muscle stimulant, an anticholinesterase, and an antispasmodic that antagonised the stimulant actions of the two previous fractions. The smooth muscle stimulant fraction was more potent towards uterine muscle.[3]

Hypoglycaemic activity has been documented for a related species *Rubus fructicosus* L. in both non-diabetic and diabetic (glucose-induced and alloxan-induced) rabbits.[4] Greatest activity was observed in the glucose-induced diabetic rabbits. The authors concluded that *R. fructicosus* possesses slight hypoglycaemic activity, which, in part, results from an increase in the liberation of insulin. Tannins are known to possess astringent properties.

In-vitro antiviral activity documented for raspberry fruit extract has been attributed to the phenolic constituents, in particular to tannic acid.[5]

Side-effects, Toxicity
None documented.

Contra-indications, Warnings
The excessive ingestion of tannins is not recommended. Hypoglycaemic activity *in vivo* has been documented for a related species.

Pregnancy and lactation Raspberry is traditionally recommended for use during labour to help ease parturition. Animal studies (*in vitro*) have reported that raspberry can reduce and initiate uterine contractions. In view of this, raspberry should not be used during pregnancy and, if taken during labour, should only be done so under medical supervision.

Pharmaceutical Comment
Limited phytochemical information is available for raspberry leaf. However, the documented presence of tannin constituents supports some of the reputed herbal uses, although it is unsuitable to use as a herbal remedy to treat eye infections such as conjunctivitis. Raspberry leaf is widely recommended to be taken during pregnancy to help facilitate easier parturition. Uteroactivity has been documented for raspberry leaf and in view of this it should not be taken during pregnancy, unless under medical supervision.

References
See General References G1,G3,G6,G9,G14,G22,G23,G29,G31, and G32.

1. Khabibullaeva LA, Khalmatov KK. Phytochemical study of raspberry leaves. *Mater Yubileinoi Resp Nauchn Konf Farm Posvyashch* 1972; (Sept) 101–2.

2. Bamford DS *et al*. Raspberry leaf tea: a new aspect to an old problem. *Br J Pharmacol* 1970; **40**: 161–2P.

3. Beckett AH *et al*. The active constituents of raspberry leaves. A preliminary investigation. *J Pharm Pharmacol* 1954; **6**: 785–96.

4. Alonso R *et al*. A preliminary study of hypoglycaemic activity of *Rubus fruticosus*. *Planta Med* 1980; **40**(Suppl): 102–6.

5. Konowalchuk JK, Speirs JI. Antiviral activity of fruit extracts. *J Food Science* 1976; **41**: 1013–17.

RED CLOVER

Species (Family)
Trifolium pratense L. (Leguminosae)

Synonym(s)
Cow Clover, Meadow Clover, Purple Clover, Trefoil

Part(s) Used
Flowerhead

Pharmacopoeial Monographs
BHP 1983
BHP 1990

Legal Category (Licensed Products)
GSL[G14]

Constituents[G2,G10,G19,G32]
Carbohydrates Arabinose, glucose, glucuronic acid, rhamnose, xylose (following hydrolysis of saponin glycosides); polysaccharide (a galactoglucomannan)
Coumarins Coumarin, medicagol
Isoflavonoids Biochanin A, daidzein, formononetin, genistein, pratensin, trifoside, calycosine galactoside,[1] pectolinarin
Flavonoids Isorhamnetin, kaempferol, quercetin, and their glycosides[2]
Saponins Soyasapogenols B–F (C–F artefacts) and carbohydrates (*see above*) yielded by acid hydrolysis[3]
Other Constituents Coumaric acid, phaseolic acid, salicylic acid, *trans*- and *cis*-clovamide (L-dopa conjugated with *trans*- and *cis*-caffeic acids), resin, volatile oil (containing furfural),[4] fats, vitamins, minerals. Cyanogenetic glycosides have been documented for a related species, *Trifolium repens*.[G13]

Food Use
Red clover is listed by the Council of Europe as a natural source of food flavouring (category N2). This category indicates that it can be added to foodstuffs in small quantities, with a possible limitation of an active principle (as yet unspecified) in the final product.[G9]

Herbal Use
Red clover is stated to act as a dermatological agent, and to possess mildly antispasmodic and expectorant properties. Tannins are known to possess astringent properties. Traditionally red clover has been used for chronic skin disease, whooping cough, and specifically for eczema and psoriasis.[G2,G3,G4,G32]

Dose
Dried flowerhead 4 g or by infusion three times daily[G2,G3]
Liquid extract (1:1 in 25% alcohol) 1.5–3.0 mL three times daily[G2,G3]
Tincture (1:10 in 45% alcohol) 1–2 mL three times daily[G2,G3]

Pharmacological Actions
Animal studies Biochanin A, formononetin, and genistein (isoflavones) are known to possess oestrogenic properties.[5] The saponin constituents are reported to lack any haemolytic or fungistatic activity.[3] A possible chemoprotective effect has been documented for biochanin A, which has been reported to inhibit carcinogenic activity in cell culture.[6]

Side-effects, Toxicity
Urticarial reactions have been documented.[G26] Infertility and growth disorders have been reported in grazing animals.[G13] These effects have been attributed to the oestrogenic isoflavone constituents, in particular to formononetin.[5]

Contra-indications, Warnings
In view of the oestrogenic constituents, excessive ingestion should be avoided. Large doses may interfere with anticoagulant and hormonal therapies (coumarin and isoflavonoid constituents).
Pregnancy and lactation In view of the oestrogenic components the use of red clover during pregnancy and lactation should be avoided.

Pharmaceutical Comment
The chemistry of red clover is well documented. Limited information is available on the pharmacological properties and no documented scientific evidence was found to justify the herbal uses. Reported oestrogenic side-effects in grazing animals have been attributed to the isoflavone constituents. Little toxicity data are available for red clover. In view of this and the isoflavone and coumarin components, excessive ingestion should be avoided.

References
See General References G2,G3,G4,G9,G10,G13,G19,G26, and G32.

1. Saxena VK, Jain AK. A new isoflavone glycoside from *Trifolium pratense. Fitoterapia* 1987; **58**: 262–3.

2. Jain AK, Saxena VK. Isolation and characterisation of 3-methoxyquercetin 7-*O*-β-D-glucopyranoside from *Trifolium pratense. Nat Acad Sci Lett* **9**: 379–80.

3. Olesek WA, Jurzysta M. Isolation, chemical characterization and biological activity of red clover (*Trifolium pratense* L.) root saponins. *Acta Soc Bot Pol* 1986; **55**: 247–52.

4. Opdyke DLJ. Furfural. *Food Cosmet Toxicol* 1978; **16**: 759–64.

5. Kelly RW *et al*. Formononetin content of 'Grasslands Pawera' red clover and its oestrogenic activity to sheep. *NZ J Exp Agric* 1979; **7**: 131–4.

6. Cassady JM *et al*. Use of a mammalian cell culture benzo(*a*)pyrene metabolism assay for the detection of potential anticarcinogens from natural products: Inhibition of metabolism by biochanin A, an isoflavone from *Trifolium pratense* L. *Cancer Res* 1988; **48**: 6257-61.

RHUBARB

Species (Family)

Rheum officinale Baill and *R.. palmatum* L. (Polygonaceae)

Synonym(s)

Chinese Rhubarb, other *Rheum* species (e.g. *Rheum tanguticum* Maxim. ex Reg., *Rheum emodi* Wall. (Indian Rhubarb), and *Rheum rhaponticum* L. (Garden Rhubarb))

Part(s) Used

Rhizome, Root

Pharmacopoeial Monographs

BHP 1990

BPC 1973

Martindale 30th edition

Pharmacopoeias—Aust., Br., Braz., Chin., Cz., Egypt., Eur., Fr., Ger., Gr., Hung., It., Jpn, Neth., Port., Rom., Rus., and Swiss. Chin. permits *Rheum tanguticum* and Jpn also permits *Rheum coreanum*. Br. and Jpn also describe Powdered Rhubarb.

Legal Category (Licensed Products)

GSL[G14]

Constituents[G1,G2,G10,G19,G24,G29,G32]

Anthraquinones Primarily anthraquinone *O*-glycosides (anthraglycosides) of aloe-emodin, emodin, chrysophanol, and physcion; dianthrone glycosides of rhein (sennosides A and B) and their oxalates; heterodianthrones including palmidin A (aloe-emodin, emodin), palmidin B (aloe-emodin, chrysophanol), palmidin C (chrysophanol, emodin), sennidin C (rhein, aloe-emodin), rheidin B (rhein, chrysophanol), and reidin C (rhein, physcion); free anthraquinones mainly aloe-emodin, chrysophanol, emodin, physcion, rhein

Tannins Hydrolysable and condensed including glucogallin, free gallic acid, (–)-epicatechin gallate, catechin

Other Constituents Calcium oxalate, fatty acids, rutin, resins, starch (about 16%), stilbene glycosides, carbohydrates, volatile oil (trace) with more than 100 components

Food Use

Rhubarb is listed by the Council of Europe as a natural source of food flavouring (category N2). This category indicates that it can be added to foodstuffs in small quantities, with a possible limitation of an active principle (as yet unspecified) in the final product.[G9] Rhubarb stems are commonly eaten as a food.

Herbal Use

Rhubarb has been used traditionally both as a laxative and an antidiarrhoeal agent.[G1,G2,G4,G32]

Dose

Rhizome/Root 0.2–1.0 g

Pharmacological Actions

The laxative action of anthraquinone derivatives is well recognised (*see* Senna). Rhubarb also contains tannins, which exert an astringent action. At low doses, rhubarb is stated to act as an antidiarrhoeal because of the tannin components, whereas at higher doses it exerts a cathartic action.[G20]

Side-effects, Toxicity

See Senna for side-effects and toxicity associated with anthraquinone-containing drugs. Rhubarb leaves are toxic because of the oxalic acid content and should not be ingested. A case of anaphylaxis following rhubarb ingestion has been documented.[G26]

Contra-indications, Warnings[G34]

See Senna for contra-indications and warnings associated with anthraquinone-containing drugs. The astringent effect of rhubarb may exacerbate, rather than relieve, symptoms of constipation.[1] It has been stated that rhubarb should be avoided by individuals suffering from arthritis, kidney disease, or urinary problems.[G20]

Pregnancy and lactation It is stated that rhubarb should be avoided during pregnancy.[G20] *See* Senna for contra-indications and warnings regarding the use of stimulant laxatives during pregnancy and lactation.

Pharmaceutical Comment

The chemistry of rhubarb is characterised by the anthraquinone derivatives. The laxative action of these compounds is well recognised and justifies the use of rhubarb as a laxative. As with all anthraquinone-containing preparations, the use of non-standardised products should be avoided because their pharmacological effect will be variable and unpredictable.

References

See General References G1,G2,G4,G7,G9,G10,G14,G19,G20,G22, G23,G24,G26,G29, G32 and G34.

1. Rohrback JA, Some uses of rhubarb in veterinary medicine. *Herbalist* 1983; **1:** 239–41.

ROSEMARY

Species (Family)
Rosmarinus officinalis L. (Labiatae)

Synonym(s)
—

Part(s) Used
Leaf, Twig

Pharmacopoeial Monographs
BHP 1983
BPC 1973
Martindale 30th edition (oil)
Pharmacopoeias (oil)—Arg, Aust., Belg., Cz., Fr., Ger., Mex., Port., Span., and Swiss.

Legal Category (Licensed Products)
GSL[G14]

Constituents[G1,G19,G35]

Flavonoids Include diosmetin, diosmin, genkwanin and derivatives, luteolin and derivatives, hispidulin and apigenin.
Phenols Caffeic, chlorogenic, labiatic, neochlorogenic and rosmarinic acids.
Volatile oil (0.5%) composed mainly of monoterpene hydrocarbons including α- and β-pinenes, camphene and limonene, together with cineole, borneol, camphor (10–20% of the oil), linalool, verbinol, terpineol, 3-octanone and isobornyl acetate
Terpenoids Carnosol (diterpene)[1]; oleanolic and ursolic acids (triterpenes).

Food Use
Rosemary herb and oil are commonly used as flavouring agents in foods. Rosemary is listed by the Council of Europe as a source of natural food flavouring (category N2). This category indicates that rosemary can be added to foodstuffs in small quantities, with a possible limitation of an active principle (as yet unspecified) in the final product.[G9]

Herbal Use
Rosemary is stated to act as a carminative, spasmolytic, thymoleptic, sedative, diuretic and antimicrobial.[G3] Topically, rubefacient, mild analgesic and parasiticide properties are documented.[G3] Traditionally rosemary is indicated for flatulent dyspepsia, headache, and topically for myalgia, sciatica, intercostal neuralgia.[G3]

Dose
Dried Leaf/Twig 2–4 g or by infusion three times daily [G3]

Liquid Extract 2–4 mL (1:1 in 45% alcohol) three times daily[G3]

Pharmacological Actions
Animal studies Antibacterial and antifungal activities *in vitro* have been reported for the oil.[G19] Rosemary herb is an effective antimicrobial agent against *Staphylococcus aureus* in meat and against a wide range of bacteria in laboratory media.[1] Antimicrobial activity has been documented for the oil towards moulds, and Gram-positive and Gram-negative bacteria[1] including *Staph. aureus, Staph. albus, Vibrio cholerae, Escherichia coli*, and corynebacteria.[2] Carnosol and ursolic acid have inhibited a range of food spoilage microbes (*Staph. aureus, E. coli, Lactobacillus brevis, Pseudomonas fluorescens, Rhodotorula glutinis*, and *Kluyveromyces bulgaricus*). Activity was comparable to that of known antioxidants butylated hydroxyanisole (BHA) and butylated hydroxytoluene (BHT), and correlated with the respective antioxidant properties of the two compounds (carnosol > ursolic acid).[1]

Rosemary oil, 1,8-cineole, and bornyl acetate have exerted a spasmolytic action in both smooth muscle (guinea-pig ileum) and cardiac muscle (guinea-pig atria) preparations, with the latter more sensitive.[3] In smooth muscle this spasmolytic effect has been attributed to antagonism of acetylcholine[4], with borneol considered the most active component of the oil.[4] The spasmolytic action of rosemary oil is preceded by a contractile action, which is attributed to the pinene components.[4] α- and β-pinenes have exhibited a spasmogenic activity towards smooth muscle, with no effect on cardiac muscle.[3]

Spasmolytic action *in vivo* has been demonstrated by rosemary oil (guinea pig, iv), via a relaxant action on Oddi's sphincter contracted by morphine. Activity increased with incremental oil doses until an optimum dose was reached (25 mg/kg) at which the unblocking effect was immediate.[5] Further increases in dose re-introduced a delayed response time.[5] Smooth-muscle stimulant and analgesic actions have been documented for a rosmaricine derivative.[G19]

Complement activation and subsequent triggering of the arachidonic acid cascade are thought to play an important role in the early phase of shock. An intact complement system is required for the formation of vasoactive prostanoids (prostacyclin, thromboxane A$_2$), arterial hypotension and thrombocytopenia.[6] The effect of rosmarinic acid on endotoxin-induced haemodynamic and haematological changes has been studied in a rabbit model of circulatory shock.[6,7] Rosmarinic acid (20 mg/kg iv) was found to suppress the endotoxin-induced activation of complement, formation of prostacyclin, hypotension, thrombocytopenia, and the release of thromboxane A$_2$.[6] Unlike NSAIDs, the mode of action by which rosmarinic acid suppresses prostaglandin formation does not involve interference with cyclo-oxygenase activity or prostacyclin synthetase.[7] Activity has been attributed to inhibition of complement factor C3 conversion to activated complement components, which mediate the inflammatory process.[7] Rosmarinic acid has inhibited carrageenin-induced paw oedema (rat, iv), and passive cutaneous anaphylaxis (rat, ID_{50} = 1 mg/kg iv, 10 mg/kg im).[8]

An antoxidant action, demonstrated by inhibition of chemiluminescence and hydrogen peroxide generation from human granulocytes, has been reported for rosmarinic acid.[7]

The complement-inhibiting and antoxidant properties of rosmarinic acid are not thought to adversely affect the chemotaxic, phagocytic and enzymatic properties of polymorphonuclear leukocytes.[9]

Pretreatment with rosmarinic acid (20 mg/kg and 10 mg/kg, iv) has been reported to inhibit the development of adult respiratory distress syndrome (ARDS) in a rabbit model.[9] This action can be attributed to both the antoxidant and anti-complement activities of rosmarinic acid.[9]

The ability to reduce capillary permeability has been described for diosmin.[G19] Activity reportedly exceeds that exhibited by rutin.[G19]

An increase in locomotor activity has been observed in mice following either inhalation or oral administration of rosemary oil.[10] The increase in activity paralleled a dose-related increase in serum 1,8-cineole level. Biphasic elimination of 1,8-cineole from the blood was observed ($t_{1/2}$ = 6 min, $t_{1/2}$ 45min).[10]

Antigonadotrophic activity (rat, im) has been documented for oxidation products of rosmarinic acid.[11] Activity was determined by suppression of pregnant mares serum-induced increase in ovarian and uterine weights.

Side-Effects, Toxicity[G35]

Rosemary oil is stated to be non-irritating and non-sensitising when applied to human skin,[G35] but moderately irritating when applied undiluted to rabbit skin.[G19] Bath preparations, cosmetics and toiletries containing rosemary oil may cause erythema and dermatitis in hypersensitive individuals.[G26] Photosensitivity has been associated with the oil.[G26]

Rosmarinic acid exhibits low toxicity (a LD_{50} mice stated as 561 mg/kg iv) and is rapidly eliminated form the circulation (iv, $t_{1/2}$ = 9 min).[8] Transient cardiovascular actions become pronounced at doses exceeding 50 mg/kg iv.[8] Acute LD_{50} values quoted include 5 mL/kg (rat, oral) and >10 mL/kg (rabbit, dermal).[2]

Diosmin is reportedly less toxic compared to rutin.[G19]

Contra-indications, Warnings

Topical preparations containing rosemary oil should be used with caution by hypersensitive individuals. Rosemary oil contains 10–20% camphor; orally, camphor readily causes epileptiform convulsions if taken in sufficient quantity.[G35]

Pregnancy and lactation Rosemary is reputed to be an abortifacient[G12] and to affect the menstrual cycle (emmenagogue).[G24] In view of its common culinary use, rosemary should not be ingested in amounts greatly exceeding those normally encountered in foods.

Pharmaceutical Comment

In addition to the well known culinary uses of rosemary, various medicinal properties are also associated with the herb. Documented antibacterial and spasmolytic actions, which support the traditional uses of the herb, are attributable to the essential oil. More recently anticomplement and antoxidant activities documented for rosmarinic acid have generated considerable interest in a potential preventative use against endotoxin shock and adult respiratory distress syndrome. A method for the isolation (TLC) and subsequent identification (HPLC) of rosmarinic acid has been proposed.[12] Rosemary should not be used by epileptic patients in doses greatly exceeding amounts used in food.

References

See General References G1, G3, G7, G9, G10, G14, G19, G24, G26, G22 and G35

1. Collin MA and Charles HP. Antimicrobial activity of carnosol and ursolic acid: two anti-oxidant constituents of *Rosmarinus officinalis* L. *Food Microbiol* 1987; **4**: 311–15.

2. Opdyke DLJ. Rosemary oil. *Food Cosmet Toxicol* 1974; **12**: 977–8

3. Hof S and Ammon HPT. Negative inotropic action of rosemary oil, 1,8-cineole, and bornyl acetate. *Planta Med* 1989; **55**: 106–7.

4. Taddei I *et al.* Spasmolytic activity of peppermint ,sage and rosemary essences and their major constituents. *Fitoterapia* 1988; **59**: 463–8.

5. Giachetti D *et al.* Pharmacological activity of essential oils on Oddi's sphincter. *Planta Med* 1988; 389–92.

6. Bult H *et al.* Modification of endotoxin-induced haemodynamic and haematological changes in the rabbit by methylprednisolone, F(ab′)₂ fragments and rosmarinic acid. *Br J Pharmacol* 1985; **84**: 317–27.

7. Rampart M *et al.* Complement-dependent stimulation of prostacyclin biosynthesis: inhibition by rosmarinic acid. *Biochem Pharmacol* 1986; **35**: 1397-1400.

8. Parnham MJ and Kesselring K. Rosmarinic acid. *Drugs Future* 1985; **10**: 756–7

9. Nuytinck JKS *et al.* Inhibition of experimentally induced microvascular injury by rosmarinic acid. *Agents and Actions* 1985; **17**: 373–4.

10. Kovar KA *et al.* Blood levels of 1,8-cineole and locomotor activity of mice after inhalation and oral administration of rosemary oil. *Planta Med* 1987; 315-18.

11. Gumbinger HG *et al.* Formation of compounds with antigonadotropic activity from inactive phenolic precursors. *Contraception* 1981; **23**: 661–5.

12. Verotta L. Isolation and HPLC determination of the active principles of *Rosmarinus officinalis* and *Gentiana lutea*. *Fitoterapia* 1985; **56**: 25–9.

SAGE

Species (Family)
Salvia officinalis L. (Labiatae)

Synonym(s)
Garden, Dalmatian and True Sage
Red sage refers to *S. haematodes* Wall.
Greek sage refers to *Salvia triloba*[5]

Part(s) Used
Leaf

Pharmacopoeial Monographs
BHP 1983
BPC 1934
Martindale 30th edition
Pharmacopoeias—Aust., Fr., Ger., Hung., Rom., Russ., Swiss, and Yug.

Legal Category (Licensed Products)
GSL[G14]

Constituents[G1,G10,G19,G31,G32,G35]
Acids Phenolic — caffeic, chlorogenic, ellagic, ferulic, gallic, rosmarinic.[1]
Tannins (3–8%). Hydrolysable and condensed.[1,2]
Volatile oils (1–2.8%). Major components are α- and β-thujones (35–50%, mainly α). Others include 1,8-cineole, borneol, camphor, caryophyllene, linalyl acetate and various terpenes.[3,4]
It has been noted that commercial sage may be substituted with *Salvia triloba*.[5] In contrast to *S. officinalis*, the principal volatile oil component of *S. triloba* is 1,8-cineole, with α-thujone only accounting for 1–5%.[5] Compared to *S. officinalis*, volatile oil yield of various *Salvia* species is lower, with lower total ketone content and higher total alcohol content.[6]

Food Use
Sage is commonly used as a culinary herb. Sage is listed by the Council of Europe as a natural source of food flavouring (category N2). This category indicates that sage can be added to foodstuffs providing the concentration of thujones (α and β) present in the final product does not exceed 0.5 mg/kg, with the exceptions of alcoholic beverages (10 mg/kg), bitters (35 mg/kg), food containing sage (25 mg/kg), and sage stuffing (250 mg/kg).[G9]

Herbal Use
Sage is stated to possess carminative, antispasmodic, antiseptic, astringent, and antihidrotic properties. Traditionally, it has been used to treat flatulent dyspepsia, pharyngitis, uvultis, stomatitis, gingivitis, glossitis (internally or as a gargle/mouthwash), hyperhidrosis, and galactorrhoea.[G1,G3,G32]

Dose
Leaf 1–4 g or by infusion three times daily[G3]
Liquid extract (1:1 in 45% alcohol) 1–4 mL three times daily[G3]

Pharmacological Actions
Animal studies Hypotensive activity in anaesthetised cats, CNS-depressant action (prolonged barbiturate sleep) in anaesthetised mice, and an antispasmodic action *in-vitro* (guinea pig ileum) have been reported for a sage extract[7] and for the essential oil.[8] 60–80% inhibition of contractions induced by acetylcholine, histamine, serotonin and barium chloride has been noted for a total sage extract, with lesser activity exhibited by a total flavonoid extract.[7] An initial spasmogenic action exhibited by low doses of sage oil has been attributed to the pinene content.[8] Antispasmodic activity *in vivo* (iv, guinea pig) has been reported for sage oil, which released contraction of Oddi's spincter induced by intravenous morphine.[4]
In-vivo studies have indicated different activities for *S. triloba* and *S. verbenaca* compared to *S. officinalis*.[7] Antimicrobial activity of the volatile oil has been attributed to the thujone content.[3] Antimicrobial activity *in vitro* was noted against *Escherichia coli*, *Shigella sonnei*, *Salmonella* species, *Klebsiella ozanae* (Gram-negative), *Bacillus subtilis* (Gram-positive), and against various fungi (*Candida albicans*, *C. krusei*, *C. pseudotropicalis*, *Torulopsis glabrata*, *Cryptococcus neoformans*)[9]. No activity was observed versus *Pseudomonas aeruginosa*.[3] Microencapsulation of the oil into gelatin-acacia capsules introduced a lagtime with respect to the antibacterial activity and inhibited the antifungal activity.[3]
Hypoglycaemic activity *in-vivo* has been reported for *S. lavandulifolia* (rabbit)[10] and for mixed phytotherapy preparations involving various *Salvia* species including *S. officinalis*.[11] Activity in normoglycaemic, hypoglycaemic and in alloxan-diabetic rabbits was observed, although no change in insulin concentrations was noted.[10]
Various activities in rats, mice and rabbits have been reported for a related species, *S. haematodes* Wall. (commonly known as red sage), including wound healing, anti-inflammatory, analgesic, anticonvulsant and hypotensive, and positive inotropic and chronotropic actions (*in vitro*).[12,13]

Side-effects, Toxicity
A case of human poisoning has been documented following ingestion of sage oil for acne.[14] Convulsant activity in both humans and animals has been documented for sage oil.[15,16] In rats, the subclinical, clinical and lethal doses for convulsant action of sage oil are estimated as 0.3, 0.5, and

3.2 g/kg.[15] This toxicity has been attributed to the ketone terpenoids in the volatile oil, namely camphor and thujone. Acute LD_{50} values for sage oil are documented as 2.6 g/kg (orally, rat) and 5 g/kg (intradermal, rabbit).[17]

Sage oil is reported to be a moderate skin irritant[17] and is not recommended for aromatherapy.[G35]

Contra-indications, Warnings

Sage oil is toxic (due to the thujone content) and should not be ingested. In view of the toxicity of the essential oil, sage extracts should be used with caution and not ingested in large amounts. Sage may interfere with existing hypoglycaemic and anticonvulsant therapies, and may potentiate sedative effects of other drugs.

Pregnancy and lactation   Sage is contraindicated during pregnancy. Traditionally, it is reputed to be an abortifacient and to affect the menstrual cycle.[G12] The volatile oil contains a high proportion of α and β thujones, which are known to be abortifacient and emmenagogic.

Pharmaceutical Comment

The characteristic components of sage to which its traditional uses can be attributed are the volatile oil and tannins. However, the oil contains high concentrations of thujone, a toxic ketone and should not be ingested. Sage is commonly used as a culinary herb and presents no hazard when ingested in amounts normally encountered in foods. However, extracts of the herb should be used with caution and should not be ingested in large amounts or over prolonged periods.

References

See General References G1, G3, G5, G9, G10, G12, G14, G19, G22, G23, G31, G32 and G35.

1.   Petri G *et al*. Tannins and other polyphenolic compounds in the genus *Salvia*. *Planta Med* 1988: **54:** 575.

2.   Murko D *et al*. Tannins of *Salvia officinalis* and their changes during storage. *Planta Med* 1974; 25: 295–300.

3.   Jalsenjak V *et al*. Microcapsules of sage oil: Essential oils content and antimicrobial activity. *Pharmazie* 1987; **42**: 419–20.

4.   Giachetti D *et al*. Pharmacological activity of essential oils on Oddi's sphincter. *Planta Med* 1988: **54:** 389–92.

5.   Tucker AO *et al*. Botanical aspects of commercial sage. *Econ Bot* 80; **34**: 16–19.

6.   Ivanic R, Savin K. A comparative analysis of essential oils from several wild species of *Salvia*. *Planta Med* 1976; **30**: 25–31.

7.   Todorov S *et al*. Experimental pharmacological study of three species from genus *Salvia*. *Acta Physiol Pharmacol Bulg* 1984; **10**: 13–20.

8.   Taddei I *et al*. Spasmolytic activity of peppermint, sage and rosemary essences and their major constituents. *Fitoterapia* 1988; **59**: 463–8.

9.   Recio MC *et al*. Antimicrobial activity of selected plants employed in the Spanish Mediterranean area. Part II. *Phytotherapy Res* 1989; **3**: 77.

10.   Jimenez J *et al*. Hypoglycaemic activity of *Salvia lavandulifolia*. *Planta Med* 1986: **52**: 260–2.

11.   Cabo J *et al*. Accion hipoglucemiante de preparados fitoterapicos que contienen especies del genero salvia. *Ars Pharmaceutica* 1985; **26**: 239–49.

12.   Akbar A *et al*. Pharmacological studies on *Salvia haematodes* Wall. *Acta Tropica* 1985; **42**: 371–4.

13.   Akbar S. Pharmacological investigations on the ethanolic extract of *Salvia haematodes*. *Fitoterapia* 1989; **60**: 270.

14.   Centini F *et al*. A case of sage oil poisoning. *Zacchia* 1987; **60**: 263–74.

15.   Millet Y. Experimental study of the toxic convulsant properties of commercial preparations of essences of sage and hyssop. *Electroencephal Clin Neurophysiol* 1980; **49**: 102P.

16.   Millet Y *et al*. Toxicity of some essential plant oils — clinical and experimental study. *Clin Toxicol* 1981; **18**: 1485–98.

17.   Opdyke DLJ. Sage oil Dalmatian. *Food Cosmet Toxicol* 1974; **12**: 987–8.

SARSAPARILLA

Species (Family)
Smilax species including
(i) *Smilax aristolochiifolia* Mill.
(ii) *Smilax regelii* Killip et Morton
(iii) *Smilax officinalis* Kunth
(iv) *Smilax febrifuga* (Liliaceae)

Synonym(s)
Ecuadorian Sarsaparilla, Sarsa, Smilax
(i) Mexican Sarsaparilla
(ii) Honduras Sarsaparilla, Jamaican Sarsaparilla
(iii) Honduras Sarsaparilla
(iv) Ecuadorian Sarsaparilla

Part(s) Used
Rhizome, Root

Pharmacopoeial Monographs
BHP 1983
BHP 1990
BPC 1949
Martindale 30th edition
Pharmacopoeias—In Chin. and Jpn, which specify *Smilax glabra*

Legal Category (Licensed Products)
GSL[G14]

Constituents[G2,G10,G19,G24,G31,G32]
Saponins (about 2%). Sarsasapogenin (parigenin), smilagenin, diosgenin, tigogenin, asperagenin, laxogenin from various species,[1] sarsasaponin (parillin), smilasaponin (smilacin), sarsaparilloside
Other constituents Caffeoylshikimic acid, ferulic acid, shikimic acid, kaempferol, quercetin, phytosterols (e.g. β-sitosterol, stigmasterol, pollinastanol), resin, starch, volatile oil (trace), cetyl alcohol

Food Use
Sarsaparilla is listed by the Council of Europe as a natural source of food flavouring (category N4). This category indicates that the use of sarsaparilla as a flavouring agent is recognised but that there is insufficient information available to further classify it into categories N1, N2, or N3.[G9] Sarsaparilla has been used as a vehicle and flavouring agent for medicaments,[G22] and is widely employed in the manufacture of non-alcoholic beverages.[G29]

Herbal Use
Sarsaparilla is stated to possess antirheumatic, antiseptic, and antipruritic properties. Traditionally, it has been used for psoriasis and other cutaneous conditions, chronic rheumatism, rheumatoid arthritis, as an adjunct to other treatments for leprosy, and specifically for psoriasis.[G2,G3,G4,G32]

Dose
Dried root 1–4 g or by decoction three times daily[G2]
Sarsaparilla Liquid Extract (BP 1898) (1:1 in 20% alcohol, 10% glycerol) 8–15 mL

Pharmacological Actions
Animal studies Anti-inflammatory[2] and hepatoprotective[3] effects have been shown in rats.
Human studies Improvement of appetite and digestion[4] as well as a diuretic[4,5] action have been reported. Limited clinical data utilising extracts indicate improvement in psoriasis;[6] the extract has also been used as an adjuvant for the treatment of leprosy.[7]

Side-effects, Toxicity
None documented for sarsaparilla. Large doses of saponins are reported to cause gastro-intestinal irritation resulting in diarrhoea and vomiting. Although haemolytic activity has been documented for the saponins,[G31] they are not harmful when taken by mouth and are only highly toxic if injected into the bloodstream.[G29]

Contra-indications, Warnings
None documented for sarsaparilla. In view of the possible irritant nature of the saponin constituents, excessive ingestion should be avoided.
Pregnancy and lactation There are no known problems with the use of sarsaparilla during pregnancy and lactation. However, in view of the possible irritant nature of the saponin components, excessive ingestion should be avoided.

Pharmaceutical Comment
Phytochemical studies on sarsaparilla have focused on the nature of the steroidal saponin constituents, with limited information available regarding additional constituents. No documented scientific evidence was found to justify the herbal uses. No toxicity data were located, although large doses may be irritant to the gastro-intestinal mucosa and should, therefore, be avoided.
Sarsaparilla saponins have been used in the partial synthesis of cortisone and other steroids. Several related *Smilax* species native to China are used to treat various skin disorders.[G19]

References
See General References G2, G3, G4, G6, G9, G10, G14, G19, G22, G23, G24, G29, G31 and G32.

1. Sharma SC *et al*. Über Saponine von *Smilax parvifolia* Wall. *Pharmazie* 1980; **35**: 646.

2.   Ageel AM *et al*. Experimental studies on antirheumatic crude drugs used in Saudi traditional medicine. *Drugs Exptl Clin Res* 1989; **15:** 369–72.

3.   Rafatullah S *et al*. Hepatoprotective and safety evaluation studies on sarsaparilla. *Int J Pharmacognosy* 1991; **29:** 296–301.

4.   Harnischfeger G, Stolze H. Smilax species — Sarsaparille. In: *Bewahrte Pflanzendrogen in Wissenschaft und Medizin*. Bad Homburg/Melsungen: Notamed Verlag. 1983; p. 216–25.

5.   Hobbs C. Sarsaparilla — a literature review. *Herbalgram* 1988; **17:** 1, 10–15.

6.   Thermon FM. The treatment of psoriasis with a sarsaparilla compound. *New Engl J Med* 1942; **227:** 128–33.

7.   Rollier R. Treatment of lepromatous leprosy by a combination of DDS and sarsaparilla (*Smilax ornata*). *Int J Leprosy* 1959; **27:** 328–40.

SASSAFRAS

Species (Family)
Sassafras albidum (Nutt.) Nees (Lauraceae)

Synonym(s)
Saxifrax, Ague Tree, Cinnamon Wood, Saloop, *Sassafras varifolium* (Salisb.) Kuntze, *Sassafras officinale* Nees et Eberm.

Part(s) Used
Inner Root Bark

Pharmacopoeial Monographs
BPC 1949
BHP 1983
Martindale 29th edition (Sassafras oil)
Pharmacopoeias (Sassafras oil)—Port., Span.

Legal Category (Licensed Products)
Sassafras is not permitted for use in medicinal products.

Constituents[G1,G10,G19,G24,G32]
Alkaloids (isoquinoline-type about 0.02%). Boldine, isoboldine, norboldine, cinnamolaurine, norcinnamolaurine, reticuline.
Volatile oils (5–9%). Safrole as major component (80–90%), others include anethole, apiole, asarone, camphor, caryophyllene, coniferaldehyde, copaene, elemicin, eugenol, 5-methoxyeugenol, menthone, myristicin, α-pinene, α- and β-phellandrene, piperonylacrolein, thujone.
Other constituents Gum, mucilage, lignans (sesamin, desmethoxyaschantin), resin, sitosterol, starch, tannins, wax.

Food Use
Sassafras oil was formerly used as flavouring agent in beverages including root beer.[G35] However, in the 1960s safrole, the major component of the volatile oil, was reported to be carcinogenic.[G35] The use of safrole in foods is now banned, and its use in toilet preparations controlled.[G22] In the USA, safrole-free sassafras extract, leaf and leaf extract are approved for food use. In 1976, the FDA banned interstate marketing of sassafras for sassafras tea.[G10]

Herbal Use
Sassafras is stated to possess carminative, diaphoretic, diuretic, dermatological agent, and antirheumatic properties. Traditionally, it has been used for cutaneous eruptions, gout, and rheumatic pains.[G1,G3,G32]

Dose
Bark 2–4 g or by infusion three times daily[G3]
Liquid extract (1:1 in 25% alcohol) 2–4 mL three times daily[G3]

Pharmacological Actions
Studies have concentrated on investigating the toxicity associated with the bark. However, aqueous and alcoholic extracts have been reported to elicit ataxia, hypersensitivity to touch, CNS depression, and hypothermia in mice.[1] Both inhibition and induction of hepatic microsomal enzymes have been documented for safrole.[2,3] Enzyme-inducing activity was found to be a transient phenomenon, with activity falling after the onset of hepatic toxicity (*see* Side-effects, Toxicity).[2] Safrole is reported to induce both cytochrome P-488 and P-450 activities. Sassafras oil has been used as a topical antiseptic, pediculicide and carminative.[4]

Side-effects, Toxicity[G35]
The toxicity of sassafras is attributable to the volatile oil, and in particular to the safrole content. It is estimated that a few drops of sassafras oil are sufficient to kill a toddler and as little as one teaspoonful has proved fatal in an adult.[5] Symptoms of poisoning are described as vomiting, stupor, collapse. High doses may cause spasm followed by paralysis.[G35] Large amounts of the oil are reported to be psychoactive with the hallucinogenic effects lasting for several days.[G10] One of the components of the oil is myristicin, the hallucinogenic principle in nutmeg. Sassafras has traditionally been used as an ingredient of beverages. To put the potential toxicity of sassafras into perspective, the following estimation has been made.[1] Extrapolation of results from animal toxicity studies indicate that 0.66 mg/kg may prove hazardous in man.[1] By comparison, a cup of sassafras tea, prepared from a 2.5 g tea bag, may provide up to 200 mg safrole, representing approximately 3 mg/kg.[1]

Safrole, the principal component of the volatile oil, was first recognised to be a hepatocarcinogen in the 1960s[6] and many animal studies have been documented concerning this toxicity.[7] Both benign and malignant tumours have developed in laboratory animals, depending on the dose of safrole administered.[2]

Both human and animal studies have shown that safrole gives rise to a large number of metabolites.[8] A sulphate ester (formed via hydroxylated metabolite) has been established as the ultimate carcinogen for safrole with tumour incidence paralleling the rate of conversion to the ester.[9] Induction of cytochrome P450 activity has been associated with mutagenic and carcinogenic activity of the inducing agent.[10] The inducing effect of safrole on certain metabolising enzymes is thought to play a role in the carcinogenic activity of safrole. The liver has a high level of cytochrome P450 activity and is therefore susceptible to induction.[10]

Acute oral LD_{50} values for safrole have been reported as 1.95 g/kg (rats) and 2.35 g/kg (mice).[2] Major symptoms of toxicity are stated as ataxia, depression, diarrhoea, followed by death within 4 hours to 7 days.[11] Rats fed safrole in their diet at concentrations of 0.25, 0.5, and 1.0% exhibited reduction in growth, stomach and testicular atrophy, liver necrosis, biliary proliferation and primary hepatomas.[G10] Animals have also developed tumours when fed safrole-free extracts.[G10]

Conflicting results have been reported from studies investigating the mutagenicity of safrole, using the Ames test and DNA repair test.[12,13] Purity of the safrole, test system employed, type of metabolic activation mix, and toxicity of the test system have been suggested as reasons for the observed variations.[12]

Contra-indications, Warnings

Sassafras should not be used internally or externally. Safrole, the major component in the volatile oil of sassafras, is hepatotoxic and even safrole-free extracts have been reported to produce tumours in animals. Sassafras essential oil is contra-indicated in internal and external use.[G35] Sassafras has been reported to inhibit and induce microsomal enzymes.

Pregnancy and lactation Sassafras is contra-indicated during pregnancy and lactation. The oil is reported to be abortifacient.[5]

Pharmaceutical Comment

In addition to its traditional herbal use for treating dermatological and rheumatic ailments, sassafras also used to be a common flavouring ingredient in beverages, in particular root beer. However, animal studies have revealed the carcinogenic and hepatotoxic potential of safrole, the major component of sassafras volatile oil. Consequently, the use of safrole is no longer permitted in foods and sassafras is not permitted as a constituent of licensed medicinal products.

Antiseptic and diuretic properties claimed for sassafras are probably attributable to the volatile oil, although no documented studies were found supporting the antirheumatic claims. Sassafras should not be used as a herbal remedy, either internally or externally.

References

See General References G1, G3, G6, G10, G19, G22, G24, G32 and G35.

1.   Segelman AB *et al*. Sassafras and herb tea. Potential health hazards. *JAMA* 1976; **238:** 477.

2.   Opdyke DLJ. Safrole. *Food Cosmet Toxicol* 1974; **12:** 983–6.

3.   Jaffe H *et al*. *In vivo* inhibition of mouse liver microsomal hydroxylating systems by methylenedioxyphenyl insecticidal synergists and related compounds. *Life Sci* 1968; **7:** 1051–62.

4.   International Agency for Research on Cancer. IARC monographs on the evaluation of carcinogenic risk of chemicals to man. Some naturally occurring substances, vol 10. WHO, 1976.

5.   Craig JO. Poisoning by the volatile oils in childhood. *Archs Dis Childh* 1953; **28:** 475–83.

6.   Homburger F, Boger E. The carcinogenicity of essential oils, flavors, and spices: A review. *Cancer Res* 1968; **28:** 2372–4.

7.   Opdyke DLJ. Sassafras oil. *Food Cosmet Toxicol* 1982; **20:** 825–6.

8.   Ioannides C *et al*. Safrole: its metabolism, carcinogenicity and interactions with cytochrome P-450. *Food Cosmet Toxicol* 1981; **19:** 657–66.

9.   Bock KW, Schirmer G. Species differences of glucuronidation and sulfation in relation to hepatocarcinogenesis. *Arch Toxicol* 1987; **10**(Suppl): 125–35.

10.   Iwasaki K *et al*. Induction of cytochrome P-448 activity as exemplified by the *O*-deethylation of ethoxyresorufin. Effects of dose, sex, tissue and animal species. *Biochem Pharmacol* 1986; **35:** 3879–84.

11.   Jenner PM *et al*. Food flavourings and compounds of related structure. I. Acute oral toxicity. *Food Cosmet Toxicol* 1964; **2:** 327–43.

12.   Sekizawa J, Shibamoto T. Genotoxicity of safrole-related chemicals in microbial test systems. *Mutat Res* 1982; **101:** 127–40.

13.   Swanson AB *et al*. The mutagenicities of safrole, estragole, eugenol, *trans*-anethole, and some of their known or possible metabolites for *Salmonella typhimurium* mutants. *Mutat Res* 1979; **60:** 143–53.

SAW PALMETTO

Species (Family)
Serenoa serrulata Hook, F. (Arecaceae/Palmae)

Synonym(s)
Sabal, Serenoa, *Serenoa repens* (Bartel.) Small

Part(s) Used
Fruit

Pharmacopoeial Monographs
BHP 1983
BPC 1934

Legal Category (Licensed Products)
GSL[G14]

Constituents[G10,G32]
Carbohydrates Invert sugar 28.2%, mannitol, high-molecular-weight polysaccharides (e.g. MW 100 000) with galactose, arabinose, and uronic acid[1] identified as main sugar components for one.
Fixed oils (26.7%). Many free fatty acids and their glycerides. Oleic acid (unsaturated) and capric acid, caproic acid, caprylic acid, lauric acid, myristic acid, palmitic acid, stearic acid (saturated)
Steroids β-sitosterol and other unidentified compounds[2,3]
Other constituents Flavonoids, pigment (carotene), resin, tannin, volatile oil 1.5%

Food Use
Saw palmetto is not used in foods. In the USA, saw palmetto is listed by the FDA as a Herb of Undefined Safety.[G19]

Herbal Use
Saw palmetto is stated to possess diuretic, urinary antiseptic, endocrinological, and anabolic properties. Traditionally, it has been used for chronic or subacute cystitis, catarrh of the genito-urinary tract, testicular atrophy, sex hormone disorders, and specifically for prostatic enlargement.[G3,G32]

Dose
Dried fruit 0.5–1.0 g or by decoction three times daily[G3]
Liquid extract (BPC 1934) 0.6–1.5 mL

Pharmacological Actions
Animal studies Anti-androgenic activity has been documented for a hexane extract (SRE) of saw palmetto. In mouse and rat studies, it has been shown that SRE opposes exogenous and endogenous stimulation of the prostate gland. Subsequent *in-vitro* studies (rat prostate, human foreskin fibroblasts) indicated that SRE competitively inhibits the binding of dihydrotestosterone to cytosolic and nuclear androgen receptor sites.[4,5] In addition, SRE was found to inhibit 5α-reductase mediated conversion of testosterone to dihydrotestosterone, and 3-ketosteroid reductase mediated conversion of dihydrotestosterone to an androgen derivative.[4,5]
In-vivo oestrogenic activity in the rat has also been documented for an alcoholic extract.[6] Activity was attributed to the high content of β-sitosterol, a known oestrogenic agent, present in saw palmetto.
In-vivo anti-oedema activity in the rat has been documented for SRE, acting by inhibition of histamine-induced increase in capillary permeability.[7] Low doses of an aqueous extract were effective in carrageenan paw oedema and pellet tests in the rat, although the extract was not found to influence the proliferative stage of inflammation.[1,8] The observed anti-inflammatory activity was attributed to a high-molecular-weight polysaccharide (approximately 100 000). Polysaccharides possessing immunostimulating activity have also been documented for saw palmetto and were stated to contain a high content of glucuronic acid.[1,8]

Human studies Numerous studies have been documented investigating the use of saw palmetto in benign prostatic hypertrophy. Two double blind trials reported a significant improvement for both objective (e.g. frequency of nocturia, urine flow rate) and subjective (e.g. intensity of dysuria, patient's and physician's self-rating) assessments in patients receiving SRE compared to those receiving placebo.[9,10] In another study, the efficacy of SRE was attributed to the anti-androgenic and anti-oedematous activities exhibited by saw palmetto in animal studies.[11]
Benign prostatic hypertrophy is stated to result from prostate accumulation of dihydrotestosterone, which is thought to be a probable mediator of the hyperplasia acting at the level of androgen receptor.[4] Most synthetic anti-androgens have been reported to inhibit dihydrotestosterone binding at androgen receptors, whilst others have been found to inhibit the action of 5α-reductase on testosterone.[4] Few synthetic androgens have been documented to exhibit both these activities.[5] SRE has been reported to inhibit both dihydrotestosterone binding at androgen receptors and 5α-reductase activity on testosterone.[5] In addition, SRE inhibits the action of 3α-ketosteroid reductase on dihydrotestosterone, which has also been implicated in the pathogenesis of prostatic hypertrophy in dogs.[5] The pharmacological actions for saw palmetto are therefore thought to indicate a possible multisite inhibition of androgen action.[5]

Side-effects, Toxicity
Documented human studies have reported saw palmetto to be well tolerated. Only one withdrawal from a study has been reported, due to gastric side-effects.[10] The results of standard blood chemistry tests were normal.

Contra-indications, Warnings

In view of the reported anti-androgen and oestrogenic activities, saw palmetto may affect existing hormonal therapy, including the oral contraceptive pill and hormone replacement therapy.

Pregnancy and lactation The safety of saw palmetto has not been established. In view of the lack of toxicity data and the documented hormonal activity, the use of saw palmetto during pregnancy and lactation should be avoided.

Pharmaceutical Comment

Available chemical data for saw palmetto are limited although much has been documented regarding its anti-androgenic activity. Results of human studies indicate that saw palmetto is a potential agent for the treatment of benign prostatic hypertrophy. In addition, *in-vivo* immunostimulant and anti-inflammatory activities have been reported. Scientific evidence supports many of the traditional uses, although these are not suitable indications for self-medication. In view of the lack of toxicity data and documented pharmacological actions, excessive use should be avoided.

References

See General References G3, G5, G10, G14, G19, and G32.

1. Wagner H, Flachsbarth H. A new antiphlogistic principle from *Sabal serrulata*, I. *Planta Med* 1981; **41:** 244–51.

2. Schöpflin G *et al.* β-Sitosterin als Möglicher Wirkstoff der Sabalfrüchte. *Planta Med* 1966; **14:** 402–7.

3. Hänsel R *et al.* Eine Dünnschichtchromatographische untersuchung der Sabalfrüchte. *Planta Med* 1964; **12:** 169–72.

4. Carilla E *et al.* Binding of permixon, a new treatment for prostatic benign hyperplasia, to the cytosolic androgen receptor in the rat prostate. *J Steroid Biochem* 1984; **20:** 521–3.

5. Sultan C *et al.* Inhibition of androgen metabolism and binding by a liposterolic extract of "*Serenoa repens* B" in human foreskin fibroblasts. *J Steroid Biochem* 1984; **20:** 515–19.

6. Elghamry MI, Hänsel R. Activity and isolated phytoestrogen of shrub palmetto fruits (*Serenoa repens* Small), a new estrogenic plant. *Experientia* 1969; **25:** 828–9.

7. Stenger A *et al.* Pharmacology and biochemistry of hexane extract of *Serenoa repens*. *Gazz Med Fr* 1982; **89:** 2041–8.

8. Wagner H *et al.* A new antiphlogistic principle from *Sabal serrulata* II. *Planta Med* 1981; **41:** 252–58.

9. Champault G *et al.* A double-blind trial of an extract of the plant *Serenoa repens* in benign prostatic hyperplasia. *Br J Clin Pharmac* 1984; **18:** 461–2.

10. Tasca A *et al.* Treatment of obstruction in prostatic adenoma using an extract of *Serenoa repens*. Double-blind clinical test v. placebo. *Minn Urol Nefrol* 1985; **37:** 87–91.

11. Carreras JO. Nuestra experiencia con extracto hexánico de *Serenoa repens* en el tratamiento de la hipertrofia benigna de próstata. *Arch Esp de Urol* 1987; **40:** 310–313.

SCULLCAP

Species (Family)

Scutellaria lateriflora L., *S. baicalensis* Georgi and other *Scutellaria* species (Labiatae)

S. baicalensis Georgi is a species commonly referred to as scullcap in Chinese herbal medicine.

Synonym(s)

Helmet flower, Hoodwort, Quaker Bonnet, Scutellaria, *Scutellaria galericulata* L., Skullcap

Part(s) Used

Herb

Pharmacopoeial Monographs

BHP 1983
BPC 1934

Legal Category (Licensed Products)

GSL[G14]

Constituents[G10,G24,G30,G32,G34]

Limited information has been documented regarding the constituents of *S. lateriflora*, although various related *Scutellaria* species have been investigated.

Flavonoids Apigenin, hispidulin, luteolin, scutellarein, scutellarin (bitter glycoside).

Iridoids Catalpol

Volatile oils Limonene, terpineol (monoterpenes); *d*-cadinene, caryophyllene, *trans*-β-farnesene, β-humulene (sesquiterpenes)

Other constituents Lignin, resin, tannin

Other Scutellaria species The related species *S. baicalensis* is reported to contain baicalein, baicalin, chrysin, oroxylin A, skullcapflavone II, and wogonin.[1–3]

S. galericulata is stated to contain apigenin, baicalein, baicalin, apigenin-7-glucoside, and galeroside (baicalein-β-L-rhamnofuranoside).[4]

Food Use

Scullcap is not used in foods. In the USA, scullcap is listed by the FDA as a Herb of Undefined Safety.[G10]

Herbal Use

Scullcap is stated to possess anticonvulsant and sedative properties[G15,G32]. Traditionally, it has been used for epilepsy, chorea, hysteria, nervous tension states, and specifically for grand mal.[G3] In Chinese herbal medicine, the roots of *S. baicalensis* Georgi have been used traditionally as a remedy for inflammation, suppurative dermatitis, allergic diseases, hyperlipidaemia and atherosclerosis.

Dose

Dried herb 1–2 g or by infusion three times daily[G3]

Liquid Extract (1:1 in 25% alcohol) 2–4 mL three times daily[G3]

Tincture (1:5 in 45% alcohol) 1–2 mL three times daily[G3]

Pharmacological Actions

Animal studies None documented for *Scutellaria lateriflora*.

Many investigations have been undertaken to study the pharmacological actions of *S. baicalensis* root. Documented actions have primarily been attributed to the various flavonoid constituents and include: *in-vitro* inhibition of mast cell histamine release comparable to disodium cromoglycate for some flavonoids;[1] *in-vitro* cytotoxicity of scullcap flavone II;[5] *in-vivo* and *in-vitro* inhibition of lipid peroxidation;[6–8] *in-vitro* inhibition of lipoxygenase and cyclo-oxygenase pathways;[9] hypocholesterolaemic activity in rats.[10] This *in-vivo* effect has been linked to *in-vitro* actions documented for various flavonoids, including prevention of ethanol-induced hyperlipidaemia,[11] catecholamine-induced lipolysis[10,11] and lipogenesis in adipose tissue;[10,11] there is no pronounced effect on blood pressure in cats and rabbits.[12] In addition, the latter study found no CNS depressant and no antispasmodic activity; marked antibacterial activity against various Gram-positive bacteria (e.g. *Bacillus subtilis*, *Escherichia coli*, *Sarcina lutea*, *Staphylococcus aureus*).[13]

Human studies Clinical trials of scutellarin involving 634 cases of cerebral thrombosis, cerebral embolism, and paralysis caused by stroke have been undertaken. An overall effective rate of more than 88% was reported following intramuscular, intravenous, or oral administration.[14]

Side-effects, Toxicity[G34]

Symptoms caused by overdosage of scullcap tincture include giddiness, stupor, confusion, and seizures.[G34] Hepatotoxic reactions have been reported after ingestion of scullcap-containing preparations.[G34,15] Adulteration of scullcap herb by *Teucrium* is recognised. Several cases of hepatitis have been associated with germander (*Teucrium chamaedrys*).[16]

Contra-indications, Warnings

None documented. In view of the possible hepatotoxicity associated with scullcap, its use is best avoided.

Pregnancy and lactation Scullcap is stated to have been used traditionally to eliminate a mother's afterbirth and to promote menstruation.[G10] Limited information is known regarding the pharmacological activity and toxicity of scullcap. In view of this and concerns over hepatotoxicity, scullcap should not be taken during pregnancy and lactation.

Pharmaceutical Comment

Limited information has been documented regarding the chemistry of scullcap. Most of the pharmacological activities reported for other *Scutellaria* species have been attributed to the flavonoid constituents. Despite the traditional uses of scullcap as a sedative and anticonvulsant, there are no documented scientific data to support these uses. Commercial scullcap is commonly recognised to be adulterated with *Teucrium* species, notably *Teucrium canadense*. Herbal preparations stated to contain scullcap may therefore contain a *Teucrium* species. Few pharmacological studies have been undertaken for *Teucrium* species. Hepatitis has been associated with germander (*Teucrium chamaedrys*). Hepatotoxicity has resulted in humans taking commercially available remedies in the UK which are stated to contain scullcap. It would seem advisable to avoid ingestion of scullcap.

References

See General References G3, G5, G10, G14, G15, G24, G30, G32 and G34

1. Kubo M *et al*. *Scutellariae radix*. X. Inhibitory effects of various flavonoids on histamine release from rat peritoneal mast cells *in vitro*. *Chem Pharm Bull* 1984; **32:** 5051–4.

2. Tomimori T *et al*. Studies on the constituents of Scutellarian species. *Yakugaku Zasshi* 1985; **105:** 148–55.

3. Tomimori T *et al*. Studies on the constituents of *Scutellaria* species. VI. On the flavonoid constituents of the root of *Scutellaria baicalensis* Georgi (5). Quantitative analysis of flavonoids in Scutellaria roots by high-performance liquid chromatography. *Yakugaku Zasshi* 1985; **105:** 148–55.

4. Popova TP *et al*. Chemical composition and medicinal properties of *Scutellaria galericulata*. *Farm Zh (Kiev)* 1972; **27:** 58–61.

5. Ryn SH *et al*. The cytotoxic principle of Scutellariae radix against L1210 cell. *Planta Med* 1985; **51:** 355.

6. Kimura Y *et al*. Studies on *Scutellariae radix*; IX. New component inhibiting lipid peroxidation in rat liver. *Planta Med* 1984; **50:** 290–5.

7. Kimura Y *et al*. Studies on *Scutellariae radix*. IV. Effects on lipid peroxidation in rat liver. *Chem Pharm Bull* 1981; **29:** 2610–17.

8. Kimura Y *et al*. Studies on *Scutellariae radix*. VI. Effects of flavanone compounds on lipid peroxidation in rat liver. *Chem Pharm Bull* 1982; **30(5):** 1792–95.

9. Kimura Y *et al*. Studies on *Scutellariae radix*; XIII. Effects of various flavonoids on arachidonate metabolism in leukocytes. *Planta med* 1985; **51:** 132–6.

10. Kimura Y *et al*. Studies on *Scutellariae radix*. III. Effects on lipid metabolism in serum, liver and fat cells of rats. *Chem Pharm Bull* 1981; **29:** 2308–12.

11. Kimura Y *et al*. Studies on *Scutellariae radix*. V. Effects on ethanol-induced hyperlipemia and lipolysis in isolated fat cells. *Chem Pharm Bull* 1982; **30:** 219–22.

12. Kurnakov BA. Pharmacology of skullcap. *Farmakol i Toksikol* 1957; **20:** 79–80.

13. Kubo M *et al*. Studies on *Scutellariae radix*. Part II: The antibacterial substance. *Planta Med* 1981; **43:** 194–201.

14. Peigen X, Keji C. Recent advances in clinical studies of Chinese medicinal herbs. 1. Drugs affecting the cardiovascular system. *Phytotherapy Res* 1987; **1:** 53–57.

15. Perharic L *et al*. Toxicological problems resulting from exposure to traditional remedies and food supplements. *Drug Safety* 1994; **11:** 284–94.

16. Larrey D *et al*. Hepatitis after germander (*Teucrium chamaedrys*) administration: another instance of herbal medicine toxicity. *Am Coll Physns* 1992; **117:** 129–32.

SENEGA

Species (Family)
Polygala senega L. and other closely related species cultivated in Western Canada and Japan. (Polygalaceae)

Synonym(s)
Polygala, Rattlesnake Root, Snake Root, *Polygala senega* var. *latifolia* (Japan), Northern Senega (Canada)

Part(s) Used
Root, Rootstock

Pharmacopoeial Monographs
BHP 1983
BHP 1990
BPC 1973
Martindale 29th edition
Pharmacopoeias—Arg., Aust., Belg., Br., Chin., Egypt., Eur., Fr., Jpn, Mex., Neth., Nord., Port., Span., and Swiss. Br. also describes Powdered Senega Root

Legal Category (Licensed Products)
GSL[G14]

Constituents[G1,G2,G18,G24,G29,G31,G32,G34]
Acids Salicylic acid and its methyl ester 0.1–0.2%; hydroxycinnamic acids (e.g. caffeic acid, ferulic acid, sinapic acid) free or esterified with saponins[1]
Carbohydrates Arabinose, fructose, glucose, melibiose, raffinose, saccharose, stachyose, sucrose; 1,5-anhydro-D-glucitol and other D-glucitol derivatives;[2,3] trisaccharides; mucilage, pectin
Terpenoids (6–10%). Saponin mixture sometimes referred to as senegin; individual components include hydroxysenegenin, polygalic acid, presenegenin, senegenin, senegenic acid (aglycones), and senegin I, senegin II (major), senegin III, and senegin IV (glycosides).[4,5] The saponins are also referred to as senegin A, B, C, and D.
Other constituents Fat, resin, sterols, valeric acid ester
Other Polygala species *Polygala paniculata* contains coumarins (aurapten, murrangatin, phebalosin, and 7-methoxy-8-(1,4-dihydroxy-3-methyl-2-butenyl)coumarin[6], pyranocoumarin).[7] *Polygala chamaebuxus* (European species) contains hydroxycinnamic acid esters involving acetic, ferulic, and sinapic acids as the ester moieties, saponins, tenuifolin (prosapogenin), rutin (flavonoid glycoside), coniferin and syringen (phenolic glycosides).[1]
Other European species (e.g. *Polygala alpestris*, *Polygala comosa*, *Polygala vayredae*) contain complex mixtures of bidesmosidic saponins, tenuifolin (prosapogenin), hydroxycinnimic acid esters similar to those reported for *P. chamaebuxus*.[8] *Polygala triphylla* contains B ring oxygen-free trioxygenated- and glucosyloxy-xanthones.[9]

Polygala polygama contains podophyllotoxin and demethylpodophyllotoxin (lignans).[10]

Food Use
Senega is listed by the Council of Europe as a natural source of food flavouring (category N2). This category indicates that senega can be added to foodstuffs in small quantities, with a possible limitation of an active principle (as yet unspecified) in the final product.[G9]

Herbal Use
Senega is stated to possess expectorant, diaphoretic, sialogogue, and emetic properties. Traditionally, it has been used for bronchitic asthma, chronic bronchitis, as a gargle for pharyngitis, and specifically for chronic bronchitis.[G1,G2,G3,G4,G32]

Dose
Dried root 0.5–1.0 g or by infusion three times daily[G2,G3]
Senega Liquid Extract (BPC 1968) 0.3–1.0 mL
Senega Tincture (BPC 1968) 2.5–5.0 mL

Pharmacological Actions
Animal studies None documented for *P. senega*. Polygalic acid and senegin are stated to be irritant to the gastro-intestinal mucosa and to cause a reflex secretion of mucus in the bronchioles.[G2,G21]
CNS-depressant properties in mice (e.g. reduction in spontaneous activity, inhibition of amphetamine stimulation, potentiation of barbiturate-induced sleeping time, and decrease in rectal temperature) were documented for *Polygala microphylla*.[11] Similar properties have been reported for *Polygala tenuifolia* and have been attributed to the saponin constituents. *Polygala erioptera* and *P. paniculata* have exhibited molluscicidal activity, and *P. paniculata* is reported to possess antifungal activity.[7]
Human studies A French patent has stated that a triterpenic acid extracted from senega possesses anti-inflammatory activity and is effective against graft rejection, eczema, psoriasis, and multiple sclerosis.[12]

Side-effects, Toxicity[G34]
Saponins are generally regarded as irritant to the gastrointestinal mucosa, and irritant properties have been documented for senega plant and for related *Polygala* species.[G26] Large doses of senega are reported to cause vomiting and purging.[G30]
The haemolytic index (HI) of senega saponins is stated to be between 2500 and 4500.[G31] Haemolytic saponins are toxic to mammals when administered intravenously, but have a low toxicity when given orally. because they do not cross the gastrointestinal mucosa.[13] Contact with damaged mucosal areas may cause a problem. Toxicity associated

with chronic exposure of the gastro-intestinal mucosa to haemolytic saponins has not been established. It has been stated that the suitability of saponins for nutritional and pharmacological use requires further investigation: free saponins in the gastro-intestinal tract may interact with the mucosal cells, causing a transient increase in the permeability of the small intestine to intraluminal solutes and inhibiting active nutrient absorption.[13] This action may consequently facilitate the entry of antigens and biologically active food peptides into the blood circulation, with adverse systemic effects.[13]

Cytotoxic lignans have been documented as constituents of a related species, *P. polygama*.[10]

Contra-indications, Warnings

Senega may exacerbate existing gastro-intestinal inflammation and excessive doses may cause vomiting.

Pregnancy and lactation Limited information is available on the chemistry, pharmacology, and toxicity of senega. In view of this, and the potential irritant properties of senega, its use during pregnancy and lactation should be avoided.

Pharmaceutical Comment

Limited chemical information is available for senega, although related *Polygala* species have been studied in more detail. No scientific evidence was found to justify the herbal uses. In view of the lack of toxicity data and uncertainty regarding the risk associated with chronic ingestion of haemolytic saponins, excessive use of senega should be avoided.

References

See General References G1, G2, G3, G4, G7, G9, G14, G18, G21, G22, G24, G26, G29, G30, G31, G32 and G34.

1. Hamburger M, Hostettmann K. Hydroxycinnamic acid esters from *Polygala chamaebuxus*. *Phytochemistry* 1985; **24**: 1793–7.

2. Takiura K *et al*. Studies on oligosaccharides. XIII. Oligosaccharides in *Polygala senega* and structures of glycosyl-1,5-anhydro-D-glucitols. *Yakugaku Zasshi* 1974; **94**: 998–1003.

3. Takiura K *et al*. Studies on oligosaccharides XVI. New trisaccharides found in *Senega radix*. *Yakugaku Zasshi* 1975; **95**: 166–9.

4. Tsukitani Y *et al*. Studies on the constituents of Senegae radix. II. The structure of senegin-II, a saponin from *Polygala senega* Linne var. *latifolia* Torry et Gray. *Chem Pharm Bull* 1973; **21**: 791–9.

5. Tsukitani Y, Shoji J. Studies on the constituents of Senegae radix III. The structures of senegin-III and -IV, saponins from *Polygala senega* Linne var. *latifolia* Torry et Gray. *Chem Bull Pharm* 1973; **21**: 1564–74.

6. Hamburger M *et al*. Coumarins from *Polygala paniculata*. *Planta Med* 1985; **51**: 215–17.

7. Hamburger M *et al*. A new pyranocoumarin diester from *Polygala panculata* L. *Helv Chim Acta* 1984; **67**: 1729–33.

8. Hamburger M, Hostettmann K. Glycosidic constituents of some European *Polygala* species. *J Nat Prod* 1986; (May-June): 557.

9. Ghosal S *et al*. 1,2,3-Trioxygenated glucosyloxyxanthones. *Phytochemistry* 1981; **20**: 489–92.

10. Hokanson GC. Podophyllotoxin and 4′-demethylpodophyllotoxin from *Polygala polygama* (Polygalaceae). *Lloydia* 1978; **41**: 497–8.

11. Carretero ME *et al*. Études pharmacodynamiques préliminaires de *Polygala microphylla* (L.), sur le système nerveux central. *Plant Méd Phytothér* 1986; **20**: 148–54.

12. Tubery P. Antiinflammatory triterpenic alcohol acids. *Fr Demande Patent* 2,202,683.

13. Johnson IT *et al*. Influence of saponins on gut permeability and active nutrient transport in vitro. *J Nutr* 1986; **116**: 2270–7.

SENNA

Species (Family)
(i) *Cassia senna* L.
(ii) *Cassia angustifolia* Vahl. (Leguminosae)

Synonym(s)
(i) Alexandrian and Khartoum senna, *Cassia acutifolia* Delite
(ii) Tinnevelly and Indian senna

Part(s) Used
Fruit (pod), Leaf

Pharmacopoeial Monographs
BHP 1983
BHP 1990
BPC 1973
Martindale 30th edition
Pharmacopoeias—Senna fruit, from Alexandrian and Tinnevelly senna is included in Arg., Aust., Belg., Br., Cz., Egypt., Eur., Fr., Ger., Hung., Ind., Int., Neth., Nord., and Swiss; some have only one monograph covering both varieties; Port. includes only Tinnevelly senna fruit.
Senna leaf from Alexandrian or Tinnevelly senna, or both, is included in Arg., Aust., Belg., Br., Braz., Chin., Egypt., Eur., Fr., Ger., Hung., Ind., It., Jpn, Mex., Neth., Nord., Port., Rus., Span., Swiss, U.S., and Yug. U.S. also includes Sennosides. Mex. includes Sennosides A and B.

Legal Category (Licensed Products)
GSL[G14]

Constituents[G1,G2,G3,G4,G10,G19,G24,G31,G32,G34]
Anthraquinones Dianthrone glycosides (1.5–3% leaf; 2–5% fruit), primarily sennosides A and B (rhein dianthrones) with sennosides C and D (rhein aloe-emodin heterodianthrones), aloe-emodin dianthrone. Sennosides A and B yield sennidin A and B respectively. Free anthraquinones including aloe-emodin, chrysophanol and rhein with their glycosides
Carbohydrates Polysaccharides (about 2.5%)[1] including mucilage (arabinose, galactose, galacturonic acid, rhamnose) and a galactomannan (galactose, mannose);[2] free sugars (e.g. fructose, glucose, pinitol, sucrose)
Flavonoids Flavonols including isorhamnetin and kaempferol
Glycosides 6-Hydroxymusizin and tinnevellin glycosides
Other constituents Chrysophanic acid, salicylic acid, saponin, resin, volatile oil (trace)

Food Use
Senna is listed by the Council of Europe as a natural source of food flavouring (Tinnevelly category N2, Alexandrian category N3). Category N2 indicates that senna can be added to foodstuffs in small quantities, with a possible limitation of an active principle (as yet unspecified) in the final product. Category N3 indicates that there is insufficient information available about Alexandrian senna, for an adequate assessment of potential toxicity.[G9]

Herbal Use
Senna is stated to possess cathartic properties (leaf greater than fruit) and has been used traditionally for constipation.[G1,G2,G3,G4,G32]

Dose
Dried pods 3–6 pods (Alexandrian) or 4–12 pods (Tinnevelly) steeped in 150 mL warm water for 6–12 hours[G2,G3]
Dried leaflets 0.5–2.0 g[G2,G3]
Leaf, liquid extract (1:1 in 25% alcohol) 0.5–2.0 mL[G2,G3]
Senna Liquid Extract (BPC 1973) 0.5–2.0 mL

Pharmacological Actions
The cathartic action of anthraquinone-containing drugs is well recognised and they have been used as laxatives for many years. However, there is still some uncertainty as to the exact mode of action of the anthraquinones.

It is thought that anthraquinone glycosides are absorbed from the gastro-intestinal tract, the aglycones liberated during metabolism and excreted into the colon resulting in stimulation and an increase in peristalsis. However, it has also been suggested that the purgative action of senna is due to the action of intestinal bacteria.[3] Using human intestinal flora, it was found that sennoside A is reduced to 8-glucosylrheinanthrone, hydrolysed to rheinanthrone and oxidised to sennidin A. The active principle causing peristaltic movements of the large intestine was thought to be rheinanthrone.[3] Sennosides A and B, and their natural metabolites sennidins A and B, have been reported to act specifically on the large intestine in the rat with the acceleration of colonic transport the major component of their laxative effect.[4] Sennosides A and B have also been reported to induce fluid secretion exclusively in the colon, following oral administration of the glycosides to rats.[5]

It has been suggested that the laxative action of the sennosides involves prostaglandins. Indomethacin has been found to partly inhibit the action of sennosides A and B, although a bolus injection of prostaglandins into the caecal lumen was stated to neither influence transit time nor to induce diarrhoea.[4] Pretreatment of mice with indomethacin and a PGE antagonist has been documented to prevent diarrhoea caused by intracaecal administration of rhein, which stimulates the production of PGE-like material specifically in the colon.[6] Indomethacin was found to depress the large intestinal propulsive activity of rhein, but did not suppress PGE_2-induced diarrhoea. The authors suggest that the action of rhein is mediated by prostaglandin biosynthesis and release.[6]

Antihepatotoxic activity has been documented for naphtho-α-pyrone and naphtho-γ-pyrone glycosides, and for the anthraquinone glycosides isolated from a related species *Cassia tora*.[7] Greatest activity was documented for the naphtho-γ-pyrone glycosides.

Significant inhibitory activity in mice against leukaemia P388 has been documented for aloe-emodin.[G19]

Side-effects, Toxicity[G34]

Senna may cause mild abdominal discomfort such as colic or cramps. Prolonged use or overdosage can result in diarrhoea with excessive loss of potassium; an atonic non-functioning colon may also develop.[G22] Excessive use and abuse of senna has been associated with finger clubbing and with the development of cachexia and reduced serum globulin concentrations.[8]

Sennosides A and B are reported to be most potent with respect to laxative action, but to be the least toxic compared to other anthraquinone fractions in senna. Similarly, fractions with a low laxative activity (e.g. rhein-8-glucoside) are reported to have the highest acute toxicity.[9] LD_{50} values in mice following intravenous injection of sennosides A and B and of rhein-8-glycoside are reported to be 4.1 g/kg and 400 mg/kg, respectively.[9] The acute oral toxicity of all senna fractions in mice has been reported to be greater than 5 g/kg, although all of the animals were stated to have died by the following week. The toxicity of total senna extracts is greater than that of the individual sennosides and it has been proposed that the laxative and toxic components of senna could be separated.[6]

In-vitro carcinogenicity testing has reported certain anthraquinones, including aloe-emodin, to be active in more than one strain of *Salmonella typhimurium*.[10] Aglycones were documented to exhibit genotoxic activity in a mammalian cell assay.[10]

Sensitising properties have been documented for emodin (*see* Aloes).[G26]

Contra-indications, Warnings

It is recommended that senna should not be given to patients with intestinal obstruction or with undiagnosed abdominal symptoms; care should also be taken by patients with inflammatory bowel disease and prolonged use should be avoided.[G22,G34] Excessive use of senna may potentiate the action of cardiac glycosides due to excessive potassium loss. Anthraquinones cause discoloration of the urine which may interfere with diagnostic tests.[G22]

Pregnancy and lactation Non-standardised anthraquinone-containing laxative preparations should not be taken during pregnancy or lactation since their pharmacological action is unpredictable. Although anthraquinone derivatives may be excreted in the breast milk, following normal dosage their concentration is usually insufficient to affect the nursing infant.[G22]

Pharmaceutical Comment

The chemistry of senna is characterised by the anthraquinone derivatives. The laxative action of these compounds is well recognised and supports the herbal use of senna as a laxative for the treatment of constipation. However, the use of non-standardised anthraquinone-containing preparations should be avoided since their pharmacological effect will be variable and unpredictable. The sennoside content of many licensed senna products is standardised and generally calculated as sennoside B.

References

See General References G1, G2, G3, G4, G7, G9, G10, G11, G14, G19, G22, G23, G24, G26, G29, G31, G32 and G34.

1.   Müller BM *et al*. Isolation and structural investigation of a polysaccharide from *Cassia angustifolia* leaves. *Planta Med* 1989; **55**: 99.

2.   Alam N, Gupta PC. Structure of a water-soluble polysaccharide from the seeds of *Cassia angustifolia*. *Planta Med* 1986; **52**: 308–10.

3.   Kobashi K *et al*. Metabolism of sennosides by human intestinal bacteria. *Planta Med* 1980; **40**: 225–36.

4.   Leng-Peschlow E. Acceleration of large intestine transit time in rats by sennosides and related compounds. *J Pharm Pharmacol* 1986; **38**: 369–73.

5.   Leng-Peschlow E. Dual effect orally administered sennosides on large intestine transit and fluid absorption in the rat. *J Pharm Pharmacol* 1986; **38**: 606–10.

6.   Yagi T *et al*. Involvement of prostaglandin E-like material in the purgative action of rhein anthrone, the intraluminal active metabolite of sennosides A and B in mice. *J Pharm Pharmacol* 1988; **40**: 27–30.

7.   Wong SM *et al*. Isolation and structural elucidation of new antihepatotoxic naphtho-gamma-pyrone glycosides, naphtho-α-pyrone glycoside and anthraquinone glycosides from the seeds of *Cassia tora*. *Planta Med* 1989; **55**: 112.

8.   Senna. *Lawrence Review of Natural Products*, 1989.

9.   Hietala P *et al*. Laxative potency and acute toxicity of some anthraquinone derivatives, senna extracts and fractions of senna extracts. *Pharmacol Toxicol* 1987; **61**: 153–56.

10.   Westendorf J *et al*. Possible carcinogenicity of anthraquinone-containing medical plants. *Planta Med* 1988; **54**: 562.

SHEPHERD'S PURSE

Species (Family)
Capsella bursa-pastoris (L.) Medic (Cruciferae)

Synonym(s)
Capsella

Part(s) Used
Herb

Pharmacopoeial Monographs
BHP 1983

Legal Category (Licensed Products)
GSL[G14]

Constituents[G1,G3,G18,G19,G32]
Amines Acetylcholine, choline, amino acids 2.33% (major component proline), histamine, tyramine, unidentified crystalline alkaloids.[1]
Flavonoids Quercetin, diosmetin, luteolin, hesperetin, and their glycosides (e.g. rutin, diosmin, hesperidin).[2]
Volatile oils (0.02%). Camphor (major); at least 74 components identified[3,4]
Other constituents Carotenoids, fumaric acid, sinigrin (mustard oil glucoside), ascorbic acid (vitamin C) and vitamin K.[4,5,G1]

Food Use
Shepherd's purse is not used in foods.

Herbal Use
Shepherd's purse is stated to possess antihaemorrhagic and urinary antiseptic properties. Traditionally, it has been used for menorrhagia, haematemesis, haematuria, diarrhoea, and acute catarrhal cystitis.[G1,G3,G32]

Dose
Dried herb 1–4 g or by infusion three times daily[G3]
Liquid extract (1:1 in 25% alcohol) 1–4 mL three times daily[G3]

Pharmacological Actions
Animal studies A variety of actions have been documented for an ethanolic extract of shepherd's purse in various animal models.[6–10] Anti-inflammatory activity has been exhibited versus carrageenan-induced and dextran-induced rat paw oedema.[7] A reduction in capillary permeability in the guinea-pig, induced by histamine and serotonin has also been observed[7] and flavonoid components isolated from shepherd's purse have been reported to reduce blood vessel permeability in mice.[2] Anti-ulcer activity has been documented in rats following intraperitoneal injection. The extract did not affect gastric secretion, but accelerated recovery from stress-induced ulcers.[7] A hypotensive effect observed in cats, dogs, rabbits, and rats, following intravenous injection, was inhibited by a β-adrenoceptor blocker but not by atropine, thus dismissing earlier reports that this action was attributable to cholinergic compounds present in shepherd's purse.[8,9]

Diuresis has been reported in mice, following oral or intraperitoneal administration. The mode of action was stated to involve an increase in the glomerular filtration rate.[7]

Documented cardiac actions include increased coronary blood flow in dogs following intra-arterial administration, and a slight inhibitory effect on ouabain-induced ventricular fibrillation in the rat following intraperitoneal injection, together with a negative chronotropic effect.[9] Studies on the isolated heart have reported negative chronotropic and inotropic actions in the guinea-pig and rabbit, and coronary vasodilatation.[9]

A CNS-depressant action in mice has been demonstrated (potentiation of barbiturate-induced sleeping time).[9]

Weak antibacterial activity mainly towards Gram-positive organisms has been reported.[11]

Antineoplastic activity in rats has been documented for fumaric acid, which prevented the development of hepatic neoplasms when co-administered with the carcinogen 3-MeDAB.[12]

Shepherd's purse seeds are stated to possess rubefacient and vesicant properties because of their isothiocyanate-yielding components.[G26]

In-vitro studies have documented stimulatory action in various smooth muscle tissues. Induced contractions of the small intestine in the guinea-pig were reported to be unaffected by atropine and diphenhydramine, but were inhibited by papaverine.[8,9] Induced uteroactivity in the rat, equivalent to the effect of oxytocin 0.1 i.u. was unaffected by atropine, but inhibited by competitive inhibitors of oxytocin.[8] Two unidentified alkaloid components of shepherd's purse have also been stated to elicit a physiological activity on the uterus.[1] Induced tracheal contractions in the guinea-pig were unaffected by adrenaline, which did inhibit acetylcholine-induced contractions.[9] These studies concluded the active substance(s) in shepherd's purse responsible for the observed actions on smooth muscle were neither acetylcholine nor histamine.[8,9]

Side-effects, Toxicity
Shepherd's purse extracts have been reported to exhibit low toxicity in mice. LD_{50} values reported are 1.5 g/kg body-weight (mice, intraperitoneal injection) and 31.5 g/kg (mice, subcutaneous injection).[9] Signs of toxicity were described as sedation, enlargement of pupils, paralysis of hind limbs, difficulty in respiration, and death by respiratory paralysis.[9] Following hydrolysis, the

constituent sinigrin yields allyl isothiocyanate which is an extremely powerful irritant and produces blisters on the skin.[G19] Isothiocyanates have been implicated in endemic goitre (hypothyroidism with thyroid enlargement) and have been reported to produce goitre in experimental animals.[G19]

Contra-indications, Warnings

Prolonged or excessive use of the herb may interfere with existing therapy for hyper- or hypotension, thyroid dysfunction, or cardiac disorder, and may potentiate sedative actions.

Pregnancy and lactation Shepherd's purse is reputed to act as an abortifacient and to affect the menstrual cycle, and tyramine is documented as a uteroactive constituent.[G12] In view of this and the reported oxytocin-like activity, the use of shepherd's purse during pregnancy should be avoided. Excessive should be avoided during lactation.

Pharmaceutical Comment

The chemistry of shepherd's purse is well documented and although a number of actions affecting the circulatory system have been observed in animal studies, these actions do not relate to the traditional herbal uses. Limited toxicity data are available. In view of this together with the demonstrated pharmacological activity of the herb, excessive use of shepherd's purse should be avoided.

References

See General References G1, G3, G12, G14, G18, G19, G21, G26 and G32.

1.   Kuroda K, Kaku T. Pharmacological and chemical studies on the alcohol extract of *Capsella bursa-pastoris*. *Life Sci* 1969; **8:** 151–5.

2.   Jurisson S. Flavonoid substances of *Capsella bursa pastoris*. *Farmatsiya (Moscow)* 1973; **22:** 34–5.

3.   Miyazawa M *et al.* The constituents of the essential oils from *Capsella bursa-pastoris* Medik. *Yakugaku Zasshi* 1979; **99:** 1041–3.

4.   Park RJ. The occurrence of mustard oil glucosides in *Lepidium hyssopifolium*, L. bonariense, and *Capsella bursa pastoris*. *Aust J Chem* 1967; **20:** 2799–801.

5.   Jurisson S. Vitamin content of shepherd's purse. *Farmatsiya (Moscow)* 1976; **25:** 66–7.

6.   Kuroda K, Takagi K. Studies on *Capsella bursa pastoris*. I. General pharmacology of ethanol extract of the herb. *Arch Int Pharmacodyn Ther* 1969; **178:** 382–91.

7.   Kuroda K, Takagi K. Studies on capsella bursa pastoris. II. Diuretic, anti-inflammatory and anti-ulcer action of ethanol extracts of the herb. *Arch Int Pharmacodyn Ther* 1969; **178:** 392–9.

8.   Kuroda K, Takagi K. Physiologically active substance in *Capsella bursa-pastoris*. *Nature* 1968; **220:** 707–8.

9.   Jurisson S. Determination of active substances of *Capsella bursa pastoris*. *Tartu Riiliku Ulikooli Toim* 1971; (270): 71–9.

10.   Kolos Pelhes E, Marczal G. Pharmacognosy of herba bursae pastoris. *Gyogyszereszet* 1966; **10:** 465–7.

11.   Moskalenko SA. Preliminary screening of far-eastern ethnomedicinal plants for antibacterial activity. *J Ethnopharmacol* 1986; **15:** 231–59.

12.   Kuroda K. Neoplasm inhibitor from *Capsella bursa pastoris*. *Japan Kokai* 77 41 207.

SKUNK CABBAGE

Species (Family)
Symplocarpus foetidus (L.) Salisb. (Araceae)

Synonym(s)
Dracontium foetidum L., Skunkweed

Part(s) Used
Rhizome, Root

Pharmacopoeial Monographs
BHP 1983

Legal Category (Licensed Products)
GSL[G14]

Constituents[G10,G32]
Reported constituents include starch, gum-sugar, fixed and volatile oils, resin, tannin, an acrid principle, iron
Other plant parts Large amounts of alkaloids (unspecified), phenolic compounds and glycosides have been isolated from all plant parts of skunk cabbage.[1] The leaves are reported to contain hydroxytryptamine;[G10] 3 anthocyanin pigments have been isolated from the flowers, namely cyanidin-3-monoglucoside, cyanidin-3-rutinoside, peonidin-3-rutinoside[2]

Food Use
Skunk cabbage is not used in foods.

Herbal Use
Skunk cabbage is stated to possess expectorant, antispasmodic, and mild sedative properties. Traditionally, it has been used for bronchitis, whooping cough, asthma, and specifically for bronchitic asthma.[G3,G32]

Dose
Powdered rhizome/root 0.5–1.0 g in honey or by infusion or decoction three times daily[G3]
Liquid extract (1:1 in 25% alcohol) 0.5–1.0 mL three times daily[G3]
Tincture (1:10 in 45% alcohol) 2–4 mL three times daily[G3]

Pharmacological Actions
Animal studies None documented for the rhizome/root. The leaf extract has haemolytic properties.[G10]

Side-effects, Toxicity
The root is reported to be bitter and acrid, with a disagreeable odour. Severe itching and inflammation of the skin has been documented.[G26] No published toxicity studies were located.

Contra-indications, Warnings
It has been stated that the fresh plant can cause blistering.[G20] In view of the acrid principle thought to be present in both the dried and fresh root,[G26] skunk cabbage should be used with caution.

Pregnancy and lactation Skunk cabbage is reputed to affect the menstrual cycle.[G10] In view of the lack of phytochemical, pharmacological, and toxicological information, and the irritant properties, the use of skunk cabbage during pregnancy and lactation should be avoided.

Pharmaceutical Comment
Little is known about the constituents, pharmacological activities or safety of skunk cabbage (even though citings as early as 1817 reported its irritant properties).[G26] No documented evidence was found to justify the herbal uses. In view of the documented irritant properties, excessive use is not recommended.

References
See General References G3, G10, G14, G20, G26, and G32.

1. Konyukhov VP *et al.* Dynamics of the accumulation of biologically active agents in *Lysichitum camtsochatcense* and *Symplocarpus foetidus. Uch Zap Khabarovsk Gos Pedagog Inst* 1970; **26**: 59–62.

2. Chang N *et al.* Anthocyanins in *Symplocarpus foetidus* (L.) Nutt. (Araceae). *Bot J Linn Soc* 1970; **63**: 95–6.

SLIPPERY ELM

Species (Family)
Ulmus fulva Michaux (Ulmaceae)

Synonym(s)
Ulmus rubra Muhl.

Part(s) Used
Bark (inner)

Pharmacopoeial Monographs
BHP 1983
BHP 1990
BPC 1949
Martindale 29th edition

Legal Category (Licensed Products)
GSL[G14]

Constituents[G2,G29,G32]
Carbohydrates Mucilage (major constituent) consisting of hexoses, pentoses, methylpentoses, at least two polyuronides, and yielding on hydrolysis galactose, glucose and fructose (trace), galacturonic acid, *l*-rhamnose and *d*-galactose
Other constituents Tannin 3.0–6.5% (type unspecified), phytosterols (β-sitosterol, citrostadienol, dolichol), sesquiterpenes, calcium oxalate, cholesterol

Food Use
It has been recommended by the FACC (Food Additives and Contaminants Committee) that the use of slippery elm as a flavouring agent in foods should be prohibited.[G21] Slippery elm is listed by the Council of Europe as a natural source of food flavouring (category N3). This category indicates that there is insufficient information available to make an adequate assessment of potential toxicity.[G9]

Herbal Use
Slippery elm is stated to possess demulcent, emollient, nutrient, and antitussive properties. Traditionally, it has been used for inflammation or ulceration of the stomach or duodenum, convalescence, colitis, diarrhoea and locally for abcesses, boils, and ulcers (as a poultice).[G2,G3,G4,G32]

Dose
Powdered bark (1:8 as a decoction) 4–16 mL three times daily[G2,G3]
Powdered bark 4 g in 500 mL boiling water as a nutritional supplement three times daily[G2,G3]
Coarse powdered bark with boiling water as a poultice[G2,G3]
Liquid extract (1:1 in 60% alcohol) 5 mL three times daily[G2,G3]

Pharmacological Actions
Mucilages are known to have demulcent and emollient properties. Mucilage is the principal constituent of slippery elm. Tannins are known to possess astringent properties.

Side-effects, Toxicity
None documented. In view of the known constituents of slippery elm it would appear to be non-toxic.

Contra-indications, Warnings
Whole bark has been used to procure abortions.
Pregnancy and lactation There are no known problems with the use of powdered slippery elm during pregnancy.

Pharmaceutical Comment
The primary constituent in slippery elm is mucilage, thereby justifying the herbal use of the remedy as a demulcent, emollient, and antitussive. There are no known problems regarding toxicity of slippery elm, although its use as a food flavouring agent has not been recommended. The supply of hole bark is controlled by regulations.[1]

References
See General References G2, G3, G4, G6, G10, G14, G21, G22, G29, and G32

1. The Medicines (Retail Sale or Supply of Herbal Medicines) Order 1977, SI 1977: 2130.

SQUILL

Species (Family)

Drimia maritima (L.) Stearn (Liliaceae)

Synonym(s)

Scilla, Urginea, *Urginea maritima* (L.) Baker, *Urginea scilla* Steinh., White Squill

Part(s) Used

Bulb (red and white varieties)

Pharmacopoeial Monographs

BHP 1983
BHP 1990. It also describes Indian Squill
BPC 1973
Martindale 29th edition
Pharmacopoeias—Arg., Br., Egypt., Ger., Port., and Span. Br. also describes Powdered Squill and Indian Squill

Legal Category (Licensed Products)

GSL[G14]

Constituents[G2,G10,G19,G24,G31,G32][1,2]

Cardiac glycosides Scillaren A and proscillaridin A (major constituents); others include glucoscillaren A, scillaridin A, scillicyanoside, scilliglaucoside, scilliphaeoside, scillicoeloside, scillazuroside, and scillicryptoside. Scillaren B represents a mixture of the squill glycosides.
Flavonoids Apigenin, dihydroquercetin, isovitexin, iso-orientin, luteolin, orientin, quercetin, taxifolin, vitexin
Other constituents Stigmasterol, tannin, volatile and fixed oils

Food Use

The Food Additives and Contaminants Committee (FACC) has recommended that squill be prohibited as a food flavouring.[G22]

Herbal Use

Squill is stated to possess expectorant, cathartic, emetic, cardioactive, and diuretic properties. Traditionally, it has been used for chronic bronchitis, asthma with bronchitis, whooping cough, and specifically for chronic bronchitis with scanty sputum.[G2,G3,G4,G32]

Dose

Dried bulb 60–200mg or by infusion three times daily[G2,G3]
Squill Liquid Extract (BPC 1973) 0.06–0.2 mL
Squill Tincture (BPC 1973) 0.3–2.0 mL
Squill Vinegar (BPC 1973) 0.6–2.0 mL

Pharmacological Actions

The aglycone components of the cardiac glycoside constituents possess digitalis-like cardiotonic properties.[G19] However, the squill aglycones are poorly absorbed from the gastro-intestinal tract and are less potent than digitalis cardiac glycosides.[1,2]

Expectorant, emetic, and diuretic properties have been documented for white squill.[G19] Squill is reported to induce vomiting by both a central action and local gastric irritation.[1,2] Sub-emetic or near-emetic doses of squill appear to exhibit an expectorant effect, causing an increase in the flow of gastric secretions.[1,2]

Antiseborrhoeic properties have been documented for methanol extracts of red squill which have been employed as hair tonics for the treatment of chronic seborrhoea and dandruff.[G19]

Squill extracts have been reported to exhibit peripheral vasodilatation and bradycardia in anaesthetised rabbits.[1,2]

Side-effects, Toxicity

Excessive use of quill is potentially toxic because of the cardiotonic constituents. However, squill is also a gastric irritant and large doses will stimulate a vomiting reflex. Red squill is toxic to rats and is mainly used as a rodenticide, causing death by a centrally-induced convulsant action.[1,2] A squill soft mass (crude extract) has been stated to be toxic in guinea-pigs at a dose of 270 mg/kg body-weight. A fatal dose for Indian squill (*Urginea indica* Kunth.) is documented as 36 mg/kg.

Contra-indications, Warnings

Squill may cause gastric irritation and should be avoided by individuals with a cardiac disorder. In view of the cardiotonic constituents, precautions applied to digoxin therapy should be considered for squill.
Pregnancy and lactation. Squill is reputed to be an abortifacient and to affect the menstrual cycle.[G12] In addition, cardioactive and gastro-intestinal irritant properties have been documented. The use of squill during pregnancy should be avoided; excessive use should be avoided during lactation.

Pharmaceutical Comment

Squill is characterised by its cardiac glycoside components and unusual flavonoid constituents. The reputed actions of squill as an expectorant, emetic, and cathartic can be attributed to the cardioactive components and squill has been used as an expectorant for many years. However, in view of the documented cardioactive and emetic properties of the aglycones, excessive should be avoided. Red squill is primarily used as a rodenticide.

References

See General References G2, G3, G4, G7, G8, G10, G12, G14, G19, G22, G24, G31, and G32.

1. Court WE. Squill — energetic diuretic. *Pharm J* 1985; **235:** 194–7.

2. Squill. *Lawrence Review of Natural Products,* 1989.

ST. JOHN'S WORT

Species (Family)
Hypericum perforatum L. (Hypericaceae)

Synonym(s)
Hypericum, Millepertuis

Part(s) Used
Herb

Pharmacopoeial Monographs
BHP 1983
Martindale 30th edition
Pharmacopoeias—Cz., Pol., Rom., and Rus.

Legal Category (Licensed Products)
GSL (for external use only)[G14]

Constituents[G1,G10,G18,G24,G31,G32]

Anthraquinone derivatives Hypericin, isohypericin, proto-hypericin. Hypericin is stated to consist of two components, hypericin and pseudohypericin.[1]
Flavonoids Flavonols (e.g. kaempferol, quercetin), flavones (e.g. luteolin) and glycosides (e.g. hyperoside, isoquercitrin, quercitrin, rutin), biflavonoids including biapigenin (a flavone) and amentoflavone (a biapigenin derivative),[3,4] catechins (flavonoids often associated with condensed tannins).[5,6] Concentrations of rutin, hyperoside, and isoquercitrin have been reported as 1.6%, 0.9%, and 0.3%, respectively.[2]
Phenols Caffeic, chlorogenic, *p*-coumaric, ferulic, *p*-hydroxybenzoic and vanillic acids, hyperfolin (3,5-dinitrobenzoate ester),[7] prenylated phloroglucinol derivatives[5,8]
Tannins (8–9%). Type not specified. Proanthocyanidins (condensed type) have been reported[G1]
Volatile oils (0.05–0.9%). Major component (not less than 30%) is methyl-2-octane (saturated hydrocarbon); others include *n*-nonane and traces of methyl-2-decane and *n*-undecane (saturated hydrocarbons),[9] α- and β-pinene, α-terpineol, geraniol, and traces of myrcene and limonene (monoterpenes), caryophyllene and humulene (sesquiterpenes).[10,11]
Other constituents Acids (isovalerianic, nicotinic, myristic, palmitic, stearic), carotenoids, choline, nicotinamide, pectin, β-sitosterol, straight chain saturated hydrocarbons (C_{16}, C_{30})[9,12] and alcohols (C_{24}, C_{26}, C_{28}).[9,12]

Food Use

St. John's wort is listed by the Council of Europe as a natural source of food flavouring (category N2). This category indicates that St. John's wort can be added to foodstuffs, provided that the concentration of hypericin does not exceed 0.1 mg/kg in the finished product. Exceptions to this are pastilles/lozenges (1 mg/kg) and alcoholic beverages (2 mg/kg).[G9]

Herbal Use

St. John's wort is stated to possess sedative and astringent properties. It has been used for excitability, neuralgia, fibrositis, sciatica, wounds, and specifically for menopausal neurosis.[G1,G3,G32] St. John's wort is used extensively in homoeopathic preparations as well as in herbal products.

Dose

Dried herb 2–4 g or by infusion three times daily[G3]
Liquid extract (1:1 in 25% alcohol) 2–4 mL three times daily[G3]
Tincture (1:10 in 45% alcohol) 2–4 mL three times daily[G3]

Pharmacological Actions

Animal studies A leaf extract has been documented to enhance the immunity of mice towards *Staphylococcus aureus* and *Bordetella pertussis*;[13] hyperforin is reported to be an antibiotic with activity against *S. aureus*.[7] Further antibiotic constituents have been isolated from St. John's wort: novoimanine, water-soluble imanine, and imanine.[14,15] Novoimanine was reported to be the most effective topical agent against *S. aureus*, with water-soluble imanine more effective than imanine or sulphanilamide.[14] Herb extracts are reported to exhibit more pronounced properties against staphylococci, shigellae, and *Escherichia coli* compared to decoctions.[15,16]

Flavonoid and catechin-containing fractions have exhibited antiviral activity, inhibiting the influenza virus by 83–100%.[17]

An extract of St. John's wort was found to suppress inflammation and leucocyte infiltration in mice, induced by carageenan and PGE_1.[18] Anti-inflammatory and anti-ulcerogenic properties have been documented for amentoflavone, a biapigenin derivative,[4] and analgesic activity in mice has been reported for the total flavonoid fraction.[19] The active principle was stated to be of the quercetin type.

A commercial extract of St. John's wort has exhibited psychotropic and antidepressant activities in mice.[20] Furthermore, virtually irreversible inhibition of monoamine oxidase type A and B in rat brain mitochondria *in vitro* has been described for hypericin with activity reported to be higher towards type B.[21]

It has been suggested that biflavonoids may be the sedative principles in St. John's wort, since CNS activity has been documented for biflavonoid constituents in another plant, *Taxus baccata*.[3] Small quantities of hypericin are stated to have a tonic and tranquillising action in humans.[G24]

Both water-soluble imanine and imanine were reported to reduce blood pressure and increase the frequency and depth of breathing following intravenous administration (50 mg/kg) to rabbits.[14] A study of the vasoconstrictor action of water-soluble imanine and imanine on the isolated rabbit ear indicated that their hypotensive action was not due to a direct effect on the vasculature.[14] When perfused through the isolated frog heart, both water-soluble imanine and imanine were found to cause cardiac systolic arrest at a dilution of 1×10^{-5}.[14] Proanthocyanidin-containing fractions isolated from St. John's wort have been reported to inhibit contractions of the isolated guinea-pig heart induced by histamine, $PGF_{2\alpha}$, and potassium chloride.[22]

A tonus-raising effect on isolated guinea-pig and rabbit uteri has been documented for a crude aqueous extract.[23] Of the group of plants investigated, St. John's wort was reported to exhibit the weakest uterotonic activity.

Tannins isolated from St. John's wort are stated to have mild astringent activity.[24] The anthraquinone derivatives documented for St. John's wort do not possess any purgative action.[G31]

Dietary administration of St. John's wort to rats was found to have no affect on various hepatic drug metabolising enzymes (e.g. aminopyrine, N-demethylase, glutathione S-transferase, epoxide hydrolase) or on copper concentrations in the liver. No major effects were observed on hepatic iron or zinc concentrations, and no significant tissue lesions were found in four rats fed St. John's wort in their daily diet for 119 days (10% for first 12 days, 5% thereafter because of unpalatability).[25]

Hypericin is a photosensitising agent and consumption can cause allergic skin reactions following exposure to UV light. A review of the photodynamic actions of hypericin has been published.[26]

In-vitro cytotoxicity against human colon carcinoma cells (CO 115) has been described for hyperforin-related constituents, isolated from *H. calycinum* and *H. revolutum*.[27]

Human studies A commercial extract of St. John's wort has been reported to improve symptoms such as anxiety, anorexia, and depression in 15 women.[28] A double blind trial in which 100 patients suffering from anxiety were either treated with a herbal product (St. John's wort and valerian) or diazepam, found that after two weeks of therapy the herbal product was more effective than diazepam.[29] A reduction in pain was experienced by up to 90% of 35 patients suffering from chronic gastroduodenitis, who were treated with a herbal combination product containing St. John's wort.[30] After therapy, gastroscopy showed that erosive and haemorrhagic mucous changes present before treatment had disappeared. However, in addition to St. John's wort the product contained agrimony, chamomile, peppermint, and plantain: the efficacy of individual herbal ingredients in combination preparations is difficult to assess.[31] A 20% St. John's wort tincture has been used in the treatment of suppurative otitis in 65 patients, and extracts are stated to have been used clinically in Russia to treat infections. The use of St. John's wort to treat vitiligo (oral administration and topical application) has also been documented.

Anti-viral activity has been reported for hypericin against HIV and hepatitis C.[32–34]

Side-effects, Toxicity

Delayed hypersensitivity or photodermatitis has been documented for St. John's wort, following the ingestion of a herbal tea made from the leaves.[35] St. John's wort is reported to have caused photosensitivity reactions in cattle and sheep.[G10,G26] Mice given 0.2–0.5 mg of the herb were found to develop severe photodynamic effects.[G10] Hypericin is stated to be the photosensitising agent present in St. John's wort.[34,G13,G36] The definitive mechanism for hypericin photosensitivity has yet to be determined although it has been confirmed that the process requires oxygen.[26] The volatile oil of St. John's wort is irritant.[36]

Cytotoxic constituents related to hyperforin have been isolated from two related *Hypericum* species (*see* Animal studies).

Contra-indications, Warnings

St. John's wort is stated to be contra-indicated in depression,[G2] although no rationale is given for this statement which appears to contradict the antidepressant actions documented for St. John's wort. Excessive doses may potentiate existing MAOI (monoamine oxidase inhibitor) therapy (*in-vitro* inhibition of MAO reported for hypericin), and may cause an allergic reaction in sensitive individuals (hypericin).

Pregnancy and lactation Slight *in-vitro* uterotonic activity has been reported for St. John's wort (*see* Animal Studies). In view of the lack of toxicity data and documented photosensitising activity, the use of St. John's wort during pregnancy and lactation is best avoided.

Pharmaceutical Comment

The chemical composition of St. John's wort is well studied. Documented pharmacological activities support some of the stated herbal uses and appear to be attributable to hypericin and to the flavonoid constituents. Hypericin is also reported to be responsible for the photosensitive reactions that have been documented for St. John's wort. In view of the lack of toxicity data and reported photosensitising ability, excessive use of St. John's wort should be avoided.

References

See General References G1, G3, G9, G10, G13, G14, G18, G22, G23, G24, G26, G31, and G32.

1. Vanhaelen M, Vanhaelen-Fastre R. Quantitative determination of biologically active constituents in medicinal plant crude extracts by thin-layer chromatography-densitometry. *J Chromatogr* 1983; **281**: 263–71.

2. Dorossiev I. Determination of flavonoids in *Hypericum perforatum*. *Pharmazie* 1985; **40**: 585–6.

3. Berghöfer R, Hölzl J. Biflavonoids in *Hypericum perforatum*; Part 1. Isolation of 13,II8-biapigenin. *Planta Med* 1987; **53**: 216–17.

4. Berghöfer R, Hölzl J. Isolation of I3',II8-biapigenin (amentoflavone) from *Hypericum perforatum*. *Planta Med* 1989; **55**: 91.

5.   Ollivier B *et al*. Separation et identification des acides phenols par chromatographie liquide haute performance et spectroscopie ultra-violette. Application à la pariétaire (*Parietaria officinalis* L.) et au millepertuis (*Hypericum perforatum* L.). *J Pharm Belg* 1985; **40**: 173–7.

6.   Hoelzl J, Ostrowski E. St John's wort (*Hypericum perforatum* L.). HPLC analysis of the main components and their variability in a population. *Deutsch Apoth Ztg* 1987; **127**: 1227–30.

7.   Brondz I *et al*. The relative stereochemistry of hyperforin — An antibiotic from *Hypericum perforatum* L. *Tetrahedron Lett* 1982; **23**: 1299–1300.

8.   Ayuga C, Rebuelta M. A comparative study of phenolic acids of *Hypericum caprifolium* Boiss and *Hypericum perforatum* L. *An Real Acad Farm* 1986; **52**: 723–8.

9.   Brondz I *et al*. *n*-Alkanes of *Hypericum perforatum*: A revision. *Phytochemistry* 1983; **22**: 295–6.

10.   Mathis C, Ourisson G. Étude chimio-taxonomique du genre *Hypericum* — II. Identification de constituants de diverses huiles essentielles d'*Hypericum*. *Phytochemistry* 1964; **3**: 115–31.

11.   Mathis C, Ourisson G. Étude chimio-taxonomique du genre *Hypericum* — IV. Repartition des sesquiterpenes, des alcools monoterpeniques et des aldehydes satures dans les huiles essentielles d'*Hypericum*. *Phytochemistry* 1964; **3**: 377–8.

12.   Mathis C, Ourisson G. Étude chimio-taxonomique du genre *Hypericum* — V. Identification de quelques constituants non volatils d'*Hypericum perforatum* L. *Phytochemistry* 1964; **3**: 379.

13.   Zakharova NS *et al*. Action of plant extracts on the natural immunity indices of animals. *Zh Mikrobiol Epidemiol Immunobiol* 1986; **4**: 71–5

14.   Negrash AK *et al*. Comparative study of chemotherapeutic and pharmacological properties of antimicrobial preparations from common St John's wort. *Fitontsidy Mater Soveshch* 1969: 198–200.

15.   Sakar MK *et al*. Antimicrobial activities of some *Hypericum* species growing in Turkey. *Fitoterapia* 1988; **59**: 49–52.

16.   Kolesnikova AG. Bactericidal and immunocorrective properties of plant extracts. *Zh Mikrobiol Epidemiol Immunobiol* 1986; **3**: 75–8

17.   Mishenkova EL *et al*. Antiviral properties of St John's wort and preparations produced from it. *Tr S'ezda Mikrobiol Ukr* 1975; 222–3.

18.   Shipochliev T *et al*. Anti-inflammatory action of a group of plant extracts. *Vet Med Nauki* 1981; **18**: 87–94.

19.   Vasilchenko EA *et al*. Analgesic action of flavonoids of *Rhododendron luteum* Sweet, *Hypericum perforatum* L., *Lespedeza bicolor* Turcz. and *L. hedysaroides* (Pall.) Kitag. *Rastit Resur* 1986; **22**: 12–21.

20.   Okpanyi SN, Weischer ML. Animal experiments on the psychotropic action of a *Hypericum* extract. *Arzneimittelforschung* 1987; **37**: 10–13.

21.   Suzuki O *et al*. Inhibition of monoamine oxidase by hypericin. *Planta Med* 1984; **50**: 272–274.

22.   Melzer R *et al*. Proanthocyanidins from *Hypericum perforatum*: Effects on isolated pig coronary arteries. *Planta Med* 1988; **54**: 572–3.

23.   Shiplochliev T. Extracts from a group of medicinal plants enhancing the uterine tonus. *Vet Med Nauki* 1981; **18**: 94–8.

24.   Grujic-Vasic J *et al*. The examining of isolated tannins and their astringent effect. *Planta Med* 1986; **52** Suppl.: 67–8.

25.   Garrett BJ *et al*. Consumption of poisonous plants (*Senecio jacobaea, Symphytum officinale, Pteridium aquilinum, Hypericum perforatum*) by rats: chronic toxicity, mineral metabolism, and hepatic drug-metabolizing enzymes. *Toxicol Lett* 1982; **10**: 183–8.

26.   Durán N, Song P-S. Hypericin and its photodynamic action. *Photochem Photobiol* 1986; **43**: 677–80.

27.   Decosterd LA *et al*. Isolation of new cytotoxic constituents from *Hypericum revolutum* and *Hypericum calycinum* by liquid-liquid chromatography. *Planta Med* 1988; **54**: 560.

28.   Müldner VH, Zöller M. Antidepressive effect of a hypericum extract standardized to the active hypericine complex/biochemistry and clinical studies. *Arzneimittelforschung* 1984; **34**: 918.

29.   Panijel M. Die behandlung mittelschwerer angstzustände. *Therapiewoche* 1985; **41**: 4659–68.

30.   Chakarski I *et al*. Clinical study of a herb combination consisting of *Agrimonia eupatoria, Hipericum perforatum, Plantago major, Mentha piperita, Matricaria chamomila* for the treatment of patients with chronic gastroduodenitis. *Probl Vatr Med* 1982; **10**: 78–84.

31.   Shaparenko BA *et al*. On use of medicinal plants for treatment of patients with chronic supurative otitis. *Zh Ushn Gorl Bolezn* 1979; **39**: 48–51.

32.   Hypericin — a plant extract with anti-HIV activity. *Scrip* 1989; (1415): 29.

33.   Anon. Hypericin improves blood safety? *Scrip* 1995; **2005**: 27.

34.   Anon. Hypericin HIV trial in Thailand. *Scrip* 1995; **2019**: 25.

35.   Benner MH, Lee HJ. *Med Lett* 1979; **21**: 29–30.

36.   Cappelletti EM *et al*. External antirheumatic and antineuralgic herbal remedies in the traditional medicine of north-eastern Italy. *J Ethnopharmacol* 1982; **6**: 161–90.

STONE ROOT

Species (Family)
Collinsonia canadensis L. (Labiatae)

Synonym(s)
Heal-All, Knob Root

Part(s) Used
Rhizome, Root

Pharmacopoeial Monographs
BHP 1983
BPC 1934
Martindale 22nd edition

Legal Category (Licensed Products)
GSL[G14]

Constituents[G18,G24,G25,G32]
Stone root is stated to contain an unidentified alkaloid, mucilage, resin, saponin glycosides, tannins, and volatile oil.

Food Use
Stone root is not used in foods.

Herbal Use
Stone root is stated to possess antilithic, litholytic, mild diaphoretic, and diuretic properties. Traditionally, it has been used for renal calculus, lithuria, and specifically for urinary calculus.[G3,G32]

Dose
Dried root 1–4 g or by decoction three times daily[G3]
Liquid extract (1:1 in 25% alcohol) 1–4 mL three times daily[G3]
Tincture (1:5 in 40% alcohol) 2–8 mL three times daily[G3]
Tincture of Collinsonia (BPC 1934) 2–8 mL

Pharmacological Actions
None documented.

Side-effects, Toxicity
None documented.

Contra-indications, Warnings
None documented.
Pregnancy and lactation The safety of stone root has not been established. In view of the lack of phytochemical, pharmacological and toxicological information, the use of stone root during pregnancy and lactation should be avoided.

Pharmaceutical Comment
Information available on the chemistry of stone root is limited and no documented scientific evidence was located to justify the herbal uses. In view of the lack of toxicity data, excessive use of stone root should be avoided.

References
See General References G3, G5, G14, G18, G24, G25, and G32.

TANSY

Species (Family)

Tanacetum vulgare L. (Asteraceae/Compositae)

Synonym(s)

Chrysanthemum vulgare (L.) Bernh., Tanacetum

Part(s) Used

Herb

Pharmacopoeial Monographs

BHP 1983
Martindale 28th edition

Legal Category (Licensed Products)

Tansy is not included on the GSL[G14]

Constituents[G10,G26,G32]

Steroids β-Sitosterol (major), campesterol, cholesterol, stigmasterol, taraxasterol[1]

Terpenoids α-Amyrin (major), β-amyrin, sesquiterpene lactones including arbusculin-A, tanacetin, germacrene D, crispolide;[2,3] tanacetols A and B[4]

Volatile oils (0.12–0.18%). Major components as β-thujone (up to 95%) and camphor, others include α-pinene, borneol, 1,8-cineole, umbellone, and sabinene. At least ten different chemotypes have been identified in which camphor was the most frequently occurring main component and thujone second.[4]

Other constituents Gum, mucilage, resin, tannins

Food Use

Tansy is listed by the Council of Europe as a natural source of food flavouring (Category N3). This category indicates that tansy can be added to foodstuffs in the traditionally accepted manner, although there is insufficient information for an adequate assessment of potential toxicity. In addition, the Council of Europe recommends that the concentration of thujones present in food products is restricted to 0.5 mg/kg.[G9] Tansy oil is prohibited from use as a food flavouring by the Food Additives and Contaminants Committee (FACC) in view of the thujone content.[G21]

In the USA, tansy is prohibited from sale by botanical dealers or by mail order as the dried herb.[G10]

Herbal Use

Tansy is stated to possess anthelmintic, carminative, and antispasmodic properties and to act as a stimulant to abdominal viscera. Traditionally, it has been used for nematode infestation, topically for scabies (as a decoction) and pruritus ani (as an ointment), and specifically for roundworm or threadworm infestation in children.[G3]

Dose

Dried herb 1–2 g or by infusion three times daily[G3]
Liquid extract (1:1 in 25% alcohol) 1–2 mL three times daily[G3]

Pharmacological Actions

Animal studies In-vitro antispasmodic activity on rabbit intestine, and *in-vivo* choleretic activity in the dog have been documented for tansy extracts.[6] The authors suggested that the choleretic action might be attributable to caffeic acid, a known bile stimulant that is present in tansy.[6] Anthelmintic activity in dogs has been described for tansy oil, an ether extract of the oil, and for β-thujone.[6] Daily intragastric doses of a tansy extract given to rabbits have been found to reduce serum-lipid concentrations and inhibit further development of hypercholesterolaemia.[6] In addition, it was noted that recovery of blood-sugar concentrations was inhibited in animals given twice daily doses. *In-vitro* antifungal activity in 15 pathogenic and non-pathogenic fungi has been reported.[6]

Human studies Aqueous infusions and alcoholic extracts have been shown to be clinically effective bile stimulants in patients with liver and gall bladder disorders.[6] The treatment alleviated pain and increased appetite and digestion.

Side-effects, Toxicity[G35]

Tansy oil contains the toxic ketone β-thujone. Symptoms of tansy oil poisoning are attributable to the thujone content and include rapid and weak pulse, severe gastritis, violent spasms, and convulsions.[G10] Documented fatalities have mainly been associated with ingestion of the oil, although fatal cases of poisoning have occurred with infusions and powders.[6,7] An oral LD_{50} value for tansy oil is stated as 1.15 g/kg body-weight.[7] The ratio of toxic to therapeutic dose has been reported as 2.5:1 and it was noted that all tansy preparations should be administered with castor oil.[6] Tansy yields potentially allergenic sesquiterpene lactones which have been implicated in the aetiology of contact dermatitis. Instances of contact dermatitis to tansy have been documented.[6,G26]

In-vitro and *in-vivo* antitumour activity has been documented for tansy.[6]

Contra-indications, Warnings

Tansy oil is toxic and should not be used internally or externally.[G35] Fatalities have been reported following ingestion of infusions and extracts. Tansy contains allergenic sesquiterpene lactones and may cause an allergic reaction. Tansy has been reported to affect blood-sugar concentrations in animals and may interfere with hypoglycaemic therapy.

Pregnancy and lactation Tansy is contra-indicated in pregnancy and lactation. Tansy is reputed to affect the menstrual cycle and uteroactivity has been documented in animal studies. The volatile oil contains β-thujone, a known hepatotoxin.

Pharmaceutical Comment

Pharmacological activities documented for tansy have been associated with the sterol and triterpene constituents. Tansy yields an extremely toxic volatile oil, which should not be used internally or externally.[G35] In view of this, the use of tansy as a herbal remedy is not justified even though documented studies have supported the traditional uses of the herb as a choleretic and anthelmintic agent.

References

See General References G3, G9, G10, G14, G21, G26, G32 and G35.

1.   Chandler RF *et al*. Herbal remedies of the Maritime Indians: Sterols and triterpenes of *Tanacetum vulgare* L. (Tansy). *Lipids* 1982; **17:** 102–6.

2.   Chandra A *et al*. Germacranolides and an alkyl glucoside from *Tanacetum vulgare*. *Phytochemistry* 1987; **26:** 1463–5.

3.   Appendino G. Crispoloide, an unusual hydroperoxysesquiterpene lactone from *Tanacetum vulgare*. *Phytochemistry* 1982; **21:** 1099–1102.

4.   Holopainen M *et al*. A study on tansy chemotypes. *Planta Med* 1987; **53:** 284–7.

5.   Appendino G *et al*. Tanacetols A and B, non-volatile sesquiterpene alcohols, from *Tanacetum vulgare*. *Phytochemistry* 1983; **22:** 509–12.

6.   Opdyke DLJ. Tansy oil. *Food Cosmet Toxicol* 1976; **14:** 869–71.

7.   Hardin JW, Arena JM, editors. Human poisoning from native and cultivated plants. 2nd edn. North Carolina: Duke University, 1974: 150–3.

THYME

Species (Family)
Thymus vulgaris L. (Labiatae)

Synonym(s)
Common Thyme, French Thyme, Garden Thyme, Rubbed Thyme

Part(s) Used
Flowering top, Leaf

Pharmacopoeial Monographs
BHP 1983
BPC 1949
Martindale 29th edition
Pharmacopoeias—Arg., Aust., Cz., Fr., Ger., Hung., Neth., Nord., Pol., and Rom. Yug. includes the leaves only.

Legal Category (Licensed Products)
GSL[G14]

Constituents[G1, G10,G19,G32,G35]
Volatile oils (0.8–2.6%). Phenols as major components (20–80%) primarily thymol and carvacrol; others include *p*-cymene and γ-terpinene (monoterpenes), linalool, α-terpineol, and thujan-4-ol (alcohols). For a more detailed analysis of the volatile oil components *see* reference [G10]
Other constituents Flavonoids, caffeic acid, oleanolic acid, ursolic acid, resins, saponins, tannins

Food Use
Thyme is commonly used as a culinary herb, and thyme oil is used in food flavouring.

Herbal Use
Thyme is stated to possess carminative, antispasmodic, antitussive, expectorant, secretomotor, bactericidal, anthelmintic, and astringent properties. Traditionally, it has been used for dyspepsia, chronic gastritis, asthma, diarrhoea in children, enuresis in children, laryngitis, tonsillitis (as a gargle), and specifically for pertussis and bronchitis.[G1,G3,G32]

Dose
Dried herb 1–4 g or by infusion three times daily[G3]
Liquid Extract of Thyme (BPC 1949) 0.6–4.0 mL
Elixir of Thyme (BPC 1949) 4–8 mL
Tincture (1:5 in 45% alcohol) 2–6 mL three times daily[G3]

Pharmacological Actions
Animal studies Antitussive, expectorant, and antispasmodic actions are considered to be the major pharmacological properties of thyme,[1] and have been associated with the volatile oils (e.g. thymol, carvacrol) and flavonoid constituents. Thyme oil has produced hypotensive and respiratory stimulant effects in rabbits following oral or intramuscular administration, and in cats following intravenous injection;[G19] an increase in rhythmic heart contraction was also observed in the rabbits.[G19] Hypotensive activity in the rat has been reported for *Thymus orospedanus* and this action was attributed to adrenaline antagonism.[2]

In-vitro antispasmodic activity of thyme and related *Thymus* species has been associated with the phenolic components of the volatile oil[3] and with the flavonoid constituents; their mode of action is thought to involve calcium-channel blockage.[1,4,5] The antispasmodic activity of the phenol components has been questioned.[3]

Analgesic and antipyretic properties in mice have been reported for a thyme extract.[6]

Thymol possesses anthelmintic (especially hookworms), antibacterial, and antifungal properties.[G19]

Human studies Thyme oil has been used for the treatment of enuresis in children.[G21]

Side-effects, Toxicity[G35]
Thyme oil is a dermal and mucous membrane irritant.[G35] Toxic symptoms documented for thymol include nausea, vomiting, gastric pain, headache, dizziness, convulsions, coma, and cardiac and respiratory arrest.[G10] Thymol is present in some toothpaste preparations and has been reported to cause cheilitis and glossitis. Hyperaemia and severe inflammation have been described for thyme oil used in bath preparations.[G26] LD_{50} values for thyme oil include 4.7 g/kg body-weight (rat, by mouth) and greater than 5 g/kg (rat, dermal).[7]

Contra-indications, Warnings
Thyme oil is toxic and should be used with considerable caution. It should not be taken internally and only applied externally if diluted in a suitable carrier oil.

Pregnancy and lactation There are no known problems with the use of thyme during pregnancy and lactation, provided that doses do not greatly exceed the amounts used in foods. Traditionally, thyme is reputed to affect the menstrual cycle and, therefore, large amounts should not be ingested.

Pharmaceutical Comment
Thyme is commonly used as a culinary herb and is characterised by its volatile oil. Documented pharmacological actions support some of the traditional medicinal uses, which have been principally attributed to the volatile oil and flavonoid constituents. However, the oil is also toxic and should not be ingested and only applied externally if diluted in a suitable carrier oil. It has been suggested that standardised thyme extracts based on the phenolic volatile compo-

nents may not be appropriate because antispasmodic actions previously attributed to these compounds may be attributable to other constituents.[3]

References

See General References G1, G3, G6, G10, G14, G19, G21, G22, G26, G32 and G35.

1.   Van Den Broucke CO. The therapeutic value of *Thymus* species. *Fitoterapia* 1983; **4:** 171–4.

2.   Jimenez J *et al*. Hypotensive activity of *Thymus orospedanus* alcoholic extract. *Phytotherapy Res* 1988; **2:** 152–3.

3.   Van Den Broucke CO, Lernli JA. Pharmacological and chemical investigation of thyme liquid extracts. *Planta Med* 1981; **41:** 129–135.

4.   Cruz T *et al*. The spasmolytic activity of the essential oil of *Thymus baeticus* Boiss in rats. *Phytotherapy Res* 1989; **3:** 106–8.

5.   Blázquez MA *et al*. Effects of *Thymus* species extracts on rat duodenum isolated smooth muscle contraction. *Phytotherapy Res* 1989; **3:** 41–2.

6.   Mohsin A *et al*. Analgesic, antipyretic activity and phytochemical screening of some plants used in traditional Arab system of medicine. *Fitoterapia* 1989; **60:** 174.

7.   Opdyke DLJ. Thyme oil, red. *Food Cosmet Toxicol* 1974; **12:** 1003–4.

UVA-URSI

Species (Family)
Arctostaphylos uva-ursi (L.) Spreng (Ericaceae)

Synonym(s)
Bearberry

Part(s) Used
Leaf

Pharmacopoeial Monographs
BHP 1983
BHP 1990
BPC 1934
Martindale 30th edition
Pharmacopoeias—Aust., Cz., Egypt, Fr., Ger., Hung., Jpn, Rus., Swiss, and Yug.

Legal Category (Licensed Products)
GSL[G14]

Constituents[G1,G2,G10,G19,G31,G32]
Flavonoids Flavonols (e.g. myricetin, quercetin) and their glycosides including hyperin, isoquercitrin, myricitrin, and quercitrin.
Iridoids Asperuloside (disputed), monotropein[1]
Quinones Total content at least 6%, mainly arbutin (5–15%) and methyl-arbutin (glycosides), with lesser amounts of piceoside[2] (a glycoside), free hydroquinone and free *p*-methoxyphenol[3]
Tannins 6–7% (range 6–40%). Hydrolysable-type (e.g. corilagin pyranoside); ellagic and gallic acids (usually associated with hydrolysable tannins)
Terpenoids α-Amyrin, α-amyrin acetate, β-amyrin, lupeol, uvaol, ursolic acid, and a mixture of mono- and di- ketonic α-amyrin derivatives[4,5]
Other constituents Acids (malic, quinic), allantoin, resin (e.g. ursone), volatile oil (trace), wax
Other plant parts The root is reported to contain unedoside (iridoid glucoside).[6]

Food Use
Uva-ursi is not used in foods.

Herbal Use
Uva-ursi is stated to possess diuretic, urinary antiseptic, and astringent properties. Traditionally, it has been used for cystitis, urethritis, dysuria, pyelitis, lithuria, and specifically for acute catarrhal cystitis with dysuria and highly acidic urine.[G1,G2,G3,G4,G32]

Dose
Dried leaves 1.5–4.0 g or by infusion three times daily[G2,G3]

Liquid Extract 1.5–4.0 mL (1:1 in 25% alcohol) three times daily[G2,G3]
Concentrated Infusion of Bearberry (BPC 1934) 2–4 mL
Fresh Infusion of Bearberry (BPC 1934) 15–30 mL

Pharmacological Actions
Animal studies Uva-ursi has exhibited antimicrobial activity towards a variety of organisms including *Staphylococcus aureus*, *Bacillus subtilis*, *Escherichia coli*, *Mycobacterium smegmatis*, *Shigella sonnei*, and *Shigella flexneri*.[7] The antimicrobial activity of arbutin towards bacteria implicated in producing urinary-tract infections, has been found to be directly dependent on the β-glucosidase activity of the infective organism.[8] Highest enzymatic activity was shown by *Enterobacter*, *Klebsiella*, and *Streptococcus* genera, and lowest by *Escherichia coli*.[8] The minimum inhibitory concentration for arbutin is reported to be 0.4–0.8% depending on the micro-organism.[8] Aqueous and methanolic extracts have demonstrated molluscicidal activity against *Biomphalaria glabrata*, at a concentration of 50 ppm.[9] The activity was attributed to the tannin constituents (condensed and hydrolysable).

Anti-inflammatory activity (rat paw oedema tests) has been documented for uva-ursi against a variety of chemical inducers such as carrageenan, histamine, and prostaglandins.[10]

Uva-ursi failed to exhibit any *in-vitro* uterotonic action when tested on rabbit and guinea-pig uteri.[11]

Hydroquinone has been reported to show a dose-dependent cytotoxic activity on cultured rat hepatoma cells (HTC line); arbutin was not found to inhibit growth of the HTC cells.[12] It was stated that hydroquinone appeared to have greater cytotoxic activity towards rat hepatoma cells than agents like azauridin or colchicine, but less than valtrate from valerian (*Valeriana officinalis*). The cytoxicity of hydroquinone has also been tested on L1210, CA-755, and S-180 tumour systems.[12]

Human studies A herbal preparation, whose ingredients included uva-ursi, hops, and peppermint, has been used to treat patients suffering from compulsive strangury, enuresis, and painful micturition.[13] Of 915 patients treated for six weeks, success was reported in about 70%. The antiseptic and diuretic properties claimed for uva-ursi can be attributed to the hydroquinone derivatives, especially arbutin. The latter is absorbed from the gastro-intestinal tract virtually unchanged and during renal excretion is hydrolysed to yield the active principle, hydroquinone, which exerts an antiseptic and astringent action on the urinary mucous membranes.[14,15] The crude extract is reported to be more effective than isolated arbutin as an astringent and antiseptic.[G24] This may be due to the other hydroquinone derivatives, in addition to arbutin, that are present in the crude extract and which will also yield hydroquinone. Furthermore, it has been stated that the presence of gallic acid in the crude extract may prevent β-glucosidase cleavage of arbutin in the gastro-intestinal tract before absorption, thereby increasing the amount of hydroquinone released during renal excretion.[G24]

Side-effects, Toxicity

No reported side-effects were located. Hydroquinone is reported to be toxic if ingested in large quantities: 1 g (equivalent to 6–20 g plant material) has caused tinnitus, nausea and vomiting, sense of suffocation, shortness of breath, cyanosis, convulsions, delirium and collapse.[G24] A dose of 5 g (equivalent to 30–100 g of plant material) has proved fatal.[G24] In view of the high tannin content, prolonged use of uva-ursi may cause chronic liver impairment.[G19]

Cytotoxic activity has been documented for hydroquinone (*see* Animal studies).

Uva-ursi herb can sometimes be adulterated with box leaves (*Buxus sempervirens*), which contain toxic steroidal alkaloids. However, no cases of poisoning as a result of such adulteration have been reported.[G13]

Contra-indications, Warnings

Uva-ursi requires an alkaline urine for it to be effective as a urinary antiseptic; an alkaline reaction is needed to yield hydroquinone from the inactive esters such as arbutin.[14] Patients have been advised to avoid eating highly acidic foods, such as acidic fruits and their juices.[14] The presence of hydroquinone may impart a greenish-brown colour to the urine, which darkens following exposure to air due to oxidation of hydroquinone.

Excessive use of uva-ursi should be avoided in view of the high tannin content and potential toxicity of hydroquinone.

Prolonged use of uva-ursi to treat a urinary-tract infection is not advisable. Patients in whom symptoms persist for longer than 48 hours should consult their doctor.

Pregnancy and lactation Large doses of uva-ursi are reported to be oxytocic,[G10] although *in-vitro* studies have reported a lack of uteroactivity. In view of the potential toxicity of hydroquinone, the use of uva-ursi during pregnancy and lactation is best avoided.

Pharmaceutical Comment

The chemistry of uva-ursi is well documented with hydroquinone derivatives, especially arbutin, identified as the major active constituents. Documented pharmacological actions justify the herbal use of uva-ursi as a urinary antiseptic. However, clinical information is lacking and further studies are required to determine the true usefulness of uva-ursi in the treatment of urinary-tract infections. Although hydroquinone has been reported to be toxic in large amounts, concentrations provided by the ingestion of therapeutic doses of uva-ursi are not thought to represent a risk to human health.[G20]

References

See General References G1, G2, G3, G4, G5, G10, G13, G14, G19, G20, G22, G24, G31, and G32.

1. Jahodár L *et al*. Investigation of iridoid substances in *Arctostaphylos uva-ursi*. *Pharmazie* 1978; **33**: 536–7.

2. Karikas GA *et al*. Isolation of piceoside from *Arctostaphylos uva-ursi*. *Planta Med* 1987; **53**: 307–8.

3. Jahodár L, Leifertová I. The evaluation of *p*-methoxyphenol in the leaves of *Arctostaphylos uva-ursi*. *Pharmazie* 1979; **34**: 188–9.

4. Droliac A. Triterpenes of *Arctostaphylos uva-ursi* Spreng. *Plant Méd Phytothér* 1980; **14**: 155–8.

5. Malterud KE. The non-polar components of *Arctostaphylos uva-ursi* leaves. *Medd Nor Farm Selsk* 1980; **42**: 15–20.

6. Jahodár L *et al*. Unedoside in *Arctostaphylos uva-ursi* roots. *Pharmazie* 1981; **36**: 294–6.

7. Moskalenko SA. Preliminary screening of far-Eastern ethnomedicinal plants for antibacterial activity. *J Ethnopharmacol* 1986; **15**: 231–59.

8. Jahodár L *et al*. Antimicrobial action of arbutin and the extract from the leaves of *Arctostaphylos uva-ursi* in vitro. *Ceskoslov Farm* 1985; **34**: 174–8.

9. Schaufelberger D, Hostettmann K. On the molluscicidal activity of tannin containing plants. *Planta Med* 1983; **48**: 105–7.

10. Shipochliev T, Fournadjiev G. Spectrum of the antiinflammatory effect of *Arctostaphylos uva ursi* and *Achilea millefolium*, L. *Probl Vutr Med* 1984; **12**: 99–107.

11. Shipochliev T. Extracts from a group of medicinal plants enhancing the uterine tonus. *Vet Med Nauki* 1981; **18**: 94–8.

12. Assaf MH *et al*. Preliminary study of the phenolic glycosides from *Origanum majorana*; quantitative estimation of arbutin; cytotoxic activity of hydroquinone. *Planta Med* 1987; **53**: 343–5.

13. Lenau H *et al*. Wirksamkeit und Verträglichkeit von Cysto Fink bei Patienten mit Reizblase und/oder Harninkontinenz. *Therapiewoche* 1984; **34**: 6054–9.

14. Frohne D. Untersuchungen zur Frage der Harndesinfizierenden Wirkungen von Bärentraubenblatt-Extrakten *Planta Med* 1970; **18**: 23–5.

15. Natural drugs with glycosides. In: Stahl E, editor. Drug Analysis in Chromatography and Microscopy. Ann Arbor: Ann Arbor Scientific Publishers, 1973: 97.

VALERIAN

Species (Family)

Valeriana officinalis L. (Valerianaceae) and related *Valeriana* species

Synonym(s)

Belgian Valerian, Common Valerian, Fragrant Valerian, Garden Valerian, All-Heal

Part(s) Used

Rhizome, Root

Pharmacopoeial Monographs

BHP 1983
BHP 1990
BPC 1963
Martindale 30th edition
Pharmacopoeias—Aust., Br., Cz., Egypt., Eur., Fr., Ger., Gr., Hung., It., Neth., Nord., Rom., Rus., Swiss, and Yug. Br. also describes Powdered Valerian.

Legal Category (Licensed Products)

GSL[G14]

Constituents[G1,G2,G10,G19,G32,G35]

Alkaloids (pyridine type). Actinidine, chatinine, skyanthine, valerianine, valerine

Iridoids (valepotriates). Valtrates (e.g. valtrate, valtrate isovaleroxyhydrin, acevaltrate, valechlorine), didrovaltrates (e.g. didrovaltrate, homodidrovaltrate, deoxydidrovaltrate, homodeoxydidrovaltrate, isovaleroxyhydroxydidrovaltrate) and isovaltrates (e.g. isovaltrate, 7-epideacetylisovaltrate). Valtrate and didrovaltrate are documented as the major components. Valerosidate (iridoid glucoside)[1]

Volatile oils (0.5–2%). Numerous identified components include monoterpenes (e.g. α- and β-pinene, camphene, borneol, eugenol, isoeugenol) present mainly as esters, sesquiterpenes (e.g. β-bisabolene, caryophyllene, valeranone, ledol, pacifigorgiol, patchouli alcohol, valerianol, valerenol and a series of valerenyl esters, valerenal, valerenic acid with acetoxy and hydroxy derivatives)[2–5]

Other constituents Caffeic and chlorogenic acids (polyphenolic), β-sitosterol, methyl 2-pyrrolketone, choline, tannins (type unspecified), gum, and resin

Food Use

Valerian is not generally used as a food. It is listed by the Council of Europe as a natural source of food flavouring (category N2). This category indicates that valerian can be added to foodstuffs in small quantities, with a possible limitation of an active principle (as yet unspecified) in the final product.[G9]

Herbal Use

Valerian is stated to possess sedative, mild anodyne, hypnotic, antispasmodic, carminative, and hypotensive properties. Traditionally, it has been used for hysterical states, excitability, insomnia, hypochondriasis, migraine, cramp, intestinal colic, rheumatic pains, dysmenorrhoea, and specifically for conditions presenting nervous excitability.[G1, G2,G3,G4,G32]

Dose

Dried rhizome/root 0.3–1.0 g or by infusion or decoction three times daily[G2,G3]
Valerian Liquid Extract (BPC 1963) 0.3–1.0 mL
Simple Tincture of Valerian (BPC 1949) 4–8 mL
Concentrated Valerian Infusion (BPC 1963) 2–4 mL

Pharmacological Actions

Animal studies Sedative properties have been documented for valerian and have been attributed to both the volatile oil and valepotriate fractions.[6,7] Screening of the volatile oil components for sedative activity concluded valerenal and valerenic acid to be the most active compounds, causing ataxia in mice at 50 mg/kg body-weight by intraperitoneal injection.[6] Further studies in mice described valerenic acid as a general CNS depressant similar to pentobarbitone, requiring high doses (100 mg/kg by intraperitoneal injection) for activity.[8] A dose of 400 mg/kg resulted in muscle spasms, convulsions, and death.[8] Valerenic acid was also reported to prolong pentobarbitone-induced sleep in mice, resulting in a hangover effect. Biochemical studies have documented that valerenic acid inhibits the enzyme system responsible for the central catabolism of GABA.[9] Increased concentrations of GABA are associated with a decrease in CNS activity and this action may, therefore, be involved in the reported sedative activity of valerenic acid.

CNS depressant activities in mice following intraperitoneal injection have been documented for the valepotriates and for their degradation products, although activity was found to be greatly reduced following oral administration of the compounds.[10] A specific valepotriate fraction, Vpt$_2$, has been documented to exhibit tranquillising, central myorelaxant, anticonvulsant, coronarodilating and antiarrhythmic actions in mice, rabbits, and cats.[11,12] The fraction was reported to prevent arrhythmias induced by Pituitrin™ vasopressin, and barium chloride, and to exhibit moderate positive inotropic and negative chronotropic effects.

Antispasmodic activity on intact and isolated guinea-pig ileum has been documented for isovaltrate, valtrate, and valeranone.[13] This activity was attributed to a direct action on the smooth muscle receptors rather than ganglion receptors. Valerian oil has been reported to exhibit antispasmodic activity on isolated guinea-pig uterine muscle[14] but proved inactive when tested *in vivo*.[15]

In-vitro inactivation of complement activation has been reported for the valepotriates.[16]

In-vitro cytotoxicity (inhibition of DNA and protein synthesis, potent alkylating activity) has been documented for the valepotriates with valtrate stated to be the most toxic compound.[17] A subsequent *in-vivo* study in which valtrate was administered to mice (by intraperitoneal injection and by mouth) did not report any toxic effects on haematopoietic precursor cells when compared with control groups.[18] The valepotriates are known to be unstable compounds in both acidic and alkaline media and it has been suggested[19] that their *in-vivo* toxicity is limited due to poor absorption and/ or distribution. Baldrinal and homobaldrinal, decomposition products of valtrate and isovaltrate respectively, have exhibited direct mutagenic activity against various *Salmonella* strains *in vitro*.[20]

Human studies A number of documented studies have described a sedative effect for valerian.[21–25] A mild hypnotic action in both normal sleepers and sufferers of insomnia has been described, as indicated by a beneficial effect on a variety of subjective sleep-disorder parameters, such as sleep latency, wake-time after sleep, frequency of waking, night-time motor activity, inner restlessness and tension, and quality of sleep. However, valerian was not found to have any effect on objective measures such as EEG sleep parameters. Sleepiness and dream recall the morning after were unaffected.

Various studies have utilised proprietary preparations, some containing a mixture of herbs including valerian.[26–30] Valerian in combination with St. Johns wort has been reported to be more effective than diazepam in treating symptoms of anxiety, when given to 100 patients for two weeks in a double blind trial.[26] A product containing valerian, camphor, cereus, and hawthorn was given to 2243 patients with functional cardiovascular disorders and/or hypotension or meteorosensitivity in an open multicentre study.[27] An improvement in 84% of treated individuals was reported. A slight increase in blood pressure and decrease in heart rate were observed. A sedative action has been described for valerian in combination with hops.[28]

Side-effects, Toxicity

There have been no reported side-effects to valerian. No published toxicity studies were located. *In-vitro* cytotoxicity and mutagenicity have been documented for the valepotriates. The clinical significance of this is unclear since the valepotriates are known to be highly unstable and, therefore, probably degrade when taken orally. The oil is unlikely to present any hazard in aromatherapy.[G35]

Contra-indications, Warnings

The documented CNS depressant activity of valerian may potentiate existing sedative therapy. Unlike many other sedative drugs, the depressant action of valerian is reported not to be synergistic with alcohol.

Pregnancy and lactation The safety of valerian during pregnancy and lactation has not been established and should, therefore, be avoided.[31] A related species, *Valeriana walli-chi*, is reputed to be an abortifacient and to affect the menstrual cycle.[G15]

Pharmaceutical Comment

The traditional use of valerian as a mild sedative and hypnotic has been supported by actions documented in studies involving both animals and humans.[G31] The sedative activity of valerian has been attributed to both the volatile oil and iridoid valepotriate fractions, but it is still unclear whether other constituents in valerian represent the active components. The valepotriate compounds are highly unstable and, therefore, probably degrade when taken orally. In view of this, the clinical significance of both the sedative and cytotoxic/mutagenic activities documented *in vitro* is unclear.

References

See General References G1, G2, G3, G4, G9, G10, G11, G14, G19, G22, G23, G32 and G35.

1.   Inouye H *et al*. The absolute configuration of valerosidate and of didovaltrate. *Tetrahedron Lett* 1974; **30**: 2317–25.

2.   Bos R *et al*. Isolation and identification of valerenane sesquiterpenoids from *Valeriana officinalis*. *Phytochemistry* 1986; **25**: 133–5.

3.   Bos R *et al*. Isolation of the sesquiterpene alcohol (–)-pacifigorgiol from *Valeriana officinalis*. *Phytochemistry* 1986; **25**: 1234–5.

4.   Stoll A *et al*. New investigations on Valerian. *Schweiz Apotheker-Zeitung* 1957; **95**: 115–20.

5.   Hendricks H *et al*. Eugenyl isovalerate and isoeugenyl isovalerate in the essential oil of Valerian root. *Phytochemistry* 1977; **16**: 1853–4.

6.   Hendricks H *et al*. Pharmacological screening of valerenal and some other components of essential oil of *Valeriana officinalis*. *Planta Med* 1981; **42**: 62–8.

7.   Wagner H *et al*. Comparative studies on the sedative action of *Valeriana* extracts, valepotriates and their degradation products. *Planta Med* 1980; **39**: 358–365.

8.   Hendriks H *et al*. Central nervous depressant activity of valerenic acid in the mouse. *Planta Med* 1985; **51**: 28–31.

9.   Riedel E *et al*. Inhibition of γ-aminobutyric acid catabolism by valerenic acid derivatives. *Planta Medica* 1982; **48**: 219–20.

10.   Veith J *et al*. The influence of some degradation products of valepotriates on the motor activity of light-dark synchronized mice. *Planta Med* 1986; **52**: 179–83.

11.   Petkov V. Plants with hypotensive, antiatheromatous and coronarodilating action. *Am J Chin Med* 1979; **7**: 197–236.

12.   Petkov V, Manolav P. To the pharmacology of iridoids. 2nd Congress of the Bulgarian Society for Physiological Sciences, Sofia, October 31–November 3, 1974.

13.   Hazelhoff B *et al*. Antispasmodic effects of *Valeriana* compounds: an *in-vivo* and *in-vitro* study on the guinea-pig ileum. *Arch Int Pharmacodyn* 1982; **257**: 274–87.

14.   Pilcher JD *et al*. The action of so-called female remedies on the excised uterus of the guinea-pig. *Arch Int Med* 1916; **18**: 557–83.

15.   Pilcher JD, Mauer RT. The action of female remedies on the intact uteri of animals. *Surg Gynecol Obstet* 1918; 97–99.

16.   Van Meer JH. Plantaardige stoffen met een effect op het complementsysteem. *Pharm Weekbl* 1984; **119**: 836–942.

17.   Bounthanh C *et al*. The action of valepotriates on the synthesis of DNA and proteins of cultured hepatoma cells. *Planta Med* 1983; **49**: 138–42.

18.   Braun R *et al*. Influence of valtrate/isovaltrate on the hematopoiesis and metabolic liver activity in mice *in vivo*. *Planta Med* 1984; **50**: 1–4.

19.   Houghton PJ. The biological activity of valerian and related plants. *J Ethnopharmacol* 1988; **22**: 121–42.

20.   Hude W *et al*. Bacterial mutagenicity of the tranquillizing constituents of Valerianaceae roots. *Mutat Res* 1986; **169**: 23–7.

21.   Leathwood PD *et al*. Aqueous extract of valerian root improves sleep quality in man. *Pharmacol Biochem Behav* 1982; **17**: 65–71.

22.   Leathwood PD, Chauffard F. Aqueous extract of valerian reduces latency to fall asleep in man. *Planta Med* 1985; **51**: 144–8.

23.   Balderer G, Borbely AA. Effect of valerian on human sleep. *Psychopharmacology* 1985; **87**: 406–9.

24.   Leathwood PD, Chauffard F. Quantifying the effects of mild sedatives. *J Psychiatr Res* 1983; **17**: 115–22.

25.   Leathwood PD *et al*. Effect of *Valeriana officinalis* L. on subjective and objective sleep parameters. In: *Sleep 1982, 6th Eur Congr Sleep Res, Zurich 1982*. Basel: Karger. 1983, 402–5.

26.   Panijel M. Die behandlung mittelschwerer angstzustände. *Therapiewoche* 1985; **41**: 4659–68.

27.   Busanny-Caspari E *et al*. Indikationen: Funktionelle Herzbeschwerden, Hypotonie und Wetterfuhligkeit. *Therapiewoche* 1986; **36**: 2545–50.

28.   Muller-Limmroth W, Ehrenstein W. Untersuchungen über die Wirkung von Seda-Kneipp auf den Schlaf schlafgёstorter Menschen. *Med Klin* 1977; **72**: 1119–25.

29.   Schmidt-Voigt J. Treatment of nervous sleep disorders and unrest with a sedative of purely vegetable origin. *Therapiewoche* 1986; **36**: 663–7.

30.   Lindhal O, Lindwall L. Double blind study of a Valerian preparation. *Pharmacol Biochem Behav* 1989; **32**: 1065–6.

31.   Houghton PJ. Valerian. *Pharm J* 1994; **253**: 95–6.

VERVAIN

Species (Family)
Verbena officinalis L. (Verbenaceae)

Synonym(s)
Verbena

Part(s) Used
Herb

Pharmacopoeial Monographs
BHP 1983

Legal Category (Licensed Products)
GSL[G14]

Constituents[G1,G10,G18,G32]
Glycosides Iridoid glycosides: hastatoside, verbenalin (verbanaloside), verbenin (aucubin). Phenylpropanoid glycosides: acetoside (verbascoside), eukovoside[1,2]
Volatile oils Monoterpene components include citral, geraniol, limonene, and verbenone.
Other constituents Adenosibe, alkaloid (unspecified), bitters, carbohydrates (stachyose, mucilage), β-carotene, invertin (sucrose hydrolytic enzymes), saponin, tannic acid

Food Use
Vervain is listed by the Council of Europe as a natural source of food flavouring (category N2). This category indicates that vervain can be added to foodstuffs in small quantities, with a possible limitation of an active principle (as yet unspecified) in the final product.[G9] In the USA, vervain is listed by the FDA as a Herb of Undefined Safety.[G10]

Herbal Use
Vervain is stated to possess sedative, thymoleptic, antispasmodic, mild diaphoretic and, reputedly, galactogogue properties. Traditionally, it has been used for depression, melancholia, hysteria, generalised seizures, cholecystalgia, jaundice, early stages of fever, and specifically for depression and debility of convalescence after fevers, especially influenza.[G1,G3,G32]

Dose
Dried herb 2–4 g or by infusion three times daily[G3]
Liquid extract (1:1 in 25% alcohol) 2–4 mL three times daily[G3]
Tincture (1:1 in 40% alcohol) 5–10 mL three times daily[G3]

Pharmacological Actions
Animal studies Galactogogue properties have been documented for vervain and attributed to aucubin.[3] A luteinising action has also been reported, and attributed to inhibition of the gonadotrophic action of the posterior lobe of the pituitary gland.[3] Extracts of vervain fruit have been used to treat dysmenorrhoea and to stimulate lactation.[3] Vervain has been documented to possess weak parasympathetic properties, causing slight contraction of the uterus.[3] Verbenalin has been reported to exhibit uterine stimulant activity.[G12] Sympathetic activity has also been documented: in small doses verbenin has been reported to act as an agonist at sympathetic nerve endings, whereas larger doses result in antagonism.[G10] Verbascoside reportedly acts as an agonist to the antitremor action of levodopa, and as an antihypertensive and analgesic.[3] A slight laxative action in mice has been documented for iridoid glycosides.[4]

Side-effects, Toxicity
None documented for vervain. High doses of verbenalin are stated to paralyse the CNS, resulting in stupor and convulsions.[G10]

Contra-indications, Warnings
None documented. Excessive doses of vervain may interfere with existing hypo- or hypertensive and hormone therapies.
Pregnancy and lactation Vervain is reputed to act as an abortifacient and oxytocic agent[G12] with *in-vivo* uteroactivity documented (*see* Animal studies). In view of this, vervain should not be taken during pregnancy.
Vervain may affect lactation in view of the reported galactogogue properties.[3]

Pharmaceutical Comment
Limited chemical, pharmacological and toxicity data are available for vervain. Documented scientific information does not justifiy the herbal uses, although galactogogue properties have been reported. No human data were located. In view of the lack of toxicity data and documented pharmacological actions in animals, excessive use of vervain should be avoided.

References
See General References G1, G3, G9, G10, G12, G14, G18, and G32

1. Lahloub MF *et al.* Phenylpropanoid and iridoid glycosides from the Egyptian *Verbena officinalis*. *Planta Med* 1986; **52:** 47.

2. Andary C *et al.* Structures of verbascoside and orobanchoside, caffeic acid sugar esters from *Orobanche rapum-genistae*. *Phytochemistry* 1982; **21:** 1123–7.

3. Oliver-Bever BEP. Medicinal plants in tropical West Africa. Cambridge: Cambridge University Press, 1986.

4. Inouye H *et al.* Purgative activities of iridoid glycosides. *Planta Med* 1974; **25:** 285–8.

WILD CARROT

Species (Family)
Daucus carota L. subsp. *carota* (Umbelliferae)

Synonym(s)
Wild Carrot, Daucus, Queen Anne's lace

Part(s) Used
Herb

Pharmacopoeial Monographs
BHP 1983
BHP 1990

Legal Category (Licensed Products)
GSL[G14]

Constituents[G2,G19,G32]
Documented constituents refer to the fruit or seeds obtained from the dried fruit unless stated.
Flavonoids Flavones (e.g. apigenin, chrysin, luteolin), flavonols (e.g. kaempferol, quercetin) and various glycosides[1]
Furanocoumarin 8-Methoxypsoralen and 5-methoxypsoralen (0.01–0.02 μg/g fresh weight) in fresh plant. Concentrations increased in the diseased plant.[2]
Volatile oils (0.66–1.65%).[3] Many components identified; relative composition varies between different cultivars.[3] Various components include α-pinene, β-pinene, geraniol, geranyl acetate, limonene, α-terpinen, *p*-terpinen, α-terpineol, terpinen-4-ol, *p*-decanolactone (monoterpenes); β-bisabolene, β-elemene, caryophyllene, caryophyllene oxide, carotol, daucol (sesquiterpenes); asarone (phenylpropanoid derivative).[3]
Other constituents Choline,[4] daucine (alkaloid), a tertiary base (uncharacterised),[5] fatty acids (butyric, palmitic), coumarin, xylitol (polyol)

Food Use
Wild carrot should not be confused with the common cultivated carrot, *D. carota* L. subsp. *sativus* (Hoffm.), which has the familiar fleshy orange-red edible root. Wild carrot has an inedible tough whitish root.[G19] Wild carrot is listed by the Council of Europe as a natural source of food flavouring (category N1, N3). Category N1 indicates that for the roots there are no restrictions on use, whereas category N3 indicates that there is insufficient information available for an adequate assessment of potential toxicity.[G9]

Herbal Use
Wild carrot is stated to possess diuretic, antilithic, and carminative properties. Traditionally, it has been used for urinary calculus, lithuria, cystitis, gout, and specifically for urinary gravel or calculus.[G2,G3,G4,G32]

Dose
Dried herb 2–4 g or by infusion three times daily[G2,G3]
Liquid extract (1:1 in 25% alcohol) 2–4 mL three times daily[G2,G3]

Pharmacological Actions
Animal studies Significant antifertility activity (60%) in rats has been reported for wild carrot.[6] In contrast, insignificant antifertility activity was observed in pregnant rats fed oral doses of up to 4.5 g/kg body-weight from day 1 to day 10 of pregnancy.[7] Aqueous, alcoholic, and petrol extracts were reported to exhibit 20%, 40%, and 10% activities respectively. Weak oestrogenic activity[6,8,9] and inhibition of implantation[6,9] has been documented for seed extracts.[8] Oestrogenic activity, demonstrated by the inhibition of ovarian hypertrophy in hemicastrated rats, has been attributed to the known constituent coumarin (a weak phytooestrogen).[10]

Central effects similar to those of barbiturates have been documented for the seed oil obtained from *D. carota* var. *sativa*.[11] The oil was reported to elicit CNS hypnotic effects in the rat, hypotension in the dog[4] leading to respiratory depression at higher doses, anticonvulsant activity in the frog, *in-vitro* smooth muscle relaxant activity reducing acetylcholine-induced contractions (ileum/uterus, rabbit/rat), antagonism of acetylcholine in isolated frog skeletal muscle, direct depressant effect on cardiac muscle in the dog.[4,11] *In-vitro* cardiotonic activity[4] and vasodilation of coronary vessels of the isolated cat heart has been reported.[12] Papaverine-like antispasmodic activity has been documented for a tertiary base isolated from wild carrot seeds.[5] Activity of approximately one-tenth compared to papaverine was noted in a number of isolated preparations: ileum, uterus, blood vessels, and trachea.[5] Cholinergic-type actions have also been reported for wild carrot with *in-vitro* spasmodic actions noted in both smooth and skeletal muscle.[4] This cholinergic activity has been attributed to choline.[13] The identity of a second quaternary base isolated was not established.

Terpinen-4-ol is a documented component of the seed oil. This constituent is considered to be the diuretic principle in juniper, exerting its effect by causing renal irritation (*see* Juniper).

Increased resistance to carbon tetrachloride-induced hepatotoxicity has been reported in rats fed carrots.[14]

Limited antifungal activity has been documented, with activity exhibited against only 1 (*Botrytis cinerea*) out of 9 fungi tested.[15]

Agglutination of *Streptococcus mutans* cells has been described for wild carrot. The agglutinin, found to be heat and trypsin stable but sensitive to dextranase, was thought to be a dextran.[16]

Side-effects, Toxicity

The oil is reported to be non-toxic.[G19,G35] Acute LD_{50} values in mice (oral) and guinea-pigs (dermal) are reported to exceed 5 g/kg.[19]

The oil contains terpinen-4-ol, which is the component associated with the renal irritancy of juniper oil.

The oil is reported to be generally non-irritating and non-sensitising.[12] However, hypersensitivity reactions, occupational dermatitis, and positive patch tests have been reported for wild carrot.[2,G26] Carrot is reported to have a slight photosensitising effect.[2] Furanocoumarins are known photosensitisers.

Contra-indications, Warnings

Fruit extracts may cause sensitivity reactions similar to those seen with celery.[2] Excessive doses of the oil may cause renal irritation in view of the terpinen-4-ol content (*see* Juniper). Excessive doses may affect existing hypo- and hypertensive, cardiac and hormone therapies.

Pregnancy and lactation The safety of wild carrot has not been established. Both spasmodic and spasmolytic actions on smooth muscle *in vitro* have been reported. In view of this, the documented mild oestrogenic activity and potentially irritant volatile oil, excessive doses of wild carrot during pregnancy and lactation should be avoided.

Pharmaceutical Comment

Phytochemical studies documented for wild carrot concentrate on the composition of the volatile oil obtained from both the fresh and dried fruits (seeds). The composition of the oil varies between different cultivars. Animal studies have documented a variety of pharmacological actions including CNS depressant, spasmodic and antispasmodic, hypotensive, and cardiac depressant activities. However, the majority of these actions were observed in *in-vitro* preparations. The principle traditional use of wild carrot is as a diuretic. This activity has not been documented in animal studies but the seed oil of wild carrot does contain terpinen-4-ol, the diuretic principle documented for juniper. Toxicity data only refer to the oil and indicate low toxicity. However, in view of the documented mild oestrogenic activity and potential for internal irritation by the oil, excessive ingestion should be avoided.

References

See General References G2, G3, G4, G9, G14, G19, G26, G32 and G35.

1.   El-Moghazi AM *et al*. Flavonoids of Daucus carota. *Planta Med* 1980; **40**: 382–5.

2.   Ceska O *et al*. Furocoumarins in the cultivated carrot, *Daucus carota*. *Phytochemistry* 1986; **25**: 81–3.

3.   Benecke R *et al*. Vergleichende Untersuchungen über den Gehalt an ätherischem Öl und dessen Zusammensetzung in den Früchten verschiedener Sorten von *Daucus carota* L. ssp. sativus (Hoffm.) Arcang. *Pharmazie* 1987 **42**: 256–9.

4.   Gambhir SS *et al*. Studies on *Daucus carota*, Linn. Part I. Pharmacological studies with the water-soluble fraction of the alcoholic extract of the seeds: a preliminary report. *Indian J Med Res* 1966; **54**: 178–87.

5.   Gambhir SS *et al*. Antispasmodic activity of the tertiary base of *Daucus carota*, Linn. seeds. *Indian J Physiol Pharmacol* 1979; **23**: 225–8.

6.   Prakash AO. Biological evaluation of some medicinal plant extracts for contraceptive efficacy. *Contracept Deliv Syst* 1984; **5**: 9.

7.   Lal R *et al*. Antifertility effect of *Daucus carota* seeds in female albino rats. *Fitoterapia* 1986; **57**: 243–6.

8.   Kant A *et al*. The estrogenic efficacy of carrot (*Daucus carota*) seeds. *J Adv Zool* 1986; **7**: 36–41.

9.   Sharma MM *et al*. Estrogenic and pregnancy interceptory effects of carrot *Daucus carota* seeds. *Indian J Exp Biol* 1976; **14**: 506–8.

10.   Kaliwal BB, Rao MA. Inhibition of ovarian compensatory hypertrophy by carrot seed (*Daucus carota*) extract or estradiol-17β in hemicastrated albino rats. *Indian J Exp Biol* 1981; **19**: 1058–60.

11.   Bhargava AK *et al*. Pharmacological investigation of the essential oil of *Daucus carota* Linn. var. *sativa* DC. *Indian J Pharm* 1967; **29**: 127–9.

12.   Carrot seed oil. *Food Cosmet Toxicol* 1976; **14**: 705–6.

13.   Gambhir SS *et al*. Studies on *Daucus carota*, Linn. Part II. Cholingergic activity of the quaternary base isolated from water-soluble fraction of alcoholic extracts of seeds. *Indian J Med Res* 1966; **54**: 1053–6.

14.   Handa SS. Natural products and plants as liver protecting drugs. *Fitoterapia* 1986; **57**: 307–51.

15.   Guérin J-C, Réveillère H-P. Antifungal activity of plant extracts used in therapy. II Study of 40 plant extracts against 9 fungi species. *Ann Pharm Fr* 1985; **43**: 77–81.

16.   Ramstorp M *et al*. Isolation and partial characterization of a substance from carrots, Daucus carota, with ability to agglutinate cells of *Streptococcus mutans*. *Caries Res* 1982; 16: 423–7.

WILD LETTUCE

Species (Family)

Lactuca virosa L. (Asteraceae/Compositae)

Synonym(s)

Bitter Lettuce, Lettuce Opium.

Related *Lactuca* species include *Lactuca sativa* (Garden Lettuce), *Lactuca scariola* (Prickly Lettuce), *Lactuca altissima* and *Lactuca canadensis* (Wild Lettuce of America)

Part(s) Used

Leaf, Latex

Pharmacopoeial Monographs

BHP 1983
BHP 1990
BPC 1934
Martindale 25th edition

Legal Category (Licensed Products)

GSL[G14]

Constituents[G2,G10,G24,G30,G32]

All parts of the plant contain a milky, white latex (sap) which, when collected and dried, forms the drug known as lactucarium.[G13]

Acids Citric, malic and oxalic (up to 1%) acids; cichoric acid (phenolic).[1]

Alkaloids Hyoscyamine, later disputed.[G13,2] *N*-methyl-β-phenethylamine, also disputed[2]

Coumarins Aesculin, cichoriin[1]

Flavonoids Flavones (e.g. apigenin, luteolin), flavonols (e.g. quercetin) and their glycosides[1]

Terpenoids Bitter principles including the sesquiterpene lactones lactucin and lactupicrin (lactucopicrin); β-amyrin, germanicol, and lactucone (lactucerin). Lactucone is a mixture of α- and β-lactucerol acetates, β-lactucerol being identical to taraxasterol

Other constituents Mannitol, proteins, resins, sugars

Food Use

Wild lettuce is not used in foods, although the related species *L. sativa* is commonly used as a salad ingredient.

Herbal Use

Wild lettuce is stated to possess mild sedative, anodyne, and hypnotic properties. Traditionally, it has been used for insomnia, restlessness and excitability in children, pertussis, irritable cough, priapism, dysmenorrhoea, nymphomania, muscular or articular pains, and specifically for irritable cough and insomnia.[G2,G3,G4,G20,G32]

Dose

Dried leaves 0.5–3.0 g or by infusion three times daily[G2]

Liquid extract 0.5–3.0 mL (1:1 in 25% alcohol) three times daily[G2]

Lactucarium (dried latex extract) 0.3–1.0 g three times daily (BPC 1934)

Soft extract 0.3–1.0 g three times daily (BPC 1934)

Pharmacological Actions

Animal studies Lactucarium has been noted to induce mydriasis.[G2] This effect may be attributable to hyoscyamine, although the dried sap is reportedly devoid of this alkaloid.

An alcoholic extract of a related species, *L. sativa*, has exhibited a sedative effect in toads, causing a reduction in motor activity and behaviour.[3] Higher doses resulted in flaccid paralysis. In addition, an antispasmodic action on isolated smooth and striated muscle, and *in–vitro* negative chronotropic and inotropic effects on normal and stressed (tachycardic) hearts were observed. The antispasmodic action was noted to be antagonised by calcium.

Lactucin, lactupicrin, and hyoscyamine have all been proposed as the sedative components in wild lettuce. However in the above study,[3] the active component was uncharacterised and acted mainly peripherally, not readily crossing the blood-brain barrier. The suggested mode of action was via interference with basic excitatory processes common to neural and muscular functions, and not via a neuromuscular block.

Low amounts (nanograms) of morphine have been detected in *Lactuca* species, although the concentrations involved are considered too low to exert any obvious pharmacological effect.[G30]

Side-effects, Toxicity

None documented for *L. virosa*. Wild lettuce contains sesquiterpene lactones which are potentially allergenic.[G33] Occupational dermatitis has been documented for *L. sativa* together with an urticarial eruption after ingestion of the leaves.[4–6,G26] The milky sap of *L. sativa* is reported to be irritant.[G26]

The toxicity of wild lettuce is stated to be low.

Consumption of large amounts of *L. scariola* has caused poisoning in cattle, who developed pulmonary emphysema, severe dyspnoea, and weakness.[8] Only the immature plants were reported to be toxic.

L. sativa has been reported to produce only negative responses when tested for mutagenicity using the Ames test (*Salmonella typhimurium* TA 98, TA 100).[7]

Contra-indications, Warnings

Overdosage may produce poisoning[G20] involving stupor, depressed respiration, coma and even death. Wild lettuce may cause an allergic reaction in sensitive individuals, in particular those with an existing sensitivity to other members of the Asteraceae/Compositae family.

Pregnancy and lactation The safety of wild lettuce has not been established. In view of the lack of toxicity data and the possibility of allergic reactions, excessive use of wild lettuce during pregnancy and lactation should be avoided.

Pharmaceutical Comment

The chemistry of wild lettuce is well documented although it is not clear which constituents represent the active components. Early reports of hyoscyamine as a constituent have not been substantiated by subsequent workers. No published information was found to support the traditional herbal uses of wild lettuce, although a sedative action in toads has been reported for a related species *L. sativa*. In view of the potential allergenicity of wild lettuce and the lack of toxicity data, excessive use should be avoided.

References

See General References G2, G3, G4, G5, G10, G13, G14, G20, G24, G26, G30, G32 and G33.

1. Rees S, Harborne JB. Flavonoids and other phenolics of *Cichorium* and related members of the Lactuceae (Compositae). *Bot J Linn Soc* 1984; **89:** 313–19.

2. Huang Z-J *et al*. Studies on herbal remedies I: Analysis of herbal smoking preparations alleged to contain lettuce (*Lactuca sativa* L.) and other natural products. *J Pharm Sci* 1982; **71:** 270–1.

3. Gonzálex-Lima F *et al*. Depressant pharmacological effects of a component isolated from lettuce, *Lactuca sativa. Int J Crude Drug Res* 1986; **24:** 154–66.

4. Krook G. Occupational dermatitis from *Lactuca sativa* (lettuce) and *Cichorium* (endive). *Contact Dermatitis* 1977; **3:** 27–36.

5. Rinkel HJ, Balyeat RM. Occupational dermatitis due to lettuce. *JAMA* 1932; **98:** 137– 8.

6. Zeller W *et al*. The sensitizing capacity of compositae plants 6. Guinea pig sensitization experiments with ornamental plants and weeds using different methods. *Arch Dermatol Res* 1985; **277:** 28–35.

7. White RD *et al*. An evaluation of acetone extracts from six plants in the Ames mutagenicity test. *Toxicol Lett* 1983; **15:** 26–31.

8. Anon. *Poisindex CD-ROM* 1995; **85.** Denver:Micromedex

WILLOW

Species (Family)
Salix species including *Salix alba* L., *Salix fragilis* L., *Salix pentandra* L., *Salix purpurea* L. (Salicaceae)

Synonym(s)
Salix

Part(s) Used
Bark

Pharmacopoeial Monographs
BPC 1934
BHP 1983
BHP 1990

Legal Category (Licensed Products)
GSL[G14]

Constituents [G1,G2,G25,G31,G32]
Glycosides (phenolic). Various phenolic glycosides including salicin, salicortin, salireposide, picein and triandrin[1] Acetylated salicin, salicortin, salireposide, and esters of salicylic acid and salicyl alcohol may also occur.
Salicylates (calculated as salicin). Vary between species, e.g. 0.5% in *S. alba*, 1–10% in *S. fragilis*, 3–9% in *S. purpurea*[2]
Tannins Condensed
Other constituents Catechins, flavonoids[2]
There is reported to be no difference between the phenolic glycoside pattern of the bark and leaf. The latter is also reported to contain flavonoids, catechins, and condensed tannins.[2,3]

Food Use
Willow is not used in foods.

Herbal Use
Willow is stated to possess anti-inflammatory, antirheumatic, antipyretic, antihidrotic, analgesic, antiseptic, and astringent properties. Traditionally it has been used for muscular and arthrodial rheumatism with inflammation and pain, influenza, respiratory catarrh, gouty arthritis, ankylosing spondylitis, and specifically for rheumatoid arthritis and other systemic connective tissue disorders characterised by inflammatory changes.[G1,G2,G3,G4,G32]

Dose
Dry bark 1–3 g or by decoction three times daily[G2,G3]
Liquid extract (1:1 in 25% alcohol) 1–3 mL three times daily[G2,G3]

Pharmacological Actions
Animal studies No documented studies were located for the herbal material. Pharmacological actions documented for salicylates include anti-inflammatory, antipyretic, dose dependent hyperglycaemic/hypoglycaemic and uricosuric/ antiuricosuric activities, an increase in blood-clotting time and plasma-albumin binding.[G23]
Tannins are known to have astringent properties.
Human studies No documented studies were located. However, the pharmacological actions of salicylates in man are well documented and are applicable to willow. Salicin is a prodrug which is metabolised to saligenin in the gastro-intestinal tract and to salicylic acid after absorption.[2]

Side-effects, Toxicity
No reported side-effects were located. Side-effects and signs of toxicity normally associated with salicylates, such as gastric and renal irritation, hypersensitivity, blood in the stools, tinnitus, nausea and vomiting, may occur. Salicin is documented to cause skin rashes.[G21]

Contra-indications, Warnings
Precautions associated with salicylate therapy are also applicable to willow. Therefore individuals with a known hypersensitivity to aspirin, with asthma, active peptic ulceration, diabetes, gout, haemophilia, hypoprothrombinaemia, kidney or liver disease should be aware of the possible risks associated with the ingestion of willow.[4,G23] Irritant effects of salicylates on the gastro-intestinal tract may be enhanced by alcohol, and barbiturates and oral sedatives have been documented to enhance salicylate toxicity as well as masking the symptoms of overdosage.[G23] Concurrent administration of willow with other salicylate-containing products, such as aspirin, should be avoided. Drug interactions listed for salicylates are also applicable to willow and include oral anticoagulants, methotrexate, metoclopramide, phenytoin, probenecid, spironolactone, and valproate.
Pregnancy and lactation The safety of willow has not been established. Conflicting reports have been documented concerning the safety of aspirin taken during pregnancy. In view of this, the use of willow during pregnancy should be avoided. Salicylates excreted in breast milk have been reported to cause macular rashes in breast-fed babies.[G23]

Pharmaceutical Comment
Willow is rich in phenolic constituents, such as flavonoids, tannins and salicylates. Pharmacological actions normally associated with salicylates are also applicable to willow which support most of the herbal uses, although no studies were located specifically for willow. In view of the lack of toxicity data on willow, the usual precautions taken with other salicylate-containing drugs are applicable. Products containing willow should preferably be standardised on their salicin content, in view of the considerable variation in

salicylate concentrations between different *Salix* species. Salicin does not irritate the stomach.[5]

References

See General References G1, G2, G3, G4, G5, G14, G23, G25, G31, and G32.

1. Meier B *et al*. Identifikation und Bestimmung von je acht Phenolglykosiden in *Salix purpurea* und *Salix daphnoides* mit moderner HPLC. *Pharm Acta Helv* 1985; **60:** 269–74.

2. Meier B *et al*. Pharmaceutical aspects of the use of willows in herbal remedies. *Planta Med* 1988: **54:** 559–60.

3. Karl C *et al*. Flavonoide aus *Salix alba*, die Struktur des terniflorins und eines Weiteren Acylflavonoides. *Phytochemistry* 1976; **15:** 1084–5.

4. Baker S, Thomas PS. Herbal medicine precipitating massive haemolysis. *Lancet* 1987; **i:** 1039–40.

5. British Pharmaceutical Codex 1954. London: Pharmaceutical Press, 1954.

WITCH HAZEL

Species (Family)
Hamamelis virginiana L. (Hamamelidaceae)

Synonym(s)
Hamamelis, Witchazel

Part(s) Used
Bark, Leaf

Pharmacopoeial Monographs
BHP 1983
BPC 1973
Martindale 30th edition
Pharmacopoeias—Egypt., Fr., It., Rom., and Swiss.

Legal Category (Licensed Products)
GSL[G14]

Constituents[G1,G10,G19,G24,G32]
Flavonoids (leaf) Flavonols (e.g. kaempferol, quercetin) and their glycosides including astragalin, quercitrin, afzelin, and myricitrin
Tannins (about 8%). Hamamelitannin (hydrolysable), lesser amounts of condensed tannins (bark) including *d*-gallocatechin, *l*-epicatechin gallate, *l*-epigallocatechin
Volatile oils (about 0.5%). Hexen-2-ol, hexenol, α- and β-ionones, eugenol, safrole, sesquiterpenes
Other constituents Fixed oil (about 0.6%), resin (hamamelin, hamamelitannin), wax, saponins, choline, free gallic acid, free hamamelose

Food Use
Witch hazel is listed by the Council of Europe as a natural source of food flavouring (category N3). This category indicates that there is insufficient information available for an adequate assessment of potential toxicity.[G9]

Herbal Use
Witch hazel is stated to possess astringent, antihaemorrhagic, and anti-inflammatory properties. Traditionally, it has been used for diarrhoea, mucous colitis, haemorrhoids, haematemesis, haemoptysis, and externally for external haemorrhoids, bruises, and localised inflamed swellings.[G1,G2,G32]

Dose
Dried leaves 2 g or by infusion three times daily[G2]
Hamamelis Liquid extract (BPC 1973)(1:1 in 45% alcohol). 2–4 mL three times daily[G2]
Hamamelis Water (BPC 1973) for local application

Pharmacological Actions
Witch hazel is known to possess astringent and haemostatic properties, which have been attributed to the tannin constituents.

Side-effects, Toxicity
None documented for witch hazel. The volatile oil contains safrole, a known carcinogen (*see* Sassafras), but in amounts too small to cause concern.

Contra-indications, Warnings
None documented for witch hazel. In view of the tannin constituents, excessive ingestion of witch hazel is not recommended.

Pregnancy and lactation There are no known problems with the use of witch hazel during pregnancy, although excessive ingestion should be avoided in view of the tannin content.

Pharmaceutical Comment
Witch hazel is characterised by its tannin constituents and astringent properties. The documented herbal uses for witch hazel are related to these astringent properties.

References
See General References G1, G3, G7, G9, G10, G14, G19, G22, G24, and G32.

YARROW

Species (Family)
Achillea millefolium L. (Asteraceae/Compositae)

Synonym(s)
Milfoil, Millefolium

Part(s) Used
Flowerhead

Pharmacopoeial Monographs
BHP 1983
BHP 1990
Martindale 30th edition
Pharmacopoeias—Aust., Cz., Fr., Hung., and Swiss. Rom. includes the oil (Aetheroleum Millefolii)

Legal Category (Licensed Products)
GSL[G14]

Constituents [G1,G2,G10,G19,G32]
Acids Amino acids (e.g. alanine, aspartic acid, glutamic acid, histidine, leucine, lysine, proline, valine),[1,2] fatty acids (e.g. linoleic, myristic, oleic, palmitic, stearic),[3,4] and others including ascorbic acid,[5] caffeic acid,[6] folic acid,[5] salicylic acid, and succinic acid.[1]
Alkaloids/Bases Betonicine and stachydrine (pyrrolidine),[1,7] trigonelline (pyridine),[1,7] betaine and choline (bases).[1,7] Uncharacterised alkaloids include achiceine, achilleine[8] (possible synonym for L-betonicine), which is stated to yield achilletine[7] on alkaline hydrolysis, and moscatine/moschatine,[7] stated to be an ill-defined glucoalkaloid.
Flavonoids Predominantly flavone glycosides apigenin- and luteolin-7-glycosides,[9] with lesser quantities of artemetin, casticin, 5-hydroxy-3,6,7,4′-tetramethoxyflavone and isorhamnetin.[6] Rutin (a flavonol glycoside).[5]
Tannins Condensed and hydrolysable,[3,10] with glucose as the carbohydrate component of the latter[2]
Volatile oils Numerous identified components include borneol, bornyl acetate (trace), camphor, 1,8-cineole, eucalyptol, limonene, sabinene, terpinen-4-ol, terpineol and α-thujone (monoterpenes), caryophyllene (a sesquiterpene), achillicin, achillin, millefin and millefolide (sesquiterpene lactones), azulene and chamazulene (sesquiterpene lactone-derived) and isoartemisia ketone. The relative composition of the components varies greatly between *Achillea* species, especially the azulene content. Azulene has been reported as the major component.[11] However, true yarrow (*A. millefolium*) is thought to be hexaploid and azulene-free, whereas closely related species, such as *Achillea lanulosa* Nutt. and *A. collina* Becker, are tetraploid and contain up to 50% azulene in their volatile oil.[5,10,11] The tetraploid species may be supplied for *A. millefolium*. The azulenes are not present in the fresh herb: they are formed as artefacts during steam distillation of the oil, from unstable precursors called proazulenes (e.g. achillin and achillicin), via equally unstable azulene-carboxylic acid intermediates.[12]
Other constituents Unknown cyanogenetic compound,[13] sugars including arabinose, galactose, dextrose, dulcitol, glucose, inositol, maltose, mannitol, sucrose[1,2]
The constituents of yarrow have been reviewed in detail.[5]

Food Use
Yarrow is listed by the Council of Europe as a natural source of food flavouring (category N2). This category indicates that yarrow can be added to foods, provided that concentrations of thujone (α and β) do not exceed 0.5 mg/kg in the final product; 5–10 mg/kg in alcoholic beverages (depending on alcohol content), and 35 mg/kg in bitters.[G9] In the USA, yarrow is only approved for use in alcoholic beverages, and the finished product must be thujone free.[G19]

Herbal Use
Yarrow is stated to possess diaphoretic, antipyretic, hypotensive, astringent, diuretic, and urinary antiseptic properties. Traditionally, it has been used for fevers, common cold, essential hypertension, amenorrhoea, dysentery, diarrhoea, and specifically for thrombotic conditions with hypertension, including cerebral and coronary thromboses.[G1,G2,G3,G4,G32]

Dose
Dried herb 2–4 g or by infusion three times daily[G2,G3]
Liquid extract (1:1 in 25% alcohol) 2–4 mL three times daily[G2,G3]
Tincture (1:5 in 45% alcohol) 2–4 mL three times daily[G2,G3]

Pharmacological Actions
Some of activities documented for yarrow are associated with the azulene constituents, although it is now thought that azulene is absent from true yarrow (see Constituents). Presumably some of the documented pharmacological studies have used *Achillea* species other than *A. millefolium*.
Animal studies Anti-inflammatory activity has been documented for an aqueous extract of yarrow using mouse[15] and rat[16] paw oedema models, with inflammation induced by yeast[15] and various inflammatory substances[16] including histamine, carrageenan, and prostaglandin. In mouse studies, the active fraction was reported as a series of protein-carbohydrate complexes. Topical anti-inflammatory activity in rabbits has also been documented for the aqueous extract.[15] In general, anti-inflammatory properties are associated with azulenes (*see* German Chamomile). Anti-inflammatory activity has been described for the azulene components documented for the volatile oil of yarrow.[5]

A diuretic effect was also noted in mice administered an aqueous extract,[15] but only at a dose more than double that required for an anti-inflammatory effect.[15] Terpinen-4-ol, the diuretic principle in juniper, has been reported as a component of yarrow volatile oil.

CNS-depressant activity has been documented for the volatile oil: a dose of 300 mg/kg decreased the spontaneous activity of mice and lowered the body temperature of rats. In addition, 300–600 mg/kg doses inhibited pentetrazole-induced convulsions and prolonged sleep induced by a barbiturate preparation.[17]

Moderate antibacterial activity has been documented for an ethanolic extract of the herb against *Staphylococcus aureus*, *Bacillus subtillus*, *Mycobacterium smegmatis*, *Escherichia coli*, *Shigella sonnei*, and *Shigella flexneri*.[18] Antimicrobial properties have been documented for the sesquiterpene lactone fraction.[5]

Achilleine 0.5 g/kg by intravenous injection has been noted to decrease the blood clotting time in rabbits by 32%.[8] The haemostatic action persisted for 45 minutes with no observable toxic effects.

Antispasmodic activity on the isolated rabbit intestine has been documented for a flavonoid-containing fraction of yarrow.[9] Antispasmodic activity is generally associated with azulene constituents (*see* German Chamomile).

Antipyretic and hypotensive actions have been reported for the basic fraction (alkaloid/base);[G19] the sesquiterpene lactone fraction is stated to possess cytotoxic activities,[5] although no further details were located. Tannins are known to possess astringent activity.

Side-effects, Toxicity

Allergic reactions to yarrow (e.g. dermatitis) have been documented and positive patch tests have been produced in individuals sensitised to other plants.[5,G26,G13] An instance of yarrow tea causing a generalised eruption in a sensitised individual was reported in 1929. The allergenic properties of some sesquiterpene lactones are well documented, although none of those present in yarrow are recognised sensitisers.[G26] Yarrow has been suspected of being a photosensitiser, although extracts have been reported to lack phototoxicity and to be devoid of psoralens, compounds with known photosensitising properties.[G26]

Yarrow is considered to be non-toxic. In mice LD_{50} values have been reported of up to 3.65 g/kg (by mouth), 3.1 g/kg (by intraperitoneal injection), and greater than or equal to 1 g/kg (by subcutaneous injection).[15,17] In the rat an LD_{50} (subcutaneous injection) has been recorded as 16.86 g/kg, with corresponding LD_0 and LD_{100} values reported as 12 and 20 g/kg, respectively.[11] By comparison, an ED_{25} for anti-inflammatory activity has been estimated as about 0.43 g/kg.[16]

Terpenoid-rich volatile oils often possess irritant properties. Terpinen-4-ol, documented as a component of yarrow volatile oil, is thought to represent the diuretic principle of juniper as a result of its irritant action on the kidneys (*see* Juniper).[12] The known toxic principle thujone has been documented as a minor component of yarrow volatile oil,

although concentrations present are probably too low to represent a risk to human health.

A single report of animal poisoning has been documented for yarrow in which a calf died following the ingestion of a single plant.[5] No additional reports of animal toxicity were located.

Contra-indications, Warnings

Yarrow may cause an allergic reaction in sensitive individuals, especially those with an existing hypersensitivity to other members of the Asteraceae/Compositae.[19] Individuals with such a known hypersensitivity should avoid drinking herbal teas containing yarrow.[G30] Excessive doses may interfere with existing anticoagulant and hypo- and hypertensive therapies, and may have sedative and diuretic effects.

Pregnancy and lactation Yarrow should not be taken during pregnancy. It is reputed to be an abortifacient and to affect the menstrual cycle,[G12] and the volatile oil contains trace amounts (0.3%) of the abortifacient principle thujone. Excessive use should be avoided during lactation.

Pharmaceutical Comment

The chemistry of yarrow is well documented although there has been some disagreement over the major component in the volatile oil. Various pharmacological actions have been reported in animal studies whic support many of the reputed herbal uses although no human data were located. Yarrow is considered to be relatively non-toxic although allergic reactions in susceptible individuals have been documented. The volatile oil is contra-indicated in pregnancy and caution should be exercised by epileptic patients.[G35]

References

See General References G1, G2, G3, G4, G9, G10, G12, G13, G14, G19, G23, G26, G30, G32 and G35.

1.   Ivanov Ch, Yankov L. Composition of *Achillea millefolium*. I. Preparation of the total extracts and composition of the part of the alcoholic extracts soluble in alcohol and water. *God Vissh Khimiko-tekhnol Inst Sofia* 1967; **14**: 195–222.

2.   Ivanov Ch, Yankov L. Composition of *Achillea millefolium*. III. Composition of the parts soluble in water and insoluble in alcohol. *God Vissh Khimikotekhnol Inst Sofia* 1967; **14**: 223–41,

3.   Ivanov Ch, Yankov L. Composition of *Achillea millefolium*. III. Composition of the acidic, water-insoluble part of the alcoholic extract. *God Vissh Khimikotekhnol Inst Sofia* 1967; **14**: 61–72.

4.   Ivanov Ch, Yankov L. Composition of *Achillea millefolium*. V. Composition and structure of the components of neutral fraction insoluble in the aqueous part of the alcoholic extract. *God Vissh Khimikotekhnol Inst Sofia* 1967; **14**: 73–101.

5.   Chandler RF *et al.* Ethnobotany and phytochemistry of yarrow, *Achillea millefolium*, Compositae. *Economic Bot* 1982; **36**: 203–23.

6.   Falk AJ *et al.* Isolation and identification of three new flavones from *Achillea millefolium* L. *J Pharm Sci* 1975; **64**: 1838–42.

7.   Zirvi KA, Ikram M. Alkaloids of some of the plants of the Compositae. *Pakistan J Sci Ind Res* 1975; **18**: 93–101.

8. Miller FM, Chow LM. Alkaloids of *Achillea millefolium* L. I. Isolation and characterization of Achilleine. *J Am Chem Soc* 1954; **76:** 1353–4.

9. Hoerhammer L. Flavone concentration of medical plants with regard to their spasmolytic action. *Congr Sci Farm Conf Commun 21st Pisa* 1961; 578–88.

10. Falk AJ *et al*. The constituents of the essential oil from *Achillea millefolium* L. *Lloydia* 1974; **37:** 598–602.

11. Haggag MY *et al*. Thin layer and gas-chromatographic studies on the essential oil from *Achillea millefolium*. *Planta Med* 1975; **27:** 361–6.

12. Sticher O. Plant mono-, di- and sesquiterpenoids with pharmacological and therapeutical activity. In: New natural products with pharmacological biological or therapeutic activity. H Wagner, P Wolff eds. Berlin: Springer Verlag, 1977; 137–176.

13. Seigler DS. Plants of the Northeastern United States that produce cyanogenic compounds. *Economic Bot* 1976; **30:** 395–407.

14. Chandler F. Maritime Indian herbal remedies. *J Ethnopharmacol* 1983; **9:** 323–7.

15. Goldberg AS *et al*. Isolation of anti-inflammatory principles from *Achillea millefolium* (Compositae). *J Pharm Sci* 1969; **58:** 938–41.

16. Shipochliev T, Fournadjiev G. Spectrum of the antiinflammatory effect of *Arctostaphylos uva ursi* and *Achilea millefolium*, L. *Probl Vutr Med* 1984; **12:** 99–107.

17. Kudrzycka-Bieloszabska FW, Glowniak K. Pharmacodynamic properties of oleum chamomillae and oleum millefolii. *Diss Pharm Pharmacol* 1966; **18:** 449–54.

18. Moskalenko SA. Preliminary screening of far-Eastern ethnomedicinal plants for antibacterial activity. *J Ethnopharmacol* 1986; **15:** 231–59.

19. Mathias CGT *et al*. Plant dermatitis — patch test results (1975–78). Note on Juniperus extract. *Contact Dermatitis* 1979; **5:** 336.

YELLOW DOCK

Species (Family)
Rumex crispus L. (Polygonaceae)

Synonym(s)
Curled Dock

Part(s) Used
Root

Pharmacopoeial Monographs
BHP 1983

Legal Category (Licensed Products)
GSL[G14]

Constituents[G10,G24,G32]
Anthraquinones (2–4%). Chrysophanol, emodin, nepodin, physcion (aglycones)[1–3]
Tannins Catechol 5% (condensed-type)
Other plants parts The plant constituents documented include oxalic acid, oxalates, chrysophanic acid, emodin, tannin, and a complex volatile oil (more than 60 components identified).[4,G26]

Food Use
Yellow Dock is not used in foods.

Herbal Use
Yellow dock is stated to possess gentle purgative and cholagogue properties. Traditionally, it has been used for chronic skin disease, obstructive jaundice, constipation, and specifically for psoriasis with constipation.[G3,G32]

Dose
Dried root 2–4 g or by decoction three times daily[G3]
Liquid extract (1:1 in 25% alcohol) 2–4 mL three times daily[G3]
Tincture (1:5 in 45% alcohol) 1–2 mL three times daily[G3]

Pharmacological Actions
Animal studies None documented for the root. Slight antibacterial activity has been reported for herb extracts, which exhibited activity towards both Gram-positive (*Staphylococcus aureus*, *Mycobacterium smegmatis*) and Gram-negative (*Escherichia coli*, *Shigella sonnei*, *Shigella flexneri*) organisms.[4]

Side-effects, Toxicity
None documented for yellow dock. In view of the documented anthraquinone constituents, side-effects generally associated with laxatives are also applicable to yellow dock. Overuse may cause abdominal cramps and diarrhoea, and prolonged use may lead to intestinal atrophy and hypokalaemia.

Dermatitis has been reported in livestock following the ingestion of plant material in large quantities.[G26] Oxalic acid is known to be a toxic plant acid that forms insoluble calcium salts which cause a disturbance in the calcium concentrations and hence affect the blood coagulation mechanism.[G13]

Contra-indications, Warnings
Warnings generally associated with stimulant laxatives are also applicable to yellow dock. Therefore, yellow dock should not be taken when there is existing intestinal obstruction, and excessive use should be avoided (*see* Side-effects).

Pregnancy and lactation In general, unstandardised stimulant laxatives are not recommended for use during pregnancy. The use of yellow dock should therefore be avoided in favour of a standardised preparation that is recommended for the treatment of constipation during pregnancy. The use of yellow dock by breast-feeding women should also be avoided, since it has been documened that anthraquinones can be secreted into the breast milk (*see* Senna).

Pharmaceutical Comment
Limited chemical, pharmacological, and toxicity information is available for yellow dock. Documented anthraquinone constituents justify the reputed purgative action. Although the purgative effect of yellow dock is reputed to be gentle, the use of unstandardised anthraquinone-containing preparations should be avoided since their pharmacological effect is unpredictable and may cause abdominal cramp and diarrhoea.

References
See General References G3, G10, G13, G14, G24, G26 and G32.

1. de Siqueira NCS *et al*. Hydroxyanthraquiones in *Rumex crispus* L. (of southern Rio Grande). *Rev Cent Cienc Biomed* 1977; **5:** 69–74.

2. Midiwo JO, Rukunga GM. Distribution of anthraquinone pigments in *Rumex* species of Kenya. *Phytochemistry* 1985; **24:** 1390–1.

3. Fairbairn JW and El-Muhtadi FJ. Chemotaxonomy of anthraquinones in *Rumex*. *Phytochemistry* 1972; **11:** 263–8.

4. Miyazawa M, Kameoka H. Constituents of essential oil from *Rumex crispus*. *Yakagaku* 1983; **32:** 45–7.

YUCCA

Species (Family)
Various *Yucca* species (Liliaceae/Agavaceae) including
(i) *Yucca schidigera* Roezl ex Ortgies
(ii) *Yucca brevifolia* Engelm.
(iii) *Yucca glauca*

Synonym(s)
(i) Mohave Yucca, *Yucca mohavensis* Sarg.
(ii) Joshua Tree, *Yucca arborescens* Trel.

Part(s) Used
Whole plant

Pharmacopoeial Monographs
None

Legal Category (Licensed Products)
Yucca is not listed in the GSL.

Constituents
Terpenoids Various saponins have been isolated from different *Yucca* species, including tigogenin and chlerogenin,[1] yuccagenin and kammogenin,[2] sarsasapogenin, markogenin, higogenin, neo-tigogenin, neo-gitogenin, hecogenin, gloriogenin, and diosgenin (trace),[3] and smilagenin.

Food Use
Yucca filamentosa L. (Bear grass) is listed by the Council of Europe as a natural source of food flavouring (category N3). This category indicates that there is insufficient information available for an adequate assessment of potential toxicity.[G9] The yucca plant has been used traditionally as a major foodstuff by Indian tribes. In the USA, both *Y. schidigera* and *Y. brevifolia* are approved for food use.[G19]

Herbal Use
Yucca has been used for the treatment of arthritis, diabetes, and stomach disorders. Concentrated plant juice has been used topically to soothe painful joints.

Dose
None documented.

Pharmacological Actions
Animal studies In the rat, anti-inflammatory activity against carrageenan-induced inflammation has been documented for a saponin-containing leaf extract from *Yucca schotti*.[2] Yucca saponin extract, from *Y. schidigera*, is reported to exhibit approximately half the haemolytic activity of commercial soap bark saponin.

Antitumour activity against B16 melanoma has been documented for a polysaccharide-containing extract of *Y. glauca*.[4] The extract was found to be inactive towards L1210 or P388 leukaemias.

Human studies A saponin-containing yucca extract has been reported to reduce symptoms of swelling, pain, and stiffness in approximately 75 of 150 arthritic patients given the extract in a double blind study.[5] The onset of a positive response was found to vary from days to weeks or months. A saponin-containing yucca extract has also been documented to reduce blood pressure, abnormal triglyceride, and high cholesterol concentrations in a double-blind study involving 212 arthritic and hypertensive patients.[6] Optimum results were obtained in conjunction with diet and exercise. Yucca extracts have also been reported to provide relief from headaches and to improve circulation and gastro-intestinal function.[5,6]

Side-effects, Toxicity
Limited toxicity data are available for yucca. A 12-week study in rats concluded that yucca was non-toxic. A saponin-containing yucca extract was given to more than 700 arthritic patients with no signs of toxicity documented. The yucca saponins are regarded to be a safe food supplement since they are not thought to be absorbed from the gastro-intestinal tract, thereby reducing the dangers of systemic haemolytic activity.[5]

Contra-indications, Warnings
Pregnancy and lactation There are no known problems with the use of yucca during pregnancy and lactation. However, it is advisable not to exceed amounts normally ingested as a food.

Pharmaceutical Comment
Limited phytochemical information is available for yucca, steroidal saponins being the only documented constituents. Human studies have reported a yucca saponin extract to have a beneficial effect on certain symptoms of arthritis such as pain and stiffness, and to reduce blood pressure and serum triglyceride and cholesterol concentrations. The traditional use of yucca as a foodstuff would indicate it to be of low toxicity.

References
See General References G9 and G19.

1. Dewidar AM and El-Munajjed D. The steroid sapogenin constituents of *Agave americana*, *A. variegata* and *Yucca gloriosa*. *Planta Med* 1970; **19**: 87–91.

2. Backer RC *et al*. A phytochemical investigation of *Yucca schotti* (Liliaceae). *J Pharm Sci* 1972; **61**: 1665–6.

3. Stohs SJ *et al*. Steroidal sapogenins of *Yucca glauca* seeds. *Lloydia* 1973; **36**: 443.

4. Ali MS *et al*. Isolation of antitumor polysaccharide fractions from *Yucca glauca* Nutt. (Liliaceae). *Growth* 1978; **42**: 213–23.

5. Bingham R *et al*. Yucca plant saponin in the management of arthritis. *J Appl Nutr* 1975; **27**: 45–51.

6. Bingham R *et al*. Yucca plant saponin in the treatment of hypertension and hypercholesterolemia. *J Appl Nutr* 1978; **30**: 127–36.

APPENDIXES

APPENDIX 1   Potential Drug/Herb Interactions

Very few herbal interactions have been reported in the medical literature, but the following **potential** drug/herb interactions are listed on the basis of known herbal constituents and their reported pharmacological actions. It should be emphasised that many drug interactions are harmless and many of those that are potentially harmful occur only in a small proportion of patients and may then vary in severity from patient to patient. Health-care professionals should be alert to undeclared use of herbal remedies as a possible cause of unexplained toxicity or lack of effect of conventional medicines.

Suspected herb/drug interactions should be reported to the regulatory authorities, as for any other suspected adverse reaction to drugs or herbs, whether licensed or not.

Drug/ Therapeutic Category Affected	Herbal Ingredients Interacting	Possible Effects
Gastrointestinal System		
Antacids, ulcer-healing drugs	Herbal ingredients irritant to gastro-intestinal tract. See appendix 13	Exacerbation of symptoms Risk of systemic side-effects
Antidiarrhoeal drugs	Herbal ingredients with laxative activity. See appendix 2	Antagonism
Laxatives	Herbal ingredients with laxative activity. See appendix 2	Potentiation; increased risk of side-effects
Cardiovascular system		
Cardiac glycosides	Cardioactive herbal ingredients. See appendix 3	Potentiation; increased risk of side-effects
Diuretics	Herbal ingredientswith diuretic activity. See appendix 4 Herbal ingredients with hypotensive activity. See appendix 5	Potentiation; increased risk of hypokalaemia Difficulty in controlling diuresis; hypertension
Anti-arrhythmic activity	Cardioactive herbal ingredients. See appendix 3 Herbal ingredients with diuretic activity. See appendix 4	Interference/antagonism with existing therapy Antagonism if hypokalaemia occurs
Beta-adrenoceptor blocking drugs	Cardioactive herbal ingredients. See appendix 3 Herbal ingredients with significant levels of amines/ sympathomimetic activity. See appendix 14	Potential antagonism Potential risk of severe hypertension
Antihypertensive therapy	Herbal ingredients with hypertensive activity. See appendix 5 Herbal ingredients with mineralocorticoid activity, e.g. bayberry, liquorice. See appendix 10 Herbal ingredients with hypotensive activity. See appendix 5 Herbal ingredients with significant levels of amines/sympathomimetic activity. See appendix 14 Herbal ingredients with diuretic activity. See appendix 4	Antagonism Antagonism Potentiation Antagonism Risk of potentiation/ interference with existing therapy
Lipid-lowering drugs	Herbal ingredients with hypolipidaemic activity. See appendix 7	Additive effect

Drug/ Therapeutic Category Affected	Herbal Ingredients Interacting	Possible Effects
Cardiovascular System (*continued*)		
Nitrates and calcium-channel blockers	Cardioactive ingredients. See appendix 3	Interference with therapy
	Blue cohosh	Interference with therapy
	Herbal ingredients with hypertensive activity. See appendix 5	Antagonism
	Herbal ingredients with anticholinergic activity	Reduced sublingual absorption of glyceryl trinitrate
Sympathomimetics	Herbal ingredients with significant sympathomimetic amines. See appendix 14	Potentiation; increased risk of hypertension
	Herbal ingredients with hypertensive activity. See appendix 5	Increased risk of hypertension
	Herbal ingredients with hypotensive activity. See appendix 5	Antagonism
Anticoagulants	Herbal ingredients with coagulant/anticoagulant activity. See appendix 6	Risk of potentiation or antagonism
	Herbal ingredients with coumarins. See appendix 15	Risk of potentiation
	Herbal ingredients with significant salicylate levels. See appendix 6	Risk of potentiation
	Garlic	Raised INR reported in 2 patients receiving warfarin
	Horse-chestnut	Plasma protein binding
Respiratory System	Herbal ingredients that are potentially allergenic. See appendix 12	Risk of allergic reaction
Terfenadine	Cardioactive herbal ingredients. See appendix 3	May increase arrhythmogenic potential of terfenadine
	Herbal ingredients with diuretic activity. See appendix 4	Electrolyte imbalance may increase arrhythmogenic potential of terfenadine
Allergic disorders	Herbal ingredients claimed to have sedative activity. See appendix 8	Potentiation of drowsiness associated with antihistamines
Central Nervous System		
Hypnotics and anxiolytics	Herbal ingredients claimed to have sedative activity. See appendix 8	Potentiation
Stimulants	Ginseng	Increased risk of ginseng side-effects
Antipsychotics	Herbal ingredients with diuretic activity. See appendix 4	Potentiation of lithium therapy; increased risk of toxicity; diuretics reported to reduce lithium clearance
	Herbal ingredients with anticholinergic activity	Risk of interference with therapy; anticholinergic drug reported to reduce plasma-phenothiazine concentrations
	Evening Primrose	Potential risk of seizure
Antidepressants	Herbal ingredients with sympathomimetic amines. See appendix 14	Risk of hypertensive crisis with monoamine-oxidase inhibitors (MAOIs)
	Ginseng	Suspected phenelzine interaction
	Herbal ingredients containing tryptophan.	Risk of CNS excitation and confusional states with MAOIs
	White Horehound	Hydroxytryptamine antagonism, *in vivo*
	Herbal ingredients with sedative activity. See appendix 8	May potentiate sedative side-effects
	Hops	
	St. John's Wort	Antagonism; contra-indicated in patients with depressive illness

Drug/ Therapeutic Category Affected	Herbal Ingredients Interacting	Possible Effects
Central Nervous System (*continued*)		
Drugs used in nausea and vertigo	Herbal ingredients with sedative activity. See appendix 8	May potentiate sedative side-effects
	Herbal ingredients with anticholinergic activity	Antagonism
Analgesics	Herbal ingredients with diuretic activity. See appendix 4	Increased risk of toxicity with anti-inflammatory analgesics
	Herbal ingredients with corticosteroid activity, e.g. bayberry, liquorice. See appendix 10	Possible reduction in plasma-aspirin concentrations
	Herbal ingredients with sedative activity. See appendix 8	May potentiate sedative side-effects
Antiepileptics	Herbal ingredients with sedative activity. See appendix 8	May potentiate sedative side-effects
	Borage	May increase risk of seizure
	Evening primrose oil	May increase risk of seizure
	Ground ivy	May increase risk of seizure
	Sage	May increase risk of seizure
	Herbal ingredients with significant salicylate levels (Meadowsweet, Poplar, Willow)	Transient potentiation of phenytoin therapy may occur
	Herbal ingredients with significant folic acid levels	Plasma-phenytoin concentration may be reduced
Drugs for parkinsonism	Herbal ingredients with anticholinergic activity	Potentiation; increased risk of side-effects
	Herbal ingredients with cholinergic activity	Antagonism
Infections		
Antifungal drugs	Herbal ingredients with anticholinergic activity	Risk of reduced absorption of ketoconazole
Endocrine System		
Antidiabetics	Herbal ingredients with hypo- or hyperglycaemic activity. See appendix 7	Potentiation/ antagonism of activity
	Herbal ingredientswith diuretic activity. See appendix 4	Antagonism
Drugs for hypo- and hyperthyroidism	Herbal ingredients with significant iodine content e.g. Fucus	Interference with therapy
	Horseradish, Myrrh	Interference with therapy
Corticosteroids	Herbal ingredients with diuretic activity. See Appendix 4	Risk of increased potassium loss
	Herbal ingredients with corticosteroid activity e.g. Bayberry, Liquorice. See appendix10	Increased risk of side-effects e.g. water and sodium retention
Sex hormones	Herbal ingredients with hormonal activity. See appendix 10	Possible interaction with existing therapy
Obstetrics and Gynaecology		
Oral contraceptives	Herbal ingredients with hormonal activity. See appendix 10	Possible interaction with existing therapy; may reduce effectiveness of oral contraceptive

Drug/ Therapeutic Category Affected	Herbal Ingredients Interacting	Possible Effects
Malignant Disease and Immunosuppression		
Methotrexate	Herbal ingredients with significant salicylate levels. See appendix7	Increased risk of toxicity
Drugs affecting immune response	Herbal ingredients with immunostimulant activity. See appendix 11	Potentiation or antagonism
Musculoskeletal and Joint Diseases		
Systemic lupus erythematosus	Alfalfa	Antagonism; contra-indicated
Probenecid	Herbal ingredients with significant salicylate levels. See appendix 6	Risk of inhibition of probenecid
Eye		
Acetazolamide	Herbal ingredients with significant salicylate levels. See appendix 6	Increased risk of toxicity
Skin	Herbal ingredients with potential allergenic activity. See appendix 12	Allergic reaction; exacerbation of existing symptoms
	Herbal ingredients with phototoxic activity. See appendix 12	Phototoxic reaction; exacerbation of existing symptoms
Anaesthetics		
General anaesthetics	Herbal ingredients with hypotensive activity. See appendix 5	Potentiation of hypotensive effect
Competitive muscle relaxants	Herbal ingredients with diuretic activity. See appendix 4	Risk of potentiation if hypokalaemia occurs
Depolarising muscle relaxants	Cardioactive herbal ingredients. See appendix 3	Risk of arrhythmias

APPENDIX 2   Laxative Herbal Ingredients

Drug	Effect
Aloes	Anthraquinone constituents
Cascara	Anthraquinone constituents
Eyebright	Iridoids, *in vivo*
Frangula	Anthraquinone constituents
Horehound, White	Large doses
Ispaghula	Bulk laxative
Plantain	Iridoids, *in vivo* (much less than senna)
Rhubarb	Anthraquinone constituents
Senna	Anthraquinone constituents
Yellow Dock	Anthraquinone constituents

APPENDIX 3   Cardioactive Herbal Ingredients

Drug	Effect
Broom	Alkaloid constituents: cardiac depressant activity
Calamus	Antiarrhythmic activity
Cereus	Tyramine: cardiotonic amine
Cola	Caffeine
Coltsfoot	Cardiac calcium-channel blocking activity
Devil's Claw	Activity *in vivo*
Fenugreek	Activity *in vitro*
Figwort	Cardioactive glycoside constituents, activity *in vitro*
Fumitory	Alkaloid constituent: cardioactive
Ginger	Activity *in vivo*

Drug	Effect
Ginseng, Panax	Activity *in vivo*
Golden Seal	Berberine: cardioactive alkaloid
Hawthorn	Tyramine: cardiotonic amine; activity *in vivo*
Horehound, White	Activity *in vivo*
Lime Flower	Activity reputed with excessive ingestion
Maté	Caffeine
Mistletoe	Viscotoxin, negative inotropic effect
Motherwort	Cardiac glycoside constituents; activity *in vitro*
Parsley	Apiole poisoning, high doses
Pleurisy Root	Cardenolides, active *in vitro* and *in vivo*
Prickly Ash, Northern	Interaction with Na+K+ ATPase
Prickly Ash, Southern	Interaction with Na+K+ ATPase
Quassia	Activity *in vitro*
Shepherd's Purse	Activity *in vitro*
Squill	Cardiac glycoside constituents
Wild Carrot	Depressant activity *in vivo*

APPENDIX 4   Diuretic Herbal Ingredients

Drug	Effect
Agrimony	Activity *in vivo*
Artichoke	Reputed action
Boldo	Irritant oil
Broom	Reputed action
Buchu	Reputed action
Burdock	Reputed action
Celery	Reputed action
Cornsilk	Human activity
Couchgrass	Activity *in vivo*
Dandelion	Activity *in vivo*
Elder	Activity *in vivo*
Guaiacum	Reputed action
Juniper	Reputed action; terpinen-4-ol
Pokeroot	Activity *in vivo*
Shepherd's Purse	Activity *in vivo*
Squill	Activity *in vivo*
Uva Ursi	Reputed action
Yarrow	Activity *in vivo*

APPENDIX 5   Hypotensive and Hypertensive Herbal Ingredients

Drug	Effect
Hypotensive	
Agrimony	Hypotensive, *in vivo*
Asafoetida	Hypotensive, *in vivo*
Avens	Hypotensive, *in vivo*
Calamus	Hypotensive, *in vivo*
Celery	Hypotensive, human and *in vivo*
Cohosh, Black	Hypotensive, human
Cornsilk	Hypotensive, *in vivo*
Cowslip	Hypotensive, then hypertensive *in vivo*
Devil's Claw	Hypotensive, *in vivo*
Elecampane	Hypotensive, *in vivo*
Fenugreek	Hypotensive
Fucus	Hypotensive
Fumitory	Hypotensive, *in vivo*
Garlic	Hypotensive, *in vivo*
Ginger	Hypotensive
Ginseng, Panax	Hypotensive, human and *in vivo*
Goldenseal	Hypotensive, alkaloid effect
Hawthorn	Hypotensive, *in vivo*
Horehound, White	Vasodilator, oil
Horseradish	Hypotensive, *in vivo*
Mistletoe	Hypotensive, *in vivo*
Nettle	Hypotensive, *in vivo*
Parsley	Hypotensive, *in vivo*
Plantain	Hypotensive, *in vivo*
Pokeroot	Hypotensive, *in vivo*
Prickly Ash, Northern	Hypotensive, *in vivo*
Prickly Ash, Southern	Hypotensive, *in vivo*
Sage	Hypotensive
Shepherd's Purse	Hypotensive
Squill	Vasodilator, *in vivo*
St John's Wort	Hypotensive, *in vivo*
Vervain	Hypotensive
Wild Carrot	Hypotensive, *in vivo*
Yarrow	Hypotensive, *in vivo*

Drug	Effect
Hypertensive	
Bayberry	Hypertensive, myricitrin mineralocorticoid side-effect
Broom	Hypertensive, alkaloid effect, stated to be contra-indicated in hypertensive individuals
Capsicum	Hypertensive, increased catecholamine secretion
Cohosh, Blue	Hypertensive, methylcytisine has nicotinic action, alkaloid effect
Cola	Hypertensive, caffeine
Coltsfoot	Hypertensive, pressor activity
Gentian	Stated to be contra-indicated in hypertensive individuals
Ginger	Hypertensive
Ginseng, Panax	Hypertensive, human and *in vivo*
Liquorice	Hypertensive, mineralocorticoid side-effect
Maté	Hypertensive, caffeine
Vervain	Hypertensive

Drug	Effect
Ginger	Inhibition of platelet activity
Ginseng, Panax	Reduction of blood coagulation
Horse-chestnut	Coumarin constituents
Horseradish	Peroxidase stimulates synthesis of arachidonic acid metabolites
Liquorice	Inhibition of platelet activity
Meadowsweet	Salicylate constituents
Poplar	Salicylate constituents
Prickly Ash, Northern	Coumarin constituents
Prickly Ash, Southern	Coumarin constituents
Quassia	Coumarin constituents
Red Clover	Coumarin constituents
Willow	Salicylate constituents
Coagulants	
Agrimony	Coagulant, human
Goldenseal	Heparin antagonist
Mistletoe	Lectins, agglutinating activity
Yarrow	Coagulant, *in vivo*

APPENDIX 6   Anticoagulant and Coagulant Herbal Ingredients

Drug	Effect
Anticoagulants	
Alfalfa	Coumarin constituents
Angelica	Coumarin constituents
Aniseed	Coumarin constituents
Arnica	Coumarin constituents
Asafoetida	Coumarin constituents, anticoagulant *in vivo*
Celery	Coumarin constituents
Chamomile, German	Coumarin constituents
Chamomile, Roman	Coumarin constituents
Clove	Eugenol powerful inhibitor of platelet activity
Fenugreek	Coumarin constituents
Feverfew	Inhibits platelet aggregation
Fucus	Anticoagulant action
Garlic	Interaction with warfarin reported

APPENDIX 7   Hypolipidaemic and Hyperlipidaemic Herbal Ingredients

Drug	Effect
Alfalfa	Hypocholesterolaemic, *in vivo*
Artichoke	Hypocholesterolaemic, *in vivo*
Cohosh, Black	Hypocholesterolaemic, *in vivo*
Fenugreek	Hypocholesterolaemic, *in vivo*, human
Garlic	Hypocholesterolaemic, *in vivo*, human
Ginger	Hypocholesterolaemic, *in vivo*
Hydrocotyle	*Hyper*cholesterolaemic, *in vivo*
Plantain	Hypocholesterolaemic, *in vivo*
Scullcap	Hypocholesterolaemic, *in vivo*
Tansy	Hypocholesterolaemic, *in vivo*

APPENDIX 8   Sedative Herbal Ingredients

Drug	Effect
Calamus	Potentiation barbiturate sleeping time
Celery	*In vivo*
Chamomile, German	Human
Couchgrass	*In vivo*
Elecampane	*In vivo*
Ginsengs	CNS depressant and stimulant
Goldenseal	*In vivo*
Hops	*In vivo*
Hydrocotyle	*In vivo*
Jamaica Dogwood	*In vivo*
Nettle	CNS depression, *in vivo*
Passionflower	*In vivo*
Sage	*In vivo*
Scullcap	Reputed action
Shepherd's Purse	Potentiation barbiturate sleeping time
St John's Wort	Traditional use, bioflavonoids
Valerian	Human, *in vivo*
Wild Carrot	*In vivo*
Wild Lettuce	*In vivo*, related species

APPENDIX 9   Hypoglycaemic and Hyperglycaemic Herbal Ingredients

Drug	Effect
Hypoglycaemic	
Alfalfa	Hypoglycaemic, manganese, human
Aloes/ Aloe vera	Hypoglycaemic, *in vivo*
Burdock	Hypoglycaemic, *in vivo*
Celery	Hypoglycaemic, *in vivo*
Cornsilk	Hypoglycaemic, *in vivo*
Damiana	Hypoglycaemic
Elecampane	Hypoglycaemic
Eucalyptus	Hypoglycaemic, *in vivo*
Fenugreek	Hypoglycaemic, human
Garlic	Hypoglycaemic, *in vivo,* human
Ginger	Hypoglycaemic, *in vivo*

Drug	Effect
Ginseng, Panax	Hypoglycaemic
Juniper	Hypoglycaemic *in vivo*
Marshmallow	Hypoglycaemic
Myrrh	Hypoglycaemic
Nettle	Hypoglycaemic
Sage	Hypoglycaemic, *in vivo*
Tansy	Hypoglycaemic, *in vivo*

Hyperglycaemic

Drug	Effect
Devil's Claw	Stated to be contra-indicated in diabetics
Elecampane	Hyperglycaemic
Figwort	*See* Devil's Claw: similar constituents
Ginseng, Panax	Hyperglycaemic
Hydrocotyle	Hyperglycaemic, human
Liquorice	Reduced K$^+$ aggravates glucose tolerance

APPENDIX 10   Hormonally Active Herbal Ingredients

Drug	Effect
Agnus Castus	Many uses in hormonal imbalance disorders
Alfalfa	Oestrogenic, *in vivo*
Aniseed	Oestrogenic
Bayberry	Mineralocorticoid
Cohosh, Black	Oestrogenic
Fucus	Hyper-/hypothyroidism reported
Ginsengs	Oestrogenic, human
Horseradish	May depress thyroid activity
Liquorice	Mineralocorticoid activity, human; oestrogenic *in vivo, in vitro*
Motherwort	Oxytocic
Pleurisy Root	Oestrogenic
Red Clover	Oestrogenic *in vivo*
Saw Palmetto	Oestrogenic and anti-androgenic *in vivo*; human use in prostate cancer
Vervain	Inhibition of gonadotrophic activity
Wild Carrot	Oestrogenic

APPENDIX 11 Immunostimulating Herbal Ingredients

Drug	Effects
Boneset	Stimulant *in vitro*
Calendula	Stimulant *in vitro*
Drosera	Stimulant and depressant (*in vitro*)
Echinacea	Stimulant *in vitro, in vivo*
Ginseng, Eleutherococcus	Stimulant, animal, human
Mistletoe	Stimulant, animal, human; suppressant (high doses), human
Saw Palmetto	Stimulant, *in vivo*

APPENDIX 12 Allergenic Herbal Ingredients

Drug	Effect
Agnus Castus	Allergic effects reported
Angelica	Furanocoumarins, photosensitivity, contact allergy
Aniseed	Furanocoumarins, photosensitivity, contact allergy
Apricot	Contact allergy, kernels
Arnica	Contact allergy
Artichoke	Sesquiterpene lactone constituents
Asafoetida	Irritant gum, contact allergy
Boneset	Sesquiterpene lactone constituents
Cassia	Allergic reactions, mainly contact
Celery	Furanocoumarins, photosensitivity
Chamomile, German	Sesquiterpene lactone constituents
Chamomile, Roman	Sesquiterpene lactone constituents
Cinnamon	Contact allergy
Cornsilk	Allergic reactions
Cowslip	Allergic reactions
Dandelion	Sesquiterpene lactone constituents
Elecampane	Sesquiterpene lactone constituents
Euphorbia	Histamine potentiating properties
Feverfew	Sesquiterpene lactone constituents
Fucus	Iodine may aggravate/trigger acne
Garlic	Sulphur-containing compounds, allergic reaction
Gravel Root	Sesquiterpene lactone constituents
Guaicum	Irritant resin
Holy Thistle	Sesquiterpene lactone constituents

Drug	Effect
Hops	Contact allergy
Hydrangea	Contact allergy
Hydrocotyle	Photosensitivity
Juniper	Contact allergy
Lady's Slipper	Contact allergy
Meadowsweet	Potentiation of histamine bronchospastic properties
Motherwort	Dermatitis, photosensitisation
Parsley	Furanocoumarins, photosensitivity
Pilewort	Contact allergy
Plantain	Contact allergy
Pleurisy Root	Contact allergy
Pulsatilla	Contact allergy, protoanemonin
Rosemary	Dermatitis, photosensitisation
St John's Wort	Photodermatitis, hypericin
Tansy	Sesquiterpene lactone constituents
Wild Carrot	Furanocoumarins, photosensitivity
Yarrow	Sesquiterpene lactone constituents

APPENDIX 13 Irritant Herbal Ingredients

Drug	Effects
Alfalfa	Irritant, canavanine in seeds
Arnica	Irritant to mucous membranes
Asafoetida	Irritant gum
Blue Flag	Irritant gum and oil
Bogbean	Irritant to GI tract
Boldo	Irritant oil
Buchu	Irritant oil
Capsicum	Capsaicinoids, mucosal irritants
Cassia	Irritant to mucous membranes, oil
Cinnamon	Irritant to mucous membranes, oil
Cohosh, Blue	Irritant to mucous membranes; spasmogenic *in vitro*
Cowslip	Irritant saponins
Drosera	Plumbagin, irritant
Eucalyptus	Irritant oil
False Unicorn	Large doses may cause vomiting
Figwort	Purgative effect
Garlic	Raw clove
Ground Ivy	Irritant oil
Guaiacum	Avoid if inflammatory condition

Drug	Effects
Horse-chestnut	Saponin constituents, contra-indicated in existing renal disease
Horseradish	Irritant oil
Hydrangea	May cause gastro-enteritis, hydrangin
Jamaica Dog-wood	Irritant to humans
Juniper	Irritant oil
Lemon Verbena	Irritant oil
Lime Flower	Irritant to kidney, oil
Nettle	Tea irritant to stomach
Parsley	Irritant oil
Pennyroyal	Toxic and irritant oil
Pilewort	Irritant sap
Pleurisy Root	Gastro-intestinal irritant
Pokeroot	Irritant saponins
Pulsatilla	Irritant to mucous membranes
Queen's Delight	Diterpene constituents
Sarsaparilla	Saponins
Senega	Saponins
Skunk Cabbage	Inflammatory and blistering to skin
Squill	Saponins

APPENDIX 14   Herbal Ingredients with Amines, Alkaloids or Sympathomimetic Action

Drug	Effects
Agnus Castus	alkaloids
Alfalfa	alkaloids
Aniseed	anethole, sympathomimetic
Arnica	betaines, choline
Bloodroot	alkaloids
Bogbean	alkaloids
Boldo	alkaloids
Borage	alkaloids
Broom	alkaloids, amines
Calamus	amines
Capsicum	sympathomimetic
Centaury	alkaloids
Cereus	tyramine
Cohosh, Black	alkaloids
Cohosh, Blue	alkaloids
Cola	alkaloids

Drug	Effects
Coltsfoot	alkaloids
Comfrey	alkaloids
Cornsilk	amines
Echinacea	alkaloids
Eyebright	alkaloids
Fenugreek	choline, trigonelline
Fumitory	alkaloids
Gentian	alkaloids
Ginseng, Panax	MAOI potentiation, suspected phenelzine interaction
Golden Seal	alkaloids
Gravel Root	alkaloids
Hawthorn	tyramine
Horehound, White	alkaloids
Hydrocotyle	alkaloids
Ispaghula	alkaloids
Jamaica Dog-wood	alkaloids
Liferoot	alkaloids
Lobelia	alkaloids
Maté	alkaloids, amines
Mistletoe	histamine release
Motherwort	alkaloids
Nettle	choline
Parsley	myristicin, sympathomimetic
Passionflower	alkaloids, MAOI activity
Plantain	alkaloids
Pleurisy Root	sympathomimetic
Pokeroot	betalains
Prickly Ash, Northern	alkaloids
Prickly Ash, Southern	alkaloids
Quassia	alkaloids
Sassafras	alkaloids
Shepherd's Purse	choline, tyramine
Skunk Cabbage	alkaloids
St. John's Wort	MAOI activity, in vitro
Stone Root	alkaloids
Valerian	alkaloids
Vervain	sympathomimetic
Yarrow	betonicine, stachydrine, betaine

APPENDIX 15   Herbal Ingredients containing Coumarins

Alfalfa, Angelica, Aniseed, Arnica, Asafoetida, Bogbean, Boldo, Buchu, Capsicum, Cassia, Celery, Chamomile (German and Roman), Fenugreek, Horse-chestnut, Horseradish, Liquorice, Meadowsweet, Nettle, Parsley, Passion Flower, Prickly Ash (Northern), Quassia, Wild Carrot, Wild Lettuce

APPENDIX 16   Herbal Ingredients containing Flavonoids

Agnus Castus, Angelica, Aniseed, Apricot, Arnica, Artichoke, Bayberry, Bogbean, Boldo, Boneset, Broom, Buchu, Burdock, Burnet, Calendula, Celery, Cereus, Chamomile (German and Roman), Chaparral, Clivers, Coltsfoot, Cornsilk, Couchgrass, Cowslip, Damiana, Devil's Claw, Drosera, Elder, Eucalyptus, Euphorbia, Eyebright, Fenugreek, Feverfew, Figwort, Frangula, Fumitory, Ginkgo, Gravel Root, Ground Ivy, Hawthorn, Hops, Horehound (Black and White), Horse-chestnut, Hydrangea, Hydrocotyle, Juniper, Lemon Verbena, Lime Flower, Liquorice, Maté, Meadowsweet, Mistletoe, Motherwort, Nettle, Parsley, Passionflower, Plantain, Pulsatilla, Raspberry, Red Clover, Rhubarb, Rosemary, Sarsaparilla, Saw Palmetto, Scullcap, Senna, Shepherd's Purse, Squill, St John's Wort, Thyme, Uva-Ursi, Wild Carrot, Wild Lettuce, Willow, Witch Hazel, Yarrow

APPENDIX 17   Herbal Ingredients containing Iridoids

Agnus Castus, Bogbean, Centaury, Clivers, Devil's Claw, Eyebright, Figwort, Gentian, Ispaghula, Motherwort, Plantain, Scullcap, Uva-Ursi, Valerian, Vervain

APPENDIX 18   Herbal Ingredients containing Saponins

Alfalfa, Aloe Vera, Bogbean, Burnet, Calendula, Chaparral, Cohosh (Blue), Cornsilk, Cowslip, False Unicorn, Fenugreek, Ginseng (Eleutherococcus and Panax), Hawthorn, Horehound (White), Horse-chestnut, Hydrangea, Hydrocotyle, Jamaica Dogwood, Lime Flower, Pokeroot, Pulsatilla, Red Clover, Sarsaparilla, Senega, Senna, Stone Root, Thyme, Yucca

APPENDIX 19   Herbal Ingredients containing Tannins

Agrimony, Apricot, Artichoke, Avens, Bayberry, Blue Flag, Boldo, Borage, Burnet, Calamus, Cascara, Cassia, Chamomile, German, Cinnamon, Clivers, Cohosh (Black), Cola, Coltsfoot, Comfrey, Cornsilk, Cowslip, Damiana, Drosera, Elder, Eucalyptus, Eyebright, Feverfew, Frangula, Gentian, Ground Ivy, Hawthorn, Holy Thistle, Hops, Horse-chestnut, Ispaghula, Juniper, Lady's Slipper, Lime Flower, Marshmallow, Meadowsweet, Mistletoe, Motherwort, Nettle, Pilewort, Plantain, Poplar, Prickly Ash (Northern and Southern), Queen's Delight, Raspberry, Rhubarb, Sage, Sassafras, Saw Palmetto, Scullcap, Slippery Elm, Squill, St John's Wort, Stone Root, Tansy, Thyme, Uva-Ursi, Valerian, Vervain, Willow, Witch Hazel, Yarrow, Yellow Dock

APPENDIX 20   Herbal Ingredients containing Volatile Oils

Agnus Castus, Agrimony, Angelica, Aniseed, Arnica, Artichoke, Asafoetida, Avens, Blue Flag, Boldo, Boneset, Buchu, Burdock, Burnet, Calamus, Calendula, Capsicum, Cassia, Celery, Chamomile (German and Roman), Chaparral, Cinnamon, Cloves, Cohosh (Black), Coltsfoot, Couchgrass, Damiana, Elder, Elecampane, Eucalyptus, Eyebright, Feverfew, Garlic, Ginseng (Eleutherococcus and Panax), Golden Seal, Ground Ivy, Holy Thistle, Hops, Horehound (Black), Horseradish, Hydrocotyle, Juniper, Lemon Verbena, Lime Flower, Liquorice, Lobelia, Meadowsweet, Motherwort, Myrrh, Parsley, Pennyroyal, Prickly Ash (Northern), Queen's Delight, Red Clover, Rosemary, Sage, Sassafras, Saw Palmetto, Senna, Skunk Cabbage, Squill, St John's Wort, Stone Root, Tansy, Thyme, Uva-Ursi, Valerian, Wild Carrot, Witch Hazel, Yarrow

INDEX

Page numbers in **bold** type refer to monographs or Appendix tables.

A

Acanthopanax senticosus 141
acetylactein 80
Achillea millefolium 271
achilleine 272
acids 21, 201
Actaeae Racemosae Radix 80
actein 80
acteina 80
adaptogen 141
aescin 166
aesculetin 166, 168
Aesculus 166
Aesculus hippocastanum 166
Agathosma betulina 51
Agathosma crenulata 51
Agavaceae 275
agglutinating activity 194
Agnus Castus **19**
agnuside 19
Agrimonia 21
Agrimonia eupatoria 21
Agrimony **21**
agropyrene 91
Agropyron 91
Agropyron repens 91
Ague Tree 235
Ajo 129
ajoene 129
alant 106
alant camphor 106
alantolactone 106
Alchemilla arvensis 205
Alchemilla vulgaris 205
Aldehydes 52
Alder Buckthorn 123
Alexandrian senna 243
Alfalfa **23**
algin 124
alginic acid 124
alkaloids 23, 42, 45, 46, 49, 50, 68, 80, 82, 84, 85, 87, 101, 117, 127, 134, 151, 153, 165, 173, 180, 187, 189, 193, 197, 206, 215, 219, 220, 223, 235, 260, 271
Alkaloids, herbal ingredients with **285**
allantoin 87, 90, 166
allergenic 34, 36, 64, 72, 90, 163, 178, 222
Allergenic herbal ingredients **284**
All-Heal 260
allicin 129
alliin 129
Allium 129

Allium sativum
allocryptopine 42
allyl isothiocyanate 246
allylisothiocyanate 168
allylpropyl disulphide 129
aloe 243
Aloe africana 25, 27
Aloe barbadensis 25, 27
Aloe capensis 27
Aloe ferox 25, 27
Aloe gel 25
Aloe spicata 25, 27
Aloe vera 25, 27
aloe-emodin 27, 228
Aloes **27**
aloin 27
Aloysia citriodora 179
Aloysia triphylla 179
Altamisa 119
Althaea 188
   Flower 188
   Leaf 188
Althaea officinalis 188
amarogentin 134
Amaryllidaceae 129
amentoflavone 176
American Elder 104
American Ginseng 145
American Mistletoe 194
American Pennyroyal 208
American Valerian 178
amides 101, 220
amines 35, 50, 55, 68, 90, 157, 189, 193, 201, 245
Amines, herbal ingredients with **285**
amino acids 23, 154, 170, 181
amoebicidal action 74
amygdalin 32
amyrin 199, 254, 258
anacardic acid 139
anagyrine 82
analgesic 268
Anemone patens 222
Anemone pratensis 222
Anemone pulsatilla 222
anemonin 209, 222
anethole 30
angelic acid esters 72
Angelica **28**
Angelica archangelica 28
Angelica koreana 28
Angelica sinensis 28
angelicin 28
angina 158
Anise 30

Aniseed **30**
Anisi Fructus 30
Anisum 30
Anisum officinarum 30
Anisum vulgare 30
anthelmintic 106, 254, 256
anthemic acid 72
Anthemis nobilis 72
anthraquinones 25, 26, 27, 62, 123, 228, 243, 250, 274
anti-allergic 69
anti-androgen 237
antibacterial 28, 250, 256
anticoagulant 24
Anticoagulant herbal ingredients **282**
antifungal 28, 256
antihaemorrhagic 245, 270
antihistamine 139
anti-inflammatory 28, 58, 69, 72, 85, 237, 268, 270, 271, 275
antimicrobial 42, 151, 229
antipyretic 268, 271
antiseptic 108
antispasmodic 231, 254, 256, 260, 263, 266
antithrombotic 130, 131
antitussive 106, 248, 256
anxiety 251
Aphanes 205
Aphanes arvensis 205
Apiaceae 28, 30, 38, 65, 203
apigenin 65, 203
Apii Fructus 65
apiin 65
apiole 203
Apium graveolens 65
Apium petroselinum 203
Apricot **32**
Apricot Vine 206
Aquifoliaceae 189
Araceae 247
Araliaceae 141, 145
arbutin 94, 258
Archangelica officinalis 28
arctigenin 160
arctiopicrin 52
Arctium lappa 52
Arctium majus 52
Arctostaphylos uva-ursi 258
Arecaceae 237
Aristolochia fangchi 6
Armoracia lopathifolia 168
Armoracia rusticana 168
Arnica **34**
Arnica montana 35

artemorin 119
arterial insufficiency 139
arthritis 119, 136, 275
Artichoke **36**
Artichoke, Globe 36
Asafetida 38
Asafoetida 38
Asant 38
asarinin 220
ascaridole 46
Asclepiadaceae 213
Asclepias 213
Asclepias curassavica 213
Asclepias engelmanniana 213
Asclepias eriocarpa 213
Asclepias glaucescens 213
Asclepias spp. 213
Asclepias tuberosa 213
asclepin 213
Ascophyllum 124
Ascophyllum nodosum 125
asiatic acid 170
Asiatic Ginseng 145
asiaticoside 170
asparagic acid 154
asparagine 188
asperuloside 78
Aster helenium 106
Aster officinalis 106
Asteraceae 35, 36, 48, 52, 69, 72, 85,
    96, 101, 106, 119, 153, 160, 180,
    254, 266, 271
asthma 139
astringent 231, 250, 258, 270, 271
atopic eczema 111
aucubin 19, 114, 122, 173, 210, 263
Avens **40**
azulene 69, 72, 271

B

Baccae Juniperi 176
Ballota 164
Ballota nigra 164
ballotenol 164
ballotinone 164
Balsamodendron Myrrha 199
barbaloin 62
Barosma betulina 51
Barosma crenulata 51
Barosma serratifolia 51
Batavia Cassia 76
Batavia Cinnamon 76
Bayberry **41**
Bear Grass 275
Bearberry 258
Bee Plant 49
Beebread 49
Benedict's Herb 40
benign prostatic hypertrophy 237

benzophenanthridine alkaloids 220
berberastine 151
Berberidaceae 82
berberine 42, 151
bergapten 28, 29, 203
betaine 35
betonicine 165, 197
Bignoniaceae 94
bilobalide 138
bilobetin 138
bilobol 139
biochanin A 227
bisabolene 135
bisabolol 69
bitter 134, 160, 165, 223
bitter acids 162
Bitter Root 134
Bitterwood 223
Black Cohosh **80**
Black Elder 104
Black Horehound **164**
Black Sampson 101
Black Snakeroot 80
Black Tang 124
Bladderwrack 124
Blazing Star 116
Blessed Thistle 160
Blond Psyllium 173
Bloodroot **42**
Blue Cohosh **82**
Blue Flag **44**
Bluegum, Tasmanian 108
Bockshornsame 117
Bogbean **45**
boldine 46, 235
Boldo **46**
   oil 46
Boldus boldus 46
Boldus 46
Boneset **48**
Borage **49**
   oil 49
Boraginaceae 49, 87
Borago officinalis 49
borneol 229
boschniakine 173
boschniakinic acid 173
box leaves 259
brahminoside 170
brahmoside 170
Brassicaceae 168
Brauneria angustifolia 101
Brauneria pallida 101
bronchitis 211, 256
Broom **50**
Buchu **51**
Buckbean 45
Burdock **52**
Burnet **54**

Burrage 49
Burseraceae 199
Buxus sempervirens 259

C

Cactaceae 68
cactine 68
Cactus grandiflorus 68
caffeic acid 254
caffeine 84, 189
Calamus **55**
Calendula **58**
Calendula officinalis 58
Calypso bulbosa 178
Campanulaceae 187
camphor 231, 245, 254
canadine 151
canavanine 24
Candleberry Bark 41
Cannabinaceae 162
canthin-6-one 223
Caprifoliaceae 104
capsaicin 60
capsaicinoids 60
Capsella 245
Capsella bursa-pastoris 245
Capsicum **60**
Capsicum spp. 60
Carbenia Benedicta 160
carbenoxolone 184
carbohydrate gum 87
cardanol 139
cardenolide glycosides 213
cardiac glycosides 197
   squill 249
Cardioactive herbal ingredients **280**
Carduus Benedictus 160
carminative 30, 79, 231, 254, 256
carnosol 229
Carrot 264
Carrot, Wild **264**
Carum petroselinum 203
carvacrol 256
caryophyllene 30,,36, 79
Caryophyllus aromaticus 79
Cascara **62**
Cascara Sagrada 62
Cascarosides A and B 62
cascarosides C and D 62
Cassia **63**
   Bark 63
   Batavia 76
   Lignea 63
   oil 63
   Saigon 76
Cassia acutifolia 243
Cassia angustifolia 243
Cassia senna 243
casticin 19

catalpol 122, 239
caulophylline 82
Caulophyllum 82
Caulophyllum thalictroides 82
caulosaponin 82
Cayenne Pepper 60
Celery **65**
    Fruit 65
    Seed 65
Centaury **67**
Centella 170
Centella asiatica 170
centelloside 170
cerebral insufficiency 139
Cereus **68**
Cereus grandiflorus 68
Ceylon Cinnamon 76
chalcones 162, 183, 184, 194
chamaelirin 116
Chamaelirium carolianum 116
Chamaelirium luteum 116
Chamaemelum nobile 72
chamazulene 69, 72, 271
Chamomile 69
    German **69**
    oil 70
    Roman **72**
Chamomilla recutita 69
Chaparral **74**
Chaste tree 19
Chasteberry 19
chelerythrine 220
Chilli Pepper 60
Chinese Cinnamon 63
Chinese Ginseng 145
Chinese Rhubarb 228
cholagogue 274
choleretic 46, 254
chrysaloin 62
Chrysanthemum parthenium 119
Chrysanthemum vulgare 254
chrysophanol 228, 274
Cimicifuga 80
Cimicifuga racemosa 80
Cimicifuga spp. 80
cimicifugin 80
cineole 108, 229, 230, 231
cinnamaldehyde 63, 76
cinnamamide 220
Cinnamomum aromaticum 63
Cinnamomum burmanii 76
Cinnamomum cassia 63
Cinnamomum japonicum 76
Cinnamomum loureirii 76
Cinnamomum obtusifolium 76
Cinnamomum sieboldii 63
Cinnamomum verum 76
Cinnamomum zeylanicum 63, 76

Cinnamon **76**
    bark 63
    Ceylon 76
    oil 76
    Saigon 76
    Wood 235
cinnzeylanin 76
cinnzeylanol 76
Cleavers 78
Clivers **78**
Clove **79**
    oil 79
cnicin 160
Cnicus 160
Cnicus benedictus 160
CNS stimulant 84
Coagulant herbal ingredients **282**
Cochlearia armoracia 168
Cohosh, Black **80**
Cohosh, Blue **82**
Cola **84**
    Seed 84
Cola acuminata 84
Cola nitida 84
Colewort 42
Collinsonia canadensis 253
Coltsfoot **85**
Comfrey **87**
    Prickly 87
    Quaker 87
    Russian 87
Commiphora 199
Commiphora abyssinica 199
Commiphora molmol 199
Commiphora mukul 199
Commiphora myrrha 199
commiphoric acids 199
commiphorinic acid 199
Common Figwort 122
Compositae 34, 36, 69, 72, 101, 106, 119, 160, 180, 266, 271
Coneflower 101
Consolidae Radix 87
constipation 243
constituents 2
contact dermatitis 48, 63
contra-indications 2
coptisine 42
Corn Silk **90**
costunolide 119
Couchgrass **91**
coumaric acid 181
coumarins 23, 28, 30, 34, 38, 45, 46, 69, 72, 78, 117, 141, 166, 168, 183, 206, 219, 223, 227, 241, 266
Coumarins, herbal ingredients containing **286**
counterirritant 60, 61
Cow Clover 227

Cowslip **92**
CQA 36
Crataegus monogyna 157
Crataegus oxyacanthoides 157
Crataegus pinnatifidia 157
Creosote Bush 74
Cruciferae 168, 245
cryptoxanthin 90
cyanide toxicity 33
cyanogenetic glycoside 32, 91, 94
Cynara scolymus 36
cynarin 36, 101
cynaropicrin 36
cypripedin 178
Cypripedium 178
Cypripedium bulbosum 178
Cypripedium calceolus 178
Cypripedium parviflorum 178
Cypripedium pubescens 178
Cytisus scoparius 50

D
Dalmatian Sage 231
Damiana **94**
Damiana aphrodisiaca 94
damianin 94
Dandelion **96**
daucosterol 141
Daucus carota 264
dehydrogingerdione 135
dehydroguaiaretic acid 156
demulcent 85, 188, 248
dermatitis 169, 197
desoxypodophyllotoxin 176
Devil's Dung 38
Devil's Claw **98**, 122
Devil's Shrub 141
diallyl disulphide 129
diallyl thiosulphinate 129
dianthrone glycosides 243
di-CQA 36
didrovaltrate 260
dihydroguaiaretic acid 74
diosgenin 117
diosmetin 51, 122, 229
diosmin 51, 122, 229
diterpenes 138, 164, 165
diuretic 51, 52, 84, 90, 91, 96, 104, 249, 258, 264, 271
Diuretic herbal ingredients **281**
Dock, Yellow 274
Dock, Curled 274
Dogs Grass 91
Dogwood, Jamaica 174
Dogwood, West Indian 174
doses 2
DPG-3-2 146
Dracontium foetidum 247
Drimia maritima 249

Dropwort 191
Drosera **100**
Drosera rotundifolia 100
Droseraeae 100
Drug/Herb Interactions, potential **277**
dyspepsia 21

E
Echinacea **101**
Echinacea angustifolia 101
Echinacea pallida 101
Echinacea purpurea 101
echinacein 101
Echinacin 102
echinacoside 101
echinatine 153
Ecuadorian Sarsaparilla 233
eczema 110
Elder **104**
Elecampane **106**
elecampane camphor 106
elemol 199
eleutherans 141
Eleutherococcus Ginseng 141
Eleutherococcus senticosus 141
eleutherosides 141
emetic 249
emodin 27, 228, 274
  glycosides 123
Endod 215
enzymes 129
EPO 110
Ericaceae 258
α-escin, 166
β-escin, 166
estragole 30
ethylmaltol 206
Eucalyptol 108
Eucalyptus **108**
  oil 108
Eucalyptus globulus 108
eudesmanolides 96, 106, 119
Eugenia aromatica 79
Eugenia caryophyllata 79
Eugenia caryophyllus 79
eugenol 76, 79
eugenyl acetate 79
euparin 153
eupatorin 153
Eupatorium 48
Eupatorium perfoliatum 48
Eupatorium purpureum 153
Eupatorium spp. 48
Euphorbia **109**
Euphorbia capitata 109
Euphorbia hirta 109
Euphorbia pilulifera 109
Euphorbiaceae 109, 225
Euphrasia 114

Euphrasia brevipila 114
Euphrasia officinalis 114
Euphrasia rostkoviana 114
European Elder 104
European Pennyroyal 208
Evening Primrose **110**
  oil 49, 110
expectorant 108, 241, 249, 256
Eyebright **114**

F
Fabaceae 23
fagaramide 220
False Cinnamon 63
False Unicorn **116**
Family 1
Farfara 85
Fenugreek **117**
fenugreekine 117
ferujol 38
Ferula assafoetida 38
Ferula communis 38
Ferula foetida 38
Ferula galbaniflua 38
Ferula jaeschkeana 38
Ferula rubricaulis 38
ferulenol 38
ferulic acid esters 38
Feverfew **119**
Fevertree 108
Feverwort 48
Ficaria 209
Ficaria ranunculoides 209
Figwort **122**
Filipendula 191
Filipendula ulmaria 191
Fish Poison Bark 174
fixed oils 90
flavones 179
flavonoids 21, 30, 35, 36, 45, 46, 48,
  50, 51, 54, 58, 65, 68, 69, 72, 74,
  85, 91, 92, 100, 104, 108, 109, 114,
  117, 119, 122, 123, 127, 138, 154,
  157, 162, 164, 165, 166, 169, 170,
  176, 179, 181, 183, 189, 191, 193,
  197, 201, 203, 206, 210, 213, 222,
  226, 227, 229, 239, 243, 245, 249,
  250, 256, 258, 264, 266, 270, 271
Flavonoids, herbal ingredients containing **286**
flavonol glycosides 154
flavonone 193
floridanine 180
florosenine 180
food use 2
formononetin 80, 183, 227
Fossil Tree 138
Frangula **123**
Frangula alnus 123

Frangula purshiana 62
frangulin A and B 123
frangulosides 123
fraxin 166
Fucaceae 124
fucoidan 124, 125
Fucus **124**
Fucus vesiculosus 124
fukiic acid 174
Fumaria officinalis 127
Fumariaceae 127
Fumitory **127**
furanocoumarins 28, 30, 65, 203, 204,
  264
furfural 44

G
G115 147
galactogogue 263
Galium 78
Galium aparine 78
gamolenic acid 25, 49, 110
Garden Burnet 54
Garden Sage 231
Garlic **129**
gastroduodenitis 21
gastrointestinal irritation 27
geijerone 176
gein 40
Genièvre 176
genistein 227
gentialutine 134
gentiamarin 134
Gentian **134**
Gentiana 134
Gentiana lutea 134
Gentiana scabra 134
Gentianaceae 134
gentianin 45
gentianine 117, 134
gentianose 134
gentiopicrin 134
gentiopicroside 134
gentisein 134
gentisin 134
German Chamomile **69**
germander 239
Geum 40
Geum urbanum 40
gin 139
Ginger **135**
  oleo-resin 135
gingerol 135
ginkgetin 138
Ginkgo **138**
Ginkgo biloba 138
Ginkgoaceae 138
ginkgolides 138

Ginseng **141, 145**
    American 145
    Asiatic 145
    Eleuterococcus 141
    extract (G115) 147
    Korean 145
    Panax 145
    polysaccharides 147
    Siberian 141
ginsenosides 145
GLA 110
glabridin 184
glabrol 184
Glechoma hederacea 154
glechomin 154
Globe artichoke 36
glucosinolates 168
glycans 141, 146
glycosides 174, 218
glycyrrhetic acid 183
glycyrrhetinic acid 183, 184
Glycyrrhiza glabra 183
glycyrrhizic acid 183
glycyrrhizin 183, 184
glycyrrhizinic acid 183
Gold-bloom 58
Golden Ragwort 180
Golden Seal **151**
Golden Senecio 180
Goosegrass 78
Gotu Kola 170
Gramineae 90, 91
Gravel Root **153**
Greater Burnet 54
Greater Plantain 210
Greek Sage 231
Grenadille 206
Ground Ivy **154**
GSL 54
GU-7 183, 184
Guaiacum **156**
Guaiacum officinale 156
Guaiacum sanctum 156
guaianolides 119
guaiaretic acid 156
guggulipid 199
Gum Asafetida 38
Gum Tree 108
Guru Nut 84

H
haemorrhoids 209
haemostatic 201
Hamamelidaceae 270
Hamamelis 270
Hamamelis virginiana 270
harman 206
harpagide 98, 122
harpagogenin 98

Harpagophytum procumbens 98, 122
harpagoside 98, 122
Hawthorn **157**
Heal-All 253
Hedeoma pulegoides 208
Hedera senticosa 141
hederagenin 222
heerabomyrrhols 199
helenalin 36
helenin 106
Helenium grandiflorum 106
Helenium microcephalum 106
Helianthus tuberosa 36
Helmet Flower 239
Helonias 116
Helonias dioica 116
Helonias lutea 116
helonin 116
Herb Bennet 40
herbal constituent 1
herbal ingredient 1
herbal remedy 1
herbal use 2
Hippocastanaceae 166
Hoarhound 165
Hoarhound, common 165
Hogweed 50
Holy Thistle **160**
Hoodwort 239
hop oil. 163
Hops **162**
hordenine 68
Horehound
    Black **164**
    White **165**
Hormonally active herbal ingredients **283**
Horse-chestnut **166**
Horseheal 106
Horseradish **168**
    peroxidase 168
Hot Pepper 60
humulone 162
Humulus 162
Humulus lupulus 162
Hungarian Chamomile 69
Hydrangea **169**
Hydrangea arborescens 169
hydrangenol 169
hydrangin 169
hydrastine 151
Hydrastis 151
Hydrastis canadensis 151
Hydrocotyle **170**
Hydrocotyle asiatica 170
hydrocotylin 170
hydrocyanic acid 104
hydroplumbagin glucoside 100
hydroquinone 258, 259

hydroxycinnamic acid esters 241
hydroxycostunolide 119
hydroxyisonobilin 72
hydroxykynurenic acid 138
hydroxyparthenolide 119
hydroxyursolic acid 154
Hyperglycaemic herbal ingredients **283**
Hypericaceae 250
hypericin 250, 251
Hypericum 250
Hypericum perforatum 250
Hyperlipidaemic herbal ingredients **282**
hyperoside 250
Hypertensive herbal ingredients **281**
Hypoglycaemic 23, 117, 130
Hypoglycaemic herbal ingredients **283**
hypolipidaemic 131
Hypolipidaemic herbal ingredients **282**
hypotensive 130, 189, 275
Hypotensive herbal ingredients **281**

I
Ichthymethia piscipula 174
ichthynone 174
Ilex 189
Ilex aquifolium 189
Ilex paraguariensis 189
Ilex pubescens 189
imanine 250
immunomodulation 102
immunostimulant 101, 141, 193, 194
Immunostimulating herbal ingredients **284**
imperatorin 28
Indian Pennywort 170
Indian Plantago 173
Indian Rhubarb 228
Indian Senna 243
Indian Squill 249
Indian Tobacco 187
Indian Water 170
indicaine 173
indoles 206, 223
insomnia 266
Interactions, potential drug/herb **277**
Inula 106
inula camphor 106
Inula helenium 106
Inula racemosa 106
inulin 106
iodine 124
Iridaceae 44
iridin 44
iridoids 45, 78, 98, 114, 122, 134, 173, 197, 210, 239, 258, 260, 263

Iridoids, herbal ingredients containing **286**

Iris caroliniana 44

Iris versicolor 44

irritant 38, 44, 45, 46, 51, 61, 82, 156, 165, 168, 174, 201, 213, 247

Irritant herbal ingredients **284**

Iscador™ 193, 194

isoalantolactone 106

isobornyl acetate 229

isobutylamides 101

isoflavones 183

isoflavonoids 23, 174, 227

isofraxidin 141

isoginkgetin 138

isoliquiritigenin 184

isoquassin 223

isoquinoline 42, 82, 127, 151, 219, 220, 235

isothiocyanate 168

isotussilagine 101

isovaltrates 260

Ispagol 173

Ispaghula **173**

J

Jamaica Dogwood **174**

Jamaican Quassia 223

jamaicin 174

Japanese Ginseng 145

Jerusalem Artichoke 36

Jesuit's Brazil Tea 189

Jintsam 145

Joe-Pye Weed 153

Joshua Tree 275

junionone 176

Juniper **176**

  oil 176

Juniperus communis 176

K

Kelp 124

Kelpware 124

Kew Tree 138

Khartoum Senna 243

King's Cureall 110

Knob Root 253

Kola Nut 84

Korean Ginseng 145

Kydney Root, 153

L

L-652,469 85

Labiatae 154, 164, 165, 197, 208, 229, 231, 239, 253, 256

labriformin 213

Lactuca sativa 266

Lactuca species 266

Lactuca virosa 266

Lactucarium 266

Lady's Mantle 205

Lady's Slipper **178**

Laetrile 32

Laminaria 124

laminarin 124

Larrea divaricata 74

Larrea mexicana 74

Larrea tridentata 74

larreantin 74

Lauraceae 63

lauriflorine 219

laxative 62, 123, 124, 173, 243

Laxative herbal ingredients **280**

lectin 104, 193, 195, 197, 201, 215

legal category 1

Leguminosae 23, 117, 174, 183, 227, 243

Lemon Verbena **179**

  oil 179

Leontodon taraxacum 96

leonurine 197

Leonurus 197

Leonurus artemisia 198

Leonurus cardiaca 197

Leonurus heterophyllus 197, 198

Leonurus sibirius 198

Leopard's Bane 35

Lesser Celandine 209

Lettuce, Wild 266

Lettuce Opium 266

Leucanthemum parthenium 119

Licorice 183

Liferoot **180**

lignans 74, 156. 160, 215, 220

Lignum Vitae 156

Liliaceae 25, 116, 129, 233, 249

Lime Flower **181**

Lime Tree 181

limonene 65

Linden Tree 181

cis-linoleic acid 110

Lion's Tooth 96

Lippia citriodora 179

Liquorice **183**

lisetin 174

lithospermic acid 160

lobelacrin 187

Lobelia **187**

Lobelia chinensis 187

Lobelia inflata 187

lobeline 187

Loranthaceae 193

Lucerne 23

Lucraceae 235

lupulone 162

Lupulus 162

lysine 117

M

Macrocystis 124

Macrotys Actaeae 80

madasiatic acid 170

madecassic acid 170

madecassoside 170

magnoflorine 82, 220

Maidenhair Tree 138

maltol 206

Malvaceae 188

mandelonitrile 33

maodongqing 189

Marigold 58

marrubiin 154, 165

Marrubium 165

Marrubium vulgare 165

Marsh Trefoil 45

Marshmallow **188**

Marybud 58

mastalgia 110, 111

Maté **189**

Matricaria chamomilla 69

matricaria oil 69

Matricaria recutita 69

matricin 69

Maypop 206

MDQ 189

Meadow Clover 227

Meadowsweet **191**

Medicago 23

Medicago sativa 23

medicagol 23

Mentha pulegium 208

menthone 208

Menyanthaceae 45

Menyanthes 45

Menyanthes trifoliata 45

methoxyphenylacetone 30

methoxypsoralen 203, 264

methyl-3-buten-2-ol 162

N-methylcytisine 80, 82

methyleugenol 63

methylpyridoxine 139

methylsalicylaldehyde 63

migraine 119

Milfoil 271

Millefolium 271

Millepertuis 250

mineralocorticoid 183

Mistletoe **193**

  berries 195

Mohave Yucca 275

Monimiaceae 46

Monk's Pepper 19

mono-CQA 36

monograph title 1

monoterpene hydrocarbons 229

monoterpenes 176

monotropein 78

Moraceae 162
Motherwort **197**
motion sickness 136, 137
Mountain Hydrangea 169
Mountain Tobacco 35
mucilage 85, 91, 173, 181, 188, 248
mustard oil glycosides 168
myrcene 176
Myrica 41
Myrica cerifera 41
Myricaceae 41
myricadiol 41
myricetin 258
myricitrin 41
myristicin 203, 204, 235
Myrrh **199**
Myrtaceae 79, 108

N

naphthoquinone 100
Nasturtium armoracia 168
'natural' remedies 1
Navelwort 170
NDGA 74
neoherculin 220
nepeta hederacea 154
Nerve Root 178
nervous excitability 260
Nettle **201**
nicotinic acid 117, 160
Night Blooming Cereus 68
Ninjin 145
nitidine 219, 220
nobilin 72
nordihydroguaiaretic acid 74
norisoguaiacin 74
Northern Prickly Ash **219**
Northern Senega 241
nortracheloside 160

O

Oenothera biennis 110
Oenothera spp. 110
oestrogenic activity 23, 30, 227, 237,
    264
oleanolic acid 229
oleo-gum resin 38, 199
oleoresin 135, 162
Onagraceae 110
oral hygiene 42
Orchidaceae 178
orexigenic 53
orientin 117
osthol 28
otosenine 180
oxypeucedanin 203
oxytocic 50

P

Padang-Cassia 76
PAF 138, 139
Paigle 92
Pale Psyllium 173
Palmae 237
palmidin C 123
Panang Cinnamon 76
Panax ginseng 145
Panax japonicus 145
Panax notoginseng 145
Panax pseudoginseng 145
Panax quinquefolius 145
Panax schinseng 145
panaxosides 145
panaxytriol 147
Papaveraceae 42
Papilionaceae 50
Papoose Root 82
Paprika 60
Paraguay Tea 189
Parsley **203**
Parsley piert **205**
part(s) used 1
parthenolide 119
Pasque Flower 222
Passiflora 206
Passiflora alata 206
Passiflora edulis 206
Passiflora incarnata 206
Passiflora spp. 206
Passifloraceae 206
Passion Vine 206
Passionflower **206**
PCF 101
Peagle 92
Pedaliaceae 98
Pennyroyal **208**
Pennywort, Indian 170
peripheral arterial insufficiency 139
peroxidase enzymes 168
Persic Oil 32
pertussis 256
Petroselinum crispum 203
Petroselinum sativum 203
Peumus 46
Peumus boldus 46
pharmaceutical comment 2
pharmacological actions 2
pharmacopoeial monographs 1
phellandrene 28
phenethyl glycosides 114
phenolic acids 193
phenolic glycosides 268
phenols 168, 250
phenylethylamine 157
phenylethylisothiocyanate 168
phenylpropanoids 141
Phoradendron sp. 194

photodermatitis 28
photosensitivity 30, 31
phototoxicity 28
phthalides 65
phytohaemagglutinins 104
Phytolacca acinosa 215
Phytolacca americana 215
Phytolacca decandra 215
Phytolacca dodecandra 215
Phytolaccaceae 215
phytolaccagenin 215
Picraena excelsa 223
Picrasma 223
Picrasma excelsa 223
Pilewort **209**
Pillbearing Spurge 109
Pimpinella anisum 30
Pinaceae 176
pinenes 229
piscerythrone 174
Piscidia 174
Piscidia communis 174
Piscidia erythrina 174
Piscidia piscipula 174
piscidic acid 174
Piscidin 174
Plantaginaceae 173, 210
Plantago lanceolata 210
Plantago major 210
Plantago ovata 173
Plantago Seed 173
Plantago spp. 211
plantagonine 173
Plantain **210**
platelet-activating factor 138
platyphylline 87
Pleurisy Root **213**
plumbagin 100
Pocan 215
Pokeroot **215**
Pokeweed 215
    antiviral protein 215
    mitogen 215
Polyacetylenes 52, 101, 160
Polyenes 160
Polygala 241
Polygala chamaebuxus 241
Polygala paniculata 241
Polygala senega 241
Polygala spp 241
Polygalaceae 241
polygalic acid 241
Polygonaceae 228, 274
polypeptides 193, 226
polysaccharides 25, 85, 101, 124,
    141, 195, 227, 237
Poplar **218**
    Buds 218
Populus Alba 218

Populus nigra 218
Populus tremula 218
Populus tremuloides 218
porphyria 21
Pot Marigold 58
preleosibirin 164
premarrubiin 165
Prickly Ash
    Northern **219**
    Southern **220**
primin 92
Primrose, Evening **110**
Primula 92
Primula officinalis 92
Primula veris 92
Primulaceae 92
primulaveroside 92
primulic acid 92
primveroside 92
proanthocyanidins 138
procumbid 122
procyanidins 157, 158
proscillaridin A 249
prostaglandin precursor 110
prostatic hypertrophy, benign 237
protoanemonin 209, 222
protopanaxadiol 145
protopanaxatriol 145
protopine 42, 127
Prunus armeniaca 32
PSF 101
psoralen 203, 264
psoriasis 171
Psyllium, Pale 173
Pulegium 208
pulegone 51, 154, 208
Pulsatilla **222**
Pulsatilla nigrans 222
purgative 45, 274
Purple Boneset 153
Purple Clover 227
Purple Medick 23
purpose and scope 1
Pyrethrum parthenium 119
pyridines 117, 260
pyrrolizidine alkaloids 49, 85, 87 101,
    153, 180

Q

Quackgrass 91
Quaker Bonnet 239
Quaking Aspen 218
Quassia **223**
quassin 223
quassinoids 223
Queen Anne's Lace 264
Queen of the Meadow 153, 191
Queen's Delight **225**
Queen's Root 225

quercetin 258
quercetin glycosides 104
quinolizidines 50, 80, 82
quinones 92, 100, 178, 258

R

Radicula armoracia 168
Radix Notoginseng 145
Ragwort, Golden 180
Ranunculaceae 80, 151, 209, 222
ranunculin 222
Ranunculus 209
Ranunculus ficaria 209
Raspberry **226**
Rattlesnake Root 241
Red Root 42
Red Clover **227**
Red Ginseng 145
Red Pepper 60
Red Plant 215
Red Sage 231
Red Squill 249
references 2
resin 38, 156, 199
Review of Medicines 7
Rhamnaceae 62, 123
Rhamni Purshianae Cortex 62
Rhamnus 62
Rhamnus frangula 123
Rhamnus purshiana 62
rhein 228
Rheum officinale 228
Rheum palmatum 228
Rheum rhaponticum 228
Rheum species 228
rheumatism 268
Rhizoma Panacis 145
Rhizoma Panacis Majoris 145
Rhubarb **228**
Rockweed 124
rodenticide 249
Roman Chamomile **72**
Root Beer 235
Roripa armoracia 168
Rosaceae 21, 32, 40, 54, 157, 191, 205,
    226
Rosemary **229**
    oil 229
rosmaricine 229
rosmarinic acid 87, 154, 229
Rosmarinus officinalis 229
rossoliside 100
rotenoids 174
rotenone 174
rubefacient 108
Rubiaceae 78
rubichloric acid 78
Rubus 226
Rubus idaeus 226

Rumex crispus 274
Rutaceae 51, 219, 220
rutin 250

S

Sabal 237
sabinene 176
safrole 76, 235
Sage **231**
Saigon Cassia 76
Saigon Cinnamon 76
Salicaceae 218, 268
salicin 218, 268
salicylaldehyde 63, 191
salicylates 191, 218, 268
saligenin 218, 268
Salix alba 268
Salix Bark 268
Salix fragilis 268
Salix pentandra 268
Salix purpurea 268
Saloop 235
Salvia haematodes 231
Salvia officinalis 231
Salvia triloba 231
Sambucus 104
Sambucus canadensis 104
Sambucus nigra 104
sambunigrin 104
Sanchi Ginseng 145
Sang 145
Sanguinaria 42
Sanguinaria canadensis 42
sanguinarine 42
Sanguisorba 54
Sanguisorba officinalis 54
sanguisorbin 54
sapogenins 145
saponin glycosides 170
saponins 23, 25, 54, 58, 82, 90, 92,
    116, 117, 141, 166, 181, 209,
    215, 222, 227, 233, 241, 275
Saponins, herbal ingredients contain-
    ing **286**
Sarothamnus scoparius 50
sarracine 87
Sarsa 233
Sarsaparilla **233**
sarsasapogenin 233
Sassafras **235**
    oil, 235
Sassafras albidum 235
Sassafras officinale 235
Sassafras varifolium 235
Saw palmetto **237**
Saxifragaceae 169
Saxifrax 235
Scabwort 106
Schinsent 145

Scilla 249
scillaren A 249
scillaren B 249
Scoparius 50
scopoletin 72, 78, 206, 223
scopolin 166
Scrophularia 122
Scrophularia nodosa 122
Scrophulariaceae 114, 122
Scullcap **239**
scutellarein 239
Scutellaria 239
Scutellaria baicalensis 239
Scutellaria galericulata 239
Scutellaria lateriflora 239
Scutellaria species 239
scutellarin 239
Seawrack 124
sedative 55, 70, 162, 206, 250, 260, 263
Sedative herbal ingredients **283**
Selenicereus grandiflorus 68
selenine 65
selinene 36
Senecio aureus 180
Senecio, Golden 180
senecionine 85, 180
Senega **241**
senegin 241
senkirkine 85, 86
Senna **243**
sennidin 243
sennoside 243
sennosides A and B 243
Serenoa 237
Serenoa repens 237
Serenoa serrulata 237
serum cholesterol 23, 36, 118
serum lipids 130
sesamin 141, 220
sesquiterpene lactones 36, 70, 106, 119, 254, 266
sesquiterpenes 48, 52, 58, 85, 108, 135, 145, 160, 170, 199
sesquiterpenoids 72
Seven Barks 169
Shepherd's Purse **245**
shikimic acid 109
shogaol 135
Siberian Ginseng **141**
side-effects 2
Simaroubaceae 223
sinigrin 245, 246
sitosterol 23
Skullcap 239
Skunk Cabbage **247**
Skunkweed 247
Slippery Elm **248**
Smallage 65

smilacin 233
Smilax 233
Smilax species 233
Smooth Hydrangea 169
Snake Root 241
Snakeroot 48
    Black 80
Snakeweed 109
Solanaceae 60
Southern Prickly Ash **220**
sparteine 50
Spartium scoparium 50
species 1
Spiraea ulmaria 191
Spogel 173
Squaw Root 82
Squaw Weed 180
Squill **249**
SRE 237
St. Bartholomew's Tea 189
St. John's Wort **250**
stachydrine 23, 197
stachyose 98
Starflower Oil 49
Starwort 116
Stephania tetranda 6
Sterculia acuminata 84
Sterculiaceae 84
steroids 160, 199
sterols 96, 109
Stigma Maydis 90
Stillingia 225
Stillingia sylvatica 225
Stillingia treculeana 225
Stinging Nettle 201
Stone Root **253**
stroke 239
sulphides 129
Sundew 100
Surinam Quassia 223
Sweet False Chamomile 69
swertiamarine 134
Sympathomimetic Action, herbal ingredients with **285**
symphytine 87
Symphytum asperum 87
Symphytum officinale 87
Symphytum peregrinum 87
Symphytum Radix 87
Symplocarpus foetidus 247
synonyms 1
syringin 141
Syzygium aromaticum 79
Syzygium cuminii 79

T
Tabasco Pepper 60
Tanacetum 254
Tanacetum parthenium 119

Tanacetum vulgare 254
tannic acid 85
tannins 21, 25, 32, 36, 40,41, 54, 63, 76, 78, 80, 84, 85, 87, 90, 92, 94, 100, 104, 108, 114, 119, 123, 157, 160, 162, 166, 176, 178, 181, 189, 191, 197, 209, 210, 218, 226, 231, 248, 250, 258, 268, 270, 271, 274
Tannins, herbal ingredients containing **286**
Tansy **254**
    Oil 254
taraxacin 96
Taraxacum 96
Taraxacum officinale 96
Taraxacum palustre 96
Taraxinic acid 96
Tasmanian Bluegum 108
terpenes 179, 181
terpenoids 34, 48, 58, 80, 96, 101, 104, 106, 109, 119, 138, 141, 145, 154, 160, 165, 170, 183, 189, 193, 197, 199, 223, 225, 241, 254, 275
terpinen-4-ol 176, 264, 272
tetraphyllin B 94
Tetterwort 42
Teucrium canadense, adulterant 240
Teucrium chamaedrys 239
theobromine 84, 189
theophylline 189
Thoroughwort 48
thujones 231, 254
Thyme **256**
thymol 34, 256
thymoleptic 263
Thymus orospedanus 256
Thymus vulgaris 256
Tienchi Ginseng 145
tiglic acid esters 72
Tilia 181
Tilia × europaea 181
Tilia cordata 181
Tilia platyphyllos 181
Tiliaceae 181
Tinnevelly Senna 243
Toothache Bark 219, 220
toothache remedy 79
Touch-Me-Not 141
toxicity 2
Trefoil 227
tricin 91
Trifolium pratense 227
Trigonella foenumgraecum 117
trigonelline 23, 117
triterpenes 21, 80, 104, 145
triterpenoid 58, 209
Triticum 91
Triticum repens 91
tryptophan 117

turicin 197
turicine 165
Turnera 94
Turnera aphrodisiaca 94
Turnera diffusa 94
Turnera microphylla 94
Turneraceae 94
tussilagine 85, 101
Tussilago farfara 85
tussilagone 85
Twitchgrass 91
tyramine 68, 195

U

Ulmaceae 248
Ulmus fulva 248
Ulmus rubra 248
Umbelliferae 28, 30, 38, 170, 203, 264
umbelliferone 69, 206
Unicorn, False **116**
Urginea 249
Urginea indica 249
Urginea maritima 249
Urginea scilla 249
urinary antiseptic 245, 258, 271
urinary calculus 264
ursolic acid 189, 197, 229
Urtica 201
Urtica dioica 201
Urticaceae 201
urticin 201
use of the book 1
Uva-ursi **258**

V

valepotriates 260
valerenal 260
valerenic acid 260
Valerian **260**
Valerian, American 178
Valeriana officinalis 260
Valeriana wallichi 261
Valerianaceae 260
vallerine 170
valtrates 260
varicose vein treatment 166
vasodilatation 80

venous insufficiency 166
Veratrum luteum 116
Verbena 263
Verbena citriodora 179
Verbena officinalis 263
Verbena triphylla 179
Verbena, lemon 179
Verbenaceae 19, 179
verbenalin 263
Vervain **263**
VHOCs 125
viscotoxins 193, 195
Viscum 193
Viscum album 193
Vitamin A 96
vitamin B_{17} 32
Vitex agnus-castus 19
vitexin rhamnoside 157
viticin 19
volatile oils 19, 28, 30, 34, 36, 38, 40, 42, 44, 46, 48, 51, 55, 58, 60, 63, 65, 69, 72, 74, 76, 79, 91, 94, 104, 106, 108, 114, 119, 135, 141, 154, 160, 162, 165, 168, 170, 176, 179, 181, 183, 191, 197, 199, 203, 222, 229, 231, 235, 245, 250, 254, 256, 260, 263, 264, 270, 271
Volatile Oils, herbal ingredients containing **286**

W

Wacholderbeeren 176
warnings 2
Wax Myrtle Bark 41
West Indian Dogwood 174
Western Ginseng 145
White Ginseng 145
White Horehound **165**
White Poplar 218
White Squill 249
Whitethorn 157
Wild Carrot **264**
Wild Chamomile 69
Wild Hydrangea 169
Wild Lettuce **266**
Wild Pepper 141

Willow **268**
Witch Hazel **270**
Witchazel 270
Wolf's Bane 34
wound healing 171

X

xanthines 84, 189
xanthones 134
Xanthorhiza simplicissima 151
Xanthoxylum 219, 220
xanthyletin 219

Y

yamogenin 117
Yarrow **271**
Yaw Root 225
Yellow Dock **274**
Yellow Gentian 134
Yellow Root 151
Yellow Starwort 106
Yerba Maté 189
Yucca **275**
Yucca arborescens 275
Yucca brevifolia 275
Yucca glauca 275
Yucca mohavensis 275
Yucca species 275

Z

Zanthoxylum 219, 220
Zanthoxylum americanum 219
Zanthoxylum clava-herculis 220
Zanthoxylum zanthoxyloides 220
Zea 90
Zea mays 90
Zimbro 176
zingerone 135
Zingiber 135
Zingiber officinale 135
Zingiberaceae 135
zingiberene 135
ziyu glycosides 54
Zygophyllaceae 74, 156